Interpersonal Relationships

Professional Communication Skills for Nurses

INTERPERSONAL RELATIONSHIPS

Professional Communication Skills for Nurses

FIFTH EDITION

Elizabeth C. Arnold, PhD, APRN-PMH, BC
Associate Professor, Retired
University of Maryland
Baltimore, Maryland

Family Nurse Psychotherapist
Montgomery Village, Maryland

Kathleen Underman Boggs, PhD, FNP-CS
Family Nurse Practitioner

Associate Professor Emeritus
College of Health and Human Services
University of North Carolina at Charlotte
Charlotte, North Carolina

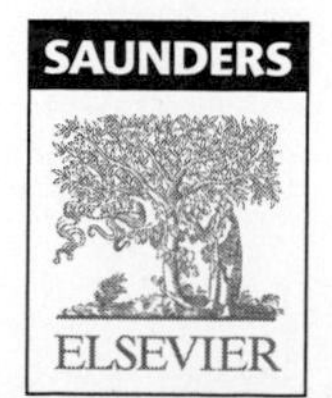

SAUNDERS
ELSEVIER

11830 Westline Industrial Drive
St. Louis, Missouri 63146

Interpersonal Relationships:
Professional Communication Skills for Nurses

ISBN-13: 978-1-4160-2913-7
ISBN-10: 1-4160-2913-3

ISBN-13: 978-1-4160-2913-7
ISBN-10: 1-4160-2913-3

Executive Editor: Tom Wilhelm
Senior Developmental Editor: Jill Ferguson
Associate Developmental Editor: Tiffany Trautwein
Publishing Services Manager: Deborah L. Vogel
Senior Project Manager: Ann E. Rogers
Design Direction: Kimberly E. Denando

Printed in the United States of America

Last digit is the print number: 9 8 7 6 5 4 3

CONTRIBUTOR

Ann Mabe Newman, RN, CS, DSN
Associate Professor of Nursing
Adjunct Associate Professor of Women's Studies
College of Nursing and Health Professions
University of North Carolina at Charlotte
Charlotte, North Carolina

Chapter 4: Self-Concept in the Nurse-Client Relationship

To the memory of my beloved husband, George B. Arnold,
a compassionate man with an undying love for his family and friends

Elizabeth C. Arnold

To my clients, students, and family

Kathleen Underman Boggs

PREFACE

Since the last edition of this text was published, our world has unfolded and expanded in ways that are both alarming and exciting. Today, we live in a world threatened by terrorism and political uncertainties, work with a health care system operating under a modern paradigm of cost containment and short-term treatments, and have unprecedented access to sophisticated global communication technologies that were virtually non-existent even a few short decades ago. We are challenged to update and incorporate fresh information about communicating with clients, peers, and other members of the multidisciplinary health care team in the context of the nurse-client relationship.

The fifth edition of *Interpersonal Relationships: Professional Communication Skills for Nurses* strives to provide a realistic framework for the study and application of therapeutic communication strategies needed for understanding, healing, and support of the clients entrusted to our care in modern health care situations. Our hope is that professional nurses will still find that developing interpersonal relationships with their clients is at the forefront of quality professional nursing care as its primary methodology. As nurses we are and will be answerable to our clients, our profession, and ourselves to communicate with clients in a therapeutic manner and to advocate for their health care and well-being in the larger political community.

Our intention is that the fifth edition will continue to serve as a primary reference source for nurses seeking to improve their communication and relationship skills across traditional and non-traditional community-based health care settings. The fifth edition has been further revised to emphasize health promotion and communication modifications in short-term treatment and community situations, provide a direct focus on end-of-life care, and describe the exponential increase in the communication use of technology in contemporary health care. A new chapter devoted to communication technology and the inclusion of evidence-based practice examples for each chapter acknowledge the importance of these variables in modern health care. Updated references and experiential exercises provide students with the opportunity to practice, observe, and critically evaluate their professional communication skills in real time.

As in previous editions, the chapters in the fifth edition of *Interpersonal Relationships: Professional Communication Skills for Nurses* can be used as individual teaching modules, as a primary text, or as a communication resource integrated across the curriculum. The text is divided into five parts, using a similar format to that of previous editions by presenting basic concepts of the chapter subject, followed by clinical applications. **Part I, Conceptual Foundations of Nurse-Client Relationships,** provides a theory-based approach to communication in nursing practice and describes the standards and professional guides that govern the relationship and examines the self as the center of the relationship. **Part II, The Nurse-Client Relationship,** provides updated information about the nature and structure of the nurse-client relationship. Chapters in this section have been reworked to reflect growing dimensions of the nurse's role and to include a comprehensive discussion of palliative care and the importance of communication in helping clients and families cope effectively with the last stage of life. **Part III, Therapeutic Communication,** explores communication strategies the nurse can use with different population groups. This material has been updated to reflect current trends in contemporary health care, particularly related to cultural competence and community-based health promotion strategies. **Part IV, Responding to Special Needs,** focuses on relating to clients with special needs. The special needs of children, the elderly, and those in crisis are addressed in greater depth. Finally, **Part V, Professional Issues,** considers the revolutionary infusion of technology into health care with the use of electronic health systems for documentation and reporting. A new chapter is specifically devoted to point-of-care communication technology.

Developing an Evidence-Based Practice boxes, new to this edition, offer a summary of a research article related to each chapter subject and are designed to stimulate awareness of the need to link research with practice. The *Ethical Dilemmas* presented at the end of each chapter offer the student an opportunity to reflect on common ethical situations, which occur on a regular basis in health care relationships.

The integration of theory-based principles and application with an experiential format is deliberately designed to encourage students to learn and develop new insights about the ways they communicate with clients and others involved with their care. Through active experiential involvement with these principles, students can develop an ease with using them in real life clinical settings. Being able to reflect on and practice communication skills in a safe learning environment with immediate constructive feedback helps build confidence as well as skill.

Instructor Resources are available on the textbook's Evolve website. Additional experiential exercises can be found in the Instructor's Manual, along with strategies for teaching and learning and brief chapter summaries with teaching tips. A revised Test Bank reflecting the updated content in the text is also included. Instructors are encouraged to contact their Elsevier sales representative to gain access to these valuable teaching tools.

Our hope is that the fifth edition of *Interpersonal Relationships: Professional Communication Skills for Nurses* will continue to serve as a primary resource for students, nurses, and faculty interested in learning more about the therapeutic responses that can calm, offer hope, and promote healing and understanding for clients and their families. As the most consistent health care provider in most clients' lives, the nurse bears an awesome responsibility in providing communication that is professional, honest, empathetic, and knowledgeable in a person-to-person relationship that is without equal. We invite you as students, nurses, and faculty to interact with the material in this text, learning from the content and experiential exercises but also seeking your own truth and understanding as professional nurses. The richness of what can happen in the nurse-client relationship can continue to grow and develop with the contributions of all nurses committed to quality in health care.

Elizabeth C. Arnold
Kathleen Underman Boggs

ACKNOWLEDGMENTS

This fifth edition carries forward the ideas and efforts of students, valued colleagues, clients, and the editorial staff at Elsevier. The evolution of this text began with an interpersonal relationship seminar developed as part of the curriculum in an upper division baccalaureate nursing program at the University of Maryland School of Nursing. The format used experiential exercises to reinforce communication concepts, which invited the students to interact with the material, thus providing them a rich, practice-oriented learning experience. To those at the University of Maryland and the University of North Carolina with whom we were privileged to be associated, whose mentorship and guidance informed and illuminated new dimensions to our understanding of interpersonal relationships in nursing practice, we express our deepest gratitude.

The material in this text also reflects the perspectives of acknowledged leaders in the field of communication, nursing, and interpersonal relationships. The contributions of their theoretical understandings provide a solid framework for the practice applications described in the text.

Over the years, faculty, students, and practicing nurses across the country have deepened the understanding of concepts presented in the text. By sharing the caring, creativity, and competence experienced in real life professional interpersonal relationships, their voices find consistent expression in each chapter. Critical linkages from current nurse researchers deserve acknowledgment for enhancing our understanding of the complex nature of communication from an evidenced-based perspective.

Ann Mabe Newman and Barbara Harrison again served as valued contributors, and we thank them for their work. We would like to acknowledge past contributors—Kristin Lynn Bussell, MS, APRN, CS-P; Verna Benner Carson, PhD, APRN, CS-P; David R. Langford, DSNc, RN; Ann O'Mara, PhD, RN; Judith W. Ryan, PhD, APRN, CRNP; and Shirley A. Smoyak, PhD, RN, FAAN—for their commitment to previous editions of this text. They each have provided a deeper and broader understanding of the communication process needed to guide professional conversations with clients across the life span and with other professionals involved with their care.

The editorial and production staff at Elsevier deserves special acknowledgment for their commitment to the preparation of this book. Jill Ferguson, senior developmental editor, and Tiffany Trautwein, associate developmental editor, each provided suggestions and unflagging support for the project as they patiently and thoroughly provided editorial support. Thanks also to Ann Rogers, senior project manager, for her very capable handling of the manuscript production, and to Tom Wilhelm, senior executive director, for his enthusiastic investment in the project. Kimberly Denando has managed the design of this text with attention to detail and quality.

Finally, we need to acknowledge the loving support of our families. We are particularly grateful to our spouses, George B. Arnold and Michael J. Boggs, for their unflagging encouragement and support.

Elizabeth C. Arnold
Kathleen Underman Boggs

INTERPERSONAL RELATIONSHIPS

Professional Communication Skills for Nurses

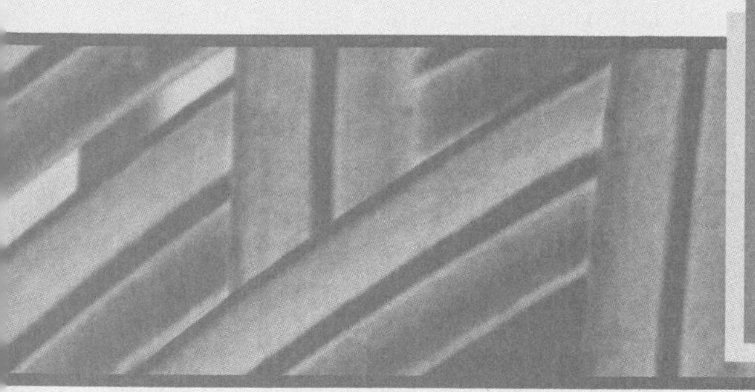

Part I
Conceptual Foundations of Nurse-Client Relationships

Chapter 1
Theoretical Perspectives and Contemporary Issues

Elizabeth Arnold

OUTLINE

OBJECTIVES

At the end of the chapter, the reader will be able to:

1. Describe the nature and purpose of nursing theory.
2. Identify the historical development of nursing theory.
3. Compare and contrast different levels of nursing knowledge.
4. Describe the implications of Peplau's nursing theory for the nurse-client relationship.
5. Analyze psychological models relevant to nurse-client relationships.
6. Specify the use of communication theory in nursing practice.

> *The unique function of the nurse is to assist the individual, sick or well, in the performance of those activities contributing to health or its recovery (or to peaceful death) that he would perform unaided if he had the necessary strength, will, or knowledge, and to do this in such a way as to help him gain independence as rapidly as possible. This part of her function she initiates and controls, of this she is master.*
>
> (Henderson, 1966)

Chapter 1 focuses on selected theoretical perspectives and contemporary issues surrounding the professional nurse-client relationship in nursing practice. Included in the chapter are the structural components of nursing knowledge and a brief, eclectic overview of theoretical perspectives drawn from nursing and other disciplines related to the nurse-client relationship. Nurses often question the relevance of nursing theory for professional practice (Kim, 1994). Nursing theory seems abstract and far removed from what nurses do every day. McKenna (1993) argues that nursing theory provides nurses with a distinct health care identity in collaborating with other members of the interdisciplinary health care team. For example, how is the nursing role different from the medical or the social work role, or distinct from paraprofessional roles in health care? Theory-based nursing care helps ensure consistency and constancy of professional nursing practice across clinical settings.

Society recognizes the expertise of the professional nurse as being distinct from that of other health care professionals. Nursing knowledge incorporates concepts and theories from many different disciplines (e.g., medicine, social work, law, sociology, and psychology). These elements are integrated into professional nursing practice (Clark, 1998). State boards of nursing and the American Nurses Association developed performance standards and scope of practice guidelines, and a code of ethics to ensure the quality of professional nursing care.

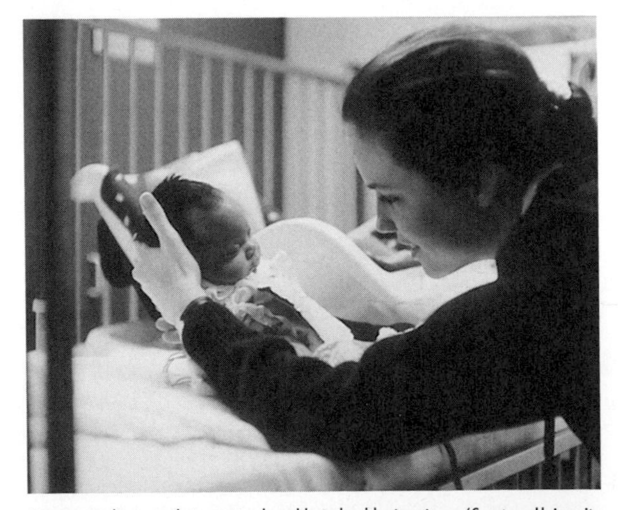

Nurses see clients at their most vulnerable in health situations. (Courtesy University of Maryland School of Nursing.)

BASIC CONCEPTS

Definition of Theory

The term theory comes from the Greek word *theoria*, which means "to see" or "a viewing" (Fawcett, Watson, Neuman et al., 2001). A **theory** represents a theorist's thoughtful examination of a phenomenon, defined as a concrete situation, event, circumstance, or condition of interest. In nursing, theory represents a well-defined view of professional nursing, which differentiates its focus and activities from those of other professions (Chinn & Kramer, 1995).

A nursing theory presents a set of principles and defines the relationships among concepts, assumptions, and propositions in a nursing model. Nurses use theoretical nursing frameworks to *describe*, *explain*, *predict*, and *prescribe* nursing practice. For example, descriptive theory frameworks describe the properties and components of nursing as a professional discipline. Explanatory theory identifies the functions of nursing and how the properties and components relate to each other. Predictive theories foretell the relationships between the components of the model, whereas prescriptive theories focus on nursing therapeutics and identify what will happen if a particular intervention is used.

All theories develop within a sociocultural context, so they are subject to adaptation as new information develops (Figure 1-1). For example, early nursing theorists such as Henderson embraced the medical model, then the gold standard of health care. Modern nursing theories broadened the definition of health to reflect the current public health focus with a stronger emphasis on health promotion and preventive nursing strategies to facilitate health and well-being.

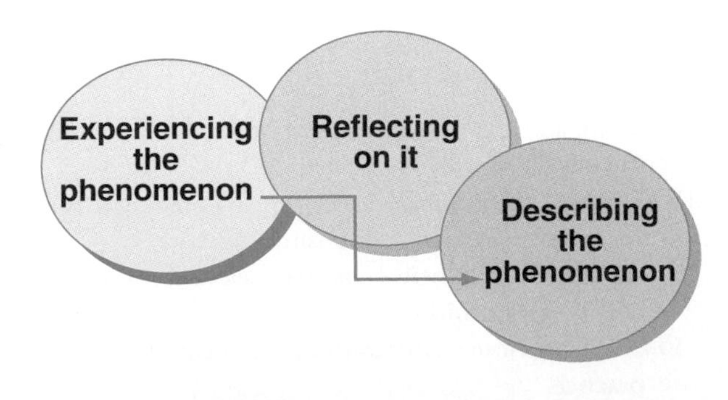

Figure 1-1 • Process of theory development.

Theory as a Guide to Practice

Nursing theory informs nursing practice by furnishing a distinct body of nursing knowledge that nurses universally recognize as being unique to their discipline. Nursing theories provide professional nurses with a systematic way to view client situations and a logical way to organize and interpret health data (Raudonis & Acton, 1997). In all nursing theory frameworks, the client is the central focus, and the goal of nursing is to promote and maintain the health and well-being of individuals, families, and communities (Doheny, Cook, & Stopper, 1997).

Nursing theories lay out the domain of the profession, establish the boundaries of professional nursing, provide a basis for research, and serve as a guide for curriculum development and clinical practice. Theory helps provide a framework for understanding the science of nursing, while patterns of knowing provide a methodology for individualizing care for the client and articulating the art of nursing. In practice, they are inseparable components of quality nursing care. Theory-based applications of the nurse-client relationship are valuable testimonials to the key role of professional nursing in today's health care arena.

To sustain critical membership as part of the interdisciplinary health care team, nurses need to view their nursing practice as a practice arena for new theory development as well as for applying nursing knowledge (Reed, 1997). Nursing theory models provide a framework for discussion, research, and the development of new thinking about the profession. Regular reading of professional journals provides nurses with explanatory and research-based applications of nursing theory in professional nursing practice, its use, and related clinical research.

Nursing Theory Development

The first nursing theorist was Florence Nightingale, with her classic work *Notes on Nursing*, first published in 1859. Nightingale believed that nurses could create environments beneficial to the restoration and preservation of health, within which the client would begin to heal. Her insistence on the importance of creating a supportive environment to facilitate the healing process continues to be relevant in today's health care arena (Dossey, Selander, Beck et al., 2005), as does her insistence on standardizing health performance information to direct quality outcomes in health care (Kudzma, 2006).

Nursing theories that guide professional practice today have a richness evolving from scholarly inquiry, as well as an integrity springing from the commitment of its primary and contributing nursing leaders to explaining the phenomenon of professional nursing. Beginning in the 1940s, nursing leaders such as Virginia Henderson, Myra Levine, Martha Rogers, Imogene King, Sister Callista Roy, Madeline Leininger, Dorothea Orem, Jean Watson, Dorothy Johnson, Patricia Benner, Margaret Newman, Betty Neuman, and Rosemarie Parse have devoted their professional lifetimes to developing theories about the body of knowledge unique to professional nursing (Fawcett, 2000, 2005). Validating theory in nursing practice and linking nursing theory to evidence-based nursing practice (Youngblut & Brooten, 2001) becomes essential as health care turns its attention to measurement of clinical outcomes.

Nursing theory continues to be relevant as curricular and practice threads for all levels of nursing. The scholarly thinking of graduate nursing students helped to further nursing theory development. Gra-duate nursing students provided ideas, struggled to understand the language and meaning of concepts, critiqued ideas, and developed important research studies to support the validity of nursing theory.

Nursing theories are classified according to their levels of abstraction, ranging from grand theories to practice theories. Most commonly, they are classified as grand theory and mid-range theory, but a more recent category is that of practice theory (Marrs & Lowry, 2006). *Grand theories* encompass thinking about nursing as a whole and are the most abstract of theoretical knowledge. Examples include Martha Rogers's theory of unitary beings and Dorothea Orem's self-care deficit theory of nursing. *Mid-range theories* cover more discrete aspects of a phenomenon specific to professional nursing, exploring them in depth rather than exploring the full phenomena of nursing (Marrs & Lowry, 2006; Meleis, 1997). To be classified as a mid-range theory, the concepts must be applicable to many nursing situations and easily recognized and operationalized in nursing practice, and the basic assumptions must fit the theory (Whall, 1996). A mid-range theory can derive from a grand theory or from inductive research methodologies

Exercise 1-1 **Critiquing a Nursing Theory Article**

Purpose: To provide students with an opportunity to understand the connection of nursing theory to clinical practice.

Procedure:

1. Select an article from a professional journal that describes the use of nursing theory or nursing concepts. Suggestions for journals include *Nursing Science Quarterly, Journal of Advanced Nursing, Journal of Professional Nursing,* and *Advances in Nursing Science.*
2. Read the article carefully and critique the article to include the following: (a) how the author applied the theory or concept; (b) relevance of the concept or theory for nursing practice; (c) how you could use the concept in your own clinical practice; and (d) what you learned from reading the article.

Discussion:

In your class group, share some of the insights you obtained from the article and engage in a general discussion about the relevance of nursing theory for the professional nursing role.

such as concept analysis or grounded theory (McKenna, 1997; Meleis, 1997). *Practice theories* present situation-producing guidelines for evidence-based practice. Walker and Avant (2005) believe that practice theories should receive greater attention in directing the direction of modern nursing. Marrs and Lowry (2006) noted that "practice theories may be as simple as a single concept that is operationalized, and may be linked to a special population or situation" (p. 47). Exercise 1-1 provides an opportunity for students to critique an article using nursing theory in clinical practice.

Nursing Knowledge

A **paradigm** is defined as a worldview with global concepts underlying the theories and methodology of a particular scientific discipline. Nursing's theoretical paradigm distinguishes the nursing profession from other disciplines and makes its functions unique (Fawcett, 2005; Marrs & Lowry, 2006; Monti & Tingen, 1999). Nursing's professional metaparadigm consists of four elements: person, environment, health, and nursing. Although each theorist views these concepts through a different lens, exploring the relationships between and among the concepts of person, health, nurse, and environment is common to all theories of professional nursing (Frisch, 2001). Despite transformational changes in the health care system from a medical model to a public health model, with the broadening of primary practice sites into the community as a first line health resource, these elements continue to define the fundamental focus of professional nursing practice.

Concept of Person

Person, defined as the recipient of nursing care, must be considered as a functional whole with unique biopsychosocial and spiritual dimensions. The term can include more than the identified client. It can encompass a family, a community, or a target population such as the elderly, adolescents, or an ethnic group at risk for a particular health care problem. Komesaroff (2005) noted that recognizing and effectively responding to the needs of people closest to the client in health care situations is an important aspect of the clinician-client relationship that often gets neglected.

Nursing activities begin with the holistic understanding that each individual client is a unique human being, even before the specific health care problem is considered (American Holistic Nurses Association, 2004). Preserving and protecting the client's basic integrity and health rights as a unique individual are the ethical responsibility of nurse to client, whether the person is a contributing member of society, a critically ill newborn, a comatose client, or a seriously mentally ill individual.

Concept of Environment

The involvement of a person with his or her environment is so interrelated that to consider a person as an isolated variable in a health care situation is impracticable. **Environment** refers to the internal and external context of the client in the health care situation. Here the nurse considers the cultural, developmental, physical, and psychosocial conditions that influence the client's perception, behaviors, growth, and development. For example, a person's religious or spiritual beliefs, type of community (rural or urban), family strengths and challenges, and access to resources are part of a client's environmental context. Even climate, space, pollution, and food choices are important dimensions of environment.

Concept of Health

The word **health** derives from the word *whole*. Weil (2004) defines health as "a dynamic and harmonious equilibrium of all elements and forces making up and surrounding a human being" (p. 51). The World Health Organization (1987) identifies health as "a positive concept emphasizing social and personal resources, as well as physical capacities" (p. iii). Nurses provide health care for individuals, families, and communities at all points along the health-illness continuum, including palliative care and a peaceful death (Fryback, 1993). Health promotion activities are an expected and significant component of the professional nursing role.

The concept of health is multidimensional, with physical, psychological, sociocultural, developmental, and spiritual elements. The spiritual domain of health emphasizes a personal relationship with a higher power and recognition of a person's mortality. Additionally, *Healthy People 2010*, the health agenda for the United States for the next decade, considers *quality of life* as an important dimension of health and an expected outcome of quality health promotion activities. Quality of life is a personal experience having to do with "life satisfaction" or "subjective well-being" that includes, but is not limited to, physical health. Exercise 1-2 provides an opportunity to explore the multidimensional meaning of health.

The concept of health in the twenty-first century requires identifiable prevention and health promotion goals (Smith, 1990). Health promotion, and emphasizing factors that influence healthy lifestyle behaviors, has become a natural part of nursing intervention regardless of personal clinical diagnosis (Antrobus, 1997; Morgan & Marsh, 1998; Polk, 1997). Meleis (1990) has further proposed that health is an even broader concept than a purely personal one. She believes health should be

Exercise 1-2 Understanding the Meaning of Health as a Nursing Concept

Purpose: To help students understand the dimensions of health as a nursing concept.

Procedure:

1. Write a one-page description about the characteristics of a healthy person that you know.
2. In small groups of three or four, read your stories to each other. As you listen to other students' stories, write down themes that you note.
3. Compare themes, paying attention to similarities and differences and developing a group definition of health derived from the stories.
4. In a larger group, share your definitions of health and defining characteristics of a healthy person.

Discussion:

1. Were you surprised by any of your thoughts about being healthy?
2. Did your peers define health in similar ways?
3. Based on the themes that emerged, how is health determined?
4. Is illness the opposite of being healthy?
5. In what ways can a nurse support the health of a client?

considered as a social concern, particularly for people who do not have personal control over their health or the necessary resources to enhance their health status. As the United States grows more diverse, nurses need to be aware of different explanatory models that other cultures use to explain cause and pathophysiology of medical disorders. They need to become well acquainted with the natural cultural healing systems used for treatment and disease prevention so that these variables can be integrated into holistic care of clients and families.

Concept of Nursing

The concept of nursing is of central importance to the development of theory for the profession. The International Council of Nursing (ICN) defines *nursing* as follows:

> Nursing encompasses autonomous and collaborative care of individuals of all ages, families, groups and communities, sick or well and in all settings. Nursing includes the promotion of health, prevention of illness, and the care of ill, disabled and dying people. Advocacy, promotion of a safe environment, research, participation in shaping health policy and in patient and health systems management, and education are also key nursing roles. (ICN, 2006)

Mead (1956) noted that nurses are invariably found wherever there is human pain and suffering. The goal of nursing is to empower clients and to provide them with the support they need to achieve health and well-being. Taken in this context, modern nursing moves away from a conceptualization of nursing as an externally applied "doing for" process to one that is intimately tied to a unique partnership with clients in health care. Nursing services are designed to build on and strengthen the natural capacities of individuals, families, and communities. Nurses provide a continuum of health care services ranging from health education to direct care and research evaluation.

Pullen, Edwards, Lenz et al. (1994) defined nursing in today's health care environment as "the provision of essential health services to promote health, prevent illness, and promote cure of/or adaptation to illness" (p. 202).

The nurse-client relationship provides the primary means for delivering quality nursing care. Central to professional nursing is the concept of the nurse-client relationship built on the core concept of caring. In examining the nature and structure of the nurse-client relationship, we start with its root definition as "a process of nourishing, of promoting the development or progress of something" (Reed, 1997, p. 76).

Caring, the element that nurses most value about their practice, is an essential characteristic of professional practice. Crowe (2000) argues that "caring does not involve specific tasks, instead it involves the creation of a sustained relationship with the other" (p. 966). Basic characteristics of professional caring in nursing include (a) giving of self; (b) involved presence; (c) intuitive knowing and empathy; and (d) supporting the patient's integrity, with (e) professional competence (Arnold, 1997). Exercise 1-3 looks at professional nursing.

Exercise 1-3 What Is Professional Nursing?

Purpose: To help students develop an understanding of professional nursing.

Procedure:

1. Interview a professional nurse; ask for descriptions of what he or she considers professional nursing to be today; in what ways he or she thinks nurses make a difference; and what he or she sees as the most significant achievement in professional nursing.
2. In small groups of three to five students, discuss findings and develop a group definition of professional nursing.

Discussion:

1. What does nursing mean to you?
2. Is your understanding of nursing different from those of the nurse(s) you interviewed?
3. As a new nurse, how would you want to present yourself?

Patterns of Knowing

Professional nursing draws from several different forms of knowledge (Berragau, 1998). In a now classic work, Carper (1995) described **four patterns of knowing** embedded in nursing practice: empirical, personal, aesthetic, and ethical (Carr, 1996; Sherman, 1997). Johnson and Webber (2001) stress the value of integrating personal, aesthetic, and ethical ways of knowing with an empirical understanding of the client as the most effective means of enabling nurses to individualize and provide quality care. Although the patterns of knowing are described as individual patterns, in practice they need to inform care as an integrated focus of knowledge, with no one pattern used in isolation from the others. Carper's work draws attention to the importance of combining knowledge gained through the less tangible aspects of clinical practice with scientific data (Fawcett et al., 2001).

Patterns of knowing also are essential elements of critical thinking and effective decision making (Radwin, 1996). The four patterns of knowing are described as follows:

- *Empirical ways of knowing* are grounded in the science of nursing and evidenced in the scientific principles a nurse consistently incorporates in all phases of the nursing process. For example, nurses use a scientific rationale as the basis for choosing skilled nursing interventions.
- *Personal ways of knowing* help nurses understand and acknowledge the humanness of another. Personal knowing occurs when a nurse is able to intuitively understand and treat individual clients as unique human beings because of the nurse's own personal experience and awareness of his or her own humanness. This allows nurses to be authentic with others (Fawcett et al., 2001).

Exercise 1-4 The Relevance of Patterns of Knowing for Clinical Practice

Purpose: To help students understand how patterns of knowing can be used effectively in clinical practice.

Procedure:

1. Break into smaller groups of three to four students. Identify a scribe for each student group.
2. Using the case study below, decide how you would use empirical, personal, ethical, and aesthetic patterns of knowing to see that Mrs. Smith's holistic needs were addressed in the next 48 hours.

Case Study:

Mrs. Jackson, an 86-year-old widow, was admitted to the hospital with a hip fracture. She has very poor eyesight due to macular degeneration and takes eye drops for the condition. Her husband died five years ago, and she subsequently moved into an assisted housing development. She had to give up driving because of her eyesight, and sold her car to another resident five months ago. Although her daughter lives in the area, Mrs. Jackson has very little contact with her. This distresses her greatly, as she describes being very close with her until eight years ago. She feels safe in her new environment but complains that she is very lonely and is not interested in joining activities. She has a male friend in the complex, but recently he has been showing less interest. Her surgery is scheduled for tomorrow, but she has not yet signed her consent form. She does not have advance directives.

Discussion:

1. In a large group, have each student scribe share their findings.
2. For each pattern of knowing, write the suggestions on the board.
3. Compare and contrast the findings of the different groups.
4. Discuss how the patterns of knowing add to an understanding of the client in this case study.

- *Aesthetic ways of knowing* allow for creative applications in the relationship designed to connect with clients in a different and more meaningful way (Chinn, Maeve, & Bostick, 1997; Johnson & Webber, 2001). Examples of aesthetic ways of knowing are found in storytelling, in which the nurse seeks to understand the experience of the client's journey through illness (Leight, 2002).
- *Ethical ways of knowing* refers to the moral aspects of nursing. These ways of knowing encompass knowledge of what is right and wrong, attention to standards and codes in making moral choices, and taking responsibility for one's actions, as well as demonstrating professional values in providing health care (Johns, 1995). Exercise 1-4 provides an application of patterns of knowing in clinical practice.

Evidence-Based Nursing Practice

Over the past decade, evidence-based practice (EBP) has emerged as a primary means to advance professional standards in nursing practice and enhance quality care for clients (Van Achterberg, Holleman, Van de Ven et al., 2006). As professional nursing keeps pace with the latest knowledge developments in clinical practice, professional nurses increasingly will be called upon to deliver quality health care according to standardized, evidence-based guidelines. This evidence will be used "to define best practices rather than to support existing practices" (Youngblut & Brooten, 2001, p. 468).

Evidence-based practice is defined as "the conscientious explicit and judicious use of current best evidence in making decisions about the care of individual patients" (Sackett, Rosenberg, Gray et al., 1996, p. 71). Evidence-based practice is informed, collaborative, and patient-centered. Evidence-based approaches can generate knowledge from a target population that can be applied to the care of other individual clients with confidence (Devery, 2006). Four components are required:

- Best practices, derived from consensus statements developed by expert clinicians and researchers.
- Evidence from scientific findings in research-based studies. The "evidence" is found in published journals of scientific clinical research studies (Sinclair, 2004).
- Clinical nursing expertise of professional nurses, including knowledge of pathophysiology, pharmacology, and psychology.
- Preferences and values of clients and family members (Sigma Theta Tau International, 2003).

Although evidence-based practice is a critical component of care planning in a managed health care environment, emphasizing provision of effective, cost-efficient, quality care outcomes, several authors caution against its exclusive use as a guideline for care (Fawcett et al., 2001; Mead, 2000). They argue that scientific evidence needs to be balanced by values-based nursing knowledge and patterns of knowing that may or may not be completely resolvable with guidelines based strictly on scientific evidence. Sources of evidence-based practice also can include philosophical texts, individual narratives, and scholarly works of criticism (Cody, 2002).

Technology plays an expanding role in directly supporting evidence-based practice in a practical way. Increasingly, nurses are using personal handheld computers to inform their clinical decision making, right at the bedside (Honeybourne, Sutton, Ward, 2006). The

Developing an Evidence-Based Practice

Hutchinson AM, Johnston L: Bridging the divide: a survey of nurses' opinions regarding barriers to, and facilitators of, research utilization in the practice setting, *J Clin Nurs* 13(3):304-315, 2004.

This survey study was designed to elicit nurse's opinions (N = 761) regarding barriers and facilitators to their utilizing research in clinical practice.

Results: Reported barriers included time constraints, lack of awareness about availability of research literature, insufficient authority and/or lack of support to make changes based on research findings, and lack of knowledge needed for critique of research studies. Facilitators included availability of time, access and support for review and implementation of research findings, and support of colleagues.

Application to Your Clinical Practice: As a profession, nurses need to develop research evidence and implement relevant study findings to help ensure the health and well-being of their clients. What steps would you need to take as an individual nurse to encourage a strong connection between research and practice in your clinical setting?

personal digital assistant (PDA) contains a critical mass of relevant information in a concise, quickly assessable clinical tool (see Chapter 24). Nurses also can find data to support evidence-based nursing practice through the website for the Agency for Healthcare Research and Quality (www.ahrq.gov). This branch of the U.S. Department of Health and Human Services sponsors and conducts evidence-based research relevant to health care outcomes, quality, safety, cost, and access.

In each chapter, a Developing an Evidence-Based Practice box related to chapter content will be presented to stimulate your thinking about using research evidence to enhance professional nursing practice (see p. 8).

APPLICATIONS

Nursing Theory in the Nurse-Client Relationship

Hildegard Peplau

Dr. Peplau was the first nurse theorist to describe the nurse-client relationship as the foundation of nursing practice. Her theory of interpersonal relationships in nursing is an example of a mid-range theory (Armstrong & Kelly, 1995) and builds on Harry Stack Sullivan's (1953) psychodynamic interpersonal theory. In shifting the focus from what nurses do to clients to what nurses do *with clients*, Peplau masterminded a major paradigm shift from a nursing model focused on medical treatments to an interpersonal model of nursing practice in which the nurse uses himself or herself as a therapeutic agent (Barker, 1998; Feely 1997; Fowler, 1995; Reynolds, 1997). She viewed nursing as a "developmental educational instrument" designed to help individuals, families, and communities achieve changes in health care status and well-being, and illness as an opportunity for improved functioning (Peplau, 1992).

According to Peplau, techniques of description, formulation, interpretation, validation, and intervention form the essence of a nurse-client relationship in which the nurse helps the client transform raw data into a meaningful shared experience that both can understand (Thelander, 1997). As a nurse observes and listens to a client, he or she develops impressions and general ideas about the meaning of the client's situation. The nurse validates these inferences by checking with the client for accuracy.

The dynamic nursing approach Peplau advocated is not that of a passive spectator. As participant-observers, nurses actively engage with their clients, simultaneously observing clients' behaviors and their own responses, and providing assistance, information, and encouragement as needed. Peplau identified six professional roles the nurse assumes in the nurse-client relationship (Box 1-1).

Box 1-1 Peplau's Six Nursing Roles

1. Stranger role: Receives the client the same way one meets a stranger in other life situations; provides an accepting climate that builds trust.
2. Resource role: Answers questions, interprets clinical treatment data, gives information.
3. Teaching role: Gives instructions and provides training; involves analysis and synthesis of the learner experience.
4. Counseling role: Helps client understand and integrate the meaning of current life circumstances; provides guidance and encouragement to make changes.
5. Surrogate role: Helps client clarify domains of dependence, interdependence, and independence, and acts on client's behalf as advocate.
6. Active leadership: Helps client assume maximum responsibility for meeting treatment goals in a mutually satisfying way.

Developmental Phases. Peplau described four developmental phases of the relationship that overlap and build on one another. She characterized the nurse-client relationship as a dynamic learning experience out of which personal-social growth can occur for both nurse and client.

In today's health care environment, nurse-client relationships are of short duration, and nursing interventions have to be brief, concise, and effective. Despite the brevity of the relationship, similar principles of building rapport, developing a working partnership, and terminating a relationship in ways that leave the client with a greater sense of well-being than before the encounter remain important. The **orientation phase** sets the stage for the rest of the relationship by offering a systematic means for gathering assessment data from the client and establishing rapport with the client. The **working phase** has two components; the *identification* component focuses on mutual clarification of ideas and expectations, setting of goals, and treatment planning to achieve identified goals. The exploitation phase helps the client work toward treatment goals, resolve health care issues and learn new coping strategies. Peplau referred to the final phase of the relationship as the **termination (resolution) phase**, in which the nurse assists the client to review progress toward goals, makes referrals, and brings closure to the therapeutic relationship (see Chapter 5 for communication skills relevant to each developmental phase).

Contributions from Other Disciplines

Selected theory contributions from psychiatry, sociology, education, and psychology reinforce the importance of the nurse-client relationship, providing a broader psychological understanding of behaviors and desired outcomes in helping relationships.

Therapeutic Conversations with Clients

Sigmund Freud. Sigmund Freud (1937, 1959) introduced the therapeutic value of talking about painful experiences as a way of reducing stress and developing a higher quality of life. Freud's ideas about **transference** (in which the client projects irrational attitudes and feelings from the past onto people in the present) are useful in understanding difficult behaviors in nurse-client relationships. For example, the client who says to the young nurse, "Get me a real nurse! You're young enough to be my daughter, and I don't want to talk with you about my personal life," may be having a transference reaction having little to do with the nurse's competence. Recognizing this statement as a transference reaction

Table 1-1 Personality Development

Age (Years)	Erikson's Psychosocial Stages	Primary Person Orientation	Strengths	Qualities	Freud's Psychosexual Stages	Jung's Psychosocial Orientation
0-2	Trust versus mistrust	Mother	Hope	To receive, to give	Oral	Largely unconscious
2-4	Autonomy versus shame-guilt	Father	Willpower	To control, to let go	Anal	
4-6	Initiative versus guilt	Basic family	Purpose	To make, to play-act	Oedipal	Beginning ego consciousness
6-12	Industry versus inferiority	Neighborhood, school	Competence	To make things, to put things together	Latency	
13-19	Identity versus identity diffusion	Peer groups	Fidelity	To be one's self	Puberty	Individual consciousness
Young adult	Intimacy versus self-absorption	Partners in marriage, friendship	Love	To share one's self with another	Geniality	Social adaptation achievement
Adult	Generativity versus self-absorption	Children, community	Care	To take care of, to create		Inner reflection, individuation
Old age	Integrity versus despair	Humankind	Wisdom	To accept being, to accept not being		Self-knowledge of the meaning of one's existence

Adapted from Erikson E: *The life cycle completed,* New York, 1982, Norton.

helps the nurse depersonalize the client's comment, allowing for a more appropriate response.

Countertransference feelings refer to unconscious attitudes or exaggerated feelings a nurse may develop toward a client. They can emerge as a negative or an overly positive response to a client's behavior. For example, feeling anger or frustration, experiencing strong attraction, or feeling like a child with a powerful client can be countertransference feelings stemming from the client's behavior, the nurse's personal needs, or even past encounters with similar behaviors. Unrecognized countertransference feelings sabotage the relationship, whereas acknowledged countertransference feelings are an important source of information.

Freud was the first clinician to identify age-related sequential stages of personality development, which he termed psychosexual development (Table 1-1). Freud believed that people who do not resolve a specific maturational stage at the appropriate age are destined to retain an immature behavioral response pattern for the rest of their lives. They remain "fixated" at that developmental stage. Behaviors and emotions out of proportion to a situation may indicate a lack of psychosocial maturity in resolving earlier developmental stages. For example, a client who experienced little parental support in early childhood may find it difficult to trust that identified caregivers, including health care professionals, will help.

Freud focused on the role of anxiety in explaining problematic behaviors and identified **ego defense mechanisms** (see Chapter 20 for definitions and examples) as unconscious methods a person uses to protect the self from experiencing anxiety. Nurses use these concepts as they strive to understand their clients' and their own behaviors in the nurse-client relationship.

Carl Jung. Jung's work (1963, 1971) helps nurses examine the complex dimensions of a person; these include gender roles, acceptance of each individual just as they are, and our universal heritage as human beings. Nurses' recognition of the common human bonds shared with all clients helps promote understanding and acceptance of people as human beings first and foremost.

Jung's concepts of adult development are useful in understanding midlife. He notes that "we cannot live the afternoon of life according to the values of life's morning" (1971). He viewed the first half of life as a search for self, and the second half of life as a search for soul.

Jung likened the role of a helping person in a therapeutic relationship to a "midwife, assisting in bringing into the light of day a natural process, the process of coming into one's self" (Von Franz, 1975). This metaphor is useful in describing the nurse-client relationship, wherein the client does the work, and the nurse assists the client in a natural life process of self-discovery, using his or her expertise to facilitate the process.

Harry Stack Sullivan. Peplau credited Sullivan's work as the theoretical base for her ideas about the nurse-client relationship. Harry Stack Sullivan (1953), an American psychoanalyst, introduced the idea of the therapeutic relationship as a human connection that heals. People learn their humanness from significant others in their environment (see Chapters 4 and 13). Having a corrective interpersonal experience in adulthood with a helping professional can help individuals find the self-security they missed in childhood.

Working mostly with schizophrenic patients, Sullivan introduced the concept that people cannot always relate easily to a helping person and may need ongoing, compassionate, supportive encouragement to make use of the therapeutic relationship. Individuals experiencing shock, panic, serious mental illness, or brain damage are particularly vulnerable. Understanding this fact allows the nurse to act empathetically with clients who are unable to relate effectively with a helping person (Peplau, 1992).

Martin Buber. The I-thou relationship described by Martin Buber (1958) captured the essence of the equal partner connection desired in the nurse-client relationship. In an **I-thou relationship**, each individual responds to the other as a unique person in a mutually respectful manner. Neither is an "object" of study. Instead, there is a process of mutual discovery. Each person feels free to be authentic.

Buber's work forms the theoretical foundation for using confirming responses in which the helping person identifies an observable strength of another person and comments on it. He described this way of responding as follows: "Man wishes to be confirmed in his being by man and wishes to have a presence in the being of the other. Secretly and bashfully, he watches for a yes which allows him to be" (Buber, 1957, p. 104). Nurses confirm the humanity of clients each time they respect their human dignity, even when clients are difficult or unappreciative.

Carl Rogers. Carl Rogers's person-centered model of therapeutic relationships emphasizes an I-thou relationship as essential to healing and points to the primacy of person as the agent of healing. According to Rogers (1961), "if I can provide a certain type of relationship, the other person will discover within himself the capacity to use that relationship for growth and change, and personal development will occur." Rogers identified three helper characteristics essential to the development of client-centered relationships: unconditional positive regard, empathetic understanding, and genuineness. He later added a fourth characteristic, a spiritual or transcendental presence as an intuitive way of being with a client (Anderson, 2001). The characteristics of the helping person that Rogers described as necessary to a successful therapeutic relationship are identified in Chapter 5, and are discussed as bridges to relationships in Chapter 6. In addition to having relevance for the nurse-client relationship, Rogers's concepts of a person-centered relationship are applicable for nurse-client health teaching formats (see Chapter 16).

Aaron Beck. Beck's (1991) cognitive behavioral therapy (CBT) model offers an evidenced-based therapeutic approach based on the premise that a person's thoughts (cognitions) are significant determinants of feelings (moods) and actions (behaviors; Figure 1-2). By changing a person's dysfunctional thoughts, beliefs, and perceptions (cognitions), it is possible to make changes in their usual pattern of behaving, resulting in a more constructive approach to a problem situation. Beck identified three variables he considered to be instrumental in maintaining dysfunctional thinking:

- Cognitive distortions
- Cognitive triad (person's negative view of him/herself, world, and the future)
- Schemata

Cognitive distortions are automatic thoughts that appear spontaneously in response to a stressful situation; seem to be valid assessments; and cause a person to interpret neutral situations in an exaggerated, personalized, negative way. These distortions can reflect negative cognitive biases (referred to as *schemata*) in a person's mind. They often represent early ingrained evaluative

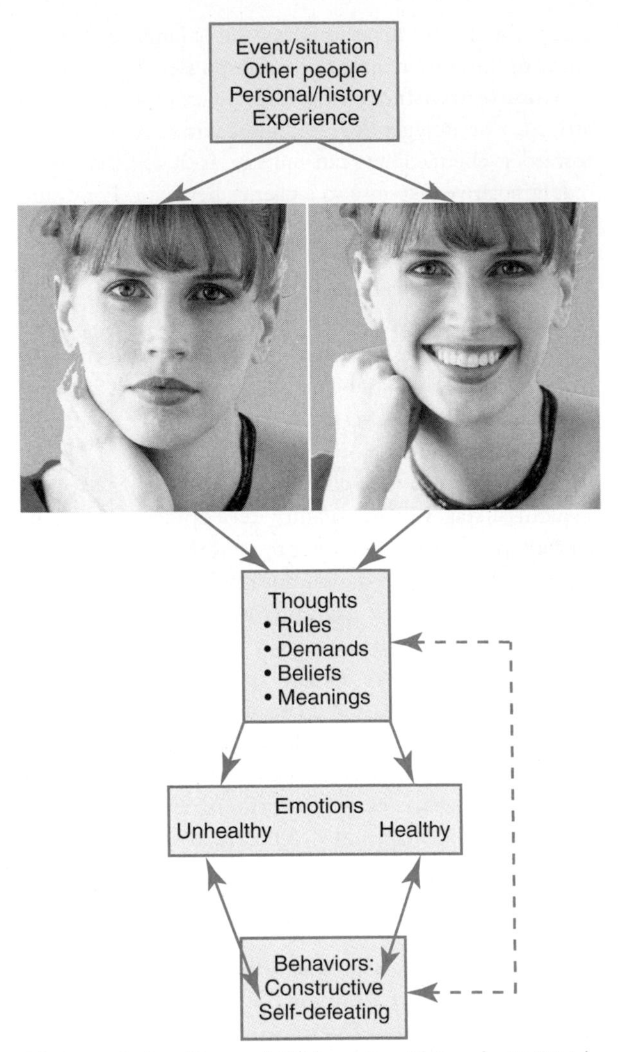

Figure 1-2 • Diagram of CBT formulation. (Photographs © 2006 by Jupiter Images Corp.)

beliefs about the person and the contextual world. Beck's theory focused on teaching people to challenge distortions and expand their thinking to include options, choices, and possibilities rather than a single and often fatalistic negative interpretation of an event or circumstance. By challenging negative distortions and rules about behaviors that narrow potential solutions to problems, people begin to take charge of the changes needed to effectively resolve difficult problems.

Developmental Theorists

Erik Erikson. Erik Erikson (1950, 1969, 1982) broadened Freud's model of psychosexual stages to include psycho*social* development. Erikson viewed identity as the central developmental life task and considered self-definition as a lifelong maturational process stimulated by age-related psychosocial crises of maturation. The first four stages of the life cycle are designed to help an individual develop identity, while the last three stages are designed to refine and expand one's personal identity. (See Table 1-1 for a listing of each life stage and Chapter 4 for a detailed description of this model.)

Erikson viewed developmental maturation as a linear process from lower to higher development, with each stage representing a more complex formation of identity development and incorporating development from previous stages. Individuals mature by developing more complex social skills as they successfully resolve psychosocial developmental crises. The transition from one developmental stage to another precipitates a psychosocial crisis, because previous patterns of psychosocial adaptation no longer work effectively. Society provides ritualistic markers of psychosocial stages in the life cycle, such as confirmations, graduations, weddings, and retirement. Developmental remnants of earlier experiences persist, to be constantly reworked and interwoven into the tapestry of life (Erikson & Erikson, 1981).

Certain life experiences and culture—for example, the death or divorce of a parent, frequent moves, and family abuse—can affect the specific timetable and expression of psychosocial development of individuals. Erikson (1982) considered unexpected life circumstances that affect appropriate mastery of developmental

Exercise 1-5 Time Line

Purpose: To give students experience with understanding psychosocial development through the life span.

Procedure:
1. Draw a time line of your life to date. Include all significant events and the age at which they occurred.
2. Insert Erikson's stages as markers in your time line.

Discussion:
1. In what ways did Erikson's stages provide information about expected tasks in your life?
2. In what ways did they deviate?
3. To what would you attribute the differences?
4. How could you use this exercise in your nursing care of clients?

Exercise 1-6 Completing the Life Cycle

Purpose: To help students understand the integration of psychosocial development through the life cycle.

Procedure:
1. Interview an adult who has reached at least the sixth decade of life.
2. Identify Erikson's psychosocial tasks, and ask the person to identify what factors in his or her life contributed to or interfered with mastery of the task for each stage.
3. Describe in short summary the factors that you believe contributed or interfered with each stage of the person's adult life.

Discussion:
1. In a larger group, share your examples.
2. For each stage, compile on the board a list of the factors identified.
3. Discuss the impact certain factors may have on the outcome of development through the life span.

life tasks (e.g., illness, job promotion, marriage, job loss) as horizontal threads in a life tapestry. When they arise in conjunction with normal developmental crises, the developmental crisis is more intense and difficult to resolve (Dowd, 1990). Exercise 1-5 provides students with a personalized understanding of psychosocial development throughout the life span. Exercise 1-6 provides an opportunity to learn about the integration of psychosocial development through the life cycle.

Abraham Maslow. Abraham Maslow (1970) describes a theory of self-development with progressive stages of personal growth needs, beginning with physiological survival needs and ending with self-actualization. At the most fundamental level of Maslow's model are basic *physiological needs*. Satisfying hunger, thirst, and sexual and sensory stimulation needs has an emotional component that requires satisfaction as well. The second level of needs, *safety and security needs*, includes physical safety and emotional security. Once a person meets safety and security needs, a person seeks to meet *love and belonging needs*, the need to be part of a family or community. As people feel part of a community, they experience self-esteem. A sense of dignity, respect, and approval by others for the self within is the hallmark of successfully meeting *self-esteem needs*.

Maslow's highest level of need satisfaction, **self-actualization**, represents humanity at its best. Self-actualized individuals are not superhuman; they are subject to the same feelings of insecurity and vulnerability that all individuals experience. However, they accept this part of their humanness and strive to share it with others. Self-actualized people take important personal stands on issues, saying no when it is appropriate, and fully committing themselves to personal goals that enrich their sense of self and contribute to the lives of others. Box 1-2 describes characteristics of self-actualized people.

Nurses use Maslow's theory to help them prioritize nursing interventions: meeting basic needs, for exam-

Box 1-2 Characteristics of Self-Actualization

- Quality of genuineness
- Passion for living
- Ability to get along well with others
- Strong sense of personal worth
- View of life situations as opportunities, not threats
- Ability to experience each moment fully
- Moments of intense emotional meaning, "peak experience"
- Full acceptance of self and others
- Identification with fellow human beings
- High sense of responsibility with a strong desire to serve humanity
- Integrity of purposes

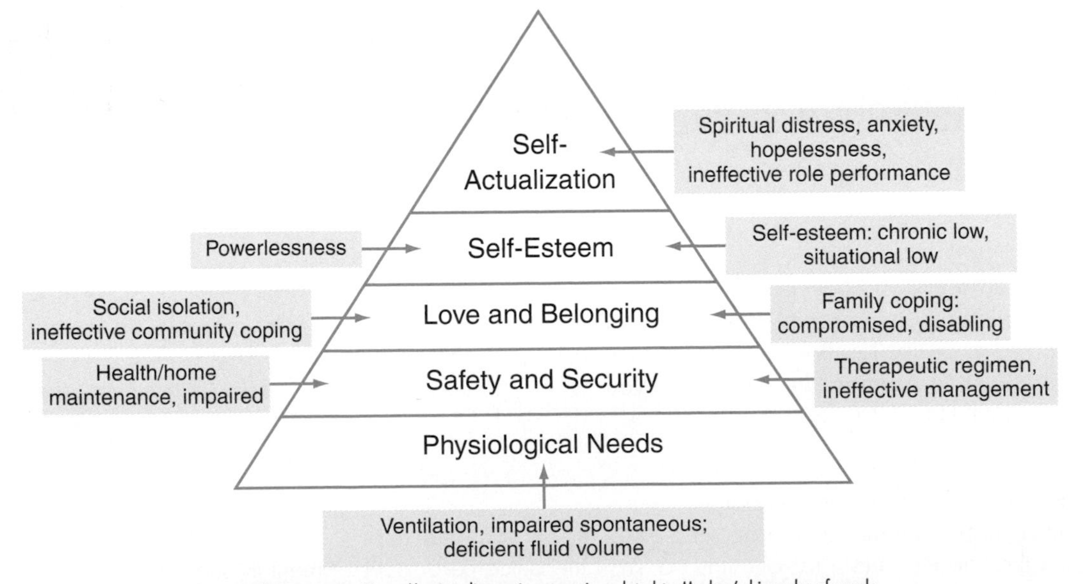

Figure 1-3 • Nursing diagnosis categories related to Maslow's hierarchy of needs.

ple, comes before helping clients meet growth needs. Figure 1-3 presents selected nursing diagnoses related to each stage of Maslow's theory. Exercise 1-7 provides the student with practice using Maslow's categories of need. Exercise 1-8 provides practice with a case study.

Communication Theory

Communication is defined as an interpersonal activity involving the transmission of messages from a source to a receiver for the purpose of influencing the receiver's behavior (Miller & Nicholson, 1976). Human com-

Exercise 1-7 Maslow's Hierarchy of Needs

Purpose: To help students understand the usefulness of Maslow's theory in clinical practice.

Procedure:

1. Divide the class into small groups, with each group assigned to a step of Maslow's hierarchy. Each group will then brainstorm examples of that need as it might present in clinical practice.
2. Identify potential responses from the nurse that might address each need.
3. Share examples with the larger group and discuss the concept of prioritization of needs using Maslow's hierarchy.

Discussion:

1. In what ways is Maslow's hierarchy helpful to the nurse in prioritizing client needs?
2. What limitations do you see with the theory?

Exercise 1-8 Case Application of Maslow's Theory

Purpose: To examine the use of Maslow's theory in a specific case.

Procedure:

In groups of three or four students, consider the following case study and apply Maslow's hierarchy of needs theory to Mr. Rodgers's case, from the time of admission to the coronary care unit until his discharge and follow-up care. Include any considerations for changing priorities because of fluctuations in his condition.

Case Study:

Mr. Rodgers was admitted to the cardiac intensive care unit with an acute myocardial infarction. He is an internationally known, middle-aged businessman, a corporate vice president of a major company, and very well liked by his employees. His blood pressure for the past two years has never fallen below a diastolic reading of 95, and he is being treated with a mild diuretic. Before this hospitalization, he had never been admitted to a hospital. Mr. Rodgers is anxious and perspiring profusely. He has many of the predisposing factors for heart problems present in his history, family, and lifestyle.

Discussion:

1. At what stage of Maslow's hierarchy is this client?
2. With what needs is the client likely to require nursing intervention during his hospitalization and after discharge?
3. In a large group, share your conclusions and recommendations for prioritizing Mr. Rodgers's care with a rationale.

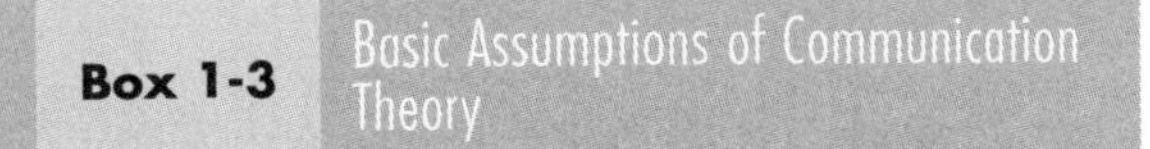

Box 1-3 Basic Assumptions of Communication Theory

- It is impossible not to communicate (Bateson, 1979).
- We only know about ourselves and others through communication.
- Faulty communication results in flawed feeling and acting.
- Feedback is the only way we know that our perceptions are valid.
- Silence is a form of communication.
- All parts of a communication system are interrelated and affect one another.
- People communicate through words and through nonverbal behaviors, both of which are necessary to interpret appropriately for complete understanding.

munication is unique. Only human beings have large vocabularies and are capable of learning new languages as a means of sharing their ideas and feelings. Communication is the primary means through which the nurse-client relationship occurs. The concept includes nonverbal behaviors as well as verbal communication. Certain basic assumptions serve as the foundation for the concept of communication (Box 1-3).

Linear Theory

Linear models refer to three components: speaker, message, receiver. The **sender** is the source or initiator of the message. The sender *encodes* the message (i.e., puts the message into verbal or nonverbal symbols that the receiver can understand). To encode a message appropriately requires a clear understanding of the receiver's mental frame of reference (e.g., feelings, personal agendas, past experiences) as well as knowledge of the desired objective of the communicated message. The sender organizes the message content to focus on key ideas that the sender wishes to convey.

The **message** consists of a verbal or nonverbal expression of thoughts or feelings transmitted from the sender to the receiver. The most effective messages are authentic and expressed in a language the receiver can understand.

The **receiver** is the recipient of the message. Once received, the receiver *decodes* it (i.e., translates the message into word symbols and internally interprets its meaning to make sense of the message). An open listening attitude and suspension of judgment strengthen the possibility of decoding the sender's message accurately (Figure 1-4).

Channels of communication refer to sensory receptors through which a person transmits information using one or more of the five senses: sight, hearing, taste, touch, and smell.

Circular Transactional Theoretical Models

A circular model is a transactional model that expands linear models to include the context of the communication, feedback loops, and validation (Figure 1-5). With this model, the sender and receiver construct a mental picture of the other, which influences the message and includes perceptions of the other person's attitude and potential reaction to the message. Two systems

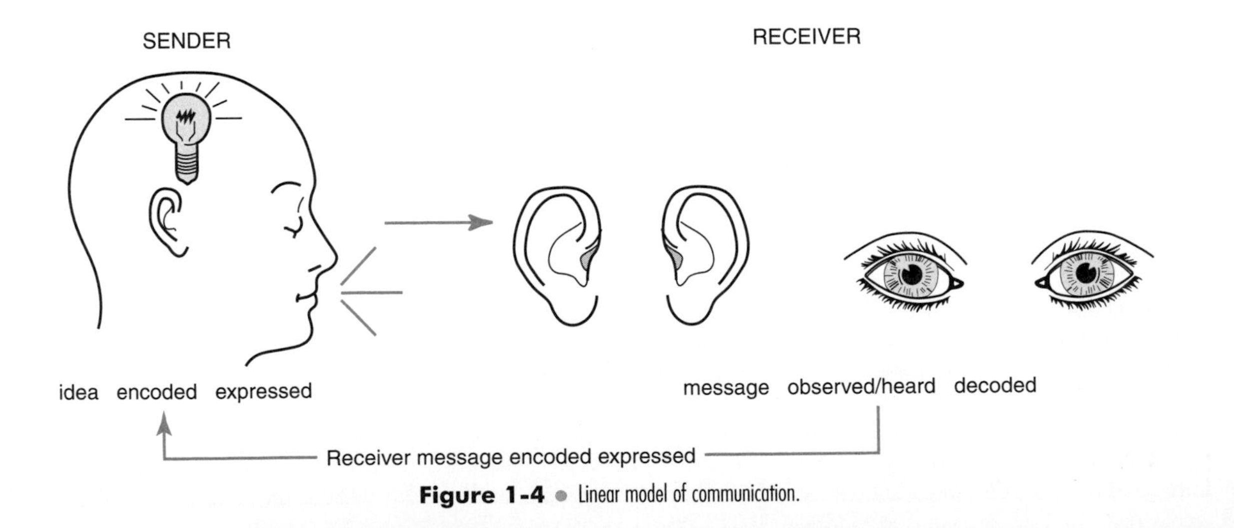

Figure 1-4 • Linear model of communication.

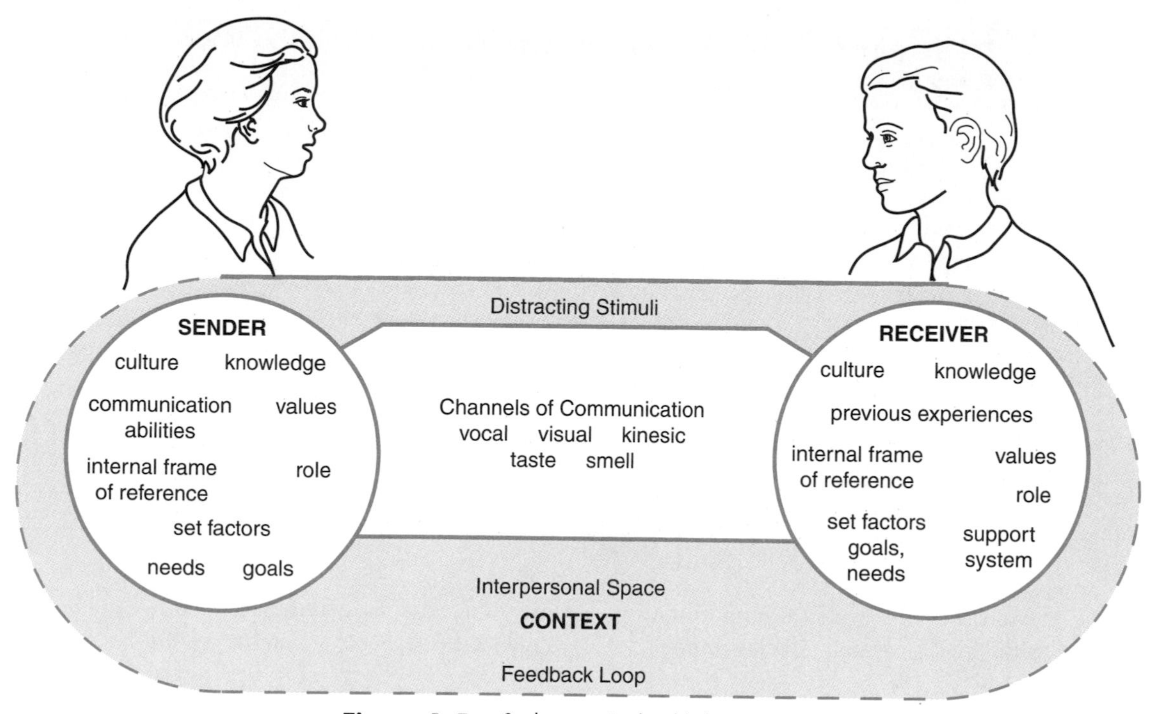

Figure 1-5 • Circular transactional model of communication.

theory concepts, *feedback* and *context*, expand linear constructs.

Circular transactional models are based on systems concepts that describe how the human system influences and is influenced by the communication it receives. Communication is conceptualized as a continuous, mutually interconnected activity in which sender and receiver influence each other in the transmission and receiving of a message. Accordingly, a human system receives information from the environment (input), internally processes the information and reacts to it based on its own internal functions (throughput), and produces new information or behavior (output) as a result of the process. Feedback allows the system to correct or sustain its original input.

Circular models also take into account the role relationships between communicators. People take either *symmetrical* or *complementary* roles in communicating. **Symmetrical role** relationships are equal, whereas **complementary role** relationships typically operate with one person holding a higher position than the other in the communication process. In health care situations, the nurse assumes the complementary role of clinical expert helping the client to achieve mutually determined health goals, and a symmetrical role in working with the client as partner on developing mutually defined goals and the means to achieve them.

Metacommunication is a nonverbal message about how the receiver should interpret the message. For example, a person may tell someone, "This is important, let's talk about it." If the person then sits down in a relaxed position with good eye contact and actively listens, the verbal and nonverbal messages are congruent. The same verbal message, delivered while looking at the clock or a watch, provides a nonverbal message that the sender doesn't have time to listen.

Feedback is the verbal or nonverbal response the receiver gives to the sender about the message. Feedback always occurs. Even by not responding, the receiver provides feedback. Feedback can focus on the content, the relationship between people and events, the feelings generated by the message, or the parts of the communication that are not clear. **Validation** is a special form of feedback that provides verbal and nonverbal confirmation that both participants have the same basic understanding of the message and the feedback (see

Exercise 1-9

Differences Between Linear and Circular Models of Communication

Purpose: To help students see the difference between linear and circular models of communication.

Procedure:

1. Role-play a scenario in which one person provides a scene that might occur in the clinical area using a linear model: sender, message, and receiver.
2. Role-play the same scenario using a circular model, framing questions that recognize the context of the message and its potential impact on the receiver, and provide feedback.

Discussion:

1. Was there a difference in your level of comfort? If so, in what ways?
2. Was there any difference in the amount of information you had as a result of the communication? If so, in what ways?
3. What implications does this exercise have for your future nursing practice?

Chapter 10). Exercise 1-9 provides an opportunity to experiment with linear versus circular models of communication.

Therapeutic Communication

Therapeutic communication (Ruesch, 1961) is a purposeful form of communication used in the helping relationship. Doheny et al. (1997) observed that "when certain skills are used to facilitate communication between nurse and client in a goal directed manner, the therapeutic communication process occurs" (p. 5). Therapeutic communication is not a method but rather a specialized application of basic communication principles designed to promote the client's health and well-being. Nurses use therapeutic communication skills to provide new information, correct misinformation, promote understanding of client responses to health problems, explore options for care, assist in decision making, and facilitate client wellbeing (Sellick, 1991).

Contemporary Issues

Today's paradigm for the health care delivery system is quite different than it was even a decade ago. Engebretson (2003) advised that the largest change in professional health care is the change in focus from diagnosis and treatment of disease to an expanded emphasis on health promotion and disease prevention.

Technological advances have advanced health care into a global enterprise, with a much stronger emphasis on promoting healthy lifestyles, personal responsibility for health, and short-term treatment. A public health framework has become a more appropriate model for care than the more traditional medical model. The emphasis in health care today is on self-knowledge and taking personal responsibility for healthy living and the utilization of health care resources.

The level and availability of Internet health care information for consumers and health care providers is unprecedented. The Internet offers immediate and, for the most part, accurate information about virtually every aspect of health care. Increased client acuity, an aging population with complex health care needs, an alarming shortage of professional nurses, and decreased financial resources are creating profound changes in how health care is delivered.

One of the most important influences on health care delivery is managed care, which was developed as a means of controlling health care costs spiraling out of control. Managed care insurance companies require evidence of medical necessity, scientific treatment efficacy, and cost effectiveness for third-party reimbursement. Not everyone benefits from the managed care paradigm; unfortunately, it has created significant issues regarding access to care for the elderly, the mentally ill, and the poor.

A variety of factors (e.g., economics, changes in demographics, multidisciplinary approaches to health care delivery, and advances in technology) are changing nursing's professional landscape (Booth, Kenrick, & Woods, 1997). These factors affect the context, goals, and strategies in the nurse-client relationship. Nursing

Table 1-2 Characteristics of the Current Health Care System

Orientation Toward Health	Coordination of services
Constrained Resources	Reconsideration of human values
Population perspective	
Intensive use of information	Expectations of accountability
Focus on the consumer	Growing interdependence
Knowledge of treatment outcomes	

From Seifer S: Recent and emerging trends in undergraduate medical education: curricular responses to a rapidly changing health care system, *West J Med* 168(5):401, 1998.

practice is becoming increasingly community-based in a health care delivery system that is market-driven, with no single discipline dominating health care delivery. In today's health care environment, the client is a consumer and an active partner in determining the focus of treatment and in planning and implementing health care measures. Seifer (1998) identifies relevant health care delivery expectations found in today's health care arena in Table 1-2.

Hospital stays today are short-term, even for major surgery. Nurses are expected to assume an expanded role in caring for complex health care needs in primary care settings. Today, community-based treatment provides a wide range of services that are coordinated by health professionals and community agencies. This requires priority setting and coordination of services to prevent duplication. The nurse in a community-based health care setting is expected to deliver comprehensive nursing care for clients with multiple health needs and to involve the informal family support system as well as formal support mechanisms. It is a networked delivery care system rather than an individual medical approach to health care. The Pew Commission (Bellack & O'Neil, 2000) set forth 21 competencies that nurses will need to incorporate into their nursing care to be successful practitioners in the twenty-first century (Box 1-4). Communication skills and the development of professional interpersonal relationships will be key to achieving and integrating these competencies into quality delivery of nursing practice.

Box 1-4 Pew Commission's Recommendations to Nursing Programs: 21 Nursing Competencies Needed for the 21st Century

1. Embrace a personal ethic of social responsibility and service.
2. Exhibit ethical behavior in all professional activities.
3. Provide evidence-based, clinically competent care.
4. Incorporate the multiple determinants of health in clinical care.
5. Apply knowledge of the new sciences.
6. Demonstrate critical thinking, reflection, and problem-solving skills.
7. Understand the role of primary care.
8. Rigorously practice preventive health care.
9. Integrate population-based care and services into practice.
10. Improve access to health care for those with unmet health needs.
11. Practice relationship-centered care with individuals and families.
12. Provide culturally sensitive care to a diverse society.
13. Partner with communities in health care decisions.
14. Use communication and information technology effectively and appropriately.
15. Work in interdisciplinary teams.
16. Ensure care that balances individual, professional, system, and societal needs.
17. Practice leadership.
18. Take responsibility for quality of care and health outcomes at all levels.
19. Contribute to continuous improvement of the health care system.
20. Advocate for public policy that promotes and protects the health of the public.
21. Continue to learn and help others learn.

From Bellack J, O'Neil E: Recreating nursing practice for a new century: recommendations and implications of the Pew Health Professions Commission's final report. *Nurs Health Care Perspect* 21(1):20, 2000.

Demographic Changes

In the twenty-first century, minority populations may well surpass the current Euro-Caucasian population majority in North America (Ketefian & Redman, 1997). Appreciation for the rapidly increasing diversity of our society is compelling in health care, not only because of differences in health-related characteristics, but also because of language, economic, and social barriers to seeking health care. The health care system in the United States is currently challenged by glaring gaps in access to care, with many segments of a growing minority population receiving inadequate or no health care. Enhancing access to care and providing culturally sensitive care to an increasingly diverse population will be major health promotion initiatives in the next decade.

Healthy People 2010 identifies "reducing health disparities" as an important goal for health care. There seems to be little question that nurses should be in the forefront of helping the nation develop prevention strategies for ethnically and economically challenged individuals, families, and communities in need of health care.

Technology

Technology advances have revolutionized health care delivery, documentation, and availability of medical information. Genome theory and scientific discoveries have increased longevity and quality of life for older adults, with the development of new diagnostics and sophisticated technological treatments such as laser and laparoscopic surgery. It is even possible to have a virtual colonoscopy. The Internet increasingly serves as a vital source of health information for consumers and health care providers, instantly linking them with current scientific and medical breakthroughs in diagnosis and treatment.

Other technological advances such as the electronic house call, Internet support groups, and the virtual health examination are still in their infancy but may well take the place of office visits and become a major health care resource in the future, particularly in remote areas. Technology makes it possible for health experts in geographically distant areas throughout the world to share information and to draw important conclusions about health care issues in real time.

Computerized medical records are replacing written records as the preferred methodology for sharing information among health care providers (see Chapter 23). Electronic record keeping, which links client information among health care providers, is already in place in large hospital systems such as Veterans Administration Hospitals, the National Institutes of Health, and the Visiting Nurses Association, as well as in remote areas of Canada.

Telehealth is fast becoming a part of the health care system, used both as a live interactive mechanism (particularly in remote areas, where there is a scarcity of health care providers) and as a way to track data about clients as a method of reducing costs (Peck, 2005). The concept is defined as "the use of telecommunications and information technology to provide access to health assessment, diagnosis, intervention, consultation, supervision, education and information across distance" (Nickelson, 1998, p. 527). Telehealth technologies have

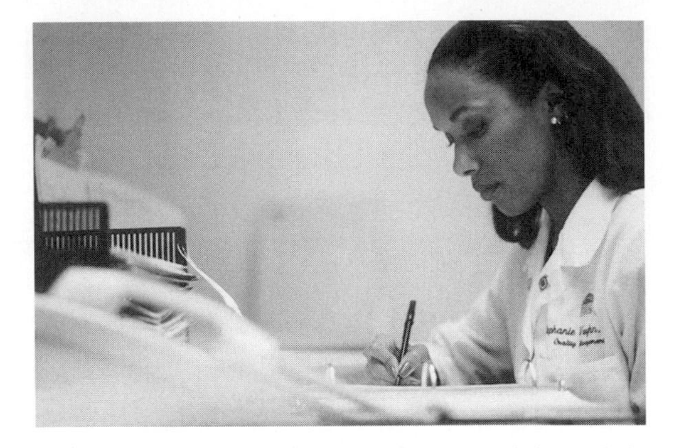

Telehealth technologies allow nurses a new level of interaction with clients and other health providers. (Courtesy University of Maryland School of Nursing.)

the capacity to bring highly trained specialists into the home through the Internet and teleconferencing. They allow nurses a level of interaction with clients and other health care providers previously not available. Telehealth educational programs can permit clients and families to learn about relevant health information on virtually every health condition, including diagnostic symptoms, recommended treatments, and health care specialists. Clark (2000) describes the integration of technology from the perspective of a Canadian nurse caring for a client in a remote area in the year 2020. In this vision, the nurse acts as both an information broker and an information generator. The case example that follows—though it may sound a little far-fetched—is possible, given that there have been more advances in communication technology over the past quarter-century than in the past millennium.

Case Example

The computer gently hums to life as community health nurse Rachel Muhammat logs into Nursenet. She asks a research partner, a cyberware specialist in London, England, for the results from a trial on neurological side effects of ocular biochips. Rachel, as part of a 61-member team in 23 countries, is studying six clients with the chips. Then it's down to local business. Rachel e-mails information on air contaminant syndrome to a client down the street whose son is susceptible to the condition, and tells her about a support group in Philadelphia. She contacts a qigong specialist to see if he can teach the boy breathing exercises and schedules an appointment with an environmental nurse specialist.

Moments before her 9:45 appointment, Rachel gets into her El-van and programs it to an address 2 kilometers away. Her patient, Mr. Chan, lost both legs in a subway accident and needs to be prepared for a bionic double-leg transplant. Together they assess his needs and put together a team of health workers, including a surgeon, physiotherapist, acupuncturist, and home care helpers. She talks to him about the transplant, and they hook up to his virtual reality computer to see and talk to another client who underwent the same procedure. Before leaving, Mr. Chan grasps her hand and thanks her for helping him. Rachel hugs him and urges him to e-mail her if he has any more questions. (Sibbald, 1995, p. 3 [quoted in Clark, 2000]).

Table 1-3 Criteria for Survival of the Nursing Profession Based on Evolutionary Principles

Criteria or Condition	Evolutionary Principle
Nursing needs to be relevant.	In nature, an organism will only survive if it occupies a niche, that is, performs a specific role that is needed in its environment.
Nursing must be accountable.	In every environment there is a limited amount of resources. Organisms that are more efficient and use the available resources more effectively are much more likely to be selected by the environment.
Nursing needs to retain its uniqueness while functioning in a multidisciplinary setting.	In nature, an organism will only survive if it is unique. If it ceases to be so it is in danger of losing its niche or role in the environment. In other words, it might lose out if the new species is slightly better adapted to the role, or if physically similar enough, it might even breed with that species and thus completely lose its identity. Successful organisms must also learn to coexist with many different species so that their role complements that of the other organisms.
Nursing needs to be visible.	In nature, organisms often are required to defend their niche and their territory usually by an outward display that allows other similar species to be aware of their presence. By being 'visible' similar species can avoid direct conflict. In addition visibility is also important for recognition by members of their own species, to allow for the formation of family and social units, based on cooperation and respect.
Nursing needs to have a global impact.	In nature, if a species is to survive, it must make its presence felt not just to its immediate neighbors but to all the members of its environment. Often, this results in a species adapting a unique presence, whether it is a color pattern, smell, or sound.
Nurses need to be innovators.	In evolution, the organisms that survive are, more often than not, innovators that have the flexibility to come up with new and different solutions to rapid changes in environmental conditions.
Nurses need to be both exceptionally competent and strive for excellence.	During evolution, when new niches open up, it is never possible for more than one species to occupy one niche. Only the best adapted and most competent among the competing organisms will survive; all others, even if only slightly less competent, will die.

From Bell (1997) as cited in Gottlieb L, Gottlieb B: Evolutionary principles can guide nursing's future development, *J Adv Nurs* 28(5):1099, 1998.

Positioning Nursing as a Key Player

The nation has moved to a model of health care delivery that, ironically, values many of the same constructs nursing has always championed. Gottlieb and Gottlieb (1998) identify nursing values important to health care in the twenty-first century as caring, holism, health promotion, continuity of care, family-based care, and working in partnership with individual and community agendas. The metaparadigm for nursing theory, with its emphasis on the interrelationship between person, environment, health, and nursing, could well be used as a template for the current focus of the health care delivery system. Nursing's strength of purpose, values, and traditions of care will need to be retained in the new visions of health care delivery.

Nursing has had a long and honorable commitment to care of poor, marginalized, and vulnerable populations consistent with the goal of reducing health disparities identified in *Healthy People 2010.* The core activities of professional nursing are well matched with national health goals related to health promotion, disease prevention, and improving quality of life. Table 1-3 identifies seven criteria or conditions and their evolutionary correlates needed to secure a key player role for nurses in the new health care delivery system.

If nursing is to survive as a unique profession in a capitated health care environment marked by blurring of roles and decreased resource allocation, nurses must take a more active part in defining their role, marking their contributions to health care with tangible examples, and developing their profession through membership and support of nursing organizations. Nurses must be prepared to learn new and expanded skills appropriate to emerging health care understandings and technology (Ludwick, 1999). The essential features of nursing practice, however, evidenced in caring relationships with clients, a holistic view of persons with a wide range of life experiences and personal responses to health care, and integration of scientific knowledge with critical thinking and clinical reasoning skills, remain unchanged. To that end, the purpose of this text is respectfully dedicated.

SUMMARY

This chapter introduces theoretical concepts that contribute to the understanding of the nurse-client relationship. Use of theoretical models in the implementation of the nurse-client relationship brings order to nursing practice, provides a cognitive structure for developing a body of knowledge identifiable with the profession, and contributes a basis for nursing research. Four elements critical to an understanding of nursing practice are person, health, nursing, and environment.

Hildegard Peplau's theory of interpersonal relationships in professional nursing practice forms the basic theory structure for the nurse-client relationship. She described three phases of the relationship: orientation, working, and resolution. Building on the work of Harry Stack Sullivan, Peplau believed that the interpersonal relationship is the crux of effective nursing practice.

Nursing integrates concepts and principles related to the development of interpersonal relationships from other disciplines. Sigmund Freud's contributions include the therapeutic value of talking about painful experiences, the concepts of transference and countertransference, and ego defense mechanisms. Carl Jung proposed several controversial ideas that today are recognized as valid regarding spirituality, the influence of culture on behavior, adult development, and gender roles. Erikson broadened the scope of earlier thinking on personality development to include humans' interaction with the larger social environment. Buber and Rogers offered basic concepts concerning the characteristics the nurse needs for developing effective interpersonal relationships with clients. Maslow's needs theory provides a basis for determining priorities in all phases of the nursing process.

Communication is the foundation and basic tool of the nurse-client relationship. Included in communication models are concepts related to the context of, as well as the participants in, the dialogue. Feedback from the environment provides additional input that makes communication a more comprehensive process.

Changes in the health care delivery system are requiring nurses to embrace new skill competencies. In the new millennium, nurses find a strong compatibility between nursing's professional goals and the emerging health promotion–oriented, community-based goals of health care. Technology, changes in demographics, and a blurring of professional health care roles in a multidisciplinary health care environment create new opportunities and new challenges for new nurses.

Ethical Dilemma ■ *What Would You Do?*

NOTE: *Refer to Chapter 3, "Clinical Judgment: Applying Critical Thinking and Ethical Decision Making" as you consider the ethical dilemmas found in each chapter.*

Craig Montegue is a very difficult client to care for. As his nurse, you find his constant argument, poor hygiene, and the way he treats his family very upsetting. It is difficult for you to provide him with even the most basic care, and you just want to leave his room as quickly as possible. What are the ethical elements in this situation, and how would you address them in implementing care for Craig?

REFERENCES

American heritage dictionary of the English language, ed 4, New York, 2000, Houghton Mifflin.

American Holistic Nurses Association: What is holistic nursing? 2004; available online: http://www.ahna.org/about/whatis.html.

Anderson H: Postmodern collaborative and person-centered therapies: what would Carl Rogers say? *J Fam Ther* 23: 339–360, 2001.

Antrobus S: Developing the nurse as a knowledge worker in health: learning the artistry of practice, *J Adv Nurs* 25(4):829–835, 1997.

Appleton C: The art of nursing: the experience of patients and nurses, *J Adv Nurs* 18:892–899, 1993.

Armstrong M, Kelly A: More than the sum of their parts: Martha Rogers and Hildegard Peplau, *Arch Psychiatr Nurs* 9(1):40–44, 1995.

Arnold E: Caring from the graduate student perspective, *Int J Hum Caring* 1(3):32–42, 1997.

Barker P: The future of the theory of interpersonal relations? A personal reflection on Peplau's legacy, *J Psychiatr Ment Health Nurs* 5(3):213–220, 1998.

Bateson G: *Mind and nature*, New York, 1979, Dutton.

Beck AT: *Cognitive therapy and the emotional disorders*, London, 1991, Penguin Books.

Bell G: *Selection: the mechanism of evolution*, New York, 1997, Chapman & Hall.

Bellack J, O'Neil E: Recreating nursing practice for a new century: recommendations and implications of the Pew Health Professions Commission's final report, *Nurs Health Care Perspect* 21(1):14–21, 2000.

Berragau L: Nursing practice draws upon several different ways of knowing, *J Clin Nurs* 7(3):209–217, 1998.

Booth K, Kenrick M, Woods S: Nursing knowledge, theory and method revisited, *J Adv Nurs* 26(4):804–811, 1997.

Buber M: Distance and relation, *Psychiatry* 20:97–104, 1957.

Buber M: *I and thou*, ed 2, New York, 1958, Scribner (Translated by R Smith).

Carper B: Fundamental patterns of knowing in nursing, *Advances in Nursing Science* 1:13–23, 1976.

Carper B: Fundamental patterns of knowing. In Nicholl L, editor: *Perspectives on nursing theory*, ed 3, Philadelphia, 1995, JB Lippincott.

Carr E: Reflecting on clinical practice: hectoring talk or reality? *J Clin Nurs* 5(5):289–295, 1996.

Chinn P, Maeve M, Bostick C: Aesthetic inquiry and the art of nursing, *Sch Inq Nurs Pract* 11(2):83–96, 1997.

Chinn PL, Kramer MK: *Theory and nursing: a systematic approach*, St Louis, 1995, Mosby.

Clark DJ: The unique function of the nurse, *Nurs Stand* 12(16):39–42, 1998.

Clark DJ: Old wine in new bottles: delivering nursing in the 21st century, *J Nurs Scholarsh* 32(1):11–15, 2000.

Cody W: Critical thinking and nursing science: Judgment or vision, *Nurs Sci Q* 15(3):184–189, 2002.

Crowe M: The nurse-patient relationship: a consideration of its discursive content, *J Adv Nurs* 31(4):962–967, 2000.

Devery K: Letter to the editor, *Palliat Med* 20:51, 2006.

Doheny M, Cook C, Stopper M: *The discipline of nursing*, Stamford, CT, 1997, Appleton & Lange.

Dossey B, Selander L, Beck D et al.: *Florence Nightingale today: healing, leadership, global action*, Silver Spring, MD, 2005, American Nurses Association.

Dowd J: Ever since Durkheim: the socialization of human development, *Hum Dev* 33:138–159, 1990.

Engebretson J: Cultural constructions of health and illness: recent cultural changes toward a holistic approach, *J Holist Nurs* 21(3):203–227, 2003.

Erikson E: *Childhood and society*, New York, 1950, WW Norton.

Erikson E: *Identity and the life cycle*, New York, 1969, WW Norton.

Erikson E: *Life cycle completed*, New York, 1982, WW Norton.

Erikson E, Erikson J: On generativity and identity: from a conversation with Erik and Joan Erikson, *Harvard Educational Review* 51:251, 1981.

Fawcett J: *Analysis and evaluation of contemporary nursing knowledge*, Philadelphia, 2000, FA Davis.

Fawcett J: *Contemporary nursing knowledge*, Philadelphia, 2005, FA Davis.

Fawcett J, Watson J, Neuman B et al.: On nursing theory and evidence, *J Nurs Scholarsh* 33(2):115–119, 2001.

Feely M: Using Peplau's theory in nurse-patient relations, *Int Nurs Rev* 44(4):115–120, 1997.

Fowler J: Taking theory into practice: using Peplau's model in the care of a patient, *Prof Nurse* 10(4):226–230, 1995.

Freud S: *The basic writings of Sigmund Freud*, New York, 1937, Modern Library (Translated and edited by AA Brill).

Freud S: *Collected papers*, New York, 1959, Basic Books (Edited by J Strachey).

Frisch N: Nursing as a context for alternative/complementary modalities, *Online J Issues Nurs* [serial online], May 31, 2001; available online: http://www.nursingworld.org/ojin/topic15/tpc15_2.htm.

Fryback P: Health for people with a terminal illness, *Nurs Sci Q* 6(3):147–159, 1993.

Gastmans C: Interpersonal relations in nursing: a philosophical-ethical analysis of the work of Hildegard E. Peplau, *J Adv Nurs* 28(6):1312–1319, 1998.

George J: *Nursing theories: the base for professional nursing practice*, ed 4, Stamford, CT, 1995, Appleton & Lange.

Gottlieb L, Gottlieb B: Evolutionary principles can guide nursing's future development, *J Adv Nurs* 28(5):1099–1105, 1998.

Henderson V: *The nature of nursing*, New York, 1966, Macmillan.

Hickman J: An introduction to nursing theory. In George J, editor: *Nursing theories: the base for professional nursing practice*, ed 4, Stamford, CT, 1995, Appleton & Lange.

Honeybourne C, Sutton S, Ward L: Knowledge in the palm of your hands: PDAs in the clinical setting, *Health Info Libr J* 23(1):51–59, 2006.

Hutchinson AM, Johnston L: Bridging the divide: a survey of nurses' opinions regarding barriers to, and facilitators of, research utilization in the practice setting, *J Clin Nurs* 13(3):304–315, 2004.

International Council of Nurses: The ICN definition of nursing [International Council of Nurses website], 2006; available online: http://www.icn.ch/definition.htm.

Johns C: Framing learning through reflection within Carper's fundamental ways of knowing in nursing, *J Adv Nurs* 22(2):226–234, 1995.

Johnson B, Webber P: *An introduction to theory and reasoning in nursing*, Philadelphia, 2001, Lippincott.

Jung CG: *Memories, dreams and reflections*, New York, 1963, Vintage (Translated by R Winston).

Jung CG: *Psychology and religion: west and east*. In Hull RFC, translator: *Collected works of CG Jung*, Princeton, NJ, 1969, Princeton University Press.

Jung CG: The stages of life. In Campbell J, editor: *The portable Jung*, New York, 1971, Viking.

Ketefian S, Redman R: Nursing science in the global community, *Image: The J Nurs Scholarsh* 29(1):11–15, 1997.

Kim HS: Practice theories in nursing and a science of nursing practice, *Sch Inq Nurs Pract* 8(2):145–158, 1994.

Komesaroff P: 'On being both professional and human': one woman's journey, *International Medical Journal* 35(11): 675–676, 2005.

Kudzma E: Florence Nightingale and health care reform, *Nurs Sci Q* 19(1):61–64, 2006.

Leight S: Starry night: using story to inform aesthetic knowing in women's health nursing, *J Adv Nurs* 37(1):108–114, 2002.

Loescher L, Merkle C: The interface of genomic technologies and nursing, *J Nurs Scholarsh* 37(2):111–119, 2005.

Ludwick R: (1999). Ethical thoughtfulness and nursing competency, *Online J Issues Nurs* [serial online]; available from: http://www.nursingworld.org/ojin/ethicol/ ethics_2.htm.

Marrs J, Lowry L: Nursing theory and practice: connecting the dots, *Nursing Science Quarterly* 19(1):44–50, 2006.

Maslow A: *Motivation and personality*, ed 2, New York, 1970, Harper & Row.

McKenna G: Unique theory—is it essential in the development of a science of nursing? *Nursing Education Today* 13(2):121–127, 1993.

McKenna H: *Nursing models and theories*, London, 1997, Routledge.

Mead P: Clinical guidelines: Promoting clinical effectiveness or a professional minefield? *J Adv Nurs* 31(1):110–116, 2000.

Meleis A: Being and becoming healthy: the core of nursing knowledge, *Nurs Sci Q* 3(3):107–114, 1990.

Meleis A: *Theoretical nursing: development and progress*, ed 3, Philadelphia, 1997, Lippincott.

Miller GR, Nicholson HE: *Communication inquiry: a perspective on process*, Reading, MA, 1976, Addison Wesley.

Monti E, Tingen M: Multiple paradigms of nursing science, *Advances in Nursing Science* 21(4):64–80, 1999.

Morgan I, Marsh G: Historic and future health promotion contexts for nursing, *Image J Nurs Sch* 30(4):379–383, 1998.

Nickelson D: Telehealth and the evolving health care system: Strategic opportunities for professional psychology, *Professional Psychology: Research and Practice* 29(6):527–535, 1998.

Peck A: Changing the face of standard nursing practice through telehealth and telenursing, *Nurs Adm Q* 29(4):339–343, 2005.

Peplau H: *Interpersonal relations in nursing*, New York, 1952, Putnam.

Peplau H: Interpersonal relations: a theoretical framework for application in nursing practice, *Nurs Sci Q* 5(1):13–18, 1992.

Peplau H: Peplau's theory of interpersonal relations, *Nurs Sci Q* 10(4):162–167, 1997.

Polk L: Toward a mid-range theory of resilience, *Adv Nurs Sci* 19(3):1–13, 1997.

Porter O'Grady P: Of hubris and hope: Transforming nursing in a new age, *Nurs Econ* 21:59–64, 2003.

Pullen C, Edwards J, Lenz C et al.: A comprehensive primary health care delivery model, *J Prof Nurs* 10(4):201–208, 1994.

Radwin LE: 'Knowing the patient': a review of research on an emerging concept, *J Adv Nurs* 23:1142–1146, 1996.

Raudonis B, Acton G: Theory-based nursing practice, *J Adv Nurs* 26(1):138–145, 1997.

Reed P: Nursing: the ontology of the discipline, *Nurs Sci Q* 10(2):76–79, 1997.

Reynolds W: Peplau's theory in practice, *Nurs Sci Q* 10(4): 168–170, 1997.

Rogers C: *On becoming a person*, Boston, 1961, Houghton Mifflin.

Ruesch J: *Therapeutic communication*, New York, 1961, Norton.

Sackett D, Rosenberg W, Gray J et al.: Evidence based medicine: what it is and what it isn't, *Br Med J* 312(7023):71–72, 1996.

Seifer S: Recent and emerging trends in undergraduate medical education, Curricular responses to a rapidly changing health care system, *Western Journal of Medicine* 168(5):401–411, 1998.

Sellick KJ: Nurse's interpersonal behaviors and the development of helping skills, *Int J Nurs Stud* 28(1):3–11, 1991.

Sherman D: Death of a newborn: Healing the pain through Carper's patterns of knowing in nursing, *Journal of the New York State Nurses Association* 28(1):4–6, 1997.

Sibbald B: 2020 Vision, *Can Nurse* 91(3):3, 1995.

Sigma Theta Tau International: Sigma Theta Tau International's position statement on evidence-based nursing [Sigma Theta Tau International's website]. 2003. Available at: http://www.nursingsociety.org/research/main.html.

Sinclair S: Evidenced-based medicine: a new ritual in medical teaching, *British Medical Bulletin* 69:179–196, 2004.

Smith MC: Nursing's unique focus on health promotion, *Nurs Sci Q* 3(3):105–106, 1990.

Sullivan HS: *The interpersonal theory of psychiatry*, New York, 1953, Norton.

Thelander B: The psychotherapy of Hildegard Peplau in the treatment of people with serious mental illness, *Perspectives in Psychiatric Care* 33(3):24–32, 1997.

Van Achterberg T, Holleman G, Van de Ven M et al.: Promoting evidence-based practice: the roles and activities of professional nurses' associations, *J Adv Nurs* 53(5):605–612, 2006.

Von Franz M: *CG Jung: his myth in our time*, Boston, 1975, Little, Brown.

Walker L, Avant K: *Strategies for theory construction in nursing*, ed 4, Upper Saddle River, NJ, 2005, Pearson Prentice Hall.

Weil A: *Health and healing*, New York, 2004, Houghton Mifflin.

Whall A: The structure of nursing knowledge: analysis and evaluation of practice, middle-range and grand theory. In Fitzpatrick J and Whall A, editors: *Conceptual models of nursing: analysis and application*, ed 3, Stamford, CT, 1996, Appleton & Lange.

World Health Organization (WHO): Ottawa charter for health promotion, *Health Promot* 1(4):iii–v, 1987.

Youngblut J, Brooten D: Evidence-based nursing practice: why is it important? *AACN Clin Issues* 12(4):468–476, 2001.

Chapter 2

Professional Guides to Action in Interpersonal Relationships

Elizabeth Arnold

OUTLINE

OBJECTIVES

At the end of the chapter, the reader will be able to:

1. Identify Standards of Care and Standards of Professional Performance.
2. Discuss current professional licensure requirements for nursing practice.
3. Discuss legal standards.
4. Discuss implications of the Code of Ethics for Nurses for the nurse-client relationship.
5. Describe the use of advance directives in professional nursing practice.
6. Describe the nursing process as a framework for professional nursing practice and the nurse-client relationship.
7. Describe the use of nursing language in standardized formats to document client care.
8. Discuss clinical pathways as a method of communication.

If a man's actions are not guided by thoughtful considerations, then they are guided by inconsiderate impulse, unbalanced appetite, caprice, or the circumstances of the moment.

(Dewey, 1933)

Chapter 2 introduces the student to the professional, legal, and ethical standards of practice that provide essential parameters for professional therapeutic activities occurring within the nurse-client relationship. Also included in the chapter are brief overviews of the nursing process and clinical pathways used to sequence nursing actions in the nurse-client relationship and to chart client progress.

Nursing, like other professional disciplines, has professional, legal, and ethical standards that identify the scope of its practice and govern its actions. These standards offer the clinician and the consumer a common means of understanding nursing as a professional service relationship (Cameron, 1997). When a client goes to a physician, the client assumes the physician will use a defined body of knowledge and will provide care consistent with discipline-specific practice and legal and ethical standards. As members of a professional discipline, nurses require similar professional, legal, and ethical standards to guide their practice.

BASIC CONCEPTS

Professional Standards

The scope and standards of professional nursing practice help define nursing's domain (American Nurses Association, 2004). The American Nurses Association (ANA) has developed Standards of Care and Standards of Professional Performance to guide nursing practice, and has made specialty practice guidelines available. These documents represent authoritative statements that describe a level of care or performance common to the profession of nursing. Standards provide a benchmark by which the quality of nursing practice can be judged. The judicial system in this country uses these standards to evaluate the appropriateness of professional nursing care provided for clients in court cases.

Professional standards of care define the diagnostic, intervention, outcome, and evaluation competencies involved in professional nursing practice. Table 2-1 presents professional standards guiding the nurse-client

Table 2-1 Professional Standards Guiding the Nurse-Client Relationship

Standards of Practice	Standards of Professional Performance
STANDARD 1. ASSESSMENT: The registered nurse collects client comprehensive data pertinent to the patient's health or the situation.	STANDARD 7. QUALITY OF PRACTICE: The registered nurse systematically enhances the quality and effectiveness of nursing practice
STANDARD 2. DIAGNOSIS: The registered nurse analyzes the assessment data to determine the diagnoses or issues.	STANDARD 8. EDUCATION: The registered nurse attains knowledge and competency that reflects current nursing practice.
STANDARD 3. OUTCOMES IDENTIFICATION: The registered nurse identifies expected outcomes for a plan individualized to the patient or the situation.	STANDARD 9. PROFESSIONAL PRACTICE EVALUATION: The registered nurse evaluates one's own nursing practice in relation to professional practice standards and guidelines, relevant statutes, rules, and regulations.
STANDARD 4. PLANNING: The registered nurse develops a plan that prescribes strategies and alternatives to attain expected outcomes.	STANDARD 10. COLLEGIALITY: The registered nurse interacts with and contributes to the professional development of peers and colleagues.
STANDARD 5. IMPLEMENTATION: The registered nurse implements the identified plan.	STANDARD 11. COLLABORATION: The registered nurse collaborates with patient, family, and others in the conduct of nursing practice.
STANDARD 5A: COORDINATION OF CARE: The registered nurse coordinates care delivery.	STANDARD 12. ETHICS: The registered nurse integrates ethical provisions in all areas of practice.
STANDARD 5B: HEALTH TEACHING AND HEALTH PROMOTION: The registered nurse employs strategies to promote health and a safe environment.	STANDARD 13. RESEARCH: The registered nurse integrates research findings into practice.
STANDARD 5C: CONSULTATION: The advanced practice registered nurse and the nursing role specialist provide consultation to influence the identified plan, enhance the abilities of others, and effect change.	STANDARD 14. RESOURCE UTILIZATION: The registered nurse considers factors related to safety, effectiveness, cost, and impact on practice in the planning and delivery of nursing services.
STANDARD 5D: PRESCRIPTIVE AUTHORITY AND TREATMENT: The advanced practice registered nurse uses prescriptive authority, procedures, referrals, treatments, and therapies in accordance with state and federal laws and regulations.	STANDARD 15. LEADERSHIP: The registered nurse provides leadership in the professional practice setting and the profession.
STANDARD 6. EVALUATION: The registered nurse evaluates progress toward attainment of outcomes.	

Reprinted with permission from American Nurses Association: *Nursing: Scope and standards of practice*, Silver Spring, Md, 2004, Nursebooks.org.

Table 2-2 Relationship of the Nursing Process to Patient Care Standards in the Nurse-Client Relationship

ASSESSMENT	
Collects data	The nurse collects data throughout the nursing process related to client strengths, limitations, available resources, and changes in the client's condition.
Analyzes data	The nurse organizes cluster behaviors and makes inferences based on subjective and objective client data and personal and scientific nursing knowledge.
Verifies data	The nurse verifies data and inferences with the client to ensure validity.
DIAGNOSIS	
Identifies health care needs/problems and formulates biopsychosocial statements	The nurse develops a comprehensive biopsychosocial statement that captures the essence of the client's health care needs/problems and validates the accuracy of the statement with the client and family; this statement becomes the basis for the nursing diagnoses.
Establishes nursing diagnosis	The nurse develops relevant nursing diagnoses and prioritizes them based on the client's most immediate needs in the current health care situation.
OUTCOME IDENTIFICATION AND PLANNING	
Identifies expected outcomes	The nurse and client mutually and realistically develop expected outcomes based on client needs, strengths, and resources.
Specifies short-term goals	The nurse and client mutually develop realistic short-term goals and choose actions to support achievement of expected outcomes.
IMPLEMENTATION	
Takes agreed-on action	The nurse encourages, supports, and validates the client in taking agreed-on action to achieve goals and expected outcomes through integrated, therapeutic nursing interventions and communication strategies.
EVALUATION	
Evaluates goal achievement	The nurse and client mutually evaluate attainment of expected outcomes and survey each step of the nursing process for appropriateness, effectiveness, adequacy, and time efficiency, modifying the plan as indicated by evaluation.

relationship; Table 2-2 outlines the relationship of the nursing process to nursing actions in the nurse-client relationship to implement those standards. Specialty practice guidelines provide an additional customized set of standards for care of specific populations (e.g., children, the elderly, and psychiatric patients) or specialty areas of clinical practice (e.g., acute care or perioperative nursing).

Professional performance standards identify the nurse's role functions in direct care, consultation, and quality assurance. They express the professional behaviors expected of the registered nurse and specify the nature of professional accountability for practice by individual nurses and by the profession as a group.

Professional Licensure

The registered nurse's professional license ensures that each individual nurse has successfully completed nursing program requirements and can demonstrate the knowledge, skills, and competencies to function as a health provider of safe, effective nursing care. The NCLEX examination, a national licensure exam, tests core nursing knowledge before granting a nurse a professional state license. This license requires anyone practicing nursing to comply with all state laws governing practice. Nursing licensure helps maintain standards for nursing.

In 2000, the National Council of State Boards of Nursing (NCSBN) developed the mutual recognition model of nurse licensure, which permits a nurse to have a professional nursing license (in his or her state of residency) and to practice in other states (both physical and electronic), subject to each state's practice law and regulation. Under mutual recognition, a nurse may practice across state lines unless otherwise restricted. The nurse practicing under the compact model of nurse licensure can only practice under the single license in those states that have adopted the RN Nurse Licensure Compact. In 2004, Utah became the first state to pass similar legislation for advanced practice registered nurse (APRN) compact state practice. This legislation is particularly helpful for nurses working in states with large rural populations and few nurses.

Nurse Practice Acts

Nurse Practice Acts are legal documents developed at the state level that define professional nursing's scope of practice and outline nurses' rights, responsibilities, and licensing requirements in providing care to individual clients, families, and communities. **Scope of practice** is a broad term that refers to the legal and ethical boundaries of practice for professional nurses established by each state and defined in written state statutes. The legal and ethical boundaries of a nurse's competence are based on the nurse's education, special skill training, supervised experience, state and national professional credentials, and appropriate professional experience. Nurse Practice Acts are the most important statutory laws governing the provision of professional nursing care through the nurse-client relationship (Betts & Waddle, 1993).

Within each Nurse Practice Act, the state or territory identifies specific nursing actions and functions defined as nursing practice, including providing direct care, effectively managing emergency and crisis situations, administering medications, monitoring changes in client conditions, teaching and coaching, prioritizing and coordinating care, supervising unlicensed personnel, and delegating. Because Nurse Practice Acts so directly affect professional nursing functions, nurses should pay close attention to legislation and state statutory definitions of nursing practice affecting their practice.

Nurse Practice Acts are written by representative nurses appointed by the governor to act as a state board of nursing. Nurse Practice Acts authorize state boards of nursing to interpret the legal boundaries of safe nursing practice and give them the authority to punish violations (ANA, 1995a). Violations of a Nurse Practice Act are serious, and professional nurses can lose their licensure to practice or have it suspended for a period of time.

Each state develops and executes its own Nurse Practice Act. Consequently, if a nurse practices in one state and then moves to another, the nurse has to apply for licensure in the new state. Because all Nurse Practice Acts reflect standards of nursing care developed by the ANA (1991), they do not usually differ significantly, but

Table 2-3 Definition and Examples of Negligent Actions

Definition of Negligent Action	Example
Performing a nursing action that a prudent nurse would not perform	Carrying out a physician's order that would have been questioned by other reasonably prudent nurses in similar circumstances
Failing to perform a nursing action that a reasonably prudent nurse would perform	Failing to report suspected physical or sexual child abuse
Failure to provide routine or customary care	Failing to check vital signs pre- and post-surgery; failing to perform postpartum checks on a client
Exhibiting conduct that a reasonably prudent nurse would recognize as posing an unreasonable risk to a client	Failing to give accurate information in a manner that the client can understand regarding choice of treatment and known side effects; sharing confidential information with a client's family or workplace without the client's permission
Failing to protect a client from unnecessary harm	Not putting up the guardrails on a bed with a newly diagnosed client suffering from a stroke; allowing unlicensed personnel to do a nursing procedure without appropriate experience or supervision

nurses are advised to have a working knowledge of the Nurse Practice Act in each state of planned employment.

Legal Standards

In addition to providing nursing care that adheres to professional nursing standards and is in accord with Nurse Practice Acts, nurses must attend to other important legal tenets that have particular relevance for the nurse-client relationship. The nurse is bound legally by the principles of tort law to provide a *reasonable standard of care*, defined as a level of care that a reasonably prudent nurse would provide in a similar situation (Cournoyer, 2001). If taken to court, this statement will be the benchmark against which the nurse's actions will be judged. Criteria for judging negligence in professional nursing practice are found in Table 2-3.

In the nurse-client relationship, the nurse is responsible for maintaining the professional conduct of the relationship. Examples of unprofessional conduct in the nurse-client relationship include the following:

- Breaching client confidentiality
- Verbally or physically abusing a client
- Assuming nursing responsibility for actions without having sufficient preparation
- Delegating care to unlicensed personnel, which could result in client injury
- Following a doctor's order that would result in client harm
- Failing to report or document changes in client health status
- Falsifying records

Confidentiality

Confidentiality is an important aspect of the nurse-client relationship. It is defined as providing only that information needed to provide care for the client to other health professionals directly involved in the care of the client. This means that the nurse must have the client's expressed permission to share private information from the nurse-client relationship, unless the withholding of information would result in harm to the client or someone else, or in cases where abuse is suspected. Chapter 6 provides further information on confidentiality in the nurse-client relationship.

In addition to protecting the client's confidentiality in the relationship, the nurse has a legal responsibility to ensure against invasion of privacy related to the following:

- Releasing information about the client to unauthorized parties
- Unwanted visitations in the hospital
- Discussing client problems in public places or with people not directly involved in the client's care
- Taking pictures of the client without consent or using the photographs without the client's permission
- Performing procedures such as testing for HIV without the client's permission
- Publishing data about a client in any way that makes the client identifiable without the client's permission (Cournoyer, 2001)

Informed Consent

Informed consent, defined as giving the client enough information on which to base a knowledgeable decision, is another aspect of legal considerations in the nurse-client relationship. Unless there is a life-threatening emergency, all clients have the right to give informed consent. For legal consent to be valid, it must contain three elements (Northrop & Kelly, 1987):

- Consent must be voluntary.
- The client must have full disclosure about the risks, benefits, cost, potential side effects or adverse reactions, and other alternatives to treatment.
- The client must have the capacity and competency to understand the information and to make an informed choice.

Only legally competent adults can give legal consent; adults who are mentally retarded, developmentally disabled, or cognitively impaired cannot give legal consent (White, 2000). Evaluation of competency is made on an individual basis (e.g., in the case of emancipated adolescents no longer under their parent's control, brain-injured clients, or clients with early dementia) to determine the extent to which they understand what they are signing. In most cases, legal guardians or parents must give legal consent for minor children, defined as those under the age of 18 (Pieranunzi & Freitas, 1992).

HIPAA Privacy Compliance

The **Health Insurance Portability and Accountability Act (HIPAA)**, which was finalized in 2001 and implemented in 2003, is designed to protect the privacy of client records. Federal regulations require all health care providers to provide clients with a written notice of their privacy practices and procedures. The HIPAA privacy rules regulate the use and disbursement of individually identifiable health information and give individuals the right to determine and restrict access to their health information. Health care providers must protect the confidentiality, accuracy, and availability of all electronic protected information that is created, received, or transmitted. Strict maintenance of written records in a protected, private environment is required. All client records are subject to HIPAA regulations (see Chapters 23 and 24 for more information about HIPAA requirements).

Documentation

Nurses are responsible for careful, accurate documentation of nursing assessments, the care given, and the behavioral responses of the client. In the eyes of the law, failure to document in written form any of these elements means the actions were not taken (Betts & Waddle, 1993). In addition, the nurse is accountable for orally informing other members of the health care team of changes in the client's condition, for appropriately supervising ancillary personnel, and for questioning unclear or controversial orders made by a physician. See Chapters 23 and 24 for a full description of documentation and its significance in professional nursing practice today.

Ethical Code for Nurses

Nurses have a moral accountability to the clients they serve that extends beyond their legal responsibility in everyday nursing situations (Erlen, 1997). The revised ANA Code of Ethics for Nurses (2001) with interpretive statements provided ethical guidelines for nurses designed to protect client rights, provide a mechanism for professional accountability, and educate professionals about sound ethical conduct. The new provisions of the Code of Ethics for Nurses are identified in Box 2-1. Similar codes of ethics for nurses exist in other nations. For example, in Canada, nursing practice is guided by the Canadian Nurses Association (CNA) Code of Ethics for Registered Nurses (1997).

The Code of Ethics for Nurses provides a broad conceptual framework outlining the principled behaviors and value beliefs expected of professional nurses in delivering health care to individuals, families, and communities. Ethical standards of behavior require a clear understanding of the multidimensional aspects of an ethical dilemma, including intangible human factors that make each situation unique (e.g., personal and cultural values or resources). Exercise 2-1 provides an opportunity to consider ethical factors in nursing care. When an ethical dilemma cannot be resolved through interpersonal negotiation, an ethics committee composed of biomedical experts reviews the case and makes recommendations (Otto, 2000). Of particular importance to the nurse-client relationship are ethical directives related to the nurse's primary commitment to the client's welfare, respect for client autonomy, recognition of each individual as unique and worthy of respect, advocacy,

Box 2-1 American Nurses Association Code of Ethics for Nurses

1. The nurse, in all professional relationships, practices with compassion and respect for the inherent dignity, worth and uniqueness of every individual, unrestricted by considerations of social or economic status, personal attributes, or the nature of health problems.
2. The nurse's primary commitment is to the patient, whether an individual, family, group, or community.
3. The nurse promotes, advocates for, and strives to protect the health, safety, and rights of the patient.
4. The nurse is responsible and accountable for individual nursing practice and determines the appropriate delegation of tasks consistent with the nurse's obligation to provide optimum patient care.
5. The nurse owes the same duties to self as to others, including the responsibility to preserve integrity and safety, to maintain competence, and to continue personal and professional growth.
6. The nurse participates in establishing, maintaining, and improving health care environments and conditions of employment conducive to the provision of quality health care and consistent with the values of the profession through individual and collective action.
7. The nurse participates in the advancement of the profession through contributions to practice, education, administration, and knowledge development.
8. The nurse collaborates with other health professionals and the public in promoting community, national, and international efforts to meet health needs.
9. The profession of nursing, as represented by associations and their members, is responsible for articulating nursing values, for maintaining the integrity of the profession and its practice, and for shaping social policy.

Reprinted with permission from American Nurses Association: *Code of ethics for nurses with interpretive statements*, Silver Spring, Md, 2001, Nursebooks.org.

Exercise 2-1 Applying the Code of Ethics for Nurses to Professional and Clinical Situations

Purpose: To help students identify applications of the Code of Ethics for Nurses.

Procedure:

1. Break into small groups of four or five students. Each student should think of a potential ethical dilemma in the clinical care of clients or an actual situation in which he or she has been involved as a caregiver, client, or family member. Write the dilemma as a short summary.
2. Share each ethical dilemma with the group and collaboratively problem-solves on how the nurse's code of ethics can be used to work through the situation.

Discussion:

1. What types of difficulty did your group encounter in resolving different scenarios?
2. What type of situation offers the most challenge ethically?
3. Were there any problems in which the code of ethics was not helpful?
4. How can you use what you learned in this exercise in your nursing practice?

and truth telling. See Chapter 3 for information about ethical decision making.

Advance Directives

In 1991, the U.S. Congress passed the Patient Self-Determination Act. This legislation requires health care institutions to inform their clients, on admission, of their right to choose whether or not to have life-prolonging treatment should they become mentally or physically unable to make this decision (Westley & Briggs, 2004). Basanta (2002) defines an **advance directive** as a written statement or document executed by a competent adult that is designed to provide medical personnel, family members, and others with information as to the person's wishes regarding the nature and extent of medical care to be provided in the future should he or she lose decision-making capacity. Advance directives allow people to put individual preferences regarding treatment options in writing, and the documents are then recognized by state law. To be valid, an advance directive must be voluntarily signed and witnessed; some states also require the document to be notarized by a notary public. An advance directive should include the client's preferences regarding pain control, use of a respirator, cardiac resuscitation, use of a feeding tube, or use of other extraordinary measures in the event that a person is near death with no chance of recovery. An advance directive can be revoked at any time by its author, if the person so chooses.

Advance directives provide a new dimension of care and respect for the autonomy of adult clients that formerly was not an explicit legal issue in nurse-client relationships. Chapter 8 provides more information about the use of advance directives in the nurse-client relationship.

Developing an Evidence-Based Practice

Shapiro S: Evaluating clinical decision rules, *West J Nurs Res* 271(5):655-664, 2005.

This study examines the role of decision support tools needed to combine different clinical evidence into bedside tools for practice.

Results: Clinical decision-making tools are similar to clinical pathways and treatment algorithms used to guide treatment and nursing care. To be effective, clinical decision rules (CDR) must follow strict protocols and be research based, valid, and reflective of multiple sources of data. The impact of CDRs on client outcomes and costs of care is measured through implementation trials and cost-effectiveness analysis.

Application to Your Clinical Practice: In today's health care arena, nurses find themselves increasingly dependent on methodologies developed to standardized practice protocols based on the best research evidence currently available. What do you see as the role of clinical decision rules for clinical practice? What would be important to consider in protecting the integrity of the rules as an evidence-based rationale for improving client outcomes?

APPLICATIONS

Nursing Process

The nursing process is a treatment management process engaged in by nurse and client as a primary means of achieving specific health goals. Health goals can relate to wellness promotion, disease and illness prevention, health restoration, and coping and altered functioning. Originally developed from general systems theory by the North American nursing profession, it serves as a primary organizing framework for sequencing, implementing, and evaluating nursing care (Mason & Attree, 1997).

The nursing process represents a consistent, comprehensive, and coordinated approach to the delivery of nursing care to clients that begins with the nurse's first encounter with a client and family and ends with discharge. The nursing process calls for an ordered sequence of activities, with each activity linked to the trustworthiness of the activity that precedes it and influencing the activity following it. Although the sequence of these activities should follow a distinctive order, each phase is flexible, flowing into and overlapping with other phases of the nursing process. This systematic process provides a clinical management framework, recognized by the profession as an organizing structure for clinical nursing practice. In 1991, the ANA expanded the nursing process to include outcome identification as a specific component of the planning phase. The nursing process consists of five progressive phases: assessment, problem identification and diagnosis, outcome identification and planning, implementation, and evaluation.

The ANA uses the progressive steps of the nursing process as a structural format for identifying measurement criteria related to the professional standards of care (see Table 2-2). The nursing process offers the nurse guidelines to identify the type of nursing a client requires and the scope of nursing activities needed to meet health goals, as well as the means to evaluate whether the individual's nursing care needs were met. Nurses are expected to develop, implement, and evaluate individualized care plans for each client. The nursing process is not complete until treatment outcomes and the client's response are documented on the client's chart using correct spelling and terminology, and the nurse has reported all pertinent data to appropriate health care personnel.

Steps in the Nursing Process

Assessment. Assessment begins with the first contact between client and nurse. The nurse uses a systematic dynamic process in gathering and analyzing data about the client seeking service from the client, family and significant others, and relevant health care providers. Intuition and empirical, personal, and aesthetic knowledge help nurses see the patient's health care needs from a broader perspective than is possible from the original, usually incomplete data.

Following a formal introduction in which the nurse informs the client of the purpose for the interaction, the nurse asks the client to tell his or her story as it relates to the current request for nursing services. A simple statement, such as, "Tell me what prompted you to seek treatment at this time" usually is sufficient to start the conversation. An intake assessment, usually completed on admission to the health care agency, should be comprehensive, because it will serve as baseline information throughout the nursing process, alerting the nurse to the resolution of nursing problems or the necessity of devising a different strategy if client needs and problems are not being addressed. As new information becomes available, the nurse refines and updates the original assessment. The nurse collects data about (a) the current problem for which the client seeks treatment; (b) the client's perception of his or her health patterns; (c) presence of other health risk and protective factors; (d) the client's past history (e.g., previous hospitalizations, family history, past medical and psychiatric treatment, and medications; (e) the client's coping patterns; and (f) level and availability of the client's support system.

Assessment data should reflect information from as many sources as needed for complete accuracy. Sources of data include interview, history, physical assessment, review of records, family interviews, and in some instances, contact with previous health care providers, schools, or other referral sources.

The nurse uses a critical-thinking format for collecting subjective and objective data from a client and the client's family, which integrates subjective with objective data into a comprehensive, coherent whole. **Subjective data** refers to the client's perception of data and what the client says about the data (e.g., "I have a severe pain in my chest"). **Objective data** refers to data that are directly observable or verifiable through physical examination or tests (e.g., an abnormal electrocardiogram). Combined, these data will present a complete picture of the client's health problem; one without the other is insufficient.

Observations of the client's nonverbal behaviors lead the nurse to make inferences. An **inference** is an educated guess about the meaning of a behavior or statement. To be sure the inference is factual, you should validate the data with the client. For example, if a client is withdrawn and distractible, the nurse may infer that the client is struggling with an internal emotional issue. To validate this inference, the nurse might comment, "You seem withdrawn, as though something is troubling you. Is that true for you right now?"

You also can use *data cues*, defined as small pieces of data that would not reveal much when taken by themselves but, when considered within the total assessment picture, can lead the nurse to ask further questions that often turn out to be important (Avant, 1991). For example, hesitancy about a certain topic, complaints of hunger or thirst, dry skin, or agitation should raise questions in the nurse's mind to look beyond the symptom for a fuller explanation. Throughout the assessment phase, the nurse should consistently validate information with the client to make sure that the information and the nurse's interpretation of it are complete and accurate.

Identify potential as well as actual problems, and ask the client for confirmation that your perceptions and problem analysis are correct. This is an important intersection between the nurse-client relationship and the nursing process.

The nurse identifies health deviations specific to the client but should not make global assumptions about a patient's situation without evidence to support the assumptions. In each clinical situation, the client's behavioral response might be assessed differently. For example, maintaining a sufficient intake of food would need to be assessed in terms of what is sufficient intake for this particular individual on the basis of age, activity, height to weight ratio, and current health status. Nutritional needs for an active teenager are greater than those for an older, sedentary adult. Having knowledge of their relevance, the nurse would ask different questions of a diabetic, anorexic, or obese client regarding nutritional intake and food choices than of those without these deviations.

Special situations also warrant more in-depth, individualized assessments. For example, the mother of a newborn with Down syndrome might know how to care for a normal infant but need help adapting care strategies for her handicapped infant. The first time a person relapses with cancer can be different from subsequent relapses. Active listening skills allow the nurse to obtain relevant data.

Once the data are complete, the nurse analyzes the data and identifies gaps in the data collection, comparing individual client data with normal health standards, behavior patterns, and developmental norms. Assessment of client strengths is an important dimension of the analysis process; it provides a sound foundation in resolving health problems. Identifying client strengths on which to build in seeking solutions to difficult health care problems is particularly important in today's health care environment, when clients have to assume much more responsibility for their health care than previously. Those health care concerns judged potentially responsive to nursing intervention form the basis for the selection of nursing diagnoses. A summary of the assessment data is put in written form so that it is easily understood and retrievable by everyone involved in the client's care.

Diagnosis. The second phase of the nursing process involves developing relevant nursing diagnoses. Written as client-centered statements, an actual diagnosis consists of three parts (North American Nursing Diagnosis Association [NANDA], 1996). The first part identifies the problem or alterations in the client's health status requiring nursing intervention. The second part of the statement specifies the causative or risk factors contributing to the existence or maintenance of the health care problem. These factors can be psychosocial, physiological, situational, cultural, or environmental in nature. The phrase "related to" (R/T) serves to connect the problem and etiology statements. The third part of the statement identifies the clinical evidence (behaviors) that support the diagnosis. An example of a nursing diagnosis statement would be, "Impaired verbal communication related to a cerebral vascular accident, as evidenced by incomplete sentences and slurred words."

Nurses need to express a nursing diagnosis in clear, precise language so that any member of the health care team can look at the statement and be able to identify relevant issues for the client. Levine (1989) suggested that "the nursing diagnosis should be as informative and useful to the physician as the medical diagnosis is to the nurse" (p. 5). Once nursing diagnoses are developed, the nurse prioritizes them with the most basic or potentially life-threatening needs to be met first. Maslow's hierarchy of needs, described in Chapter 1, provides an excellent hierarchal framework for prioritizing nursing actions. Nurses may address more than one nursing diagnosis at a time, because attention to several interconnected nursing diagnoses can often serve the same outcome. By communicating the results of this decision-making process to other health care providers involved in the treatment of the client, the nurse ensures continuity and an ordered approach to meeting the individualized needs of the client (Carpenito, 1999). Exercise 2-2 gives practice in writing nursing diagnoses. Chapter 23 elaborates on appropriate documentation of assessment and diagnostic data.

Another way of working with assessment data and the development of relevant diagnoses to direct care of clients is through the use of a care map. The care map combines medical and nursing data into a comprehensive whole, individualized to each client's needs. Exercise 2-3 provides the opportunity to develop a care map for a client.

Outcome Identification. Shaughnessy (1997) defines a **health care outcome** as "the change in health status between a baseline time point and a final time point" (p. 1225). Outcomes should be client-centered (e.g., "The client will...") and described in specific, measurable terms. Outcome criteria are stated as long- and short-term treatment goals. Each treatment outcome specifies the action or behavior that the client will demonstrate once the health problem is resolved. The ANA (1991) specified that outcomes should be

- Based on diagnoses.
- Documented in measurable terms.
- Developed collaboratively with the client and other health providers.
- Realistic and achievable.

Measurable action verbs are key to describing outcomes; for example, "The client will take his medicine as prescribed." The client either takes his medicine or he

Exercise 2-2 Writing Nursing Diagnoses

Purpose: To help students develop skill in writing nursing diagnoses.

Procedure:

1. In small groups of two or three students, develop as many nursing diagnoses as possible for each of the following clinical situations, based on the information you have. Indicate what other types of information you would need to make a complete assessment.
   a. Michael Sterns was in a skiing accident. He is suffering from multiple internal injuries, including head injury. His parents have been notified and are flying in to be with him.
   b. Lo Sun Chen is a young Chinese woman admitted for abdominal surgery. She has been in this country for only 8 weeks and speaks very little English.
   c. Maris LaFonte is a 17-year-old unmarried woman admitted for the delivery of her first child. She has had no prenatal care.
   d. Stella Watkins is an 85-year-old woman admitted to a nursing home after suffering a broken hip.

Discussion:

1. What common diagnoses emerged in each group?
2. In what ways were the diagnoses different? How would you account for the differences?
3. Were there any common themes in the types of information each group decided it needed to make a complete assessment?
4. How could you use what you learned from this exercise in your clinical practice?

Exercise 2-3 Developing Care Maps*

Purpose: To provide students with experience developing care maps based on client assessment data.

Procedure:

1. For a client you have been assigned to work with, develop a skeleton diagram of the client's health problems from the assessment data from the client, the client's chart, and other key informants.
2. Analyze and categorize specific assessment data.
   a. Indicate relationships between nursing and medical diagnoses.
3. Develop relevant, individualized nursing diagnoses.
4. Specify client goals, outcomes, and nursing interventions for each nursing diagnosis in order of priority.

Discussion:

In small groups of three to five students, discuss your findings and compare rationales for the care map you developed.

*Note: This exercise can also be done with a selected case study.

doesn't; his behavior is easy to measure. Other measurable verbs include perform, identify, discuss, and demonstrate. Broad-spectrum verbs such as understand, know, and learn are not easily measurable and should not be used.

Outcome criteria take into account the client's culture and life situation, past medical and psychological history, present mental status, intellectual and emotional capabilities, strengths and limitations, and available resources. Important client values and preferences should be factored into the development of relevant outcome criteria. Time limits need to be realistic so that the client can be successful. Outcomes provide direction for documentation of client response. For example, the following treatment outcome would be appropriate for a client post-surgery:

Client will show no signs of infection as evidenced by incision well-approximated and free of redness and swelling, normal temperature, and WBC within normal limits by 9/21/07.

Planning. The Joint Commission on Accreditation of Healthcare Organizations (JCAHO) requires that each client seeking health care treatment have an individualized treatment plan that describes specific planned nursing interventions needed to achieve therapeutic outcomes (JCAHO, 1991). Developing the treatment plan is a mutual individualized process that requires the client's active involvement with the nurse in establishing and prioritizing appropriate treatment goals (Hensen, 1997). Lifestyle, values, economics, and personal preference will influence individualized goals and the client's ability to meet them. The treatment plan provides for continuity of care and supplies a concrete framework for supporting documentation of client response. JCAHO has identified six interrelated elements required of the nursing care plan; these are presented in Box 2-2. The treatment plan should be sequential, with priority attention focused on the most immediate, life-threatening problems. It also needs to be dynamic, meaning that it needs to be continuously updated as the client's condition and needs change.

Box 2-2 JCAHO Requirements for Nursing Care Plans

1. Initial assessment, modified as needed
2. Nursing diagnosis of patient care needs
3. Specified nursing interventions that address client health care needs
4. Provision of appropriate nursing interventions
5. Documentation of the client's response and achievement of treatment outcomes
6. Discharge plan providing direction to client and others involved in care to manage continuing health care needs post discharge

From Joint Commission on Accreditation of Healthcare Organizations: *Accreditation manual for hospitals,* Chicago, 1991, Author.

Treatment plans begin with short- and long-term goals related specifically to expected outcomes. Short-term goals represent the progressive steps needed to reach each long-term goal. Corresponding nursing interventions are listed as actions the nurse will take to help the client meet identified goals related specifically to identified outcome criteria. For example, "The client will achieve dietary control of his diabetes" might be a long-term outcome for a diabetic client; "The client will identify a sample American Dietetic Association (ADA) diet plan for one week" might be a short-term outcome. The nurse should identify a specific target date/time for goal achievement (e.g., "by discharge" or "by 9/08/07").

Implementation. During the implementation phase, the client and nurse carry out the care plan through clearly specified nursing interventions. McCloskey and Bulechek (1996) define nursing intervention as "any treatment, based upon clinical judgment and knowledge, that a nurse performs to enhance patient/client outcomes. Nursing interventions include both direct and indirect care, nurse-initiated, physician-initiated, and other provider-initiated treatments" (p. xvii). Interventions appropriate to the purposes of the nurse-client relationship include giving physical, psychological, social, and spiritual support; health teaching; collaborating with other health professionals on behalf of the client; continuing to make ongoing assessments; documenting client responses; and updating or revising the care plan as needed.

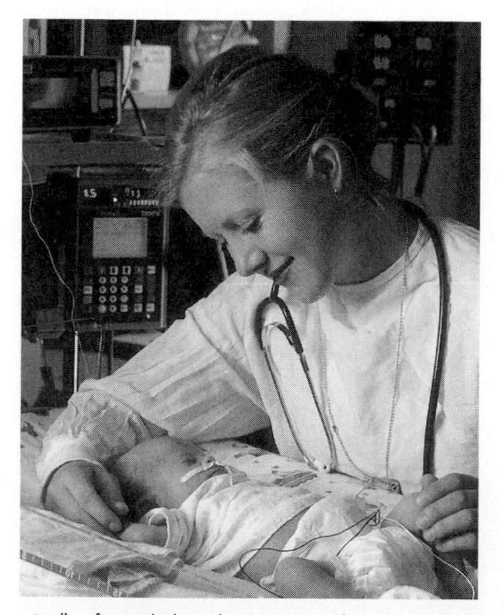

The nurse, in all professional relationships, practices with compassion and respect for the inherent dignity, worth, and uniqueness of every individual. (Courtesy of the University of Maryland School of Nursing.)

Nursing interventions are often classified as independent, dependent, or collaborative (Snyder, Egan, & Nojima, 1996). **Independent nursing interventions** are interventions that nurses can provide without a physician's order or direction from another health professional. Independent nursing interventions are permitted under Nurse Practice Acts and are protected through professional licensure and law. Many forms of direct care assistance, health education, health promotion strategies, and counseling fall into this category, and nurses are particularly well equipped to provide these functions. **Dependent nursing interventions** require an oral or a written order from a physician to implement. For example, in most states, staff nurses cannot administer a medication without having a physician order it. The nurse is accountable for using appropriate knowledge, judgment, and competence in administering the medication a physician orders—and for questioning a physician about a problematic medical order. Thus, a nurse would not automatically carry out a physician's order without considering first the appropriateness of the medication or without knowing appropriate dosage, mode of action, side effects, and potential adverse reactions. Collaborative nursing interventions are those performed by the nurse and other health care team members with the mutual goal of providing the most appropriate and effective care to clients (McCloskey & Bulechek, 2000). Box 2-3 identifies factors the nurse should consider in developing nursing interventions.

Evaluation. The nurse uses the evaluation phase of the nursing process to compare projected behavioral responses and outcomes with what actually occurred.

Box 2-3 Factors for Consideration When Choosing a Nursing Intervention

- Desired client outcomes
- Characteristics of the nursing diagnosis
- Research base for the intervention
- Feasibility of doing the intervention
- Acceptability to the client
- Capability of the nurse

The nurse and client together assess the client's progress or lack of progress toward identified goals. When there is a lack of progress, the nurse needs to ask the following questions:

- Was the assessment data collected appropriate and complete?
- Was the nursing diagnosis appropriate?
- Were the treatment outcomes realistic and achievable in the time frame allotted?
- Were the nursing interventions chosen appropriate to the needs of the situation and the capabilities of the client?
- Was there any variable within the client, situation, or family that was overlooked and should have been addressed?

Nurses need to analyze the effectiveness, time efficiency, appropriateness, and adequacy of the nursing actions

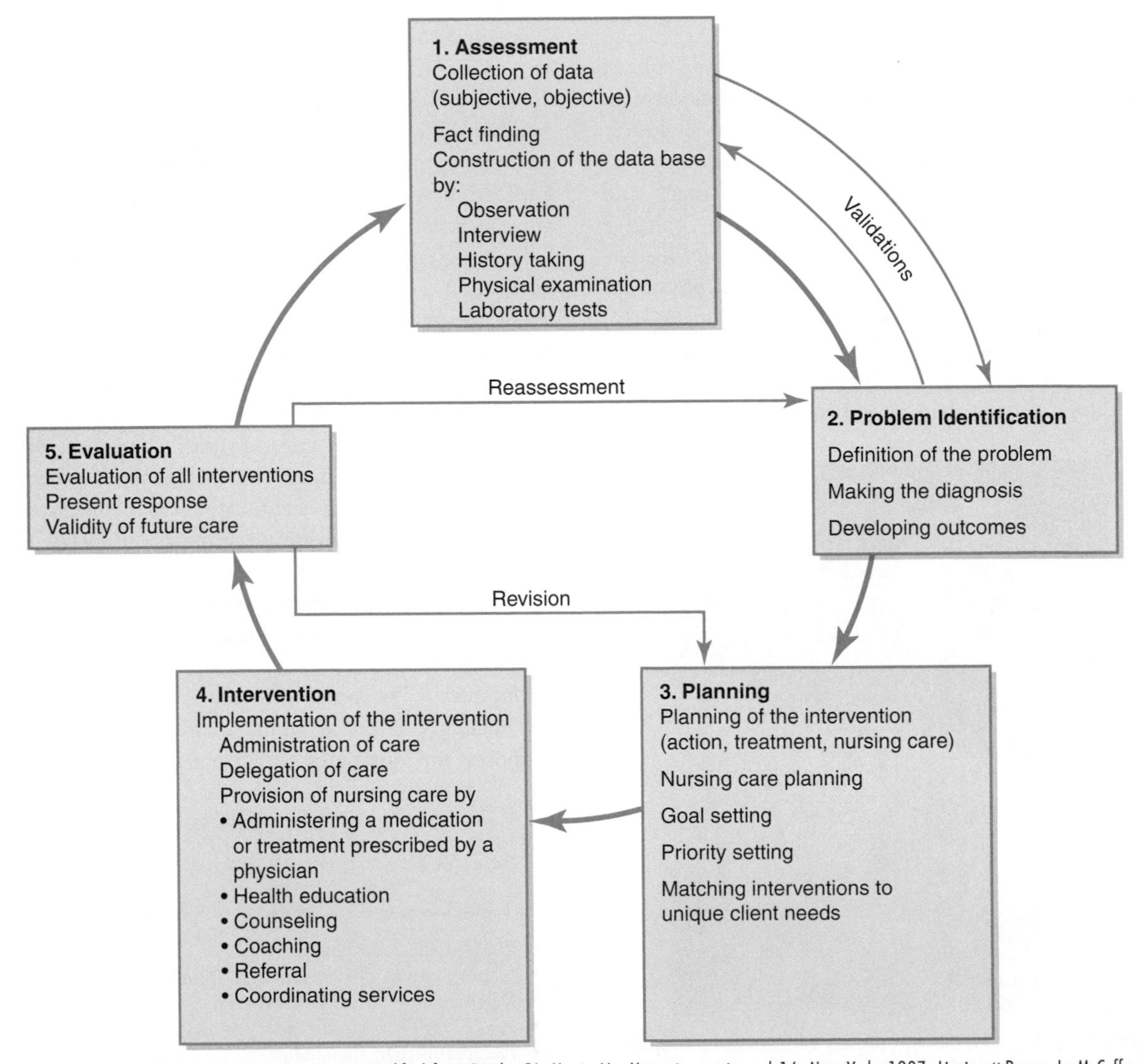

Figure 2-1 ● Steps in the nursing process. (Modified from Reeder SJ, Martin LL: *Maternity nursing*, ed 16, New York, 1987, Lippincott-Raven. In McCaffery M, Beebe A: *Pain: clinical manual for nursing practice*, St Louis, 1989, Mosby.)

selected for implementation. Paying attention to the reality of the situation, the motivation of the client, and the setting in which the interventions need to be accomplished can prevent unnecessary frustration on the part of both nurse and client. The client gives input regarding actions perceived as helpful or not useful. Mutually agreed-on modification follows in any area of the nursing process requiring it. Figure 2-1 diagrams the steps of the nursing process.

Nursing Process and Professional Relations

The nurse-client relationship affects every aspect of the nursing process, which in turn provides the basic format for all activities carried out in the relationship. The relationship acts as a continuous feedback system for nursing interventions, incorporating a thoughtful process of analysis, synthesis, and critical thinking about the individualized needs of clients (Taylor, 1997).

The assessment and nursing diagnosis phases of the nursing process correspond with the orientation phase of the relationship. The client should be the *primary* source of information. *Secondary* sources of information include the client's chart, family or significant others, referral notes, teachers and counselors, and other health team members. In the orientation phase, the nurse tries to understand the client as a person responding to an alteration in health status. Data collection includes a description of the health problem or need from the client's perspective, the client's expectations for treatment, strengths and resources available to the client, and a working diagnosis that will serve as the basis for planning and therapeutic intervention.

The outcome identification and planning phase of the nursing process correspond to the identification component of the working phase of the relationship. Here the nurse and client develop goals that will direct further work together. Implementation strategies correspond to the exploitation part of the working phase and consist of client activities toward goal achievement and nursing interventions needed to support them. Evaluation strategies are a significant focus in the resolution phase of the nurse-client relationship as nurse and client review progress, determine necessary modifications, and terminate the relationship. The goals of communication as they relate to the nursing process are directed toward the following:

- Helping clients to promote, maintain, or restore health or to achieve a peaceful death
- Facilitating client management of difficult health care issues
- Providing quality nursing care in an efficient manner

Developing a Common Language to Document the Nursing Process (NNN Terminology)

As health care moves into the technological age, there is a strong impetus to standardize documentation of the nursing process so that it can be entered into electronic patient care records. To accomplish this task, the ANA established a Steering Committee on Databases to Support Clinical Nursing Practice (SCD) to monitor and support the development and evolution of the use of multiple vocabularies and classification schemes reflective of nursing outcomes and interventions (ANA, 1995b). Referred to as taxonomies of nursing practice, the best-known is the NANDA Classification of Nursing Diagnoses (2001). Approved outcome classification systems (Wilkinson, 2000) linked to the nursing process include the **Nursing Interventions Classification (NIC)** and the **Nursing Outcomes Classification (NOC)** systems. Table 23-1 displays the integrated domains of NANDA, NIC and NOC classifications, which are referred to collectively as **NNN terminologies** (Von Krogh, Dale, & Naden, 2005). (See Chapter 23 for more information on the use of these systems with electronic documentation.)

These new systems expand on the original NANDA classification system, providing a standardized vocabulary that can be used across clinical settings and in nursing outcome studies (Johnson, Bulechek, Dochterman et al., 2001; Marrs & Lowry, 2006). The new classification systems allow for the development of aggregate data sets for comparisons at the local, regional, national, and international levels. These systems are intended to enhance data collection *about* the nursing process rather than to guide the nursing process. Frisch (2001) observed, "Nurses documenting practice using these systems are accomplishing three important things: appropriate documentation of care, identification of work as within the scope of professional nursing, and building a body of knowledge for nurses on the use of specific interventions" (pp. 11-12).

Clinical Pathways

In the twenty-first century, managed care has dramatically shortened hospital stays and treatment, forcing the development of clinical management tools that extend beyond the nursing process (Walsh, 1997). Care in today's health care arena is multidisciplinary and focused on outcome management. **Clinical pathways** represent a standardized, integrated multidisciplinary care plan, which includes the assessment and care given by all disciplines involved with a client's care. Its purpose is to help coordinate health care services and to decrease costs associated with duplication of effort (Schuster, 2002). Using a clinical pathway helps to optimize quality, efficiency, and organization of health care delivery services. A clinical pathway requires the active understanding of care principles and participation of members of the health care team, including the client.

Each clinical pathway puts forth a set of comprehensive, predetermined interdisciplinary benchmarks of care for a specific diagnosis, condition, or population. Relevant clinical assessment data are the basis for developing a holistic comprehensive care plan for the "average" client. The link between process of care and expected outcome is made more explicit with standardized guidelines for care applicable to the average client. This clinical management tool identifies expected outcomes, associated health care provider interventions, expected treatment time, and appropriate allocation of resources. Clinical pathways can help collect valuable information about effective treatments and can help reduce redundancy with routine organizational tasks.

Ideally, clinical pathways represents a consensus about the optimal ways to clinically manage a homogeneous group of medical care. Developed by the interdisciplinary team using best-practice guidelines, the entire health team should accept the standard guidelines as the management tool for all clients with a particular diagnosis (e.g., diabetes, stroke, coronary heart disease, or depression) or for a particular procedure (e.g., surgery or dialysis).

The team begins with a desired client outcome based on clinical diagnosis, rather than with individualized client needs. Each clinical pathway identifies pathway goals, inclusion and exclusion criteria, and pathway alteration criteria. Benchmark standards focus on the clinical elements and events necessary to achieve predetermined treatment outcomes, with specific responsibility for health care services identified for physicians, nurses, physical therapists, nutritionists, occupational therapists, and social workers, if applicable. In the hospital, clinical pathways use days as time frames; in home care, the time frames are developed around visits. Since clinical pathways represent general care guidelines, they can never replace clinical judgment for individual care needs, which require a specialized focus. Any deviations from the pathway's standardized schedule of clinical assessments, interventions, or outcomes, usually in the form of complications, are recorded as "variations." These variations should be reported using a detailed narrative format.

The actual care given to the client is documented on a written clinical record for each client. This record is a multidisciplinary document, constructed as a flow sheet that provides a composite guide to treatment and account of outcome achievement. All care givers are expected to record their part of the care given.

Clinical pathways have implications for the nurse-client relationship. The nurse commonly is in charge of coordinating the clinical pathway and of explaining treatment expectations and the client's role in the process of goal achievement. The role of the client is active and focused on the treatment process. From the start of treatment, the client knows the anticipated short- and long-term outcomes, and just what is expected of him or her as a partner in the clinical pathway to a successful outcome.

The nursing process helps the nurse organize nursing care within the clinical pathway. Clinical pathways spell out desired nursing interventions related to specific medical and nursing diagnoses in precise but global terms. The nurse can still individualize the application. For example, health teaching about symptom and medication management for a diabetic would be a standard nursing intervention for a benchmark outcome (e.g., of the client being able to personally administer insulin, or having knowledge of symptoms warranting medical attention). The actual process of teaching, however, would be different for different newly diagnosed clients, such as a teenager who doesn't want to accept her condition or a man with late-onset diabetes whose father also had diabetes.

SUMMARY

Chapter 2 focuses on the nurse's need to have a basic knowledge of the legal and ethical variables that influence the nurse's choice of actions in the nurse-client relationship. The chapter provides a brief overview of the nursing process as a framework for the actions taken in the relationship. Knowledge of practice guidelines and ethical principles is necessary for implementing an effective nurse-client relationship.

The nurse-client relationship is contained within the scope of nursing practice as defined by the Nurse Practice Acts. Standards of professional practice provide a measurement standard that guides the activities of professional nursing. The nurse-client relationship is bound legally by the principles of tort law to provide a reasonable standard of care. This means that the nurse is obligated to provide a level of care that a reasonably prudent nurse would provide in a similar situation. The ANA Code of Ethics for Nurses provides a broad conceptual framework for identifying the moral dimensions of nursing practice and is an important guide to choices of actions in nurse-client relationships.

The nursing process serves as a clinical management framework. It is recognized by all nursing theorists as an organizing structure for clinical nursing practice and involves five phases: assessment, diagnosis, outcome criteria and planning, implementation, and evaluation. The nursing diagnosis is established at the end of the assessment phase and forms the basis for the remaining phases of the nursing process. During the implementation phase, the client and nurse carry out the care plan through clearly specified nursing interventions. The nurse uses the evaluation phase of the nursing process to compare projected behavioral responses and outcomes with what actually occurred.

As health care moves further into the technological age, there is a strong impetus to standardize documentation of the nursing process so that it can be entered into electronic patient care records. Two new models include the Nursing Outcomes Classification (NOC) and Nursing Interventions Classification (NIC) systems.

Clinical pathways have emerged as an interdisciplinary clinical management framework because of radical changes in the health care system and the introduction of managed care. Clinical pathways merge medical and nursing care plans, offering a standardized format for ordering and evaluating treatment from admission to discharge.

Ethical Dilemma ■ *What Would You Do?*

As a student nurse, you observe a fellow nursing student making a medication error. She is a good friend of yours and is visibly upset by her error. She also is afraid that if she tells the instructor, she could get a poor grade for clinical, and she needs to have a good average to keep her scholarship. The client was not actually harmed by the med error, and your friend seems sufficiently upset by the incident to convince you that she wouldn't make a similar error again. What would you do?

REFERENCES

American Nurses Association: *Code for nurses with interpretative statements*, Kansas City, MO, 1985, Author.

American Nurses Association: *Nursing: a social policy statement*, Washington, DC, 1995a, Author.

American Nurses Association: *ANA's position statement on national nursing databases to support clinical nursing practice*, Washington, DC, 1995b, Author.

American Nurses Association: *ANA's position paper on implementation of the patient self-determination act*, Washington, DC, 1995c, Author; available online: http://www.nursingworld.org/readroom/position/ethics/etsdet.htm.

American Nurses Association: *Code of ethics for nurses with interpretive statements* (approved revised), Washington, DC, 2001, Author.

American Nurses Association: *Nursing: scope and standards of practice*, Washington, DC, 2004, Author.

Avant K: Paths to concept development in nursing diagnosis, *Nurs Diagn* 2(3):105–110, 1991.

Basanta WE: Advance directives and life sustaining treatment: A legal primer, *Hematol Oncol Clin North Am* 16(6):1381–1396, 2002.

Betts V, Waddle F: Legal aspects of nursing. In Chitty K, editor: *Professional nursing: concepts and challenges*, Philadelphia, 1993, WB Saunders.

Cameron ME: Legal and ethical issues: professional boundaries in nursing, *J Prof Nurs* 13(3):142, 1997.

Canadian Nurses Association: *The code of ethics for registered nurses*, Alberta, Canada, 1997, Author; available online http://www.cna-nurses.ca/CNA/practice/ethics/code/default_e.aspx.

Carpenito LJ: *Handbook of nursing diagnoses*, ed 7, Philadelphia, 1999, JB Lippincott.

Cournoyer C: Legal relationships in nursing practice. In Creasia J, Parker B, editors: *Conceptual foundations: the bridge to professional nursing practice*, St Louis, 2001, Mosby.

Creasia J, Parker B: *Conceptual foundations: the bridge to professional nursing practice*, St Louis, 2001, Mosby.

Dewey J: *How we think: a restatement of the relation of reflective thinking to the educative process*, Boston, 1933, DC Health.

Erlen J: Everyday ethics, *Orthop Nurs* 16(4):60–63, 1997.

French B: The process of research use in nursing, *J Adv Nurs* 49(2):125–134, 2005.

Frisch N: Nursing as a context for alternative/complementary modalities, *Online J Issues Nurs* [serial online] 6(2):2, 2001; available online: http://www.nursingworld.org/ojin/ topic15/ tpc15_2.htm.

Haynes RB: bmjupdates+, a new free service for evidence-based clinical practice, *Evid Base Nurs* 8(2):39, 2005.

Hensen R: Analysis of the concept of mutuality, *Image* 29: 77–79, 1997.

Johnson M, Bulechek G, Dochterman J, et al.: *Nursing diagnoses, outcomes, and interventions: NANDA, NOC, and NIC linkages*, St Louis, 2001, Mosby.

Johnson M, Maas M: *Nursing outcomes classification (NOC)*, ed 2, St Louis, 2000, CV Mosby.

Joint Commission on Accreditation of Health Care Organizations: *Accreditation manual for hospitals*, Chicago, 1991, Author.

Levine M: The ethics of nursing rhetoric, *Image* 21(1):4–6, 1989.

Marrs J, Lowry L: Nursing theory and practice: Connecting the dots, *Nurs Sci Q* 19:44–50, 2006.

Mason G, Attree M: The relationship between research and the nursing process in clinical practice, *J Adv Nurs* 26(5):1045–1049, 1997.

McCloskey JC, Bulechek GM, editors: *Nursing interventions classification (NIC)*, ed 2, St Louis, 1996, Mosby.

McCloskey JC, Bulechek GM, editors: *Nursing interventions classification (NIC)*, ed 3, St Louis, 2000, Mosby.

North American Nursing Diagnosis Association: *Nursing diagnosis: definitions and classification, 2001-2002*, Philadelphia, 2001, Author.

Northrop C, Kelly M: *Legal issues in nursing*, St Louis, 1987, Mosby.

Otto S: A nurse's lifeline: a nursing ethics committee offers the chance to review and learn from ethical dilemmas, *Am J Nurs* 100(12):57–59, 2000.

Pieranunzi V, Freitas L: Informed consent with children and adolescents, *J Child Adolesc Psychiatr Ment Health Nurs* 31(6):9–12, 30–31, 1992.

Schuster PM: *Concept mapping: a critical-thinking approach to care planning*, Philadelphia, 2002, FA Davis.

Shaughnessy P: Outcomes across the care continuum: home health care, *Med Care* 35(12):1225–1226, 1997.

Snyder M, Egan EC, Nojima Y: Defining nursing interventions, *Image J Nurs Sch* 28(2):137–141, 1996.

Taylor C: Problem solving in clinical nursing practice, *J Adv Nurs* 26(2):329–336, 1997.

Von Krogh G, Dale C, Naden D: A framework for integrating NANDA, NIC, and NOC terminology in electronic patient records, *J Nurs Scholarsh* 37(3):375–381, 2005.

Walsh M: Will clinical pathways replace the nursing process? *Nursing Standard* 11(52):39–42, 1997.

Westley C, Briggs L: Stages of change model to improve communication about advance care planning, *Nurs Forum* 39(3):5–12, 2004.

Westra B: *Clinical pathways in home care*, 1997; available online: http://carefacts.com/articles/criticalPathways.htm

White G: Informed consent, *Am J Nurs* 100(9):83, 2000.

Wilkinson JM: *Nursing diagnosis handbook with NIC interventions and NOC outcomes*, Upper Saddle River, NJ, 2000, Prentice-Hall.

Chapter 3

Clinical Judgment: Applying Critical Thinking and Ethical Decision Making

Kathleen Underman Boggs

OUTLINE

OBJECTIVES

At the end of the chapter, the reader will be able to:

1. Define terms related to thinking, ethical reasoning, and critical thinking.
2. Describe the 10 steps of critical thinking.
3. Identify criteria necessary for acquisition of a value.
4. Discuss the application of ethics in nurse-client relationships.
5. Analyze the critical thinking process used in clinical judgments with clients.
6. Apply the critical thinking process to decision making in clinical nursing situations.
7. Demonstrate use of an organized critical thinking/decision-making process to make a clinical decision.
8. Discuss use of findings from a research study in clinical practice.

Critical thinking, content knowledge, and practice experience are the three essential components of the development of expertise in clinical judgment.

(Facione and Facione 1996)

Your standards for practice get shaped each time [your] values are tested.

(Zeigler 2005)

Chapter 3 examines the role of ethical decision making and critical thinking in clinical judgment. Considerable evidence indicates that much professional decision making is not based on *the best evidence* but instead on an individual's subjective intuitive judgments concerning the appropriate actions to take for a given clinical challenge (Lamond & Thompson, 2000). Traditionally, nurses learned to develop their clinical judgment skills by acquiring experience in caring for clients in a variety of situations. Analysis has shown that experienced nurses employ a critical thinking process. The steps in this process can be taught. Nursing studies show that introducing decision-making information to novices can help them reach decisions similar to those of experienced nurses (Lamond & Thompson, 2000). Information and application simulations provided in this chapter can improve nursing proficiency.

Additionally, nurses often face ethical dilemmas in their effort to give quality care to clients. A nurse frequently has to act in value-laden situations. For example, you may have clients who request abortions or who want "do not resuscitate" ("no code") orders. Your decisions affect the client's rights and the client's quality of life. Meeting a client who holds very different values about culture, sexuality, or religion may stir feelings in you that can be destructive in a therapeutic relationship. Instead of learning to make clinical judgments by trial and error on the job as a novice nurse, you can learn while still a student nurse how to systematically apply critical thinking and ethical decision-making skills.

THINK
Total Recall
Habit
Inquiry
New Ideas
Knowledge of Self

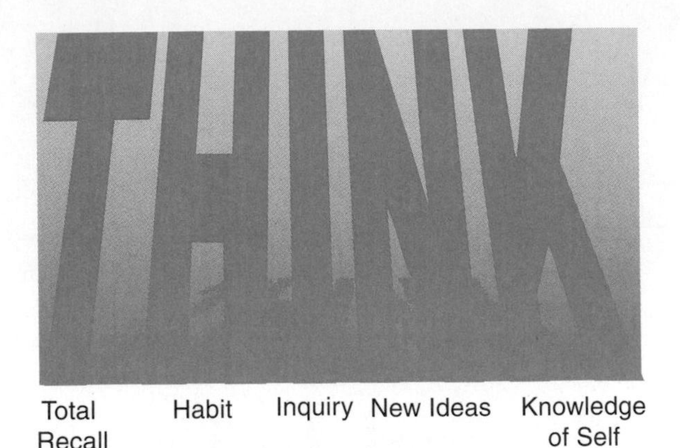

Figure 3-1 • Mnemonics can be useful tools.

BASIC CONCEPTS

Types of Thinking

There are many ways of thinking about how we think. The mnemonic listed in Figure 3-1 illustrates several of these ways. Students often attempt to use total recall by simply memorizing a bunch of facts (e.g., memorizing the cranial nerves by using a mnemonic such as "On Old Olympus' Towering Tops . . ."). At other times, nursing students rely on developing habits by repetition, such as practicing cardiopulmonary resuscitation techniques. More structured methods of thinking, such as inquiry, have been developed in disciplines related to nursing. For example, you are probably familiar with the scientific method. As used in research, this is a logical, linear method of systematically gaining new information, often by setting up an experiment to test an idea. The nursing process has been developed after this sort of method of systematic steps: assessment before planning, planning before intervention, and so on.

Knowing about your individual thinking style is vital not only for your own learning but also because your values affect the quality of relationships you are able to establish with clients. This chapter focuses on only a few of the more important concepts to help you develop your clinical judgment abilities. Completing the exercises will help you develop your skills.

Critical or Analytical Thinking

Critical thinking is a purposeful reasoning process that uses specific thinking skills (Bethune & Jackling, 1997). In other words, critical thinking is a method of thinking about thinking. An ability to engage in self-reflective inquiry is required to reflect on one's own thinking process. Besides developing knowledge and skills, the nurse who is a critical thinker needs to develop an attitude of open-mindedness. When you use this method, you improve and clarify your thinking process so that you are more accurately able to solve problems based on available evidence. The process of critical thinking is systematic, organized, and goal-directed.

Characteristics of a Critical Thinker. Critical thinkers are open-minded, able to consider alternatives, and able to recognize gaps in available information (Schank, 1990). They recognize that priorities change continually, requiring constant assessment and alternative interventions. An analysis of the decision-making process of expert nurses demonstrated that they all used the critical thinking steps described in this chapter when they made their clinical judgments (Boggs, 1997). However, they were not always able to verbally state the components of their thinking processes. The expert nurses organized each input of client information and quickly distinguished relevant from irrelevant information. They seemed to categorize each new fact into a problem format, obtaining supplementary data and arriving at a decision about diagnosis and intervention. Often, they commented about comparing this new information with prior knowledge, sometimes from academic sources but usually from information gained from preceptors. The most striking aspect of the analyses was the constant scanning for new information and constant reassessment of the client's situation. The critical thinking of these experts was not linear; rather, they constantly added new input. This contrasts with the thinking attributed to the novice nurse who tends to think a problem straight through to its solution; who has a collection of facts that is not as efficiently organized into a logical structure; and who makes fewer connections with past knowledge. Novice nurses' assessments are more generalized and less focused, and they tend to jump too quickly to a diagnosis without recognizing the need to obtain more facts.

Employing agencies periodically retest staff nurses for competencies. Mostly, this procedure has been done to retest or recertify technical skills, such as cardiopulmonary resuscitation. Some agencies are adding evaluation of critical thinking skills (Maloy & Mattas, 2005).

Barriers to Thinking Critically and Reasoning Ethically. Barriers that decrease a nurse's ability to think critically have been well described in the literature (Rubenfeld & Scheffer, 1995). Attitudes such as "my way is better" tend to interfere with our ability to empower clients to make their own decisions. Our thinking habits can also impede communication with clients or families making complex bioethical choices. Examples of such thinking habits include becoming accustomed to acknowledging "only one right answer" or selecting only one option. Behaviors that act as barriers include automatically responding defensively when challenged, resisting changes, and desiring to conform to expectations. Cognitive barriers, such as thinking in stereotypes, also interfere with our ability to treat a client as an individual.

Cognitive Dissonance. In psychology class, you learn that **cognitive dissonance** refers to the mental discomfort you feel when there is a discrepancy between what you already believe and some new information that does not go along with your view. In this book, we use the term to refer to the holding of two or more conflicting values at the same time.

Personal Value System and Professional Value System

We all have a **personal value system** developed over a lifetime that has been extensively shaped by our family, our religious beliefs, and our years of life experiences. Additionally, our education as nurses helps create a **professional value system**. Awareness of our own value system is essential to developing an ability to think critically. Later in this chapter, you will have an opportunity to focus on application of the values clarification process.

Of course, clients bring their own set of values, including personal biases, to any interaction. Clients may not even be aware of biases that are actively affecting a current situation. For example, a male client's attitudes toward people of the opposite gender may interfere with his ability to accept advice about his condition or needed changes in lifestyle from female physicians and nurses.

An important first step in values clarification is to know your own personally held values. For example, think about how you would respond if someone of significance to you asked you to steal a watch from an open case in a jewelry store. Would you do it? How about taking a monogrammed towel from a hotel at which you were staying, or claiming charitable donations on your tax return that, in fact, you never made? The nursing process offers many opportunities to incorporate values clarification into care of the client. During the assessment phase, the nurse can obtain an assessment of the client's values with regard to the health system. For example, the nurse might interview a client for the first time and learn that he has obstructive pulmonary disease and is having difficulty breathing. The client insists on smoking. As the nurse caring for the client, is it appropriate to intervene? If so, to what extent? This is an example of having knowledge that smoking is detrimental to a person's health and, as a nurse, finding the value of health in conflict with the client's value of smoking. In this case, it is important to examine your own values and to try to identify and understand your client's values. Although your values differ, whenever possible, you must attempt to care for this client within his realm of value. A client has the right to make decisions that are not always congruent with those of the health care system. These decisions may cause the nurse to feel uneasy unless there is a commitment to respect the rights of the client (Steele & Harmon, 1983).

When identifying specific nursing diagnoses, it is important for the nurse to continue to reflect on his or her own values and on those of the client so that the diagnoses reflect a specific problem and are not biased by the nurse's values. When caring for a client from another culture, diagnoses may involve potential or actual problems. Examples of conflicts indicating differences in values orientation might be spiritual distress related to a conflict between spiritual beliefs and prescribed health treatments, or ineffective family coping related to restricted visiting hours for a family in which full family participation is a cultural value.

In the planning phase, it is important to identify and understand the client's value system as the foundation for developing the most appropriate interventions. Care plans that support rather than discount the client's health care beliefs are more likely to be received favorably.

The intervention used identifies values as guidelines for care. The nurse can also use the values clarification process as a therapeutic technique. The process may be used to help clients sort out feelings, identify conflict areas, examine and choose from alternatives, set goals, and act in a manner consistent with their value systems and according to their physical and emotional health. During the evaluation phase, the results of therapeutic intervention can be examined in terms of how well the nursing and client goals were met while keeping within the guidelines of the client's value system.

In a conflict that involves incompatible points of view, people often form opinions prematurely based on their emotional reactions. The ability to make decisions based on values becomes blurred. Most people do not pay much attention to their values until called on to do so by actions that conflict with their personal values. For example, what would you do if you witnessed a fellow student cheating on an examination? Some people would immediately call attention to the situation by summoning the examination proctor. Others might tell the proctor after the examination was over. Still others might wait several days and tell the proctor that "some student" was cheating the other day during the examination. Still others might choose not to do anything, believing that cheating will hurt the student in the long run. The ultimate decision on which action to take often directly relates to the person's value system. Personal values are developed as part of your upbringing and your exposure to values held by important influences such as your family and your religion. Many of the things you value may have had an impact on why you decided to become a nurse in the first place. At this time, take a few minutes to contemplate your reasons for wanting to become a nurse. Next, think about aspects of your life that you value a great deal. Examples might include health, friends, and socialization.

One important component of both moral reasoning and critical thinking is the ability to identify personal values and to separate these from the professional clinical situation. **Values** are a set of personal beliefs derived from life experiences, interwoven with each other. Our values change as we mature in our ability to think critically, logically, and morally. When analyzing values, it is important to examine them not only in terms of what a person *says*, but also in what the person *does* in situations that involve an element of choice. For example, an individual who values honesty would probably give back the extra change that a cashier gave by mistake.

The intensity of one's values can be measured in several ways. One measurement is the amount of time and energy a person is willing to expend to preserve or act on a value. A nursing student might value high grades and be willing to give up weekend recreational

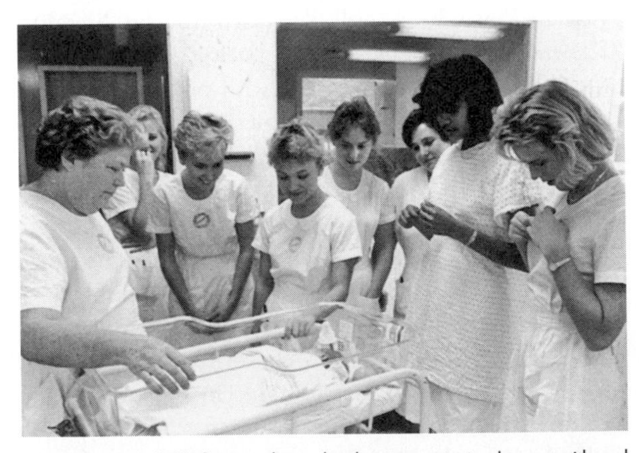

The values people hold often are observed in their interest in, involvement with, and commitment to people, places, and things. (Courtesy University of North Carolina Charlotte College of Nursing.)

time with friends to spend more time in the library, whereas another student might choose to party with friends. Another measure of intensity is the amount of satisfaction or guilt that is derived from holding on to a particular value. Many times, nursing students hold values that are belittled by their peers. The amount of satisfaction the student gets from staying faithful to his or her value system may determine the level of commitment to it. Strongly held values become a part of selfconcept.

Values acquisition, however, is the conscious assumption of a new value. In nursing school, as you advance through your clinical experiences, you begin to take on some of the values of the nursing profession. Five core values of professional nursing have been identified by the American Association of Colleges of Nursing (AACN):

- Human dignity
- Integrity
- Autonomy
- Altruism
- Social justice

You are acquiring these values as you learn the nursing role. The process of this role socialization is discussed in Chapter 7. Fahrenwald, Bassett, Tschetter et al. (2005) feel that the embodiment of these five professional values best demonstrates the concept of caring discussed in this book. Maintaining client confidentiality is another example of a professional value, with both a legal and a moral requirement, that nursing students and all health professionals acquire.

Ethical Reasoning

Ethics and bioethics both deal with moral choices. Discussions in this book focus on the current literature in bioethics as held in western society. Habel (2000) notes that ethical dilemmas are encountered with increasing frequency. In 1991, 79% of nurses surveyed by the ANA reported facing ethical issues daily or weekly (Miller, Beck, & Adams, 1991). This occurrence has increased with the rapid explosion in technology associated with health care in recent years. When various professionals answered questions about ethical dilemmas presented to them in a study, physician responses were correctly ethically based 49.2% of the time, nurse responses 46.3%, and adult citizens 40% (Johnson, 2005). As nurses you will be faced with many ethical issues requiring you to perform or abstain from some action. Examples include issues involving client choice, quality of life, end-of-life decisions, and a variety of other matters. Until recently, nurses have had little academic preparation for dealing with ethical problems (Zaher, 2000). As recently as 2000, experts wrote that nurses have a relatively low level of sensitivity to ethical issues other than those concerned with client autonomy, even though the ANA first published its Code of Ethics for Nurses in 1950 (Habel, 2000). While an agency's ethics committee often is the primary party involved with the client or family in resolving difficult ethical dilemmas, on many other occasions you, the nurse, will be called on to make ethical decisions.

Ethical Theories and Decision-Making Models

Ethical theories provide the bedrock from which we derive the principles that guide our decision making. There is no one "right" answer to an ethical dilemma: the decision may vary depending on which theory the involved people subscribe to. The following section briefly describes the most common models currently used in bioethics. They are, for the most part, representative of a western European and Judeo-Christian viewpoint. As we become a more culturally diverse society, other equally viable viewpoints may become acculturated. For our discussion, we focus on three decision-making models: utilitarian or goal-based, duty-based, and rights-based.

The **utilitarian** or **goal-based model** says that the "rightness or wrongness" of an action is always a function of its consequences. Rightness is the extent to which performing or omitting an action will contribute to the overall good of the client. Good is defined as maximum welfare or happiness. The rights of clients and the duties of a nurse are determined by what will achieve maximum welfare. When a conflict in outcome occurs, the correct action is the one that will result in the greatest good for the majority. An example of a decision made according to the goal-based model is forced mandatory institutionalization of a client with tuberculosis who refuses to take medicine to protect other members of the community. The client's hospitalization produces the greatest balance of good over harm for the majority. Thus "goodness" of an action is determined solely by its outcome.

The **deontological** or **duty-based model** is person-centered. It incorporates Immanuel Kant's deontological philosophy, which holds that the "rightness" of an action is determined by other factors in addition to its outcome. Respect for every person's inherent dignity is also a consideration. For example, a straightforward implication would be that a physician (or nurse) may never lie to a client (Mappes & DeGrazia, 1996). Decisions based on this duty-based model have a religious-social foundation. Rightness is determined by moral worth, regardless of the circumstances or the individual involved. In making decisions or implementing actions, the nurse cannot violate the basic duties and rights of individuals. Decisions about what is in the best interests of the client require consensus among all parties involved. Examples are the medical code "do no harm" or the nursing duty to "help save lives."

The **human rights–based model** is based on the belief that each client has basic rights. Our duties as health care providers arise from these basic rights. For example, a client has the right to refuse care. Conflict occurs when the provider's duty is not in the best interest of the client. The client has the right to life and the nurse has the duty to save lives, but what if the quality of life is intolerable and there is no hope for a positive outcome? Such a case might occur when a neonatal nurse cares for an infant with anencephaly (born without brain tissue in the cerebrum) in whom even the least invasive treatment would be extremely painful and would never provide any quality of life.

Ethical dilemmas arise when an actual or potential conflict occurs regarding principles, duties, or rights. Of course, many ethical or moral concepts held by western society have been codified into law. Laws may vary from state to state, but a moral principle should be universally applied. Moral principles that are shared by most members of a group, such as physicians or nurses, represent the professional values of the group. Conflict arises when a nurse's professional values differ from the law in his or her state of residence. Conflict may also arise when a nurse has not come to terms with situations in which his or her personal values differ from the profession's values. One example is doctor-assisted suicide (euthanasia). *Legally*, at the turn of the twenty-first century, such an act was legal in Oregon but illegal in Michigan. *Professionally*, the ANA Code of Ethics guides you to do no harm. *Personally*, your belief about whether euthanasia is right or wrong may be at variance with either of the above.

To practice nursing in an ethical manner, you must be able to recognize the existence of a moral problem.

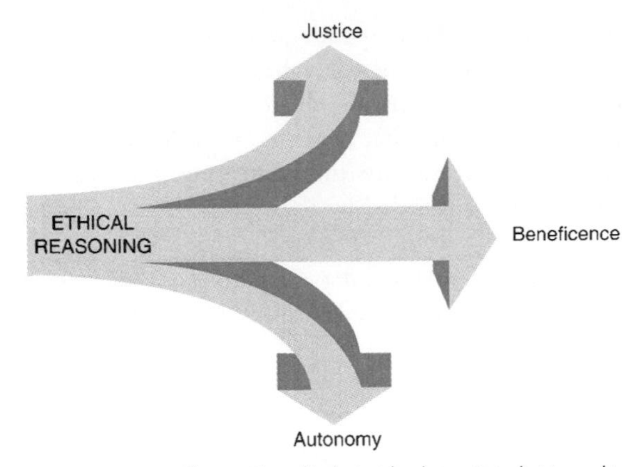

Figure 3-2 ● Three guiding ethical principles that assist in decision making.

Once you recognize a situation that puts your client in jeopardy, you must be able to take action. Three essential, guiding ethical principles have been developed from the theories cited above. The three principles that can assist us in decision making are autonomy, beneficence, and justice (Figure 3-2).

Bioethical Principles: Autonomy Versus Medical Paternalism. **Autonomy** is the client's right to self-determination. Zeigler (2005) cites a colleague who says that in one generation, the medical profession went from having a paternalistic relationship with clients to letting them decide everything, but feels that this concept will swing back to a more middle-of-the-road position. In the past, nurses and physicians often made decisions for clients based on what they thought was best for the client. This paternalism successfully discounted the voices of women and other disadvantaged groups internationally, according to Dodds (2005). The ethical concept of client autonomy has so strongly emerged as a client right in the United States and other western countries that aspects involved in an individual's right to participate in medical decisions about own care have become law (Schattner, 2002).

This moral principle of autonomy means that each client has the right to decide about his or her health care. Clients who are empowered to make such decisions are more likely to comply with your treatment plan, according to Karlowicz (2004). It is the client's body, and the client has the freedom to choose what will be done to it. As a nurse, you and your employer must legally obtain the client's permission for all treatment procedures. Under provisions of the Patient Self-Determination Act, passed in 1991 as part of the Omnibus Budget Reconciliation Act, all clients of agencies receiving Medicaid funds in the United States must receive written information about their rights to make decisions about their medical care. In a position paper, the ANA states that it is the nurse's responsibility to assist clients to make these decisions. Client consent must be informed consent, that is, they must be told all of the possible harm as well as possible benefits. The law views any touching not consented to by the client as "battery"; this is a tort, a personal injury for which the client may file a lawsuit seeking civil damages, even if the person's condition was improved by the procedure. Refer to Chapter 23 for more information. Informed choice is increasingly recognized as important in supporting client autonomy (Jepsen, Hewison, Thompson et al., 2005). What happens when the client says no? Having the right to refuse treatment does not mean that the client *should* refuse, but it gives the client room to make a wise decision (Gunderson, 2004).

Many of the nursing theories incorporate concepts about autonomy and empowering the client to be responsible for self-care, so you may find this easy to accept as part of your nursing role. However, what happens if the client's right to autonomy puts others at risk? Whose rights take precedence?

Case Example

A pregnant woman's fetus can survive only with surgical intervention; however, the mother refuses surgery on religious grounds. The hospital obtains a court order forcing the woman to undergo surgery on her fetus.

Case Example

A child is admitted to the emergency department with life-threatening blood loss after an automobile accident. The father refuses transfusion on religious grounds. The hospital obtains a court order, and the physician gives the transfusion.

Case Example

A 62-year-old woman refuses physician-assisted suicide after being diagnosed with Alzheimer's disease. She also refuses entry into a long-term care facility, deciding instead to rely on her aged, disabled spouse to provide her total care as she deteriorates physically and mentally.

The concept of autonomy has also been applied to the way we practice nursing, but our professional autonomy has some limitations. For example, the American Medical Association's Principles of Medical Ethics says a physician can choose whom to serve, except in an emergency; however, the picture is a little different in nursing practice. According to the ANA Committee on Ethics, nurses are ethically obligated to treat clients seeking their care. For example, you could not refuse to care for a client with AIDS who is assigned to you.

A nurse has autonomy in caring for a client, but this is somewhat limited because legally he or she must also follow physician orders and be subject to physician authority. Before the nurse or physician can override a client's right to autonomy, they must be able to present a strong case for their point of view based on either or both of the following principles: beneficence and justice.

Beneficence and Nonmaleficence. **Beneficence** implies that a decision results in the greatest good or produces the least harm to the client. This is based on the Hippocratic oath and its concept of "do no harm." Avoiding actions that bring harm to another person is known as nonmaleficence. An example is the Christian belief of "do not kill," which has been codified into law but has many exceptions (e.g., soldiers sent to war are expected to kill the enemy).

In health care, beneficence gives care providers the moral obligation to act at all times for the benefit of their clients. Again, nursing theorists have incorporated this into the nursing role, so you may find this easy to accept. Helping others may be why you chose to become a nurse. In nursing you not only have the obligation to avoid harming your clients, but you also are expected to advocate for your clients' best interests. For example, if your client is in pain, you are expected to assess for it and treat it. Yet it is estimated that over 50% of conscious clients spend their last week of life in moderate to severe pain. Who is advocating for them?

Beneficence is challenged in many clinical situations (e.g., requests for abortion or euthanasia). Currently, some of the most difficult ethical dilemmas involve situations where decisions may be made to withhold treatment. For example, decisions are made to justify such violations of beneficence in the guise of permitting merciful death. Is there a moral difference between actively causing death and withholding treatment, when the outcome for the client is the same death? There are clear legal differences. In most states, a health care worker who intentionally acts to cause a client's death is legally liable.

Other challenges to beneficence occur when the involved parties hold different viewpoints about what is best for the client. Consider a case in which the family of an elderly, post-stroke, comatose, ventilator-dependent client wants all forms of treatment continued, but the health care team doesn't believe it will benefit the client. The initial step toward resolution may be holding a family conference and really listening to the viewpoints of family members, asking them whether the client ever expressed wishes verbally or in writing in the form of an advance directive. Maintaining a trusting, open, mutually respectful communication may help avoid an adversarial situation (Haddad, 2000a; 2000b).

Justice. **Justice** is actually a legal term; however, in ethics it refers to being fair or impartial. A related concept is equality (e.g., the just distribution of goods or resources, sometimes called social justice or distributive justice). Within the health care arena, this distributive justice concept might be applied to scarce treatment resources. As new and more expensive technologies that can prolong life become available, who has a right to them? Who should pay for them? If resources are scarce, how do we decide who gets them? Should a limited resource be spread out equally to everyone? Or should it be allocated based on who has the greatest need?

Unnecessary Treatment. Decisions made based on the principle of justice may also involve the concept of unnecessary treatment. Are all operations that are performed truly necessary? Why do some clients receive antibiotics for viral infections, when we know they do not kill bacteria? Are unnecessary diagnostic tests ever ordered solely to document that a client does not have Condition X, just in case there is a malpractice lawsuit?

Social Worth. Another justice concept to consider in making decisions is that of social worth. Are all people equal? Are some more deserving than others? If a client Dan is 7 years old instead of 77 years old, and the expensive medicine would cure his condition, would these factors affect the decision to give him the medicine? Should they? If there is only one liver available for transplant today, and there are two equally viable potential recipients—Larry, age 54, whose alcoholism destroyed his own liver; or Kay, age 32, whose liver was destroyed by hepatitis she got while on a life-saving mission abroad—who should get the liver?

Veracity. Truthfulness is the bedrock of trust. And trust is an essential component of the professional nurse-client relationship. Not only is there a moral injunction

Table 3-1 Moral Decision-Making Guide

Moral Component	Data	Evaluation
Claim	Clear statement of the claim or dilemma. Issues and values are clearly identified.	Are values of all parties represented? Who has a stake in the outcome? Are there any ethical conflicts between two or more values?
Evidence	Clarify the facts; list the grounds, statistics, and so on.	Are they true? Relevant? Sufficient?
Warrant	Agency policy, professional standards of care, written protocols, legal precedents.	Are they general? Are they appropriate?
Basis	Identify the moral basis for each individual's claim. List backing, such as ethical principle of autonomy, beneficence, or justice.	Is the backing recognizable? Impressively strong?
Rebuttal	List the benefit and the burdens. Weigh them for each alternative in terms of possible consequences for each of the parties involved.*	How strong and compelling is the rebuttal argument? Is the decision in accord with or in conflict with the law?

*Benefits might include profit for one of the parties. Burden might include causing physical or emotional pain to one of the parties or imposing financial burden on them.

against lying, but it is also destructive to any professional relationship (Goold, 2001). Should veracity be listed as a basic ethical principle? Generally, nurses would agree that a nurse should never lie to a client. However, there is still controversy in the health care literature about withholding information from a client. Surveys show that most nurses feel a need for more information about truth telling (National Rural Bioethics Project, 2003). Health care providers exercise some judgment about to whom to disclose information. There is an obligation to protect potentially vulnerable clients from information that would cause emotional distress. Hamilton (2005) suggests that disclosing results of genetic testing might even lead to discrimination by insurance companies. While it is never acceptable to lie, nurses have evaded answering questions by saying, "You need to ask your physician about that." What do you think?

Steps in Ethical Decision Making

The process of moral reasoning and making ethical decisions has been broken down into steps. These steps are only a part of the larger model for critical thinking. Table 3-1 summarizes a model useful for nurses that was adapted from John Lincourt's model. This model covers the most essential parts of an ethical reasoning process. If the nurse is the moral agent making this decision, he or she must be committed and skillful enough to implement the actions in a morally correct way. Consider the following situation discussed by Veatch and Fry (1987, pp. 84-85):

Case Example

Cora is working alone at night with four critical clients on a medical unit. Mrs. Rae, 83, is post-stroke and semicomatose. She will inevitably die, but now needs suctioning every 10 minutes. Mr. Jones, 47, has been admitted for observation and has been having severe bloody stools. Mr. Hernandez, 52, is a newly diagnosed diabetic with intravenous drip insulin who requires monitoring of vital signs every 15 minutes. Mr. Martin, 35, is suicidal and has been told today he has inoperable cancer.

In deciding how to spend her limited time with these clients, does Cora base her decision entirely on how much good she can do each one?

Once she has made a commitment to care for more than one client, under distributive justice, what should happen when the needs of these four conflict?

Beneficence can be used to decide on the greatest good for the most clients, but this is a very subjective judgment. Would one of these clients benefit more from the nurse's time than the others?

In using both the ethical decision-making process and the critical thinking process, nurses must be able to tolerate ambiguity and uncertainty (Schank, 1990). One of the most difficult aspects for the novice nurse to accept is that there often is no one "right" answer; rather, there usually are several options that may be selected, depending on the person or situation.

Developing an Evidence-Based Practice

Martin P, Yarbrough S, Alfred D: Professional values held by baccalaureate and associate degree nursing students, *J Nurs Scholarship* 35(3):291-296, 2003.

A nonrandom sample of 1450 seniors from 23 BSN and 16 ADN programs completed the Nurses Professional Values Scale (NPVS) questionnaire, which covers the 11 values of the ANA Code of Ethics. The purpose was to determine if professional values held by associate degree student nurses differ from those held by baccalaureate students.

Results: ADN students did not differ significantly overall from BSN students, but out of 11 subscales, they did score higher on the five measuring values related to clients' right to privacy, nurse accountability, use of informed judgment, implementing nursing standards, and collaborating with others. BSN students were more likely to be Caucasian, younger, and never married. Approximately 13% of each group was male. The greatest differences in some of the subscale scores were lower scores for male students and for members of ethnic minorities.

Application to Your Clinical Practice: Acquisition of professional values occurs as students progress through both types of nursing curriculums, yet this study found better professional value-based decisions being made by ADN students. Analysis of demographics suggests that these students have more life experiences. Do ADN programs teach students to better implement professional-value decision making? Do ADN students' personal value systems affect their choices? Reflect on what professional values you have acquired so far. Where in your curriculum are ANA values taught? Should BSN curricula increase their focus on professional values?

APPLICATIONS

Participation in Clinical Research

You or your clients may be called upon at some time to participate in clinical research trials. The focus of this book is examining ethical dilemmas faced in nursing practice, and it does not encompass the ethical aspect of conducting or participating in research studies. To examine what makes clinical research ethical, study a nursing research book or review the seven ethical requirements as listed in the *Journal of the American Medical Association (JAMA)* (Emanuel, Wendler, & Grady, 2000).

Values Clarification

Values clarification is a technique that can help you identify and prioritize your values. Values clarification is a valuable tool for nurses because it serves as a base for helping clients identify the values they hold as important. The way your clients respond to the health care system, to their individual diagnoses, and to your therapeutic interventions is influenced by their personal value systems. Unless you are able to identify your client's values and can appreciate the validity of those values, you run the risk of imposing your own values. It is not necessary for your values and your client's values to coincide; this is an unrealistic expectation. However, whenever possible, the client's values should be taken into consideration during every aspect of nursing care.

Professional Values Acquisition

Professional values or ethics consist of the values held in common by the members of a profession (Roufail, 1999). During your time as a student you are exposed to and hopefully acquire the values held by the profession. Professional values are formally stated in professional codes. One example is the ANA Code of Ethics for Nurses. Often professional values are transmitted by tradition in nursing classes and clinical experiences. They are modeled by expert nurses and assimilated as part of the role socialization process during your years as a student and new graduate. Exercise 3-1 will help you begin to identify professional values.

Values are a strong determinant in making selections between competing alternatives. Consider whether the nursing profession holds values regarding the following situation: What if you observed a nurse charting that a medicine was given to a client when you know it was not? What professional value should guide your response? Exercise 3-2 is designed to help you further distinguish between your personal values and the values of the nursing profession.

As mentioned, professional values are acquired over time through interaction with expert nurses. Professional values acquisition should perhaps be the result of conscious choice by a nursing student. This is the first of seven steps in values acquisition. Can you apply it to your own life? It may also help you understand the value system of your clients.

Exercise 3-1 Defining Values

Purpose: To help students clarify professional values.

Procedure:

Complete the following statements:

1. In giving care to a dying 18-year-old client, the most difficult aspect of care for me would be . . .
2. If I were asked to administer a narcotic medication for pain relief to a client who clearly was not having any pain, I would . . .
3. If I were assigned to care for a client with a contagious disease, and my employer did not provide protective equipment, I would . . .
4. If I observed a colleague's unsafe practice, I would . . .

Discussion:

What happens when your personal values are in conflict with your professional values?

Exercise 3-2 Professional Values Clarification

Purpose: To learn another way to clarify values.

Procedure:
Refer to the Code of Ethics for Nurses in Chapter 2. Please indicate your belief in the values presented by placing the number from the continuum below that most closely represents your feelings next to the statement. This exercise is to be completed before class.

Strongly Disagree	Disagree	Ambivalent	Agree	Strongly Agree
1	2	3	4	5

_______ 1. I should be able to help every client.
_______ 2. The client's needs are more important than mine.
_______ 3. If I make a medication error, I probably should look into a profession other than nursing.
_______ 4. I consider it my responsibility to challenge my client's value system if it does not seem to be in the client's best interest.
_______ 5. If a client's condition is terminal, I believe the choice to use extraordinary measures is not mine to make; it belongs to the family.
_______ 6. I can be most effective with clients who have a similar value system.
_______ 7. It is not possible to express caring without having time to sit down and talk with a client.
_______ 8. I would find it difficult to be empathetic with a child abuser.
_______ 9. Severely ill clients should be encouraged to make a living will, which allows the medical and nursing staff to withhold life-saving treatment.
_______10. Nurses have an ethical responsibility to tell clients of the limits of confidentiality.

Discussion:
Share responses to the exercise in a brief class discussion.

The seven criteria for acquisition of a value are as follows. The value must be

1. Freely chosen.
2. Chosen from alternatives.
3. Chosen after careful consideration of each alternative.

There must be

4. Pride in and happiness with the choice.
5. Willingness to make the values known to others.

It must be acted upon

6. In response to the choice.
7. In a pattern of behavior consistent with the choice (value is incorporated into the individual's lifestyle).

Exercise 3-3 will give you an opportunity to practice explaining which of your choices are based on the profession's values.

Applying Critical Thinking to the Clinical Decision-Making Process

The following section discusses a procedure for developing critical thinking skills as applied to solving clinical

Exercise 3-3 Professional Nurses' Values

Purpose: To begin to focus thinking on professional role values.

Procedure:

Read the following statements. Think about each situation carefully. How would you want to respond if you were the primary nurse in the situation?

1. An 8-year-old girl is admitted to the emergency room, immaculately dressed, with many bruises and welts on her arms and legs. Her mother states she was hurt on the playground.
2. You note that your student partner has alcohol on her breath when she picks up her assignments. This has happened on more than one occasion.
3. A client has been told his bone scan shows metastatic lesions. He tells you not to tell his wife because she will just worry.

Discussion:

Share the responses to this exercise in a class discussion.

1. How did your answers compare with those of your peers?
2. In what ways did your values enter into your choices?

problems. A number of different paradigms illustrate the reasoning process developed by several disciplines. Unfortunately, each discipline has its own vocabulary. Table 3-2 shows that we are talking about concepts with which you are already familiar. It also contrasts terms used in education, nursing, and philosophy to specify 10 steps to help you develop your critical thinking skills. For example, the nurse performs a client assessment, which in education is referred to as "collecting information" or in philosophy is possibly called "identifying claims."

Table 3-2 Reasoning Process

Generic Reasoning Process	Diagnostic Reasoning in the Nursing Process	Ethical Reasoning	Critical Thinking Skill
Collect and interpret information	Gordon's functional patterns of health assessment	Parties, claim, basis	1. Clarify concepts 2. Identify own values and differentiate
Identify problem	Statement of nursing diagnosis	Statement of ethical dilemma	3. Integrate data and identify missing data 4. Collect new data 5. Identify problem 6. Apply criteria 7. Look at alternatives 8. Examine skeptically 9. Check for change in context 10. Make decision
Plan for problem solving	Prioritization of problems/interventions	Prioritized claims and action plan	
Implement plan	Nursing action	Moral action	
Evaluate	Outcome evaluation	Moral evaluation	Reflect/evaluate

The process of critical thinking is systematic, organized, and goal-directed. An extensive case application follows. During your learning phase, the critical thinking skills are divided into 10 specific steps. Each step includes a discussion of application to the clinical case example provided.

To help you understand how to apply critical thinking steps, read the following case and then see how each of the steps can be used in making clinical decisions. Components of this case are applied to illustrate the steps and stimulate discussion in the critical thinking process; many more points may be raised. From the outset, understand that whereas these are listed as steps, they do not occur in a rigid, linear way in real life. The model is best thought of as a circuit, or circular model. New data are constantly being sought and added to the process.

Case Example

Day 1—Mrs. Vlios, a 72-year-old widowed teacher, has been admitted to your unit. Her daughter Sara lives 2 hours away from her mother, but she arrives soon after admission. According to Sara, her mother lived an active life before admission, taking care of herself in an apartment in a senior citizens' housing development. Sara noticed that for about 3 weeks now, telephone conversations with her mother did not make sense or she seemed to have a hard time concentrating, although her pronunciation was clear. The admitting diagnosis is dehydration and dementia, rule out Alzheimer's disease, organic brain syndrome, and depression. An IV of 1000 ml dextrose/0.45 normal saline is ordered at 50 drops/hour. Mrs. Vlios's history is unremarkable except for a recent 10-pound weight loss. She has no allergies and is known to take acetaminophen regularly for minor pain.

Day 2—When Sara visits her mom's apartment to bring grooming items to the hospital, she finds the refrigerator and food pantry empty. A neighbor tells her that Mrs. Vlios was seen roaming the halls aimlessly 2 days ago and could not remember whether she had eaten. As Mrs. Vlios's nurse, you notice that she is oriented today (to time and person). A soft diet is ordered, and her urinary output is now normal.

Day 5—In morning report, the night nurse states that Mrs. Vlios was hallucinating and restraints were applied. A nasogastric tube was ordered to suction out stomach contents because of repeated vomiting. Dr. Green tells Sara and her brother Todos that their mother's prognosis is guarded; she has developed a serious systemic infection, is semicomatose, is not taking nourishment, and needs antibiotics and hyperalimentation. Sara reminds the doctor that her mother signed a living will in which she stated she refuses all treatment except IVs to keep her alive. Todos is upset, yelling at Sara that he wants the doctor to do everything possible to keep their mother alive.

Step 1: Clarify Concepts

The first step in making a clinical judgment is to identify whether a problem actually exists. Poor decision makers often skip this step. To figure out whether there is a problem, you need to think about what to observe and what basic information to gather. If it is an ethical dilemma, you not only need to identify the existence of the moral problem, but you need to also identify all the interested parties who have a stake in the decision. Figuring out exactly what the problem or issue is may not be as easy as it sounds.

Look for Clues. Are there hidden meanings to the words being spoken? Are there nonverbal clues?

Identify Assumptions. What assumptions are being made?

Case Discussion. This case is designed to present both physiological and ethical dilemmas. In clarifying the problem, address both domains.

- Physiological concerns: Based on the diagnosis, the initial treatment goal was to restore homeostasis. By Day 5, is it clear whether Mrs. Vlios's condition is reversible?
- Ethical concerns: When is a decision made to initiate treatment or to abide by the advance directive and respect the client's wishes regarding no treatment?
- What are the wishes of the family? What happens when there is no consensus?
- Assumptions: Is the diagnosis correct? Does the client have dementia? Or was her confusion a result of dehydration and a strange hospital environment?

Step 2: Identify Your Own Values

Having just completed the exercises given above should help your understanding of your own personal values and the professional values of nursing. Now apply this information to this case.

Case Discussion. Identify the values of each person involved:

- Family: Mrs. Vlios signed an advance directive. Sara wants it adhered to; Todos wants it ignored. Why? (Missing information: Are there religious beliefs? Is there unclear communication? Is there guilt about previous troubles in the relationship?)
- Personal values: What are yours?
- Professional values: The ANA says nurses are advocates for their clients; beneficence implies nonmaleficence ("do no harm") but autonomy means the client has the right to refuse treatment. What is the agency's policy? What are the legal considerations? Practice refining your professional values acquisition by completing the values exercises in this chapter.

In summary, you need to identify which values are involved in a situation or which moral principles can be cited to support each of the positions advocated by the involved individuals.

Step 3: Integrate Data and Identify Missing Data

Think about knowledge gained in prior courses and during clinical experiences. Try to make connections between different subject areas and clinical nursing practice.

- Identify what data are needed. Obtain all possible information and gather facts or evidence (evaluate whether data are true, relevant, and sufficient). Situations are often very complicated. It is important to figure out what information is significant to this situation. Synthesize prior information you already have with similarities in the current situation. Conflicting data may indicate a need to search for more information.
- Compare existing information with past knowledge. Has this client complained of difficulty thinking before? Does she have a history of dementia?
- Look for gaps in the information. Actively work to recognize whether there is missing information. Was Mrs. Vlios previously taking medications to prevent depression? For a nurse, this is an important part of critical thinking.
- Collect information systematically. Use an organized framework to obtain information. Nurses often obtain a client's history by asking questions about each body system. They could just as systematically ask about basic needs.
- Organize your information. Clustering information into relevant categories is helpful. For example, gathering all the facts about a client's breathing may help focus your attention on whether or not the client is having a respiratory problem. In your assessment, you note rate and character of respirations, color of nails and lips, use of accessory muscles, and grunting noises. At the same time, you exclude information about bowel sounds or deep tendon reflexes as not being immediately relevant to his respiratory status. Categorizing information also helps you notice whether there are missing data. A second strategy that will help you organize information is to look for patterns. It has been indicated that experienced nurses intuitively note recurrent meaningful aspects of a clinical situation.

Case Discussion. Rely on prior didactic knowledge or clinical experience. Cluster the data. What was Mrs. Vlios's status immediately before hospitalization? What was her status at the time of hospitalization? What information is missing? What additional data do you need?

- Physiology: Consider pathophysiological knowledge about the effects of hypovolemia and electrolyte imbalances on the systems such as the brain, kidneys, and vascular system. What is her temperature? What are her laboratory values? What is her 24-hour intake and output? Is she still dehydrated?
- Psychological/cognitive: How does hospitalization affect older adults? How do restraints affect them?
- Social/economic: Was weight loss a result of dehydration? Why was she without food? Could it be due to economic factors or mental problems?
- Legal: What constitutes a binding advance directive in the state in which Mrs. Vlios lives? Is a living will valid in her state, or does the law require a health power of attorney? Are these documents on file at the hospital?

Step 4: Obtain New Data

Critical thinking is not a linear process (Boggs, 1997; Fraser & Strang, 2004). Constantly consider whether you need more information. Establish an attitude of inquiry and obtain more information as needed. Ask questions; search for evidence; and check reference books, journals, the ethics sources on the Internet, or written professional or agency protocols.

Evaluate conflicting information. There may be time constraints. If a client has suspected "respiratory problems," you may need to set priorities. Obtain data that are most useful or are easily available. It would be useful to know oxygenation levels, but you may not have time to order laboratory tests. But perhaps there is a device on the unit or in the room that can measure oxygen saturation.

Sometimes you may need to change your approach to improve your chances of obtaining information. For example, when the charge nurse caring for Mrs. Vlios used an authoritarian tone to try to get the sister and brother to provide more information about possible drug overdose, they did not respond. However, when the charge nurse changed his approach, exhibiting empathy, the daughter volunteered that on several occasions her mother had forgotten what pills she had taken.

Case Discussion. List sources from which you can obtain missing information. Physiological data such as temperature or lab test results can be obtained quickly; some of the ethical information, however, may take longer to consider.

Step 5: Identify the Significant Problem

- Analyze existing information: Examine all the information you have. Identify all the possible positions.
- Make inferences: What might be going on? What are the possible diagnoses? Develop a working diagnosis.
- Prioritize: Which client problem is most urgently in need of your intervention? What are the appropriate interventions?

Case Discussion. A significant physiological concern is sepsis, regardless of whether it is an iatrogenic (hospital-acquired) infection or one resulting from immobility and debilitation. A significant ethical concern is the conflict among family members and client (as expressed through her living will). At what point do spiritual concerns take priority over a worsening physical concern?

Step 6: Examine Skeptically

Thinking about a situation may involve weighing positive and negative factors, and differentiating facts that are credible from opinions that are biased or not grounded in true facts.

- Keep an open mind.
- Challenge your own assumptions.
- Consider whether any of your assumptions are unwarranted. Does the available evidence really support your assumption?
- Discriminate between facts and inferences. Your inferences need to be logical and plausible, based on the available facts.
- Are there any problems that you have not considered?

In trying to evaluate a situation, consciously raising questions becomes an important part of thinking critically. At times there will be alternative explanations or different lines of reasoning that are equally valid. The challenge is to examine your own and others' perspectives for important ideas, complicating factors, other plausible interpretations, and new insights to see "the big picture" (Jones & Brown, 1993). Some nurses believe that examining information skeptically is part of each step in the critical thinking process rather than a step by itself.

Case Discussion. Challenge assumptions about the cause of Mrs. Vlios's condition. For example, did you eliminate the possibility that she had a head injury caused by a fall? Could she have liver failure as a result of acetaminophen overdosing? Have all the possibilities been explored? Challenge your assumptions about outcome: are they influenced by expected probable versus possible outcomes for this client? If she indeed has irreversible dementia, what will the quality of her life be if she recovers from her physical problems?

Step 7: Apply Criteria

In evaluating a situation, think about appropriate responses.

- Laws: There may be a law that can be applied to guide your actions and decisions. For example, by law certain diseases must be reported to the state. If you suspect physical abuse, there is a state statute that requires professionals to report abuse to the Department of Social Services.
- Legal precedents: There may have been similar cases or situations that were dealt with in a court of law. Legal decisions do guide health care practices. In end-of-life decisions, when there is no legally

binding health care power of attorney, the most frequent hierarchy is the spouse, then the adult children, then the parents (Lang & Quill, 2004).
- Protocols: There may be standard protocols for managing certain situations. Your agency may have standing orders for caring for Mrs. Vlios if she develops respiratory distress, such as administering oxygen per face mask at 5 L/min.

Case Discussion. Many criteria could be used to examine this case, including the Nurse Practice Act in the area of jurisdiction, the professional organization code of ethics or general ethical principles of beneficence and autonomy, the hospital's written protocols and policies, state laws regarding living wills, and prior court decisions about living wills. Remember that advance directives are designed to take effect only when clients become unable to make their own wishes known.

Step 8: Generate Options and Look at Alternatives

- Evaluate the major alternative points of view.
- Involve experienced peers as soon as you can to assist you in making your decision.
- Use clues from others to help you "put the picture together."
- Can you identify all the arguments—pro and con—to explain this situation? Almost all situations will have strong counterarguments or competing hypotheses.

Case Discussion. The important concept is that neither the physician nor the nurse should handle this alone; rather, others should be involved (e.g., the hospital bioethics committee, the ombudsman client representative, the family's spiritual counselor, and other medical experts such as a gerontologist, psychologist, and nursing clinical specialist).

Step 9: Consider Whether Factors Change if the Context Changes

Consider whether your decision would be different if there were a change in circumstances. For example, a change in the age of the client, in the site of the situation, or in the client's culture may affect your decision.

Case Discussion. If you knew the outcome from the beginning, would your decisions be the same? What if you knew Mrs. Vlios had a terminal cancer? What if Mrs. Vlios had remained in her senior housing project and you were the home health nurse? What if Mrs. Vlios had remained alert during her hospitalization and refused IVs, hyperalimentation, nasogastric tubes, and so on? What if the family and Mrs. Vlios were in agreement about no treatment? Would you make more assertive interventions to save her life if she were 7 years old, or a 35-year-old mother of five young children?

Step 10: Make the Final Decision

After analyzing available information in this systematic way, a judgment or decision needs to be made. An important part of your decision is your ability to communicate it coherently to others and to reflect on the outcome of your decision for your client.

- Justify your conclusion.
- Evaluate outcomes.
- Test out your decision or conclusion by implementing appropriate actions.

The critical thinker needs to be able to accept that there may be multiple solutions that can be equally acceptable. In other situations, a decision may need to be made even when there is incomplete knowledge. Be able to cite your rationale or present your arguments to others for your decision choice and interventions.

After you implement your interventions, examine the client outcomes. Was your assessment correct? Did you obtain enough information? Did the benefits to the client and family outweigh the harm that may have occurred? In retrospect, do you know you made the correct decision? Did you anticipate possibilities and complications correctly? This kind of self-examination can foster self-correction. It is this process of reflecting on one's own thinking that is the hallmark of a critical thinker.

Case Discussion. The most important concept is to forget the idea that there is one right answer to the dilemmas raised by discussion of this case. Accept that there may be several equally correct solutions depending on each individual's point of view.

Summarizing the Critical Thinking Learning Process

The most effective method of learning these steps in critical thinking results from repeatedly applying them to clinical situations. This can occur in your own clinical care. Del Bueno (1994) stated that a new graduate nurse must at a minimum be able to identify essential clinical data, know when to initiate interventions, know why a particular intervention is relevant, and differentiate between problems that need immediate intervention versus problems that can wait for action. Repeated practice in applying critical thinking can help a new graduate fit into the expectations of employers.

Students have demonstrated that critical thinking can be learned in the classroom as well as through clinical experience (Boggs, 1997). Effective learning can occur when opportunities are structured that allow for repeated in-class applications to client case situations. This includes using real-life case interviews with experienced nurses, which allow you to analyze their decision-making process. The interview and analysis of an expert nurse's critical thinking described in Exercise 3-4 explains how this is done using a 10-minute recording.

If recording an expert nurse's experience is not possible, you may help increase your critical thinking and clinical problem solving skills by discussing the following additional case examples. Remember that most clinical situations requiring decision making will not involve the types of ethical dilemmas discussed earlier in this chapter.

Case Example

Mr. Xia, age 42 years, has been admitted for surgical repair of his right knee, scheduled for tomorrow. When you enter his room, he complains of being short of breath. Respirations are 22/min and regular. Skin color is pink. Vital signs are normal. Mr. Xia has an anxious facial expression. You stay with him a few minutes to make sure he is oxygenating adequately. After 1 minute, his color is tinged with gray, and respirations are now 30/min and labored (Farrell & Bramadat, 1993).

What were you thinking at first?
What are you thinking now?
How do you sort out this situation?
What do you do first (e.g., assess for pain, provide reassurance, administer oxygen, sit him up in bed)?
Are you accustomed to doing this?
Where did you learn it?

Exercise 3-4 Your Analysis of an Expert's Critical Thinking: Interview of Expert Nurse's Case

Purpose: To develop awareness of critical thinking in the clinical judgment process.

Procedure:

Find an experienced nurse in your community and record him or her describing a real client case. You can use a computer or cell phone with recording capability, videotape, or audiotape to record an interview that takes less than 10 minutes. During the interview, have the expert describe an actual client case in which there was a significant change in the client's health status. Have the expert describe the interventions and thinking process that took place during this situation. Ask what nursing knowledge, lab data, or experience helped the nurse make his or her decision. You can work with a partner. Remember to protect confidentiality by omitting names and other identifiers.

Discussion:

Analyze the tape using an outline of the 10 steps in critical thinking. Discussion should first include citation examples of each step noted during their review of the taped interview, followed by application to the broad principles. Discussion of steps missed by the interviewed expert can be enlightening, as long as care is taken to avoid any criticism of the guest "expert."

Case Example

Mr. Gonzales has terminal cancer. His family defers to the attending physician who prescribes aggressive rescue treatment. The hospice nurse is an expert in the expressed and unexpressed needs of terminal clients. She advocates for a conservative and supportive plan of care (Jones & Brown, 1993). A logical case could be built for each position.

Solving Ethical Dilemmas in Nursing

Nurses, especially those in rural areas, have reported a great need for information about dealing with the ethical dilemmas they encounter, yet most report receiving no education in doing so (National Rural Bioethics Project, 2003). Exercises 3-5 (autonomy), 3-6 (beneficence), and 3-7 (justice) will give you the opportunity denied to the rural nurses who were surveyed! All nurses commonly encounter ethical dilemmas in and out of clinical settings. Ethical issues may include anything from euthanasia, to who should receive an organ transplant, to caring for a client with AIDS. With expanded technological advances in health care, there is an ever-increasing need for ethical decisions to accompany these advances. As a result, nurses may feel a growing pressure to be proficient in ethical decision making.

The ethical issues that nurses commonly face today can be placed in three general categories: moral uncertainty, moral or ethical dilemmas, and moral distress. **Moral uncertainty** occurs when a nurse is uncertain as to which moral rules (i.e., values, beliefs, or ethical principles) apply to a given situation. For example, should a terminally ill client who is in and out of a coma and

Exercise 3-5 Autonomy

Purpose: To stimulate class discussion about the moral principle of autonomy.

Procedure:
In small groups, read the three case examples on page 49 and discuss whether the client has the autonomous right to refuse treatment if it affects the life of another person.

Discussion:
Prepare your argument for an in-class discussion.

Exercise 3-6 Beneficence

Purpose: To stimulate discussion about the moral principle of beneficence.

Procedure:
Read the following case example and prepare for discussion:

Dawn, a staff nurse, answers the telephone and receives a verbal order from Dr. Smith. Ms. Patton was admitted this morning with ventricular arrhythmia. Dr. Smith orders Dawn to administer a potent diuretic, Lasix 80 mg, IV, STAT. This is such a large dose that she has to order it up from pharmacy.

As described in the text, you are legally obliged to carry out a doctor's orders unless they threaten the welfare of your client. How often do nurses question orders? What would happen to a nurse who questioned orders too often? In a research study using this case simulation, nearly 95% of the time the nurses participating in the study attempted to implement this potentially lethal medication order before being stopped by the researcher!

Discussion:
1. What principles are involved?
2. What would you do if you were this staff nurse?

Exercise 3-7 Justice

Purpose: To encourage discussion about the concept of justice.

Procedure:
Consider that in Oregon several years ago, attempts were made to legislate some restrictions on what Medicaid would pay for. A young boy needed a standard treatment of bone marrow transplant for his childhood leukemia. He died when the state refused to pay for his treatment.

Read the following case example and answer the discussion questions:

Mr. Diaz, age 74, has led an active life and continues to be the sole support for his wife and disabled daughter. He pays for health care with Medicare government insurance. The doctors think his cancer may respond to a very expensive new drug, which is not paid for under his coverage.

Discussion:
1. Does everyone have a basic right to health care as well as to life and liberty?
2. Does an insurance company have a right to restrict access to care?

chooses not to eat or drink anything be required to have intravenous therapy for hydration purposes? Does giving IV therapy constitute giving the client extraordinary measures to prolong life? Is it more comfortable or less comfortable for the dying client to maintain a high hydration level? When there is no clear definition of the problem, moral uncertainty develops, because the nurse is unable to identify the situation as a moral problem or to define specific moral rules that apply. Strategies that might be useful in dealing with moral uncertainty include using the values clarification process, developing a specific philosophy of nursing, and acquiring knowledge about ethical principles.

Ethical or **moral dilemmas** arise when two or more moral issues are in conflict. An ethical dilemma is a problem in which there are two or more conflicting but equally right answers. Organ harvesting of a severely brain-damaged infant is an example of an ethical dilemma. Removal of organs from one infant may save the lives of several other infants. However, even though the brain-damaged child is definitely going to die, is it right to remove organs before the child's death? It is important for the nurse to understand that in many ethical dilemmas there is often no single "right" solution. Some decisions may be "more right" than others, but often what one nurse decides is best differs significantly from what another nurse would decide.

The third common kind of ethical problem seen in nursing today is **moral distress**. Moral distress results when the nurse knows what is "right" but is bound to do otherwise because of legal or institutional constraints. When such a situation arises (e.g., a terminally ill client who does not have a "do not resuscitate" medical order and for whom, therefore, resuscitation attempts must be made), the nurse may experience inner turmoil.

Nurses in the National Rural Bioethics Project reported that three of their most commonly encountered ethics problems had to do with resuscitation decisions for dying clients with unclear, confusing, or no code orders; patients and families who wanted more aggressive treatment; and colleagues who discussed clients inappropriately.

Because values underlie all ethical decision making, nurses must understand their own values thoroughly before making an ethical decision. Instead of responding in an emotional manner on the spur of the moment (as people often do when faced with an ethical dilemma), the nurse who uses the values clarification process as a tool can respond rationally. It is not an easy task to have sufficient knowledge of oneself, of the situation, and of legal and moral constraints to be able to implement ethical decision making quickly. Expert nurses still struggle. Taking time to examine situations can help you develop skill in dealing with ethical dilemmas in nursing, and the exercises in this book will give you a chance to practice. Each chapter in this book has also included at least one ethical dilemma, so you can discuss what you would do.

Finally, in thinking about your own ethical practice, reflect on how important it is for your client to be able to always count on you. Consider the following client journal entry (Milton, 2002):

> *...I ask for information, share my needs, to no avail. You come and go...*
> *"Could you find out for me?" "Sure I'll check on it."*
> *[But] check on it never comes...*
> *Who can I trust? I thought you'd be here for me...*
> *You weren't. What can I do?*
> *Betrayal permeates...*

SUMMARY

Critical thinking is the ability to think about your thinking. It is not a linear process. Analysis of the thinking processes of expert nurses reveals that they continually scan new data and simultaneously apply these steps in clinical decision making. They monitor the effectiveness of their interventions in achieving desired outcomes for their client. A nurse's values and critical thinking abilities often have a profound effect on the quality of care given to a client, even affecting client mortality outcomes. Functioning as a competent nurse requires that you have knowledge of medical and nursing content, an accumulation of clinical experiences, and an ability to think critically. Almost daily, we confront ethical dilemmas and complicated clinical situations that require expertise as a decision maker. We can follow the 10 steps of the critical thinking process described in this chapter to help us respond to such situations. Developing skill as a critical thinker is a learned process, one requiring repeated opportunities for application to clinical situations. Reflecting on one's own thinking about case example situations provided in this chapter can assist such learning.

Ethical Dilemma ■ *What Would You Do?*

Rosa Sanchez, RN, is a case manager for 20 clients with severe chronic health problems in her community. Within the limitations on her time and budget, she makes decisions daily about distribution of equipment, staff to provide direct care in the home, or assistance to a family member who could provide needed care. In this rural county, one client lives nearly 100 miles away. Providing home care to him every day would mean his nurse could not provide care to two clients who live in town.

1. Which of the following factors should be most heavily weighed in making this decision: clients' ages, ability to pay, projected recovery based on standardized care plan such as clinical pathway (see Chapter 23), level of services needed, and inability of any family member to provide care?
2. Is this a business decision or an ethical one?

For further information, read Fraser KD, Strang V: Decision-making and nurse case management, *Adv Nurs Sci* 27(1):32-43, 2004.

REFERENCES

Bethune E, Jackling N: Critical thinking skills: the role of prior experience, *J Adv Nurs* 26:1005–1012, 1997.

Boggs KU: *Addendum to final report (CID grant)*, Charlotte, NC, 1997, UNCC Foundation.

Del Bueno D: Why can't new grads think like nurses? *Nurse Educ* 19:9–11, 1994.

Dodds S: Gender, aging, and injustice: social and political contexts of bioethics, *J Med Ethics* 31:295–298, 2005; available online: http://jme.bmjjournals.com/cgi/content/ful/31/5/295.

Emanuel EJ, Wendler D, Grady C: What makes clinical research ethical? *JAMA* 283(20):2701–2711, 2000; available online: http://jama.ama-assn.org/cgi/content/full/283/20/ 2701.

Facione NC, Facione PA: Externalizing the critical thinking in knowledge development and clinical judgment, *Nurs Outlook* 44(3):129–136, 1996.

Fahrenwald NL, Bassett SD, Tschetter L, Carlson PP et al.: Teaching core nursing values, *J Prof Nurs* 21(1):46–51, 2005.

Farrell P, Bramadat I: Paradigm case analysis and simulated recall, *Clin Nurse Spec* 4:153–157, 1993.

Fraser KD, Strang V: Decision-making and nurse case management, *Adv Nurs Sci* 27(1):32–43, 2004.

Goold SD: Trust and the ethics of health care institutions, *Hastings Cent Rep* 31(6):26–33, 2001.

Gunderson M: Being a burden: reflections on refusing medical care, *Hastings Cent Rep* 34(5):37–43, 2004.

Habel M: Bioethics: strengthening nursing's role, 2000; available online: www.nurseweek.com.

Haddad A: Ethics in action, *RN* 63(9):25–28, 2000a.

Haddad A: Ethics in action, *RN* 63(11):21–23, 2000b.

Hamilton RJ, Bowers BJ, Williams JK: Disclosing genetic test results to family members, *J Nurs Scholarship* 37(1):18–23, 2005.

Jepson RG, Hewison J, Thompson AGH, Weller D: How should we measure informed choice? The case of cancer screening, *J Med Ethics* 31:192–196, 2005.

Johnson P: US journalists fare well on test of ethics, study finds, *USA Today* 5D, February 2, 2005.

Jones SA, Brown LN: Alternative views on defining critical thinking through the nursing process, *Holist Nurs Pract* 7(3):71–76, 1993.

Karlowicz KA: Making tough decisions, *Urol Nurs* 24(6):460–461, 2004.

Lamond D, Thompson C: Intuition and analysis in decision making and choice, *J Nurs Scholarsh* 32(4):411–414, 2000.

Lang F, Quill T: Making decisions with families at the end of life, *American Family Physician* 70(4):719–723, 2004.

Lincourt J: Private conversations, 2006.

Maloy L, Mattas C: Clinical competencies: a program designed to optimize critical thinking skills, care delivery and collaborative practice, *Clin Nurse Spec* 19(2):77, 2005.

Mappes TA, DeGrazia D: *Biomedical ethics*, ed 4, New York, 1996, McGraw-Hill.

Martin P, Yarbrough S, Alfred D: Professional values held by baccalaureate and associate degree nursing students, *J Nurs Scholarsh* 35(3):291–296, 2003.

Miller BK, Beck L, Adams D: Nurses' knowledge of the code for nurses, *J Contin Educ Nurs* 22(5):198–200, 1991.

Milton C: Ethical implications for acting faithfully in nurse-person relationships, *Nurs Sci Q* 15:21–24, 2002.

National Rural Bioethics Project: Research studies and updates, 2003; available online: http://www2.umt.edu/bioethics/research_studies/completed.htm.

Roufail WM: The spheres of medical ethics, *Forum: NC Medical Board* 1:7–8, 1999.

Rubenfeld MG, Scheffer B: *Critical thinking in nursing: an interactive approach*, Philadelphia, 1995, JB Lippincott.

Schank MJ: Wanted: nurses with critical thinking skills, *J Contin Educ Nurs* 21(2):86–89, 1990.

Schattner A: Truth telling and patient autonomy: the patient's point of view. *Am J Med* 113(1):66–69, 2002.

Steele SM, Harmon VM: *Values clarification in nursing*, ed 2, Norwalk, CT, 1983, Appleton-Century-Crofts.

Veatch RM, Fry ST: *Case studies in nursing ethics*, Boston, 1987, Jones & Bartlett.

Zaher SJ: Ethics content in community health nursing textbooks, *Nurse Educ* 25(4):186–194, 2000.

Zeigler J: Weighty decisions, *New Physician* 54(3):17–22, 2005.

Part II

The Nurse-Client Relationship

Chapter 4

Self-Concept in the Nurse-Client Relationship

Ann Mabe Newman

OUTLINE

OBJECTIVES

At the end of the chapter, the reader will be able to:

1. Define self-concept.
2. Describe the characteristics and functions of self-concept.
3. Identify the psychosocial stages of self-development.
4. Identify nursing interventions relevant to nursing diagnoses of alteration of self-concept.
5. Describe the role of self-awareness in the nurse-client relationship.
6. Discuss factors related to self-concept: body image, personal identity, self-esteem, and spiritual distress.

The greatest gift I can conceive of having from anyone is to be seen by them, heard by them, to be understood and touched by them. The greatest gift I can give is to see, hear, understand and to touch another person. When this is done, I feel contact has been made.

(Satir, 1976)

The content of Chapter 4 explores the meaning of self and self-concept as it affects interpersonal relationships. Characteristics of self-concept and factors affecting formation of self-esteem are described. Understanding of these principles leads to more effectiveness in relating with clients. Applying content discussed in this chapter and skills gained from participating in the accompanying exercises should help develop the building blocks essential for establishing therapeutic nurse-client relationships.

BASIC CONCEPTS

The self is the most complex of all human attributes. While most theorists agree that infants do not have an awareness of self at birth, mothers who peer into the faces of their tiny, squirming newborns report a feeling of "knowing." From a biopsychosocial and spiritual standpoint, however, infants are essentially biological beings, containing drives, predispositions, and tendencies waiting to develop in ways determined by their heritage, human socializing agents, and environment. An understanding of the concept of self is essential to the understanding of the behavior of our clients and of ourselves as nurses. Thus it is not an overstatement to say that understanding a client's self-concept must be a component of all nursing care.

Self, **self-concept**, and self-system are used interchangeably in the human developmental and psychological literature. Harry Stack Sullivan (1892-1949), considered to be the father of the interpersonal theory of psychiatry, wrote widely about how self develops and what processes mediate its development. Hildegard Peplau (1909-1999), considered to be the mother of psychiatric nursing, studied Sullivan's work and extended it.

The self, self-concept, or self-system is an organized network of ideas, feelings, and actions that every person has as a consequence of experiences and interactions with other people (parents being the most important in the development process). **Self-esteem** reflects the degree to which one feels valued, important, or satisfied with the concept of self.

Development of Self

Peplau (1952) described four steps that clearly spell out how the self develops:

Appraisals are made by significant others about the self. Mothers and other significant others make appraisals or evaluative statements about the very young infant. Generally these appraisals are very warm, positive, or complimentary (e.g., "good girl," "good boy," "beautiful baby," "how wonderful") and said in pleasant tones. The infant cannot comprehend the words but does absorb the affect and general meaning.

The appraisal is not based on anything the infant does, but on the expectations of the evaluator or appraiser. For example, when an infant is burped properly and expels air while keeping the milk down, the evaluator (mother or caretaker) says, "Good baby!" When the evaluator burps the infant incorrectly, and the infant spits up milk along with the air, what is said is "Oh, messy baby." In the first instance, the statement really should be, "Good burper!" and in the latter, "Bad burper!" If the burper does not get the air up after a feeding and the infant later has gas pains, the statement made is, "Oh, what a colicky baby."

Appraisals are repeated, become a pattern, and become incorporated into the self. As the infant grows, appraisals take on regularity and become patterns. Mothers who feel competent about being mothers generally feel positively toward their infants. Mothers who are ill or stressed, or who are having many problems of their own, will tend to see their infants in a less positive light. Their appraisals will be more negative. Expectations held by significant others, even if not in full awareness, are very critical to this process. If the infant's feeding clock is set at 2 hours and the mother thinks infants should eat every 4 hours, negative appraisals will be made about the infant's signal for hunger, which is crying.

Behavior emerges to match the appraisals. Even before speech emerges, infants react to the appraisals. Infants can be observed as generally satisfied, pleasant, or happy little beings; or unhappy, unpleasant beings. When speech emerges, validation of this appraisal is evident by the child's language. Generally, children begin referring to self in the third person, such as, "Johnny good," or by pointing to self and smiling after doing something positive. Later, the first person is used and we hear, "I ate it all up!"

With each new era of development, the self is open for reappraisal. The self joins the process of appraisal by becoming a vital part of the appraisal work. For instance, the self might not agree with a negative appraisal and might correct it: "I'm not naughty; I'm trying to discover things," or, "I am not sleepy, or hungry," or, "I am ______." Refining one's sense of self or self-concept is never completely finished. Similarly, one's self-esteem can be damaged at times but then repaired and enhanced.

Because they touch and confirm the self-concept, caring human connections often are as healing as medication and specific treatments in influencing human responses to an illness. Even when the nurse is unable to promote healing through physical measures, the interpersonal process of understanding the meaning of the illness in a person's life provides a different type of healing.

Characteristics of Self-Concept

The self-concept is a dynamic mental construct reflecting a person's interaction with the larger social community as well as intrapersonal characteristics. More than the sum of its parts, the self-concept acts as an inner snapshot of a person. It helps people experience who they are and what they are capable of becoming physically, emotionally, intellectually, socially, and spiritually in a community with others.

The self-concept is a dynamic process, increasing in both diversity and complexity as the child develops (Stuart, 2005). Throughout his or her life a person develops and defines self-concepts as generalizations about the self: "I am shy"; "I have excellent mathematical skills"; "I am a born loser." As the person develops from child to adult, the self-concept becomes increasingly complex, reflecting responses of the self to new challenges in the life cycle. Attitudes about the self are modified by all of life's experiences.

Exercise 4-1 Who Am I?

Purpose: To help students understand some of the self-concepts they hold about themselves.

Procedure:

This exercise may be done as homework exercise and discussed in class. The class should sit face to face in a circle.

Fill in the blanks to complete the following sentences. There are no right or wrong answers.

The thing I like best about myself is ____________________.
The thing I like least about myself is ____________________.
My favorite activity is ____________________.
When I am in a group, I ____________________.
It would surprise most people if they knew ____________________.
The most important value to me is ____________________.
I like ____________________.
I most dislike ____________________.
I am happy when ____________________.
I feel sad when ____________________.
I feel most self-confident when I ____________________.
I am ____________________.
I feel committed to ____________________.
Five years from now I see myself as ____________________.

Discussion:

1. What were the hardest items to answer? The easiest?
2. Were you surprised by some of your answers? If so, in what ways?
3. Did anybody's answers surprise you? If so, in what ways?
4. Did anyone's answers particularly impress you? If so, in what ways?
5. What did you learn about yourself from doing this exercise?
6. How would you see yourself using this self-awareness in professional interpersonal relationships with clients?

Self-concepts allow roles to change and enlarge as a person matures. The self-concept of a child broadens through social interactions. As the emerging person develops close associations with others, the self-concept eventually becomes that of adult, marriage partner, or parent. James (1891) and others feel that a person has as many different social selves as there are distinct groups of persons about whose opinion he or she cares. Appropriate psychosocial development requires the emerging adult to incorporate the self-identities of worker, contributor to the community, spouse, and parent in an evolving spectrum of self-identifying concepts. One can think of the self-concept basically as the response to the question, "Who am I?" (Exercise 4-1).

Functions of Self-Concept

Self-concepts do the following:

- Help explain behavior
- Provide a conceptual framework for decision making
- Shape expectations for the future
- Provide bridges to meaning

Self-concept acts as a decision-making framework within which the individual can evaluate current behaviors and weigh the legitimacy of feelings. Decisions congruent with self-concept affirm the sense of self-identity. Decisions that conflict with understandings of self diminish self-worth and negatively affect the quality of a person's relationships with others.

Self-concept serves to shape future expectations through the concept of "possible selves" (Markus & Nurius, 1986). Possible selves unfold in the form of thoughts about goals, dreams, and fears about events still to come. Future thoughts provide either positive or negative input to the self-concept. For example, the nursing student might think, "I am a nursing student, but I can see myself one day as a nurse practitioner." Such thoughts help the novice nurse work harder to achieve professional goals. Possible selves have the capacity to prompt behaviors and aspirations, bringing about a self-fulfilling prophecy (Markus & Nurius, 1986).

Crises and illnesses provide the stage for considering possible selves that would not occur without these life interruptions. This concept is particularly important in health care, because possible selves offer clients the hope that the current self-concept can be enlarged to include more positive possibilities. At the same time, negative possible selves (e.g., failure, incompetence, and powerlessness) can work against the person, providing a negative context for evaluating the current self-concept (Sneed & Whitbourne, 2005). The nurse-client relationship provides support for positive possibilities of self and helps clients reframe the negative possible selves.

Self-concept provides interpersonal bridges to meaning. The journey to becoming completely one's own unique self is an intensely personal experience. At different points, the terrain appears dark, lonely, and unfamiliar. The nurse offers the client an interpersonal bridge between external events and internal perceptions, aiding the client in search of the deeper meaning of life or providing that interpersonal bridge simply by one's presence and valuing of the client. For example, a nursing student reported to her instructor that her encounter with her severely depressed client was spent tossing a ball, mostly in silence. "I know she felt my presence, but she never spoke," said the student. At the end of the rotation, the client kissed her on the cheek, with tears in her eyes, but never spoke. In the fall, when the instructor returned to the unit with a different group of students, the depressed client had been readmitted in a vegetative state. She had not spoken, but when she saw the instructor, she smiled and said, "Leslie." That was the name of the nursing student who had worked with her. For both participants, the interaction had meaning. The client felt caring. The instructor called Leslie and told her of the experience. For the student, it was a peak experience, reaffirming her self-concept as a professional nurse. There were no words that made this meeting memorable; it was the genuine presence of the participants that gave this conversation its I-thou qualities. Exercise 4-2 helps the nurse identify personality variations that contribute to self-concept.

Erikson's Model of Psychosocial Development

Erik Erikson's (1963, 1982) seminal work on personality development is a primary developmental construct used by nurses in the nurse-client relationship. Erikson's model labels a stage of personality development, names the ego strength to be developed during the stage, defines the stressors experienced in the developmental stage, and defines the behavior necessary to successfully move on to the next stage. Concepts related to Erikson's model are described in Table 4-1.

Exercise 4-2 Contribution of Life Experiences to Self-Concept

Purpose: To help students identify some of the many personality variations contributing to self-concept. There are no right or wrong responses.

Procedure:
1. Pair off with another student, preferably one with whom you are not well acquainted.
2. Student A spends 5 minutes questioning Student B to collect a biography of facts, including such information as ethnic background, number of siblings, place of birth, job or volunteer experiences, unusual life experiences, types of responsibilities, and favorite leisure activities. The process is then reversed, and Student B interviews Student A.
3. Each student introduces the other to the class, using the information gained from the interview.

Discussion:
1. Were you surprised by any of the information you found out?
2. How did your perception of other students change in light of the information shared?
3. In what ways were your perceptions different from your initial impression of your partner after the interview portion of the exercise?
4. What did you learn about yourself from doing this exercise?
5. How do you think what you learned might apply to nursing practice?

Nurses use Erikson's model as an important part of client assessment. Exercise 4-3 can help apply Erikson's concepts to client situations. Analysis of behavior patterns using this framework can identify age-appropriateness or arrested development of interpersonal skills (see Table 4-1).

APPLICATIONS

Figure 4-1 identifies the characteristics of a healthy self-concept. NANDA (2005) separates the nursing diagnosis related to self-concept into four discrete elements: body image, personal identity, self-esteem, and

Exercise 4-3 Erikson's Stages of Psychosocial Development

Purpose: To help students apply Erikson's stages of psychosocial development to client situations.

Procedure:
This exercise may be done as a homework exercise with the results shared in class.
To set your knowledge of Erikson's stages of psychosocial development, identify the psychosocial crisis or crises each of the following clients might be experiencing:
1. A 16-year-old unwed mother having her first child.
2. A 50-year-old executive "let go" from his job after 18 years of employment.
3. A stroke victim paralyzed on the left side.
4. A middle-aged woman caring for her mother who has Alzheimer's disease.
5. A 17-year-old high school athlete suddenly paralyzed from the neck down.

Discussion:
1. What criteria did you use to determine the most relevant psychosocial stage for each client situation?
2. What conclusions can you draw from doing this exercise that would influence how you would respond to each of these clients?

role performance. The first three elements are described here. Role relationships are described in Chapter 7, because they have a dual function as an interpersonal bridge between the inner and the outer world of health care.

Although self-concept can be described as the separate processes of body image/physical self, personal identity/personal self, self-esteem, and role performance, the separation is artificial. In the Roy Conceptual Model

Table 4-1 Erikson's Stages of Psychosocial Development, Clinical Behavior Guidelines, and Stressors

Stage of Personality Guidelines	Ego Strength or Virtue	Clinical Behavior Guidelines	Stressors
Trust versus mistrust	Hope	Appropriate attachment behaviors. Ability to ask for assistance with an expectation of receiving it. Ability to give and receive information related to self and health. Ability to share opinions and experiences easily. Ability to differentiate between how much one can trust and how much one must distrust.	Unfamiliar environment or routines. Inconsistency in care. Pain. Lack of information. Unmet needs (e.g., having to wait 20 minutes for a bedpan or pain injection). Losses at critical times or accumulated loss. Significant or sudden loss of physical function (e.g., a client with a broken hip being afraid to walk).
Autonomy versus shame and doubt	Willpower	Ability to express opinions freely and to disagree tactfully. Ability to delay gratification. Ability to accept reasonable treatment plans and hospital regulations. Ability to regulate one's behaviors (overcompliance, noncompliance, suggest disruptions). Ability to make age-appropriate decisions.	Overemphasis on unfair or rigid regulation (e.g., putting clients in nursing homes to bed at 7 p.m.). Cultural emphasis on guilt and shaming as a way of controlling behavior. Limited opportunity to make choices in a hospital setting. Limited allowance made for individuality.
Initiative versus guilt	Purpose	Ability to develop realistic goals and to initiate actions to meet them. Ability to make mistakes without undue embarrassment. Ability to have curiosity about health care. Ability to work for goals. Ability to develop constructive fantasies and plans.	Significant or sudden change in life pattern that interferes with role. Loss of a mentor, particularly in adolescence or with a new job. Lack of opportunity to participate in planning of care. Overinvolved parenting that doesn't allow for experimentation. Hypercritical authority figures. No opportunity for play.
Industry versus inferiority	Competence	Work is perceived as meaningful and satisfying. Appropriate satisfaction with balance in lifestyle pattern, including leisure activities. Ability to work with others, including staff. Ability to complete tasks and self-care activities in line with capabilities. Ability to express personal strengths and limitations realistically.	Limited opportunity to learn and master tasks. Illness, circumstance, or condition that compromises or obliterates one's usual activities. Lack of cultural support or opportunity or training.

Continued.

Table 4-1 Erikson's Stages of Psychosocial Development, Clinical Behavior Guidelines, and Stressors – *Cont'd.*

Stage of Personality Guidelines	Ego Strength or Virtue	Clinical Behavior Guidelines	Stressors
Identity versus identity diffusion	Fidelity	Ability to establish friendships with peers. Realistic assertion of independence and dependence needs. Demonstration of overall satisfaction with self-image, including physical characteristics, personality, and role in life. Ability to express and act on personal values. Congruence of self-perception with nurse's observation and perception of significant others.	Lack of opportunity. Overprotective, neglectful, or inconsistent parenting. Sudden or significant change in appearance, health, or status. Lack of same-sex role models.
Intimacy versus solation	Love	Ability to enter into strong reciprocal interpersonal relationships. Ability to identify a readily available support system. Ability to feel the caring of others. Ability to act harmoniously with family and friends.	Competition. Communication that includes a hidden agenda. Projection of images and expectations onto another person. Lack of privacy. Loss of significant others at critical points of development.
Generativity versus stagnation and self-absorption	Caring	Demonstration of age-appropriate activities. Development of a realistic assessment of personal contributions to society. Development of ways to maximize productivity. Appropriate care of whatever one has created. Demonstration of a concern for others and a willingness to share ideas and knowledge. Evidence of a healthy balance among work, family, and self demands.	Aging parents, separately or concurrently with adolescent children. Obsolescence or layoff in career. "Me generation" attitude. Inability or lack of opportunity to function in a previous manner. Children leaving home. Forced retirement.
Integrity versus despair	Wisdom	Expression of satisfaction with personal lifestyle. Acceptance of growing limitations while maintaining maximum productivity. Expression of acceptance of certitude of death as well as satisfaction with one's contributions to life. Lack of opportunity.	Rigid lifestyle. Loss of significant other. Loss of physical, intellectual, and emotional faculties. Loss of previously satisfying work and family roles.

of Nursing, Driever (1976a) noted that "self-concept is the composite of beliefs and feelings that one holds about one's self at a given time" (p. 169). Throughout this chapter, the student must keep in mind that the division of self-concepts into detached dimensions is for discussion purposes only.

Body Image or Physical Self

Body image represents the physical dimension of self-concept and a person's first awareness of self. The perceptions of the body and its associated elements, not its reality, make up body image. Physical structures associated with body image include not only the actual

Developing an Evidence-Based Practice

Rowland JH, Desmond KA, Meyerowitz BE, Belin TR et al.: Role of breast reconstructive surgery in physical and emotional outcomes among breast cancer survivors, *J Natl Cancer Inst* 92(17):1422-1429, 2000.

A self-report questionnaire was twice administered to 1957 breast cancer survivors in order to compare whether type of surgery influenced the psychosocial outcomes, including body image and feelings of attractiveness.

Results: 45.4% of women who had a mastectomy with reconstructive surgery reported that the breast cancer had had a negative impact on their sex lives. These negative outcomes were far greater than for women whose breast cancer was treated with a lumpectomy (29.8%), and more even than the women who had a mastectomy without reconstruction (41.3%). However, beyond the first year after diagnosis, the women's quality of life was more likely to be influenced by her age and exposure to adjuvant therapy than by her type of breast surgery.

Application to Your Clinical Practice: More studies are needed on the effects of breast cancer surgical treatments on self-image, but based on results from this study, your counseling about treatment choices might need to consider age and surgical invasiveness as important factors in the clients' decision-making process about treatment choices.

material body but also all somatic sensations of pain, fatigue, pleasure, heat, and cold. The physical self-concepts include the senses as well as physical attributes, functioning, sexuality, wellness-illness state, and appearance (Driever, 1976a).

Functions of Body Image

Schontz (1974) described four functions of body image: (a) a sensory image; (b) an instrument for action and source of drives; (c) a stimulus to self and others; and (d) an expressive instrument. As a sensory register, the body recognizes important information through one or more of its sensory receptors.

The physical self functions as a major instrument for action. Through a remarkable network of muscle, nerve, and cellular interactions, the human body can perform an infinite variety of independent actions. No other physical structure can autonomously decide to move on its own, be able to complete the action, reflect on the meaning of it, and discuss the meaning of it with another.

As a stimulus to self, the mental picture of a person's body and associated feelings (e.g., body weight, shape, and size) affect the value we place on ourselves. Consider how you feel about yourself when you have not showered, shaved, brushed your teeth, or combed your hair; then think how you feel when you know you look your best. Some mental disorders (e.g., major depression, schizophrenia, and eating disorders) reflect disturbed body image as part of their symptomatology.

Finally, body image serves as an expressive instrument, giving interpersonal signals and information about the self to others. People who are dressed well and are well groomed generally command more respect than those who are not.

Alterations in Body Image

Types of Alterations. Most people think of body image as describing visible changes in physical characteristics. However, the concept includes more subtle variations related to loss of body function, loss of control, and deviations from the norm.

Loss of Body Function. Loss of body function is an aspect of body image that can be either very obvious or well hidden by the client. The inability to move freely, infertility, impotence, and loss of bladder or bowel function are examples of functional loss. The loss is only part of the problem: many people experience shame about their condition and avoid social situations because of their embarrassment. The mind and body interface so tightly that real or perceived inability to function biologically both affects and is affected by psychological factors. Worrying can further compromise functioning. Talking about loss of function with a sympathetic listener makes it more acceptable and more manageable for the client.

Loss of Control. Similar in impact to loss of function are alterations in control and loss of sensation. Clients in pain and those subject to seizures, alcoholism, cardiac arrhythmias, or periodic depressions may exhibit few obvious changes in body image; however, the repeated loss of control over the body leaves the client with similar feelings of insecurity and uncertainty. Being able to talk about these realities that dominate some people's feelings about themselves can be enormously reassuring.

Deviations in Physical Characteristics. Body image is affected by subtle reactions of others. Those who are too thin or too fat, or who look considerably older or younger than they are, often are judged on the basis of

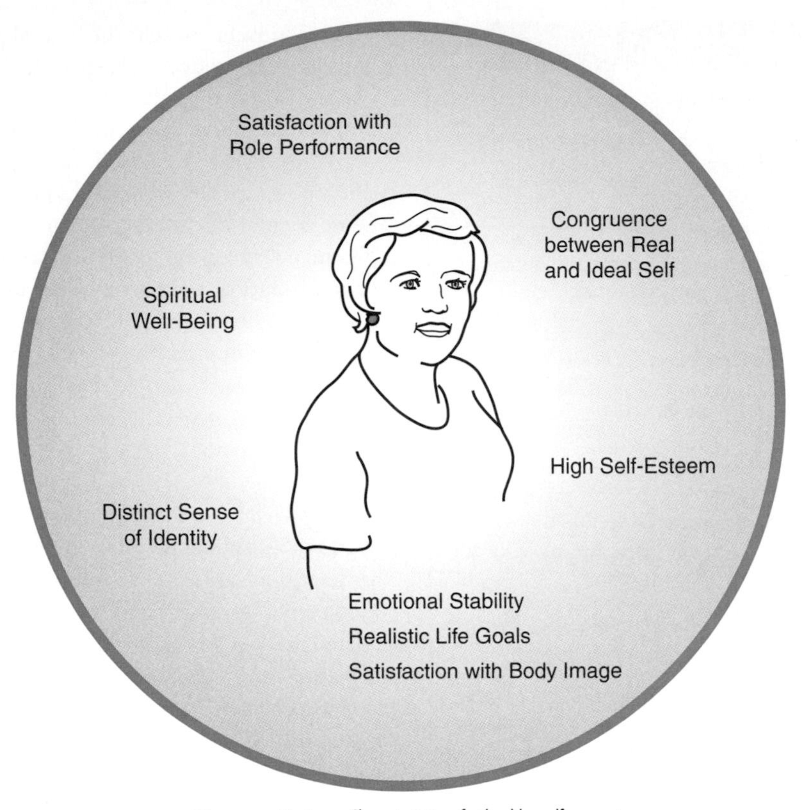

Figure 4-1 • Characteristics of a healthy self-concept.

their looks. Physical attractiveness and conformity to the norm unfortunately result in special treatment, and those who are different or unattractive are not treated so well. People who are different speak of feeling invisible, receiving subtle discrimination, and being misunderstood.

Significant deviations in physical characteristics have a profound effect on self-concept and self-esteem (Driever, 1976b). Understanding differences and working with clients to develop effective coping strategies enhance self-esteem and self-efficacy.

A common response to people with longstanding physical deviations is to ignore them or to assume they have gotten used to being different. Lifelong experience with significant deviations in body image does not necessarily make the person unaware of it or any more comfortable with it. Sensitivity to the impact of physical differences is essential to effective communication. Otherwise, nurses can overlook or minimize chronic alterations in body image that are of great importance in assessing the meaning of client behaviors.

Culture and Body Image. Culture plays a significant role in our perception of body image by emphasizing some physical characteristics as positive and others as negative. For example, in the United States, a slim, trim figure is admired (Thomas & Ricciardelli, 2000). The overweight individual is thought of as unhealthy, whether or not this is true. In other cultures, obesity may be viewed as a sign of prosperity.

Assessment Strategies. Alterations in body image always require some type of adaptation. The extent of adjustment is determined partially by the nature and magnitude of the alteration and partially by the degree to which the alterations interfere with functioning or lifestyle. Highly visible changes usually require more of an adjustment. Likewise, sudden changes in body image may be more difficult to absorb than changes in appearance that occur over time. Important in the human response to alterations in body image are the feelings and attitudes of others, the potential capacity of the client to cope with change, and the availability of sources of support.

Beginning with the first encounter, the nurse seeks to understand the meaning behind the symptoms. The value placed on body image differs from person to person. Some individuals, like Helen Keller and Ray Charles, are able to adapt an objectively negative physical feature of self in ways that benefit not only themselves but also all whom they encounter. Others let a physical deviation so dominate self-image that it becomes their only defining characteristic.

The same medical treatment or surgical procedure stimulates different body images. For some women, the prospect of a hysterectomy is viewed with relief; for others, it has serious psychological implications related to attractiveness and physical enjoyment of sex. Understanding these variations in the meaning of physical changes enables the nurse to respond effectively. Instead of simply accepting a single behavioral response as a given, the nurse takes into consideration the personalized meaning of the change for each client in planning care. Assessment data for a nursing diagnosis of self-concept disturbance in body image might include one or more of the following behaviors:

- Verbal expression of negative feelings about the body
- No mention of changes in body structure and function, or preoccupation with changed body image
- Reluctance to look at or touch a changed body structure
- Expression of worthlessness or hopelessness related to changes in body structure or appearance
- Social isolation and loss of interest in friends

The nurse can seek supporting data through open-ended questions or circular questioning related to the client's perception of altered body structure or function. Examples of these questions include, "What has it been like for you since you had your operation?" or, "Who do you think could be most helpful to you in making the transition back to work?" Often the concerns of clients relate not only to their perception of the changed appearance or function but also to perceptions of possible reactions of significant others. For example, a client with a speech impediment resulting from surgery or a stroke may not talk because he is anxious about the way his speech sounds to others, or a cancer victim may fear how she looks to others without her wig.

Other data should include the client's identified strengths and limitations, expressed needs and goals, the nature and accessibility of the client's support system, and the impact of body image change on lifestyle.

Planning and Intervention. Sensitivity to the client's need to absorb the implications of a change in body image is a critical component of support. Most clients need time to absorb physical changes. Interventions to modify alterations in body image might include the following:

- Providing information and support
- Modeling acceptance
- Introducing adaptive functioning
- Encouraging the client to share experiences with others
- Enhancing social support

Providing relevant information and creating opportunities for the client to ask questions make it acceptable for the client to explore an anticipated or actual change in body image. In the case of a new diagnosis, it is important for the nurse to go over information more than once, even if it appears that the client understands it initially. Validation checks, asking whether the client has any questions, and suggesting realistic responses can facilitate communication when the client seems very anxious.

Modeling acceptance starts with the nurse. Showing the client that a physical change does not frighten the nurse reduces the fear and panic that a significant change in appearance often produces. Nurses see clients with serious body image changes on a regular basis; for the client, it is a unique and potentially horrifying experience. Finding that a significant physical change does not cause the nurse to recoil in disgust allows the client to reframe the situation and to see that the person within remains intact. For example, one client with extensive head and neck surgery would deliberately unwrap his wound to see how each new nurse would react. He needed to know that his nurse would not turn away from him because of his appearance.

As the client demonstrates beginning acceptance through inquiry or a willingness to talk about the physical change, the nurse can slowly introduce the idea of resuming normal functions appropriate to the client's age and developmental level. A warm, supportive, yet tactfully objective interpersonal approach encourages expressions of feelings. For example, the nurse can help a client anticipate and respond with dignity to the reactions of others. Sharing the experience with others who have gone through a similar ordeal recognizes the legitimacy of having feelings that otherwise might go unexpressed. For example, having a "Reach for Recovery" volunteer visit a mastectomy client to share feelings, hopes, alternative options, and practical suggestions for adapting to change is a very simple intervention that helps increase the client's adjustment and acceptance of the change. With children, the nurse can act as an advocate in explaining alterations in body image to peers who otherwise might ridicule or avoid a child with a significant physical, cognitive, or emotional deficit.

Finally, the importance of social support from family and friends cannot be overestimated. Social support does as much or more than medication and technical skill for the person with altered self-concept related to body image. The client needs to know that his or her altered appearance will not disturb relationships. The nurse can suggest that the client call family or friends. Sometimes just a suggestion is enough to put the client in contact with others. At other times the nurse needs to provide encouragement and support to help the client take this step. Anticipatory guidance with visitors to prepare them for dramatic changes in their family member's or friend's appearance helps promote acceptance.

Evaluation. Throughout the relationship, the nurse and client mutually evaluate the effectiveness of the rehabilitation process. Confirming statements about client effort and small steps taken, as well as goals attained, encourage the client to acknowledge short-term goals and point out areas of development that require further modification of the nursing care plan. Appropriate adjustments, if needed, are mutually determined and implemented.

Personal Identity or Personal Self

Personal identity is more difficult to characterize than the physical aspects of self-concept because the nurse cannot actually see it.

Personal identity consists of all the psychological beliefs and attitudes people have about themselves: the perceptual, cognitive, emotional, and spiritual elements of self-concept. Driever (1976a) identifies the components of self-concept as the personal self, and further divides it into the moral-ethical self, self-consistency, and self-ideal/self-expectancy.

The moral-ethical self is the aspect of the personal identity that functions as an observer, standard setter, dreamer, and evaluator of who one says one is. The moral-ethical self makes judgments that influence one's self-evaluation (Carson & Trubowitz, 2006).

Self-consistency deals with the component of the self-identity that tries to maintain a consistent self-image. Even if the image is negative, one resists letting go of the image because of this need for self-consistency.

Self-ideal/self-expectancy relates to one's perception of what one wants to do, be, or become. This ideal self arises out of the perception one has of the expectations of others. Perception becomes one's reality.

Perception

Perception is a personal identity construct by which a person transforms external sensory data into personalized images of reality. As an intrapersonal process, perception allows a person to choose among sensory images and to cluster sensory images into a meaningful design. Perception is the first gatekeeper of self-concept.

Perception is a function of the mind and not of the senses. Consider the image in Figure 4-2. Depending on how one's eyes focus on the picture, it is possible to draw quite different conclusions about the images. The same

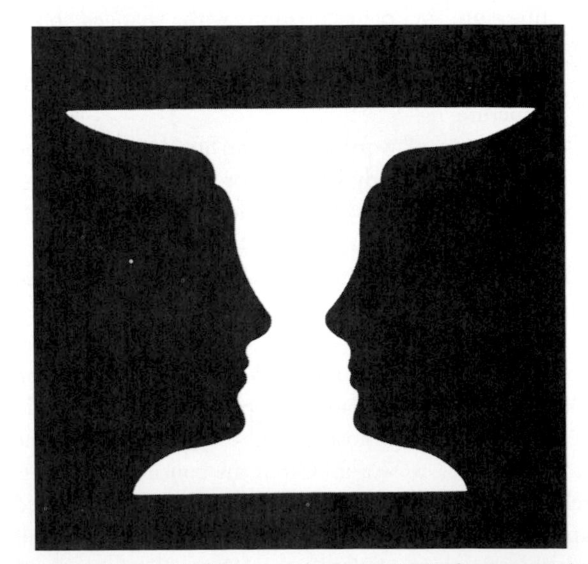

Figure 4-2 • The figure-ground phenomenon. Are the figures presented in white against a black background or in black against a white background? Does it make a difference in your perception of the figures? (From the Westinghouse Learning Corporation: *Self-instructional unit 12: perception,* 1970. Used with permission.)

phenomenon is true in life: reality lies in the eye of the beholder. Perceptions differ because people develop mindsets that automatically alter sensory data in specific personal ways. Validation of perceptual data is needed because the nurse and the client may not be looking at the same phenomenon.

Types of Perceptual Alterations in Self-Concept

Distorted Reality. Perceptual processes contribute significantly to the self-concept in the way individuals think about themselves and others. When perceptions are colored by unresolved past conflicts or by simple misunderstandings, they contribute to a sense of self not based in reality. For example, a young boy with artistic abilities and little interest in sports might think of himself as odd or as not fitting in with his more aggressive, sports-minded schoolmates if there is no support from the environment for his more aesthetic inclinations. A sympathetic teacher or school art club, however, can dramatically reshape his self-concept.

Perceptual distortions of reality are found in many mental and neurological disorders. People can create their own personal world that has little to do with reality. Usually, if the perceptual distortions are significant, the client is unable to maintain independent living.

Selective Attention. This is a less serious interpersonal perceptual process by which a person hears selected parts of a message and fails to absorb other parts because of defensive self-needs. A person who has heard only part of the message is unlikely to respond appropriately. For example, people who are depressed hear only the negative comments a person makes and fail to register the positive comments made in the same conversation (Cutler, 2001). Some common perceptual filters associated with selective attention include culture, sex, age, physical condition, mood, past experience, similarity of problem, stereotyping, expectations, and interpersonal differences.

Selective attention focuses on behavior extremes. People pay more attention to stimuli that are attention-grabbing, and also remember them longer. Often it is difficult to erase the perceptual image created by a particularly intense or painful stimulus, even if new information contradicts it or if the image was only a peripheral aspect of a larger situation. Interestingly, negative impressions are retained longer than favorable impressions.

First impressions contribute to a subtle form of selective attention by blocking subsequent information that would contradict the initial assessment. For example, a co-worker tells you that Mr. Mabe in Room 200 is difficult and cantankerous, and as you enter his room, he glares at you. Mr. Mabe may be having a bad day, and his behavior may not really reflect his normal behavioral responses. However, the next time you work with him you may approach him as a "difficult" client. Reframing Mr. Mabe's angry symptoms as a cry for help could prevent this stereotyping action on your part.

Self-Fulfilling Prophecy. When a person's perceptions of a certain outcome actually influence the person's present and future behaviors, the process is referred to as a self-fulfilling prophecy. For example, Martha receives an evaluation indicating a need for improved confidence. Martha interprets the instructor's comments as meaning she is awkward. Instead of seeing the instructor's comment as related to a behavior that is simple to correct, Martha perceives it as a personal commentary on her self. This perception colors Martha's behavior, and from that point on she performs awkwardly and freezes when asked questions in the clinical area.

Assessment Strategies. A nursing assessment of perceptual difficulty is based on knowledge of the expected developmental level of a particular client and observation of unsatisfactory behavioral responses to stress. Disturbances in perception can be inferred when the client seems to block out parts of his or her experience, projects the blame for personal frustration onto the environment, or is hypercritical of self or others. Hopelessness expressed as an inability to see alternative options also indicates limited perceptual functioning.

Health status, intelligence, life experience, and age are important considerations in assessing the client's perceptual capacity. For example, anxiety, brain trauma or dysfunction, disease, reaction to medication, certain abnormal blood values, sheltered living experiences, and the age-related evolution of thinking in childhood all have a significant impact on perceptual ability.

Assessment of perceptual patterns should take into account the environmental context in which the interaction takes place. People "edit" their behaviors to meet their perceived expectations of the other person and the appropriateness of their communication to the current situation. They tend to be more guarded in unfamiliar and exposed settings. If the interview takes place in a less-than-ideal setting, this should be noted as an environmental variable.

Assessment data should incorporate the cultural diversity of clients. Major and minor language differences between client and nurse can affect the perception of the intent of the message sender or receiver. People are sometimes insulted by comments, gestures, and emblems they perceive as intrusive or degrading when this was not the intent of the message sender. Different cultures have culture-specific norms about the use of eye contact and deference to others. Without an understanding of cultural diversity, the nurse may unintentionally misinterpret a client's response or offend a client. Asking clients about their cultural world helps prevent insensitivity.

Perceptions of both nurse and client may be colored by interests, emotions, or needs that either party carries into the conversation. For example, if the nurse is worried about something that happened that morning in his or her own family, it is likely that some of the client's data may go unnoticed or may be distorted because of the nurse's distraction.

Hospitalization by its very nature narrows perceptual ability. Adjusting to a physical impairment and a different living situation simultaneously may prove overwhelming to clients and significantly affect their perceptual acuity (Kurlowicz, 2001).

Case Example

Mrs. New, a fiercely independent elderly woman, has suddenly been immobilized with a broken hip. After a short hospital stay, she is sent to a nursing home because she can no longer take care of herself. She is bewildered and acts slightly confused.

To reorient herself to the meaning of her new situation, Mrs. New might have some of the following concerns: "In what ways am I like or unlike the other nursing home residents? Will I fit in? Is this a temporary or permanent arrangement?" Mrs. New finds herself in a whole new social milieu. Furthermore, physically helpless elderly clients who have all of their mental faculties are sometimes treated as though they are mentally incompetent because of stereotypes about aging. The nursing staff needs to understand that just because Mrs. New is 90 does not mean she has significant memory problems. She has the same needs as they do: to be valued and treated with dignity. How can Mrs. New be helped to communicate her needs without being seen as demanding or out of line?

The art of nursing involves protecting the integrity of Mrs. New's self-concept while giving her the emotional support and assistance she needs. Providing information and cues for action are structural interventions the nurse can use. The nurse can also encourage the client to take advantage of activities with gentle verbal support.

Planning and Intervention. When perceptions are clouded, the nurse may intentionally provide a calm, unhurried, interpersonal atmosphere for therapeutic conversations. Timing and interpersonal space are critical in planning interventions. For example, the suspicious client needs shorter and more objective verbal interactions until trust is established. Sometimes the undemanding presence of a nurse allows the client to move closer without fear of reprisal. In the hospital, taking time to make sure the newly admitted client or family is comfortable, offering a beverage, and introducing yourself are simple actions that reduce the anxiety most clients feel in this unfamiliar setting. An uncomplicated game or small talk about a neutral topic can be useful bridges in working with psychotic clients, for whom perceptions and the relationship are intertwined.

Tone of voice, choice of words, and nonverbal gestures create perceptual barriers if the person experiencing them feels devalued. The person receiving the message may not know the reason for being devalued, but the underlying communication is likely to affect every aspect of the nurse-client relationship and of goal accomplishment.

Perceptual Checks: A Useful Nursing Strategy. The interpersonal relationship offers an excellent means of reformulating false perceptions through perception checks. Adler and Rodman (1999) offer a three-step process for checking the validity of perceptual inferences:

- *Describe precisely the behavior of concern.* All aspects of the problem, including the reasons the problem is of major concern at this time and possible causes, are considered.
- *Offer two alternative explanations for the problem.* In most situations, the nurse asks only one question at a time to avoid confusing the client; however, the client with perceptual problems may need alternative suggestions. Adler and Rodman advocate using two possible cause-effect explanations rather than one interpretation as a way of broadening their perspective.

Most situations are multidetermined. Offering alternate explanations models the idea that most situations in life carry more than one possible explanation and more than one solution, or perhaps none.

- *Request feedback.* Feedback forces the client to interact with the helping person in checking reality. It reduces the chances of misinterpretations and false assumptions. This three-step process helps a person maintain an accurate picture of reality. In the process of developing shared meanings, people draw closer together. The knowledge that another individual cares enough to find out what is going on within the person affirms the value of the interpersonal relationship for both participants.

Case Example

Nurse: Mr. Sutphin, I notice that you didn't use the Ames glucose monitor this morning to test your blood for sugar. *(Focused description of behavior.)* Is that because you need more practice in what we went over yesterday, or is it difficult for you to consider using it for other reasons? *(Two alternative logical explanations of behavior.)*

Client: The idea of pricking myself all the time isn't appealing.

Nurse: So it is the needle stick that disturbs you. Can you tell me more about your reluctance to test your blood? *(Asking for feedback.)*

From the client's response, the nurse now knows that use of the glucose monitor, rather than a misunderstanding of instructions, is the major concern for the client. This perceptual check means that further instruction, support, and feedback will center on those parts of the problem of greatest import to the client. Equally important, the client feels heard.

Perceptual checks, combined with well-thought-out inferences about the meaning of client behaviors, enhance the quality of decision making in the nurse-client relationship. They allow the nurse to use perceptual data in a conscious, deliberate way to facilitate the relationship process. Because the client feels heard and because communication focuses on matters of interest and concern to the client, mutuality occurs with greater frequency. Nursing interventions are more likely to fit the client's needs, resulting in deeper satisfaction and a more successful outcome.

The nurse-client relationship is not the only source of perceptual checks. Referent groups, defined as groups of persons having common interests and concerns, are a form of social support. These informal support groups allow people who perceive that they are alone to find others who have similar physical, emotional, and spiritual situations.

Evaluation. Behaviors indicating broader perceptual flexibility include the ability to develop different perspectives on the same subject. Willingness to enter a support group and to try different options also suggests perceptual adaptability.

Cognition

Thinking is a complex, creative, cognitive process stimulated by conscious data, internal as well as external. Cognitive processes take perceptual images and categorize them into new informational sets through the process of reflective thinking. Through cognitive thinking processes, a person determines the accuracy of perceptual data and assesses the possible outcomes of alternate options. Without the ability to process the meaning of perceptual images cognitively, people would be unable to develop realistic goals, implement coherent patterns of behavior, and evaluate their efforts.

The cognitive aspects of self-concept are best characterized by the level, clarity, and logic of thinking. New cognitive images are stored in long- or short-term memory, and are able to be retrieved when needed. When illness, genetic factors, pain, accident, or injury affects cognition, there is also a profound effect on a person's overall sense of personal identity. Although images may enter the psyche, the normal cognitive processes directing behavior can no longer make sense of them.

Assessment Strategies. The information-processing characteristics of each client are different. Because people think differently about the same issues, it is logical to assume that individuals' cognitive approaches to problem solving differ. Efforts to accurately assess and respond appropriately to the individual learning characteristics of the client save time for the nurse and minimize frustration for the client.

Assessment data that might lead the nurse to suspect a disturbance in cognition start with the client's knowledge about his or her illness, treatment protocols, and expectations of therapy. Other information includes the client's knowledge of risk factors; previous illnesses;

motivation; orientation to time, place, and person; and memory assessment.

Cognition can be compromised at any time by alterations in an individual's physiological and emotional state. For example, low blood sugar affects cognition in a very direct and immediate way. Pain, hunger, and hormone or chemical imbalances in the body influence cognitive functioning adversely. Strong emotions and intense psychological states can temporarily reduce the level of cognitive function and awareness.

It is not unusual to see an Alzheimer's disease patient clutching his head as if to make sense out of a meaningless world. Taking into account the agony that loss of cognition creates in its victims enhances the development of appropriate nursing strategies.

When assessing cognition, it is important to differentiate transient memory loss from more permanent loss in the elderly. Elderly clients can appear acutely confused when confronted with the unfamiliar context of a hospitalization, yet the disorientation may completely disappear when they return home, as happened in the case of Mrs. New.

Planning and Intervention. Reflective thinking and the ability to express thoughts clearly contribute to effective functioning. Not all thinking processes are clear. Cognitive distortions occur as a result of thoughts about the meaning of a situation that have little to do with reality (Box 4-1). Faulty perceptions lead to cognitive distortions, but it is the thinking about them that leads to disordered behavior. When this occurs, the nurse looks for the cause of the distortion and links the intervention to the nursing diagnosis.

Box 4-1 Examples of Cognitive Distortions

- "All or nothing" thinking—the situation is all good or all bad; a person is trustworthy or untrustworthy.
- Overgeneralizing—one incident is treated as if it happens all the time; picking out a single detail and dwelling on it.
- Mind-reading and fortune-telling—deciding a person does not like you without checking it out; assuming a bad outcome with no evidence to support it.
- Personalizing—seeing yourself as flawed, instead of separating the situation as something you played a role in but did not cause.
- Acting on "should" and "ought to"—deciding in your mind what is someone else's responsibility without perceptual checks; trying to meet another's expectations without regard for whether or not it makes sense to do so.
- "Awfulizing"—assuming the worst; every situation has a catastrophic interpretation and anticipated outcome.

Special modifications of the nurse-client relationship allow for individual differences in cognitive capacities. Clients with dementia have limited functioning because their ability to use knowledge constructively and to put facts together in a systematic way is no longer available to them. Mentally ill clients often are unable to use cognitive problem-solving skills.

Keeping communication simple; breaking instructions down into smaller, sequential steps; presenting ideas one at a time; and using touch to emphasize directions or guide the client all can help compensate for cognitive deficits. Unless there is a pronounced cognitive deficit, knowledge of the client's educational level influences the type of language the nurse uses. Clients with flexible thinking styles may need less direct structural support from the nurse to assimilate new ideas than clients with more rigid thinking patterns. Older and chronically mentally ill individuals may need more time to process information. Sensory overload can compromise the assimilation of unfamiliar information in clients of all ages.

Self-Talk. It is difficult to separate thoughts from feelings, and much of the reason that people feel bad about themselves has to do with negative self-talk. **Self-talk** is a cognitive process that produces a thought or thoughts that then lead to a feeling about a situation. Feelings attach a value to a person's thoughts, characterizing them as good or bad testimony about the self. When the thought carries a negative value connotation, it can affect the individual as though the thought represented the whole truth about the person. The thought, "I stuttered in the interview" becomes emotionally translated into, "I had a terrible interview," and, "I know I probably won't get the job." If the person thinks about it long enough, negative thoughts and associated feelings escalate to, "I'm never going to get a job. I don't ever interview well. I'm no good." One part of one interview suddenly becomes a major defining statement of self. The pervading thoughts create a decrease in self-esteem. Changing the self-talk resets the thinking process. With positive self-talk as a therapeutic strategy, the person chooses the feeling he or she will have about a situation or person.

Through self-talk, a person can question the legitimacy of cognitive distortions, and often their irrationality becomes apparent. The nurse's comments can support the client's questioning. This can be done with direct challenge when appropriate, such as, "Is it really true that you have never been successful at anything?" or it can be done with humor, as in the following case example.

Case Example

Grace Ann Hummer is a 65-year-old widow with arthritis, a weight problem, and failing eyesight. She looks older than she is. Admitted for a minor surgical procedure, Ms. Hummer tells the nurse she does not know why she came. Nothing can be done for her because she is too old and decrepit.

Nurse: As I understand it, you came in today for removal of your bunions. Can you tell me more about the problem as you see it? *(Asking for this information separates the current situation from an overall assessment of ill health.)*

Client: Well I've been having trouble walking, and I can't do some of the things I like to do that require extensive walking. I also have to buy "clunky" shoes that make me look like an old woman.

Nurse: So you are not willing to be an old woman yet? *(Taking the client's statement and challenging the cognitive distortion presented in her initial comments with humor allows the client to view her statement differently.)*

Client (laughing): Right, there are a lot of things I want to do before I'm ready for a nursing home.

Nurse: What are some of the things you would like to do that will be possible after the surgery? *(Questions relating the shared experience of the surgery to shared possible outcomes of the surgery stimulate the client to think about possible options and subtly diminish the validity of the client's overgeneralized negative thinking about life being over for her.)*

Exercise 4-4 gives practice in recognizing and responding to cognitive distortions.

Developing a Prevention Plan. A therapeutic intervention that combines self-talk strategies with social support forms the basis for a prevention plan designed to correct cognitive distortions. First, it is important to separate the person from the problem. This thinking process allows the client to step back and view the situation as an objective observer might, before beginning to resolve it. A certain amount of emotional distance is required to resolve difficult issues. When this condition is met, the client is able to develop and evaluate concrete strategies to cope with the issues. Even when the solutions chosen are appropriate and effective, however, the client may need to have ongoing support to implement them. Enlisting the help of others for support and advice gives rise to more effective problem solving.

Exercise 4-4 Correcting Cognitive Distortions

Purpose: To provide students with practice in recognizing and responding to cognitive distortions.

Procedure:

This exercise may be done in small groups of four or five students.

Using the definitions of cognitive distortions presented in the text, identify the type of cognitive distortion and the response you might make in each of the following situations:

1. I shouldn't feel anxious about making this presentation in class.
2. I am boring and people don't like to talk to me.
3. I shouldn't get upset when people don't approve of me.
4. If I hadn't been raised in a dysfunctional family, I would be a different person.
5. If I don't get high grades, my family will think less of me.
6. I can't experience true satisfaction unless I do things perfectly.

Discussion:

1. How do cognitive distortions affect behavior?
2. In what ways can you use this exercise to enhance your nursing practice and personal relationships?

Feedback and social support are powerful antidotes to cognitive distortions about responsibility. Although a plan to correct cognitive distortions is easier to articulate than to implement, these guidelines have proved useful in helping people to relinquish faulty thinking patterns and to take constructive action instead.

Emotion

Emotions are an important part of personal identity. They clarify the nature of relationships as, for example, happy, sad, fearful, or angry. The person who is feeling angry and despondent because he has just lost a job and the person who is ecstatic because she has had a promotion are each expressing their self-consistent reactions to the relationship between self and the job. To the extent that a person, object, or situation has positive or negative value, there is always emotional involvement. Emotions color a person's perceptions and thinking processes through an additional filter of value-laden feelings.

Feeling awareness of self profoundly affects how we experience another person's humanity. Feelings allow people to experience compassion and sensitivity for another's experience even if they do not fully understand it. Feelings may also contribute to negative actions. Much of the brutality and inhumanity that occur in society relate to a suppression of feeling or to strong negative feelings about the value of others.

Emotions are an inseparable part of all human experience. In nursing, emotions are an important part of the commitment to caring. Nursing actions performed with genuine feeling for a client are qualitatively different from those executed without feeling. A touch that communicates empathy for the client's situation differs from one that occurs without compassion. Conversations that value and respect the uniqueness of the client contrast markedly with halfhearted communications. The difference lies in the presence or absence of feeling for the client or one's work.

Almost without exception, feelings are significant pieces of information in the nurse-client relationship. Often, it is the emotional sharing in the therapeutic relationship that stands out as most meaningful to both nurse and client. The emotional encounters are remembered with intensity, positively or negatively, long after the tangible nurse-client relationship has terminated.

Emotions as Social Responses. Expressions of feeling are influenced by culture as well as by the personal characteristics of the individual. They do not occur in a vacuum but in the form of a social response to a situation. To understand happiness, sadness, and anger, one must also understand the situations that precipitate these emotions. How people handle emotions depends on the intensity of the experience stimulating the emotion, cultural norms, genetic temperament, and family constellation. Cultures express sadness, shame, guilt, and other feelings in many different ways. Until recently in our culture, men were socialized to repress feelings of emotional fragility. Exposing vulnerable feelings by crying or showing pain was not considered manly. Some cultures, such as Latin and Mediterranean cultures, seemingly permit free expression of emotions. Others, such as Asian and British cultures, seem to restrict the use of spontaneous, openly expressed emotion.

Family rules in dysfunctional families often prevent members from understanding and accepting legitimate emotions. Unacceptable feelings are automatically replaced with an emotional void or more socially acceptable emotions. Rules about emotional expression are very difficult to understand without knowing the "script" of the family.

Interplay with Physical and Cognitive Processes. Although expression of emotion can occur verbally, it is more often and more truly communicated nonverbally through facial expression and behaviors such as smiling, laughing, frowning, striking out, and crying. Specific physiological changes in the body, such as a quickening of the heartbeat, blushing, headache, muscle tension, or relaxation, accompany the experience and expression of strong emotion. Thus, there is a close connection between physical and emotional expressions of personal identity.

Complexity of Emotions. Emotions can occur as simple expressions of a momentary feeling. They can also be so complicated that even the person experiencing the emotions is neither fully aware of their existence nor able to describe them. People may know what they feel but not why. A person may feel conflicting emotions about someone or something simultaneously (e.g., outrage, fear, and love all at once). Nurses are an important resource in helping clients clarify their emotions and develop productive ways of expressing them.

Unhealthy Emotional Expression. Feelings are dangerous only when they get out of control and serve to diminish the self or another person. Unresolved feelings tend to distance partners in a relationship. Behavior usually is an indicator that something is wrong, but if the reason for the behavior is not apparent, feelings have no chance of being clarified. "Unacceptable" feelings can be camouflaged by a calm exterior demeanor or hidden behind a mask of superrationality. Feelings that have been strongly repressed are sometimes expressed with an intensity that is significantly out of proportion to the situation. When the receiver of a communication feels angry about a neutral message and there is no personal reason for having such a response, the receiver may be picking up strong hostile feelings about which the sender has little awareness.

Assessment Strategies. The emotions the nurse is most likely to encounter in health care settings include helplessness, frustration, hopelessness, powerlessness, anger, inadequacy, joy, anxiety, peacefulness, fearfulness, and apathy. In assessing the health of emotional self-concepts, the nurse considers several factors. Does the emotion fit the nature of the stimulus? Does it reflect a correct understanding of a situation or circumstances? When feelings do not match the nature of the behavioral stimulus (e.g., are too much, too little, contradictory, or unrelated), there may be an emotional block.

Does communication get blurred, or are tasks left unfinished for no known reason? For example, a client who refuses to take medication as instructed may be experiencing emotional barriers of anger or anxiety rather than a cognitive lack of understanding.

Do the emotions support the communicated message and match the body language of the participants? Emotions are important message carriers. Besides the actual verbal message, the sender and receiver steadily exchange emotionally laden, nonverbal communication signals through facial expression, tone of voice, choice of words and gestures, emphasis, omissions, and timing of the communication.

The receiver of the message may hear only part of the message through an additional emotional filter that has little to do with the ongoing conversation. Feelings about the sender, as well as about the content of the message, influence how the message is received and interpreted. If the receiver feels threatened by the sender of the message or by the message itself, the receiver may read into the situation things that are not meant. The margin of distortion hides the true meaning of an experience to the client; factors contributing to this are presented in Figure 4-3. Exercise 4-5 helps develop skill in clarifying feelings.

Planning and Intervention. Feelings do not obey the rules of logic, so arguing the legitimacy of a feeling wastes time and energy. The presence of emotions needs no justification; feelings simply exist, in all people. However, acting on emotions is not always in the best interest of the person experiencing the emotions. For example, it may be inappropriate to express anger to one's boss in the same way one might express anger to a friend.

Understanding that the language of emotion is telling you how the client is experiencing a life event or relationship is the key to giving a sensitive response. In highly charged emotional situations, for instance, the nurse commonly encounters angry, belligerent, out-of-control clients and families, and much of the emotion is projected onto the nurse or innocent family members. Armed with an understanding of the underlying feelings (e.g., intense fear, anguish about an anticipated loss, and lack of power in an unfamiliar situation), the nurse provides the

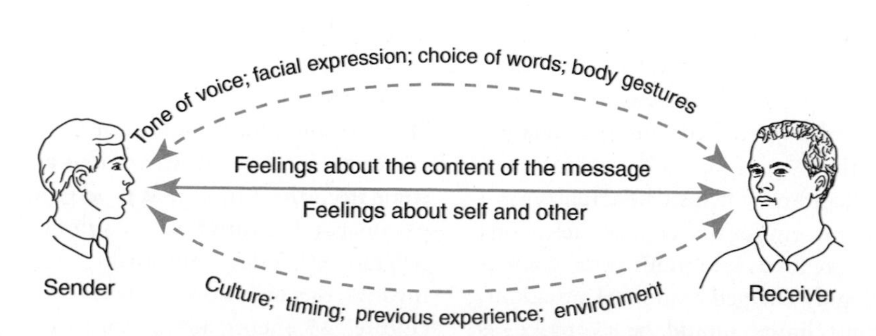

Figure 4-3 • Affective margin of distortion in communication.

Exercise 4-5 Clarifying Feelings

Purpose: To provide an opportunity to develop skill in recognizing underlying emotions and responding effectively to them.

Procedure:

This exercise should be done in small groups of three to five students.

A class has been assigned a group project for which all participants will receive a common group grade. Each group consists of six students. Develop a group understanding of the feelings experienced in each of the following situations as well as a way to respond to each. Consider the possible consequences of your intervention in each case.

1. Don tells the group that he is working full time and will be unable to make any group meetings. There are so many class requirements that he also is not sure he can put much effort into the project, although he would like to help and the project interests him.
2. Martha is very outspoken in group. She expresses her opinion about choice of the group project and is willing to make the necessary contacts. No one challenges her or suggests another project. At the next meeting, she informs the group that the project is all set up and she had made all the arrangements.
3. Joan promises she will have her part of the project completed by a certain date. The date comes, and Joan does not have her part completed.

Discussion:

1. What are some actions the participants can take to move the group forward?
2. How can you use this exercise as a way of understanding and clarifying feelings in clinical work situations?

opening for the client to tell his or her story. The nurse might identify a legitimate feeling by saying, "It must be frustrating to feel that your questions go unanswered," and then saying, "How can I help you?" From a non-reactive position, the nurse can demonstrate caring about the client as a person by helping the client obtain needed information and seeking validation of legitimate client concerns.

Clients caught up in the emotion of an event may need the nurse's permission to take a break. A simple comment from the nurse, such as, "Why don't you go down to the cafeteria and get something to eat? We'll contact you immediately if your mother's condition changes," gives the family needed respite from an overly intense emotional involvement. Recognizing escalating emotions before they get out of control and acknowledging their legitimacy helps relieve tension.

When setting limits on out-of-control behaviors, how the limit is presented is as important as the content of the message. In highly charged emotional situations, communication about limits should be expressed as clear, definite expectations: "Mr. Sutphin, I can see that you are really upset about the doctor not being here. Would you come with me, please, so that we can straighten this out?" Expectations should be clear and not open to interpretation. Nurses who display a calm approach by not making the angry person feel "backed into a corner" (e.g., by giving opportunities for face-saving alternatives) are more likely to be able to help resolve the situation (Gillmore-Hall, 2001).

Spiritual Aspects of Personal Identity

Spiritual aspects of personal identity are sometimes spoken of as spiritual perspectives. Like other aspects of personal identity, they are intangible and are inferred from behaviors. McSherry (2000) defines spirituality as "a mysterious and complex dimension of our being and existence" (p. 24). The mysterious aspects of spirituality come from the notion that it pervades our life in deeply personal and sensitive ways, as through our religion and religious affiliation. Spirituality is complex in that it involves the interwoven aspects of beliefs, values, and culture. McSherry admonishes that caution must be used when attempting to define the concept of spirituality because each individual interprets spirituality differently, and there is always a danger of applying our own definition of spirituality when caring for clients.

Fowler (1995) viewed spiritual perspectives as faith, "a patterned process or structure underlying and giving form to the contents of believing, valuing, knowing, and committing" (p. 135). Spiritual self-concepts help us answer vital questions about what is human, which human events have depth and value, and what are imaginative possibilities of being. Spiritual dimensions of self make significance possible and sustain a person's belief that he or she is worthy of respect as a human being. Although spiritual perspectives can occur within the framework of an organized religion, many deeply spiritual people do not embrace any organized religious group.

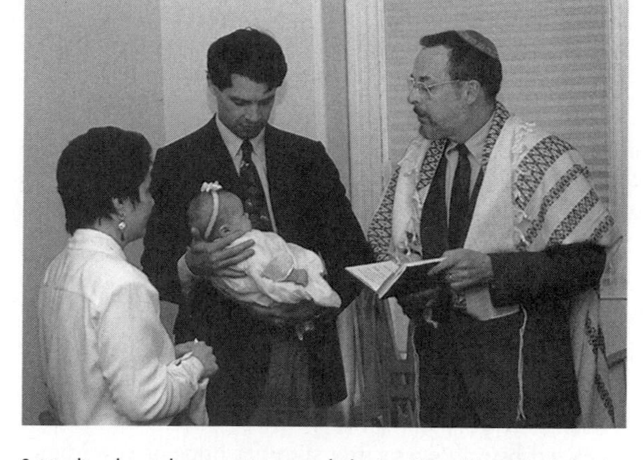

Spirituality plays a large part in personal identity. (From Wong DL, Hockenberry-Eaton M: *Wong's essentials of pediatric nursing*, ed 6, St Louis, 2001, Mosby.)

Having the courage and determination to do and say what one believes to be right rather than what is easy or currently fashionable is a benchmark for determining spiritual health. For the person with integrity, the goals or outcomes are important. The means by which the goals are achieved are equally significant. A person with integrity is motivated by a desire to create and to do things that matter to others as well as to self. The language of the soul is found not only in words and actions but also in music, poetry, and art, media that stir our inner depths and create new and broader meanings in life.

Spirituality in Health. The literature in health care increasingly demonstrates an important positive relationship between spirituality and health (Ameling & Provilonis, 2001). The crisis of illness can be a time of spiritual renewal, when one discovers new inner resources, strengths, and capacities never before tested. In contrast, it can be a time of spiritual desolation, leaving the individual feeling powerless to control or change important life circumstances (Krebs, 2001).

The realization that there are some things beyond our control, some realities and circumstances that can leave us temporarily immobilized, perhaps never to be settled to our satisfaction, can be overwhelming. Because human spiritual nature touches on the innermost core of an individual, the depth of a spiritual need is not always readily observable either to the nurse or to the client.

Unlike physical pain, spiritual pain can only be inferred from the client's behavior and from what the client is willing to share verbally. Spiritual well-being and being able to see the purpose and meaning of one's life are particularly important concepts when one is ready to leave this life. If the nurse can assist a client to find a connectedness with the meaning of his or her life, the client can find healing and acceptance (Baldacchino & Draper, 2001).

For the holistic nurse, the challenge in nurturing spirituality will be learning the tools of spiritual assessment, developing ways of praying, and being attentive to developing caring relationships.

Assessment Strategies. Spiritual distress can occur in the form of pain experienced through loss; separation from a faith community; or treatments that create spiritual anxiety, guilt, anger, or despair. Carson (1989) referred to four areas of spiritual concern as a framework for assessment:

- A person's personal concept of God
- Personal sources of energy and hope
- Relevance of specific religious practices to the individual
- Areas of spiritual concern activated by the illness

Assessing a Person's Personal Concept of God. The client's personal concept of God and spiritual needs may be quite obvious and initially responsive to clergy and pastoral counselors and to readings. The nurse notes the client's comments about God, a higher power, or "the man upstairs." Often, however, the spiritual needs of the client are ambivalent, cloaked in feelings of anger and disappointment toward a God who let this illness happen.

For example, a lack of faith in the value of humanity may represent a need to find a spiritual meaning for life. Other clients may express the need in the form of anger. C. S. Lewis (1976), the noted author of traditionally spiritual books, calls his God "the cosmic sadist" as he experiences his personal grief following the death of his wife. Yet few would doubt the depth of his spirituality.

Personal Sources of Hope. It is well known that hope is critical in maintaining the spirit of a person in health care settings. How else can one explain the will to live or the complete serenity of some individuals in the face of life's most adverse circumstances? Jourard (1964) suggests that "it is probably the spirit-response which is mobilized by any event that signifies hope or confidence in self or in the future; it is probably the spirit-response which, when weakened, permits illness to flourish." Societal sources of hope may be found in organized religion, in self-help books, in support groups, and in poetry and music. The nurse might ask the client, "What do you see as your primary sources of strength at the present time?" and, "In the past, what have been sources of strength for you in difficult times?" as ways of focusing attention on sources of hope and energy in the current situation.

Current Spiritual Practices. When assessing the current spiritual preferences of the client, the nurse also needs to consider past religious affiliations. It is not unusual for the religion listed on the client's chart to be quite different from the religious practices the client actually follows. Cultural orientation and practices influence not only beliefs but also the way beliefs are expressed. Questions the nurse might ask during the nursing assessment interview include the following:

- Are there special spiritual practices that are particularly important to you now?
- Would it be helpful for me to arrange a visit from the hospital chaplain or your pastor? (There should be client data to warrant this question.)

The nurse also explores areas of special concern the client has expressed. Inquiring about religious rituals important to the client can be very helpful. Baptisms, last rites, and ethnic practices in preparing the body can occur within the hospital setting and can provide peace for a client experiencing spiritual and emotional pain.

Planning and Intervention. Carson (1989) suggested that the compassionate presence of the nurse in the nurse-client relationship is the most important tool the nurse has in helping the client reinforce and confirm spiritual self-concepts. From the moment the client enters the hospital, orientation to available religious services should be an essential component of the relationship. It is important, however, for the nurse to be aware of his or her own spiritual beliefs and not to impose them on the client. This can be particularly tempting in times of

Exercise 4-6 Responding to Issues of Spiritual Distress

Purpose: To help students understand responses in times of spiritual distress.

Procedure:

Review the following case situations and develop an appropriate response to each.

1. Mary Trachter is unmarried and has just found out she is pregnant. She belongs to a fundamentalist church in which sex before marriage is not permitted. Mary feels guilty about her current status and sees it as "God punishing me for fooling around."
2. Linda Carter is married to an abusive, alcoholic husband. Linda reads the Bible daily and prays for her husband's redemption. She feels that God will turn the marriage around if she continues to pray for changes in her husband's attitude. "My trust is in the Lord," she says.
3. Bill Compton tells the nurse, "I feel that God has let me down. I was taught that if I was faithful to God, He would be there for me. Now the doctors tell me I'm going to die. That doesn't seem fair to me."

Discussion:

1. Share your answers with others in your group.
2. Give and get feedback on the usefulness of your responses.
3. In what ways can you use this new knowledge in your nursing care?

crisis or when death seems imminent. Client autonomy requires that the client give the nurse permission for the pastoral counselor or clergy to visit.

Praying with a client, even when the client is of a different faith, can be soothing. However, the nurse again is cautioned not to impose any spiritual ritual on the client just to meet his or her own spiritual beliefs. If the client professes no faith, the nurse can help the client identify actions that bring peace and meaning in times of stress without praying with a client. Exercise 4-6 helps in understanding spiritual responses to distress.

Developing the Next Step. Long-term goals are not always the primary focus in promoting, maintaining, or restoring spiritual health. Only the "next step" is important. Breaking down potentially overwhelming problems into manageable steps makes the problem seem workable and stimulates hope. The hopeful person also trusts in a transcendent source to show itself in the form of suggestion and direction about the next step.

Social Support. Social support can have spiritual as well as emotional and social effects on a client. Usually other people in the immediate situation play a critical role in the stimulation of hope through their encouragement and practical suggestions, or sometimes simply through their presence during a stressful time. Carson (1989) offered the following example of a caring intervention with a 16-year-old athlete with a bilateral amputation. Exercise 4-7 may increase your appreciation of the role of social support.

Case Example

One morning after shift report, Mrs. Johnson walked into Robert's room and found him crying. Her first response was to leave the room as she thought, "I can't handle this today." However, she was able to stop herself and she went over to Robert and touched his shoulder. He continued to sob and said, "What am I going to do? I wish I were dead. My whole life is sports. I would have qualified for an athletic scholarship if this hadn't happened. I feel like my life is over at 16."

Mrs. Johnson recognized the feelings of despair that Robert was expressing, and said to him, "It doesn't seem like life has any meaning at all. You are feeling that this is such an unfair thing to have happened to you. I agree with you, it is. But let's talk about it. We can't change what has happened, but maybe we can start to look at where to go from here." (Carson, 1989, p. 167)

Evaluation. Client outcomes suggestive of resolution of spiritual distress include reconnection with a higher power, decreased guilt, forgiveness of others, expressions of hope, and evidence that the client finds meaning in his or her current situation.

Self-Esteem

Self-esteem is not the same as self-concept, but it is intimately related to it (Sundeen, 2005). It refers to the value and significance people place on their self-concepts. It is an emotional process of self-judgment, an orientation to the self, ranging on a continuum from feelings of self-efficacy and respect to a feeling of being fatally flawed as a person.

Self-esteem is subjective. It develops from individuals' perceptions of their personal being and achievements, particularly in interpersonal relations. It is possible

Exercise 4-7 Social Support

Purpose: To help students understand the role of social support in significant encounters.

Procedure:

1. Describe a "special" situation that had deep meaning for you.
2. Identify the person or people who helped make the situation meaningful for you.
3. Describe the actions taken by the people or person identified above that made the situation memorable.

Discussion:

1. What did you learn about yourself from doing this exercise?
2. What do you see as the role of social support in making memories?
3. How might you use this information in your practice?

to have many objective achievements and to have low self-esteem. People with few achievements but with the knowledge that they have conducted themselves as well as possible can have high self-esteem. Although self-esteem can be reinforced by confirming relationships, the inner worth of a person can be experienced only by that person.

Self-esteem reflects a delicate balance between fitting into a larger social community and retaining the support and affirmation of others for being unique. Wanting the approval of others at the expense of personal integrity decreases self-respect, which in turn affects the admiration of others and leads to social alienation.

A relationship exists between self-esteem and the level of psychological adaptation (Driever, 1976c). People who value themselves become freer to know and to cherish the intrinsic value of others. Energy is not wasted on self-defensive behavior. People with high self-esteem have a strong emotional as well as intellectual conviction that they are worthy of respect and recognition, with something unique and useful to offer to society. When individuals do not feel there is much value to who they are as human beings or what they are able to contribute to others, they experience low self-esteem. Box 4-2 identifies characteristic behaviors related to self-esteem.

Self-esteem is not a fixed concept; it fluctuates whenever the self-concept is challenged by life transitions or crises, illnesses, or changes in status or role. Turning points of self-meaning related to developmental, situational, relational, and spiritual circumstances affect self-esteem. Sources of low self-esteem include loss of a job; loss of an important relationship; negative change in appearance, role, or status; and criticism by significant others.

Perceptions of the opinions and feelings of significant others have a profound effect on self-esteem. Contrast, for example, a social situation in which you are considered an authority or a prized guest with one in which you clearly are on a different social level and have less life experience or fewer credentials than most of the other people present. Most probably there is a significant difference in the value you felt you have in each of these situations. If people feel valued by others, they begin to experience themselves as being worthy. Criticism, disconfirming comments, and devaluing by others through insensitive actions usually have the opposite effect.

Self-Esteem in Health Care. Epstein (1973) suggested that a sudden decrease in self-esteem is experienced as a greater loss than a more gradual decline. In most chronic or major illnesses, there is a lowering of self-esteem because the individual is no longer able to function as before in ways that inspired higher levels of self-esteem. In many cases, there is also no real reason to believe there will be a return to normal activities or a positive change in functioning. Yet high levels of self-esteem can accompany even the most debilitating illness if the client is given enough social support.

When illness occurs, at least two outcomes are possible. The client may become emotionally immobilized by the threat to self-identity that a symptom imposes, and the result is loss of self-esteem. Alternatively, the client may feel challenged by the illness to develop new coping skills, and there is an increase in self-esteem. The nurse, in providing support and confirmation of the client's efforts, plays an important role in the client's decisions and subsequent actions.

Box 4-2 Self-Esteem Characteristics

People with High Self-Esteem	People with Low Self-Esteem
Expect people to value them	Expect people to be critical of them
Are active self-agents	Are passive or obstructive self-agents
Have positive perceptions of their skills, appearance, sexuality, and behaviors	Have negative perceptions of their skills, appearance, sexuality, and behaviors
Perform equally well when being observed as when not	Perform less well when being observed
Are nondefensive and assertive in response to criticism	Are defensive and passive in response to criticism
Can accept compliments easily	Have difficulty accepting compliments
Evaluate their performance realistically	Have unrealistic expectations about their performance
Are relatively comfortable relating to authority figures	Are uncomfortable relating to authority figures
Express general satisfaction with life	Are dissatisfied with their lot in life
Have a strong social support system	Have a weak social support system
Have a primary internal locus of control	Rely on an external locus of control

Assessment Strategies. Assessment of self-esteem tends to be observational: the nurse notes what the client says about himself or herself. Does the client devalue accomplishments, project blame for problems on others, minimize personal failures, or make self-deprecating remarks? Does the client express shame or guilt? Does the client seem hesitant to try new things or situations or express concern about ability to cope with events? Lack of culturally appropriate eye contact, poor hygiene, self-destructive behaviors, hypersensitivity to criticism, need for constant reassurance, and an inability to accept compliments are behaviors associated with low self-esteem.

Planning and Intervention. When people have low self-esteem, they feel they have little worth and that no one really cares enough to bother with them. The nurse helps clients increase self-esteem by being psychologically present as a sounding board. Just the process of engaging with another human being who offers a different perspective can have the effect of enhancing self-esteem. The implicit message the nurse conveys with personal presence and interest, information, and a guided exploration of the problem is twofold. The first is confirmation of the client: "You are important and I will stay with you through this uncomfortable period." The second is the introduction of the possibility of hope: "There may be some alternatives you haven't thought of that can help you cope with this problem in a meaningful way." Once a person starts to take charge of his or her life, a higher level of well-being can result.

Self-esteem affects the ability to weather stress without major changes in self-perception. With a positive attitude about self, an individual is more likely to view life as a glass that is half full rather than half empty.

The nurse can use several strategies to help a client experience deeper levels of self-esteem. Modeling is very effective. The nurse can convey a positive self-image, which is contagious. In addition, the nurse's questions can be deliberately designed to assist clients in reflecting on their strengths and accomplishments. The nurse can say, "Tell me the achievement you are most proud of," or, "Tell me some things you like about yourself." The nurse can give the client positive feedback: "The thing that impresses me about you is . . ." or, "What I notice is that although your body is so much weaker, it seems as if your spirit is stronger. Is that your perception as well?" Such questions help the client focus on positive strengths. Exercise 4-8 strengthens the nurse's skill in this area.

When the nurse helps the client make independent judgments about health care, the process strengthens the client's self-esteem. The act of taking charge and choosing among alternatives indirectly suggests that the client can cope with difficult problems. Communication, combined with compassionate health care inform-

Exercise 4-8 **Positive Affirmations: Contributions to Self-Esteem**

Purpose: To help students experience the effects of interpersonal comments on self-esteem.

Procedure:

This exercise may be done in a group or used as a homework assignment and later discussed in class.

1. List a positive affirming comment you received recently, something someone did or said that made you feel good about yourself.
2. List a disconfirming comment you received recently, something someone did or said that made you feel bad about yourself.
3. What have you done recently that you feel helped enhance someone else's self-esteem?

Discussion:

1. In general, what kinds of actions help enhance self-esteem?
2. What are some things people do or fail to do that diminish self-esteem?
3. What are some specific things you might be able to do in a clinical setting that might help a client develop a sense of self-worth?
4. What did you learn about yourself from doing this exercise?

ation and actions, confirms the value of a person as worthwhile.

Evaluation. Self-esteem behaviors are evaluated by comparing the number of positive self-statements with those originally observed. Behaviors suggestive of enhanced self-esteem include the following:

- Taking an active role in planning and implementing self-care
- Verbalizing personal psychosocial strengths
- Expressing feelings of satisfaction with self and ways of handling life

Self-Awareness

Self-awareness is the means by which a person gains knowledge and understanding of all aspects of self-concept. An interpersonal approach focusing on human responses in the client and the nurse is quite different from one approaching self-understanding from a behaviorist or psychoanalytic perspective. In professional relationships with clients and colleagues, the nurse engages with other human beings from a position in which all that a person is capable of being becomes stretched to the utmost.

The nurse's self-concept in the nurse-client relationship is as important as that of the clients (Box 4-3). Nurses who are comfortable with themselves can help clients use a similar process of self-reflection in understanding themselves. Creating an interpersonal environment that heals is possible only if self-awareness skills are built into the communication process.

Self-awareness provides an inner frame of reference for connecting emotionally with the experiences of another. Self-awareness occurs through the mechanism of intrapersonal communication, defined as communication taking place within the self, in contrast to interpersonal communication, which takes place between people. The two concepts are very much interwoven in most interpersonal relationships.

Self-awareness provides an external structure for inquiring into and interpreting important behavioral inferences related to illness. Throughout the therapeutic relationship the questions "How is this illness affecting the client?" and "What is the meaning of the treatment process for this client?" frame the interpersonal experience. Describing the meaning of an illness and one's human responses to it is an interpersonal process that relies heavily on the client as a self-interpreting being.

Box 4-3 Questions to Encourage Self-Awareness in the Nurse-Client Relationship

1. Can I behave in some way that will be perceived by the other person as trustworthy, dependable, or consistent in some deep sense?
2. Can I be expressive enough as a person that what I am will be communicated unambiguously?
3. Can I let myself experience positive attitudes toward this other person: attitudes of warmth, caring, liking, interest, and respect?
4. Can I be strong enough as a person to be separate from the other?
5. Am I secure enough within myself to permit the client separateness?
6. Can I let myself enter fully into the world of the client's feelings and personal meanings and see these as the client does?
7. Can I receive the client as he or she is? Can I communicate this attitude?
8. Can I act with sufficient sensitivity in the relationship that my behavior will not be perceived as a threat?
9. Can I free the client from the threat of external evaluation?
10. Can I meet this other individual as a person who is in the process of becoming, or will I be bound by his or her past and by my past?

Adapted from Rogers CR: The characteristics of the helping relationship, *Person Guid J* 37(1):6-16, 1958.

Self-Reflection

Nurses learn about themselves through self-reflection and the feedback of others. Self-reflection is a mental process by which we are able to consciously examine the meaning of our motives and actions. It is a mental faculty available only to humans. Taking time alone to explore and to discover what is happening or what has happened in human relationships puts the pain and human suffering a nurse encounters on a daily basis into better perspective. Cowin (2001a) has developed an instrument that measures a nurse's self-concept. Cowin (2001b) reports that the tool will be available soon and should be helpful for nurses in the self-reflective process.

Self-reflection increases the nurse's capacity to be genuine. Knowing personal motivations, prejudices, strengths, and limitations helps the nurse connect with clients in a straightforward manner. Self-awareness helps the nurse avoid using the therapeutic interpersonal relationship with clients to meet personal rather than client needs (Eckroth-Bucher, 2001). Consider, for example, the nurse who strongly believes that breast-feeding is more beneficial than bottle-feeding. Without self-awareness, the nurse may unconsciously project her personal values about breast-feeding on a teenage mother who has no desire to breast-feed her infant.

Role Modeling. To be role models for clients in a professional relationship, nurses need first to recognize their own needs and find ways to meet them in their personal lives. It is difficult for nurses to be considerate and sensitive to the needs of others if they are unable to be gentle and understanding of similar needs within themselves. "To give to others, nurses need to nourish all aspects of the self. Therefore, giving of self requires self-nurturance of the physical, mental, emotional, and spiritual aspects" (Burkhardt & Nagai-Jacobson, 2001).

Becoming Centered. The basic goal of any constructive relationship is to help the participants enlarge self-knowledge and enhance their potential by integrating disowned, neglected, unrecognized, or unrealized parts of the self into the personality. This process is referred to as being centered. Expected outcomes include the following:

- Enhanced self-respect
- Increased resourcefulness and sense of what the person can do
- Greater productivity
- Increased personal satisfaction

Attainment of these goals is impossible without a personal experiential knowledge of the self-concept and its effect on the development and maintenance of relationships.

SUMMARY

The self is the most complex of all human attributes. At birth, infants do not have an awareness of the concept of "self." Self emerges from the appraisals of significant others and is reappraised with each new era of development.

Self-concept is a major nursing diagnosis that involves four components: body image, personal identity, self-esteem, and role performance. Body image alterations encompass loss of function and control as well as physical changes. Included in personal identity are the spiritual, cognitive, emotional, and perceptual dimensions of self-concept. Erikson's model of psychosocial development is the framework used to assess client attainment of normal psychosocial tasks.

Self-concept influences communication through perceptual and cognitive processes such as selective attention and self-fulfilling prophecy. Spiritual self-concepts add meaning.

Self-esteem, described as the emotional valuing of the self-concept, stems from perceptual images viewed by the person as good or bad assessments of self. A healthy self-concept results in behaviors reflective of satisfaction with body image, a realistic relationship between actual and ideal self, high self-esteem, general satisfaction with role performance, and a distinct sense of identity and spiritual well-being. Strategies to enhance the development of a positive self-concept result in higher self-esteem.

As nurses see themselves worthy of being cared for, they are more capable of giving to others. Becoming centered enhances the nurse's ability for helping clients to develop their self-concept in developing to their highest potential.

Ethical Dilemma ■ *What Would You Do?*

Sarah Best, a 16-year-old ice-skater, is brought into the emergency room after being in a car accident. The physician examines Sarah and determines that her right leg needs to be amputated below the knee. Sarah's parents are traveling in Europe and cannot immediately be located. Sarah refuses surgery. The physician asks Sarah's nurse, Ann, to get Sarah's consent. If you were in Ann's position, what would you do?

REFERENCES

Adler R, Rodman L: *Understanding human communication*, ed 7, New York, 1999, Holt, Rinehart & Winston.

Ameling A, Provilonis M: Spirituality, meaning, mental health, and nursing, *J Psychosoc Nurs Ment Health Serv* 39(4):15-20, 2001.

Baldacchino D, Draper P: Spiritual coping strategies: a review of the literature, *J Adv Nurs* 34(6):833-841, 2001.

Burkhardt M, Nagai-Jacobson I: Nurturing and caring for the self, *Nurs Clin North Am* 36(1):23-32, 2001.

Carson V: *Spiritual dimensions in nursing practice*, Philadelphia, 1989, Saunders.

Carson V, Trubowitz J: Relevant theories and therapies for nursing practice. In Varcarolis E, Carson V, Shoemaker N, editors: *Foundations of psychiatric mental health nursing*, St Louis, 2006, Saunders.

Cowin L: Measuring nurses' self-concept, *West J Nurs Res* 23(3):313-325, 2001a.

Cowin L: Personal communication, September 4, 2001b.

Cutler C: Self-care agency and symptom management in patients treated for mood disorders, *Arch Psychiatr Nurs* 15(1):24-31, 2001.

Driever M: Theory of self-concept. In Roy C, editor: *Introduction to nursing: an adaptation model*, Englewood, Cliffs, NJ, 1976a, Prentice-Hall.

Driever M: Problems of low self-esteem. In Roy C, editor: *Introduction to nursing: an adaptation model*, Englewood Cliffs, NJ, 1976b, Prentice-Hall.

Driever M: Development of self-concept. In Roy C, editor: *Introduction to nursing: an adaptation model*, Englewood Cliffs, NJ, 1976c, Prentice-Hall.

Eckroth-Bucher M: Philosophical basis and practice of self-awareness in psychiatric nursing, *J Psychosoc Nurs Ment Health Serv* 39(2):32-39, 2001.

Ellis-Hill C, Horn S: Change in identity and self-concept: a new theoretical approach to recovery following a stroke, *Clin Rehabil* 14(3):279-287, 2000.

Epstein S: The self-concept revisited: or a theory of a theory, *Am Psychol* 5:414, 1973.

Erikson E: *Childhood and society*, ed 2, New York, 1963, Norton.

Erikson E: *The life cycle completed: a review*, New York, 1982, Norton.

Fowler J: *Stages of faith: the psychology of human development and the quest for meaning*, San Francisco, 1995, Harper.

Gillmore-Hall A: Violence in the workplace, *The Am J Nurs* 101(7):55-56, 2001.

James W: *The principles of psychology*, New York, 1891, Henry Holt.

Jourard S: *The transparent self*, New York, 1964, Van Nostrand Reinhold.

Krebs K: The spiritual aspect of caring: an integral part of health and healing, *Nurs Adm Q* 25(3):55-60, 2001.

Kurlowicz L: Benefits of psychiatric consultation-liaison nurse interventions for older hospitalized patients and their nurses, *Arch Psychiatr Nurs* 15(2):53-61, 2001.

Lewis CS: *A grief observed*, New York, 1976, Bantam Books.

Markus H, Nurius P: Possible selves, *Am Psychol* 41:954-969, 1986.

McSherry W: *Making sense of spirituality in nursing practice*, New York, 2000, Harcourt.

North American Nursing Diagnosis Association: *Nursing diagnoses: definition and classification 2005-2006*, Philadelphia, 2005, Author.

Peplau H: *Interpersonal relations in nursing*, New York, 1952, Putnam.

Satir V: *Conjoint family therapy*, Palo Alto, 1976, Science & Behavior Books.

Schott G, Bellin W: The relational self-concept scale: a context-specific self-report measure for adolescents, *Adolescence* 36(141):86-105, 2001.

Schontz F: Body image and its disorders, *Int J Psychiatr Med* 5:464, 1974.

Shaw J, Ebbeck V, Snow C: Body composition and physical self-concept in older women, *J Women Aging* 12(3/4):59–75, 2000.

Sneed J, Whitbourne S: Models of the aging self, *J Social Issues* 61(2):375, 2005.

Stuart G: Self-concept responses and dissociative disorders. In Stuart G, Laraia M, editors: *Principles and practices of psychiatric nursing*, ed 8, St Louis, 2005, Mosby.

Sundeen S: Psychiatric rehabilitation and recovery. In Stuart G, Laraia M, editors: *Principles and practices of psychiatric nursing*, ed 8, St Louis, 2005, Mosby.

Thomas K, Ricciardelli I: Gender traits and self-concept as indicators of problem eating and body dissatisfaction among children, *Sex Roles* 43(7/8):441-459, 2000.

Chapter 5

Structuring the Relationship

Elizabeth Arnold

OUTLINE

OBJECTIVES

At the end of the chapter, the reader will be able to:

1. Discuss key concepts in the nurse-client relationship.
2. Identify the four phases of the therapeutic relationship.
3. Contrast tasks in each of the four phases of the relationship.
4. Specify effective nursing interventions in each phase of the relationship.

Something, however imperceptible, happens between the two, no matter whether it is marked at the time by any feeling or not. The only thing that matters is that for each . . . the other happens as the particular other, that each becomes aware of the other and is thus related to him in such a way that he does not regard and use him as his object, but as his partner in a living event.

(Buber, 1965)

Chapter 5 focuses on the structure and functional processes of a therapeutic nurse-client relationship. Certain guiding principles (e.g., purpose, mutuality, authenticity, empathy, active listening, confidentiality, and respect for the dignity of the client) strengthen the therapeutic relationship (McGrath, 2005). Although some therapeutic relationships extend over weeks in home care or public psychiatric settings, most therapeutic relationships in health care today will take place in a much shorter period of time.

Nurses see clients at their most vulnerable in health care situations. The relationship between nurse and client in such situations is unique and intensely personal. Nursing interventions carried out through the nurse-client relationship cover the spectrum of care ranging from health promotion to caring for clients in the home; caring for critically ill clients in the hospital; caring for clients in prisons and nontraditional settings; and caring for dying clients in hospice, hospital, or at home.

Several authors point to nurses helping clients achieve a sense of meaning from their illness and suffering as one of the most important and rewarding aspects of relationship in nursing practice (Frankl, 1955; Travelbee, 1971). In health care, human connections are essential to the healing process and effective health care delivery.

BASIC CONCEPTS

Characteristics of a Therapeutic Relationship

A therapeutic relationship is a professional alliance (Williams, 2001) in which the nurse and client join together for a defined period of time to achieve health-related treatment goals. The client enters this relationship with a health care need that is potentially responsive to nursing intervention. The nurse enters the relationship with a certain body of knowledge, a genuine desire to help others, and an openness to experiencing the client as a special and unique person worthy of personal as well as professional attention and respect (Henson, 1997).

The relationship starts with the conscious commitment of the professional nurse to understand how an individual client and his or her family perceive, feel, and respond to their world. From beginning to end, listening closely to verbal and nonverbal messages, focusing on the client's concerns, and attempting to understand the client as a unique person reinforce the client's value as a human being. The underlying theme in all nursing actions is a respect for the human dignity of the client.

The goal of the therapeutic relationship is always promotion of the client's health and well-being. This is true, even when the client is dying, or is uncooperative. The nurse-client relationship is an interdependent relationship. Each health care relationship offers a special opportunity for the personal growth of both parties. In the process of giving excellent nursing care, nurses can learn a great deal about themselves from their clients.

Because each of the participants has a distinctive personality, each human interaction between nurse and client is unique (Chauhan & Long, 2000). Therapeutic relationships share many of the human caring characteristics of a social relationship.

There are, however, distinct structural and functional differences between a social and professional relationship. These include the following:

- A client-centered approach focused on identified actual or potential health care needs
- Professional therapeutic boundaries that both link and separate the participants
- Health-related goals of empowering clients to achieve maximum health and well-being
- A defined beginning and end, dictated by a health-related purpose and realistic interventions to serve that purpose

The relationship can be a well-intentioned but ineffectual process if it lacks a planned direction to guide the participants (Forchuk, 1994b). Therapeutic relationships require thoughtful attention. The *purposeful thinking* behind the actions taken in the relationship best distinguishes the nurse's role from other types of relationships. Activities to establish and maintain healing relationships related to the care of the client are threaded through all stages of therapeutic relationships. Table 5-1 presents the differences between a therapeutic helping relationship and a social relationship.

Client-Centered Approach

A client-centered approach, first described by Carl Rogers, requires a collaborative process in which the nurse and client join together their personal and professional expertise to resolve health care problems. (See Box 5-1 for key questions for reflection in a client-

Table 5-1 Differences Between Helping Relationships and Social Relationships

Helping Relationships	Social Relationship
Helper takes responsibility for the conduct of the relationship and for maintaining appropriate boundaries.	Both parties have equal responsibility for the conduct of the relationship.
Relationship has a specific purpose and a health-related goal.	Relationship may or may not have a specific purpose or goals.
Relationship terminates when the identified goal is met.	Relationship can last a lifetime or terminate without goal achievement.
Focus of the relationship is on needs of the helpee.	The needs of both partners should receive equal attention.
Relationship is entered through necessity.	Relationship is entered into spontaneously, accompanied by feelings of liking.
Choice of who to be in relationship is not available to either helper or helpee.	Behavior for both participants is spontaneous; people choose companions.
Self-disclosure is limited for the helper, encouraged for the helpee.	Self-disclosure for both parties in the relationship is expected.
Understanding should always be put into words.	Understanding does not necessarily need to be put into words.

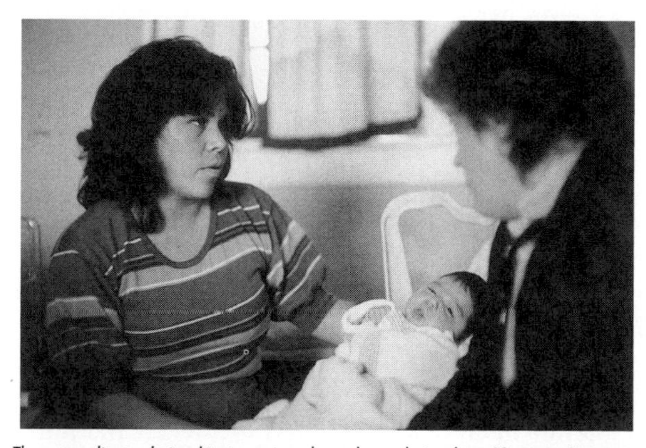

The nurse-client relationship is an interdependent relationship. (Courtesy University of Maryland School of Nursing.)

centered interaction.) The client is considered the expert on his or her life; the nurse the expert on health care matters in therapeutic relationships. For the client, this can include cultural, spiritual, and personal beliefs about health care and his or her personal situation. The client always has the right to choose personal goals and courses of action, even when they are at odds with the nurse's ideas. This helping attitude respects the client's right to self-determination and the ethical principle of autonomy. In today's health care arena, with its emphasis on increased client participation in care, full client and/or family involvement is an essential component of effective clinical decision making (Schoot, Proot, Meulen et al., 2005).

Box 5-1 Key Questions for Reflection in a Client-Centered Interaction

- Can I behave in some way that will be perceived by the other person as trustworthy as dependable or consistent in some deep sense?
- Can I be expressive enough as a person that what I am will be communicated unambiguously?
- Can I let myself experience positive attitudes toward this other person—attitudes of warmth, caring, liking interest, and respect?
- Can I be strong enough as a person to be separate from the other?
- Can I let myself enter fully into the world of my client's feelings and personal meanings and see these as he or she does?
- Can I act with sufficient sensitivity that my behavior will not be perceived as a threat in the relationship?
- Can I meet this other individual as a person who is in the process of becoming, or will I be bound by his or her past and by my past?

From Rogers C: The characteristics of a helping relationship. In Rogers C, editor, *On becoming a person*, Boston, 1961, Houghton-Mifflin.

The nurse's expertise derives from an integrated empirical, personal, aesthetic, and ethical knowledge base, evidenced in listening to the client, helping the client to reflect and clarify what is important in the dialogue, and offering professional insights that the client may not have considered previously.

Client-centered approaches start with the client perspective. According to Delbanco (1992), consideration of a client's perspective should include each client's

- Values, preferences, and expressed needs.
- Perception of coordination and integration of care.
- Communication and education needs of the patient.
- Physical comfort level.
- Available emotional supports.
- Level of involvement of family and friends.

The client's perspective will be different for different clients, even if they have a similar health diagnosis. Each therapeutic relationship should be uniquely tailored to the client involved. Godkin (2001) reported that being treated as a unique individual is an important dimension of the nurse-client relationship, specifically identified as a "caring presence." No matter how challenging the client behavior is, there is always the potential for change.

There is no one way to approach a client, and no single interpersonal strategy that works equally well with every client. Some clients clearly are more emotionally accessible and attractive to work with than others. When a client seems unapproachable or uninterested in human contact, it can be quite disheartening for the nurse. It is not uncommon for the nurse to report the kind of initial contact with a client seen in the following case examples.

Case Example

"I tried, but he just wasn't interested in talking to me. I asked him some questions, but he didn't really answer me. So I tried to ask him about his hobbies and interests. It didn't matter what I asked him. He just turned away. Finally, I gave up because it was obvious that he just didn't want to talk to me."

Although, from the nurse's perspective, this client's behavior may represent a lack of desire for a relationship, in most cases the rejection is not personal. It can reflect boredom, insecurity, or physical discomfort. Anxiety expressed as anger or unresponsiveness may be the only way a client can control fear in a difficult situation. Rarely does it have much to do with the personal approach used by the nurse unless the nurse is truly insensitive to the client's feelings or the needs of the situation. In this situation, the nurse might say, "It seems to me that you just want to be alone right now. But I would like to help you, so if you don't mind, I'll check back later with you. Would that be OK with you?" Most of the time, clients appreciate the nurse's willingness to stay involved.

For novice nurses, it is important to recognize that all nurses have experienced some form of client rejection at one time or another. The nurse needs to explore whether the timing was right, whether the client was in pain, and what other circumstances might have contributed to the client's attitude. Behaviors that initially seem maladaptive may appear quite adaptive when the full circumstances of the client's situation are understood. As nurses become more expert, they are better able to appreciate the feelings conveyed through an individual's response to his or her illness (Benner, 1984).

Case Example

A third-year student nurse, Joan Thoms, stops at the hospital to pick up her next day's assignment. Mrs. Groot, her client, is scheduled for a radical mastectomy. Joan enters Mrs. Groot's room to introduce herself but finds her client in tears and unable to talk. Joan gives her a tissue and sits with her, holding her hand. After about 5 minutes, Joan asks, "Would you like to talk for a while? You seem really upset." Mrs. Groot replies, "I'd rather be alone." Realizing that talking about her fears with a nurse she is meeting for the first time is uncomfortable for Mrs. Groot, Joan states, "There are times when we all need to have some time alone, and there is a lot to think about. I'll close the door now to give you some privacy, and I will be back to see you later, before I leave the unit."

Meeting the client's needs nonverbally when the client is reluctant to communicate verbally demonstrates respectful interest without pressure. When the nurse returns later, the client may find the nurse's presence very helpful.

Note that the nurse respects the client's immediate need while leaving the door open for further dialogue. Observing the client's nonverbal cues can often tell you more than his or her words about a feeling state. Exercise 5-1 examines nonverbal cues in relationships.

Role of the Nurse

Self-Awareness

To be truly effective, the nurse must have a keen sense of **self-awareness** that provides direction and acts as a barometer of the relationship process. Bonnivier (1996) suggests, "nurses are 'safe' but real people on whom to try out new social skills, modify dysfunctional relationship patterns, and reveal emotional vulnerabilities" (p. 38).

Exercise 5-1 Nonverbal Messages

Purpose: To provide practice in validation skills in a nonthreatening environment.

Procedure:

1. Each student, in turn, tries to communicate the following feelings to other members of the group without words. They may be written on a piece of paper, or the student may choose one directly from the following list.
2. The other students must guess what behaviors the student is trying to enact.

Pain	Anxiety	Shock	Disinterest
Anger	Disapproval	Disbelief	Rejection
Sadness	Relief	Disgust	Despair
Confidence	Uncertainty	Acceptance	Uptightness

Discussion:

1. Which emotions were harder to guess from their nonverbal cues? Which ones were easier?
2. Was there more than one interpretation of the emotion?
3. How would you use the information you developed today in your future care of clients?

The psychological mindset of the nurse influences his or her emotional availability for developing the relationship. For example, if the nurse resents being on night duty or is preoccupied with personal matters, it is difficult to be truly present with the client. The process of self-awareness requires that nurses examine their personal value positions so personal biases and prejudices are not projected onto their clients (Eckroth-Bucher, 2001).

Remaining centered and confident is difficult when clients are confronted with life-altering health conditions. Self-awareness allows nurses to treat each client with respect (i.e., as a person having value) even if the nurse cannot understand or approve of certain behaviors. Self-awareness is about discovery—learning new information about the self as well as being aware of existing biases and prejudices. Peplau (1997) notes that nurses must observe their own behavior as well as the client's with "unflinching self-scrutiny and total honesty in assessment of their behavior in interactions with patients" (p. 162). By critically and simultaneously examining the behaviors of the client and the nurse and what is going on in the relationship, nurses can create a safe, trustworthy, and caring relational structure (Benner, 1984; Lowry, 2005).

Professional Boundaries

Consistent boundaries are an essential component of establishing and maintaining an effective nurse-client relationship. **Boundaries** are defined as interpersonal limits on what is acceptable behavior in a professional alliance. **Professional boundaries** in a therapeutic relationship represent invisible structures imposed by legal, moral, and professional standards of nursing that respect nurse and client rights. Examples include defining the time, purpose, and length of contact; maintaining confidentiality regarding what the client says; and providing an appropriate setting for the relationship, including which people may be involved in various interactions. Relationship boundaries protect the client's vulnerability and enhance the functional integrity of the relationship in health care by managing the power differential that exists in every professional alliance with a client. Boundaries help define the professional conduct of the nurse in relating to the client as a helping person—not as a friend, not as a judge, but as a skilled professional companion committed to helping the client achieve mutually defined health care goals (Briant & Freshwater, 1998).

The boundaries of a professional relationship make it a safe relationship for the client. Just as guardrails protect the public from falling into danger when observing a tourist attraction, professional boundaries protect the client from becoming injured in the relationship with the health care provider. The client must be able to trust that all kinds of feelings are possible without fear of misunderstanding or retaliation (Gallop, 1998). Professional boundaries require the nurse to continually reflect on his or her personal and professional involvement in the relationship. Katherine (2000) notes "*[the nurse] is in the position of mentor, steward, authority, employer, or parent to another. Those with power have certain responsibilities toward the people they serve, assist, teach, supervise, or lead. The person who has power carries an ethical mandate not to exploit their position, not to abuse a subordinate in order to extract personal gain."*

The nurse is ethically bound to observe the boundaries needed to make a relationship therapeutic (Sheets, 2001). When clients seek health care in good faith from licensed professionals, they are in a vulnerable position as persons in need of help. They have every right to expect that the professionals who care for them will be active, responsive participants and guides in the client's progress toward optimal health and well-being (Forchuk, 1994b). An important aspect of the concept of boundaries is the nurse's level of involvement.

Level of Involvement

To be effective, nurses must maintain emotional objectivity. Heinrich (1992) notes that nurses constantly walk a fine line between having compassion for a client and developing a relationship that is too close, resulting in a friendship with potential serious complications for the client as well as the nurse.

Overinvolvement is a form of countertransference (O'Kelly, 1998). It can happen when positive feelings about the relationship override objectivity, when the client is needy and/or effusively grateful, or when the client reminds the nurse of a similar previously unresolved care situation.

Whenever overinvolvement occurs, the nurse loses the necessary detachment and objectivity needed to support the client in meeting health goals (Kines, 1999). Lost is the needed balance between compassion and professionalism, a primary ingredient in successful nurse-client relationships. Ethical commitments made to the client to serve as protector and facilitator of the client's personal growth are placed in serious jeopardy.

Overinvolvement can have unexpected outcomes that extend beyond the individual client. It can compromise the nurse's obligation to the institution, professional commitment to the treatment regimen, collegial relationships with other health team members, and professional responsibilities to other clients (Morse, 1991).

Warning signs that the nurse is becoming overinvolved include the following:

- Giving extra time and attention to certain clients
- Visiting the client in off hours
- Doing things for clients that the clients could do for themselves
- Discounting the actions of other professionals
- Feeling resentment about the ways other health team members care for the client
- Persistently thinking about the client while off duty

Maintenance of professional boundaries is always the responsibility of the professional nurse. Carmack (1997) suggests the following actions that the nurse can take to regain perspective:

- Assume full responsibility for the process of care while acknowledging that the outcome may not be within your control.
- Focus on the things that you can change while acknowledging that there are things over which you have no control.
- Be aware and accepting of your professional limits and boundaries.
- Monitor your reactions and seek assistance when you feel uncomfortable about any aspect of the relationship.
- Balance giving care to a client with taking care of yourself, without feeling guilty.

The opposite extreme, disengagement, occurs when nurses find themselves withdrawing from clients because of the client's behavior or because they cannot bear to witness the client's suffering. Clients who fail to progress, who suffer intensely or who have a lingering death, or who have significant changes in appearance or condition drain the nurse emotionally. Sometimes nurses will detach from relationship with the client because they cannot bear to watch a patient struggle unsuccessfully or lose hope. When this occurs, the client is left to suffer alone, which further intensifies their emotional pain (Rodgers & Cowles, 1997). Morse et al. (1992) note that "sufferers watch for any signs of rejection, dismay, or horror in their caregivers' faces. If the caregiver does reveal these feelings, and if the patient recognizes these feelings, he/she may become alarmed and lose hope" (p. 818). Support groups for nurses working in high-stress situations and the mentoring of new nurses help to offset lack of balance in the nurse-client relationship.

Nurses tend to detach from clients who are sexually provocative, complaining, hostile, or extremely anxious or depressed. Physical characteristics such as poor hygiene, marked physical disability, socially stigmatized illness, or an unusual or altered appearance can negatively affect the nurse's willingness to engage with a client. It is much harder to stay present with such clients because they trigger uncomfortable feelings in us. Signs of disengagement include withdrawal, limited perfunctory contacts, minimizing the client's suffering, and defensive or judgmental communication. Sometimes processing these reactions with another health professional helps restore the needed empathy in difficult client situations.

Therapeutic Use of Self

The Nurse as a Healing Presence. The most striking quality of the therapeutic use of self is the nurse's ability to be fully and uniquely present with another human being (Carpenito, 2000; Covington, 2003). Miller (2001) defines *healing presence* as "the condition of being consciously and compassionately in the present moment with another or with others, believing in and affirming their potential for wholeness, wherever they are in life" (p. 12). Presence involves the capacity to know when to provide help and when to stand back; when to speak frankly, and when to withhold comments because the client is not ready to hear them. Being fully present with another brings comfort and strength to the client (Morse, 2000), but it is not always comfortable or pleasant for the nurse. Sometimes it is one of the hardest caring acts a nurse can perform for another human being, because to do so creates intense feelings of helplessness or vulnerability. Yet the relationship may be the only stable element in the client's life, so the nurse's presence becomes an extremely significant component of the healing process (Taylor, 1992). For the nurse willing to engage in such a relationship, it can be like none experienced before, filling the nurse with awe and respect for the humanness of suffering and the magnificence of humanity.

Authenticity is a precondition for the therapeutic use of self in the nurse-client relationship. "To be authentic is to be true to oneself or to one's being" (Daniels, 1998, p. 191). It is not always easy to be authentic in professional situations where clients, peers, and supervisors look to the nurse to have the answers in even the most complicated situation. Being authentic requires recognizing your own vulnerabilities, strengths, and limitations—and working within this knowledge in the service of the client. It means allowing yourself to really engage with a client, knowing that parts of the relationship may be painful, uncomfortable, and yet rewarding because you have allowed yourself to be vulnerable. Daniels suggests that when nurses recognize parts of themselves in their clients, they humanize the nurse-client relationship.

Because they are human, nurses will have all sorts of feelings about working closely with their clients. There are some clients that nurses simply don't like working with (Erlen & Jones, 1999). Our humanity is what makes us good nurses, but it also makes nurses more vulnerable to caring too much or too little. Nurses need to acknowledge overinvolvement, avoidance, anger, frustration, or detachment from a client when it occurs, and then begin to work on developing a deeper understanding of the underlying interpersonal issues. The ethical principle "First, do no harm" should be foremost in the nurse's mind throughout the relationship.

Therapeutic use of self requires the nurse to be authentic and clear about his or her personal values, feelings, and thoughts in responding to a client—without making the client assume responsibility for the nurse's position. For example, a homeless client may tell the nurse, "I know you want to help me, but you can't understand my situation because you have money and a husband to support you. You don't know what it is like out on the streets." Instead of feeling defensive, the nurse might say, "You are right, I don't know what it is like to be homeless, but I would like to know more about your experiences. Can you tell me what it has been like for you?" With this listening response, the nurse invites the client to engage in a dialogical conversation, defined as "a two-way conversation, a back-and-forth, give-and-take, in-there-together process in which people talk *with* rather than *to* each other" (Anderson, 2001, p. 348). After this discussion, the nurse might address the loneliness, fear, and helplessness the client is experiencing. These are universal feelings that the nurse can relate to, even if the experience of homelessness is not a part of his or her personal life experience.

Even mistakes can be a forum for genuine communication. For example, a nurse may promise a client to return immediately with a pain medication and then forget to do so because of other pressing demands. When the nurse brings the medication, the client might accuse the nurse of being uncaring and incompetent. It would be appropriate for the nurse to apologize for forgetting the medication and for any extra discomfort suffered by the client.

Empathy

Empathy should be a core component of all phases of the therapeutic relationship; it assures a client that the nurse has truly heard and understood the client's perspective (Myers, 2000). The concept was first described in 1887 by Lipps, a German psychologist, as being able to fully understand the experience of another without loss of self (Olsen, 1991). Katz (1963) describes it as the capacity "to see with the eyes of another, to hear with the ears of another, and feel with the heart of another" (p. 1). Empathy is closely aligned to the concept of presence; it is impossible to be fully present to another person without being empathetic. Empathy allows the nurse to fully perceive the depth of a client's anger, fear, and anxiety without being overwhelmed by it. Empathy also requires a response from the listener. An accurate empathetic response captures the essence of the client's feelings and assures both parties that they are talking about the same phenomena. Empathetic responses allow clients to feel respected, understood, and validated. They should be expressed tentatively, for example: "I sense that you feel really overwhelmed by this news." Be brief and use your own words, asking for validation of what you are observing. Even if you are incorrect, your efforts to understand will not go unnoticed by the client. Sometimes a gentle touch delivered simultaneously can enhance the effect of an empathetic response. Egan (2002) provides some suggestions for increasing empathic understanding, which have been incorporated into Box 5-2. Chapter 6 further details empathy.

Box 5-2 Suggestions for Facilitating Empathy

- Actively listen carefully to the client's concerns.
- Tune into physical and psychological behaviors that express the client's point of view.
- Do self-checks often for stereotypes or premature understanding of the client's issues.
- Set aside judgments or personal biases.
- Be tentative in your listening responses and ask for validation frequently.
- Mentally picture the client's situation and ask appropriate questions to secure information about areas or issues you are not clear about.
- Give yourself time to think about what the client has said before responding or before asking the next question.
- Mirror the client's level of energy and language.
- Be authentic in your responses.

Modified from Egan G: *The skilled helper*, ed 7, Pacific Grove, CA, 2002, Brooks Cole Publishing.

Self-Disclosure

Self-disclosure by the nurse refers to the intentional revealing of personal experiences or feelings that are similar to or different from those of the client. Appropriate self-disclosure can facilitate the relationship, providing the client with information that is both immediate and personalized (Deering, 1999). Self-disclosure can be relevant when it fits the goals of the conversation at hand, when it is used to model self-disclosure and educate the client, or when it provides a concrete reflection that encourages reality testing. On the other hand, nurses should not share intimate details of their life with their clients. The nurse, not the client, is responsible for regulating the amount of disclosure needed to facilitate the relationship. If the client asks a nonoffensive, superficial question, the nurse may answer briefly with a minimum of information and return to a client focus. Simple questions such as, "Where did you go to nursing school?" and, "Do you have any children?" may represent the client's effort to establish common ground for conversation (Morse, 1991). Answering the client briefly and returning the focus to the client is appropriate. If the client persists with questions, the nurse can say simply, "I'd really like to talk about you. Can you tell me about . . .?"

Requests for intimate information about the nurse do not need to be answered. If the client is persistent, the nurse may need to redirect the client by saying, "I'd like to spend this time talking about you," or simply indicate that personal questions are not relevant to understanding the client's health care needs. Deering (1999) suggests the following guidelines for keeping self-disclosure at a therapeutic level: (a) use self-disclosure to help clients open up to you, not to meet your own needs; (b) keep your disclosure brief; and (c) don't imply that your experience is exactly the same as the client's. Exercise 5-2 provides an opportunity to explore self-disclosure in the nurse-client relationship.

Empowerment

Empowerment in the nurse-client relationship becomes even more important in today's health care arena with its shortened hospital stays and the need to maximize the care given in the hospital (Rogan & Timmins, 2004). McQueen (2000) defines **empowerment** in health care

Exercise 5-2 Recognizing Role Limitations in Self-Disclosure

Purpose: To help students differentiate between a therapeutic use of self-disclosure and spontaneous self-revelation.

Procedure:

1. Make a list of three phrases that describe your own personality or the way you relate to others, such as the following:
   I am shy.
   I get angry when criticized.
   I'm nice.
   I'm sexy.
   I find it hard to handle conflicts.
   I'm interested in helping people.
2. Mark each descriptive phase with one of the following:
   A = Too embarrassing or intimate to discuss in a group.
   B = Could discuss with a group of peers.
   C = This behavior characteristic might affect my ability to function in a therapeutic manner if disclosed.
3. Share your responses with the group.

Discussion:

1. What criteria were used to determine the appropriateness of self-disclosure?
2. How much variation is there in what each student would share with others in a group or clinical setting?
3. Were there any behaviors commonly agreed on that would never be shared with a client?
4. What interpersonal factors about the client would facilitate or impede self-disclosure by the nurse in the clinical setting?
5. What did you learn from doing this exercise that could be used in future encounters with clients?

as helping people develop the knowledge skills and other resources they need to set their own health agendas and to take a primary role in their health care. Rodwell (1996) describes empowerment as "enabling people to choose to take control over and make decisions about their lives" (p. 309). (See Chapter 6 and Chapter 15 for more about this concept in contemporary health care.)

Empowerment encompasses the concept of being with a client as a guide and providing direction, rather than doing things to a client (Oudshoorn, 2005; Pearson, Borbasi, & Walsh, 1997). Nurses empower clients every time they foster their client's self-direction in choosing treatment options, setting goals, and devising effective problem-solving strategies for difficult health problems. Providing relevant information (D'Alessandro & Dosa, 2001), validating the client's personal strengths, and helping clients and families recognize opportunities for choice are therapeutic strategies that help empower clients. For example, giving the client information about what to expect after surgery, who to contact if experiencing side effects, and what to look for with medications empowers the client. Allowing clients to do as much for themselves as possible while providing enough support necessary for them to feel successful empowers clients and enhances self-esteem.

APPLICATIONS

Phases of the Relationship

In 1952, Peplau described four sequential phases of a nurse-client relationship, each characterized by specific tasks and interpersonal skills: preinteraction, orientation, working (active intervention), and termination. Each phase serves to broaden as well as deepen the scope of emotional connection with clients. Peplau maintained that the **orientation phase** sets the stage for the rest of the relationship. This phase correlates with the assessment phase of the nursing process. Once the nurse

Developing an Evidence-Based Practice

Sahlsten M, Larsson I, Lindencrona C et al.: Patient participation in nursing care, *J Clin Nurs* 14:35-42, 2005.

This qualitative study, using a grounded theory method, was designed to clarify the registered nurse's understanding of patient participation in nursing care by studying staff nurses' interpretations of patient participation and how it occurred. A purposive sample of 31 registered nurses providing inpatient nursing care in five different hospitals participated in focus groups.

Results: Study results revealed four different approaches and procedures involved with patient participation: interpersonal procedure (mutual interaction between nurse and patient), therapeutic approach (understanding and being understood, contact, respect), focus on resources (exchange of information and knowledge), and opportunities for influence (information, choices, decisions).

Application to Your Clinical Practice: As health consumers become active partners in their personal health care, their participation with nurses to achieve desired outcomes becomes an integral component of their nursing care. How would you see the factors identified in this study applied to your nursing care of clients?

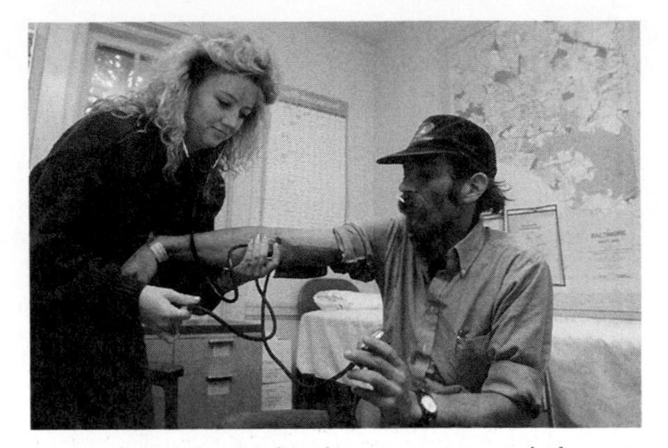

Concepts of the therapeutic relationship are present even in brief encounters. (Courtesy University of Maryland School of Nursing.)

and client together define the problem in the orientation phase, they move into the **working phase**, which is subdivided into two aspects: identification and exploitation. The *identification* component focuses on mutual clarification of ideas and expectations, and corresponds to the planning phase of the nursing process. The *exploitation* component, using the client's personal strengths and community resources to help the client resolve health care issues, parallels the implementation phase. Peplau referred to the final phase of the relationship as the **termination (resolution) phase**, which corresponds to the evaluation phase of the nursing process. The nurse assists the client in evaluating the resolution of issues that initially brought the client into treatment.

The therapeutic relationship is a potentially fragile alliance if not handled with care. In any phase of the developing relationship, the process can break down. Remaining at the superficial, social level of the orientation phase hampers the active problem-solving process needed for successful resolution of health care issues identified in the working phase. Developing a strong rapport with a client in the orientation and working phases, and then failing to terminate adequately with a client, calls into question much of the effectiveness of the nurse's efforts during the earlier phases. The chances of the client trusting in the value of future relationships diminish when termination is treated casually.

Flexibility in returning to more superficial levels may be necessary when the client is not ready to discuss sensitive issues. For example, a difficult diagnosis or beginning awareness of a terminal condition may cause the client to become silent. The client may need more time to internally absorb disturbing changes before using the therapeutic relationship to work through potentially overwhelming feelings about a situation.

Preinteraction Phase

Creating the Psychological Environment. Careful preparation usually makes the first encounter with a client go more smoothly (Forchuk, 1994a). Having a clear knowledge of the theoretical principles and role responsibilities associated with the relationship does not guarantee a successful outcome, but it does prevent the "lost" feeling that comes from not knowing what one is doing or what one hopes to accomplish through one's efforts. Developing professional goals helps the nurse select concrete, specific nursing actions that are purposeful and aligned with individualized client needs.

The goals of a professional relationship dictate that the client is always the architect of the content; the nurse supplies the coaching framework necessary for understanding the nature of the problem-solving process. Having professional goals communicates to the client that the nurse is knowledgeable, in control of nursing role responsibilities, and ready to focus on the needs of the client. Professional goals rarely are communicated directly to the client, but they are implicit in all that the nurse does and says with a client.

Making the interpersonal environment a safe place in which to explore feelings and to work through painful issues is of critical importance in the beginning stages of the relationship (Forchuk, 1995). For example, the nurse on a maternity floor should have a different perspective in approaching a client whose infant is in the neonatal intensive care unit because of respiratory distress than in approaching a client who is rooming in with a healthy infant. The few minutes it takes to obtain a quick overview of client status before the initial meeting can make quite a difference in the choice of interpersonal approaches and in the success of the initial encounter. This is what is meant by individualized nursing care. Treating critical yet sometimes subtle differences in individual circumstances as important information in the initial encounter respects the uniqueness of the person experiencing them.

Timing is important. Select times for longer discussions when the client is physically comfortable and free of pain. In the home, the client should select an appropriate time that does not conflict with the nurse's other responsibilities. Offering the client several different times helps with this process. Nurses should set times with the client when they can give the client undivided attention for the full duration of the visit. The client needs to feel comfortable and unhurried. If the relationship is to be ongoing, the nurse should share initial plans related to time, purpose, and other details with staff. Failure to involve staff in the initial planning stages can sabotage the most careful and creative plan.

Creating the Physical Environment. When the interview takes place at the client's bed in a hospital setting, the curtain should be drawn and the nurse can sit at an angle facing the client. One-on-one relationships with psychiatric clients commonly take place in a designated, noiseless room apart from the client's bedroom. In the client's home, the nurse is always the client's guest, and

Table 5-2 Interviewing and Relationship Skills

Phase	Stage	Purpose	Skills
Orientation Phase			
Engagement, assessment	Gathering information, defining the problem, identifying strengths	To determine how the client views the problem and what client strengths might be used in their resolution	Basic listening and attending; open-ended questions, verbal cues and leads
Working (Implementation) Phase			
Planning (Identification Component)	Determining outcomes: What needs to happen to reduce the self-care demand? Where does the client want to go?	To find out how the client would like to be; how things would be if the problems were solved	Attending and basic listening; influencing; feedback
Implementation (Exploitation Component)	Explaining alternatives and options	To work toward resolution of the client's self-care needs	Influencing; feedback balanced by attending and listening
Termination Phase			
Evaluation	Generalization and transfer of learning	To enable changes in thoughts, feelings, and behaviors; to evaluate the effectiveness of the changes in modifying the self-care need	Influencing; feedback; validation

Modified from Ivey A, Ivey M: Ivey's five stage model of interviewing. In Ivey A, editor, *Intentional interviewing and counseling,* Monterey, CA, 2002, Brooks/Cole; and Richmond V, McCroskey J, Payne S: *Nonverbal behavior in interpersonal relations,* Englewood Cliffs, NJ, 1987, Prentice Hall; Peplau H: Peplau's theory of interpersonal relations, *Nurs Sci Q* 10:(4): 162–167, 1997.

the client plays a stronger role in selecting the most appropriate place for the relationship.

Specific client needs can dictate the most appropriate interpersonal setting. For example, a rape victim in a busy emergency room should be accorded privacy in a private room with a staff member even before the interview begins. Although rape may not represent the most physically urgent triage situation, it is one of the most profound psychological emergency situations a woman can experience. The client needs privacy and someone to stay with her. An adolescent or elderly client may appreciate a "walking interview" on the grounds rather than in his or her room. Each time a nurse considers such factors in a nurse-client relationship, the nurse models thoughtfulness, respect, and empathy.

Orientation Phase

The nurse-client relationship formally begins with the orientation phase and ends with the termination phase. Table 5-2 identifies interviewing strategies associated with each phase of the nurse-client relationship. All beginnings are important, because they set the tone for the relationship. Caring communication validates the uniqueness of each individual client (Reynolds, 1997). Introductions are important even with clients who are confused, aphasic, or unable to make an objective response because of mental illness or coma. In this case, the introduction should be simply your name and that you are a nurse who will be taking care of the patient. Address the introduction to the client, as well as to family members who may be present.

The nurse enters the relationship in the stranger role and begins the process of developing trust by providing the client with basic information about the nurse (e.g., name and professional status) and essential information about the purpose, nature, and time available for the relationship (Peplau, 1997). This can be a simple introduction: "I am Susan Smith, a registered nurse, and I am going to be your nurse on this shift." Nonverbal supporting behaviors of a handshake, eye contact, and a smile reinforce the spoken words. Tell clients that you will be asking them a lot of questions in order to give them the best care possible, but that they should tell you if anything makes them feel uncomfortable. Assure them that personal information will be treated as confidential (Heery, 2000).

The nurse can continue with an invitation to the client to share similar information, "How would you prefer to be addressed?" and follow with some other basic questions to put the client at ease.

Clarifying the Purpose of the Relationship. Nurse and client must develop a working partnership before the work on health care problems takes place, so you should provide basic information about the purpose and nature of the interview or relationship, including what information is needed, how the client can participate in the process, what the client can expect from the encounter, and how the information will be used. For example, you can say, "I'd like to talk with you about how I can help you in the hospital, and I will need to ask you for some information about your health and what you expect here in the hospital." The nurse will need to inform the client that it may be necessary for the nurse to disclose certain information relevant to clinical decisions that must be made by other members of the health care team.

The goals of the relationship dictate the depth of the orientation to the purposes of the relationship. A basic orientation given to a client by a nurse assigned for a day would be different from that given to a client when the nurse assumes the role of primary care nurse. When the relationship is to be of longer duration, the nurse should be prepared to discuss the parameters of the relationship (e.g., length of sessions, frequency of meetings, and role of the nurse).

Initial meetings should have two outcomes. First, the client should emerge from the encounter with a better idea of some of the beginning health issues and possible goals. Second, the client should feel that the nurse is interested in him or her as a person. At the end of the contact, the nurse should thank the client for his or her participation and indicate what will happen next.

When you initially use this introductory strategy, the words may feel mechanical, and you might prefer to be more informal and spontaneous in your communication. Obviously, you can vary the words, but the verbal message needs to contain this combination of data. Having an idea of what you will say to a client at the beginning of your relationship should decrease your anxiety. Exercise 5-3 is designed to give you practice in making introductory statements.

Spontaneity can be expressed in the way you present yourself. Are you smiling and relaxed in manner? Do your posture and gestures support your genuine desire to get to know this client? Are you truly receptive to hear-

Exercise 5-3 Introductions in the Nurse-Client Relationship

Purpose: To provide experience with initial introductions.

Procedure:

The introductory statement forms the basis for the rest of the relationship. Effective contact with a client helps build an atmosphere of trust and connectedness with the nurse. The following statement is a good example of how one might engage the client in the first encounter:

"Hello, Mr. Smith. I am Sally Parks, a nursing student. I will be taking care of you on this shift. During the day, I may be asking you some questions about yourself that will help me to understand how I can best help you."

1. Role-play the introduction to a new client with one person taking the role of the client; another, the nurse; and a third person, an involved family number, with one or more of the following clients:
2. Mrs. Dobish is a 70-year-old client, admitted to the hospital with a diagnosis of diabetes and a question about cognitive impairment.
3. Thomas Charles is a 19-year-old client admitted to the hospital following an auto accident in which he broke both legs and fractured his sternum.
4. Barry Fisheis is a 53-year-old man who has been admitted to the hospital for tests. The physician believes he may have a renal tumor.
5. Marion Beatty is a 9-year-old girl admitted to the hospital for an appendectomy.
6. Barbara Tangiers is a 78-year-old woman living by herself. She has multiple health problems including chronic obstructive pulmonary disease and arthritis. This is your first visit.

Discussion:

1. In what ways did you have to modify your introductions to meet the needs of the client and/or circumstances?
2. What were the easiest and hardest parts of doing this exercise?
3. How could you use this experience in your clinical practice?

ing what the client has to share with you? Your accompanying actions are no less important than the words you use. Both your actions and your words are data the client needs to begin trusting you.

Assessing Client Needs. The nurse and the client can have different perceptions of reality, and the nurse needs to begin the assessment process with an open mind. How the client perceives his or her health status, reasons for seeking treatment at this time, and expectations for health care are critical data that will form the basis for all nursing interventions.

Initially, the nurse focuses on the immediate crisis of the hospitalization or clinic visit and begins to identify factors with the client and the client's family that will facilitate or hinder the treatment process. Asking the client to tell you what brought him or her to the hospital (clinic) or to seek treatment elicits the client's perspective on the illness. See Chapter 10 for ways to best communicate with your clients. Planning questions to follow a logical sequence and asking only one question at a time helps orient the clients and provide more complete data.

Participant Observation. Peplau describes the role of the nurse throughout the relationship as being that of a participant observer. This means that the nurse is observing the client's behavior, as well as his or her personal responses, while at the same time interacting with the client. Nurses mentally form impressions about the client's behavior, mental status, and anxiety level from the moment that they enter the client's room. These impressions, when validated with the client, serve as guides for subsequent actions in the relationship. For the nurse to obtain the full picture, learning as much as possible about a client through data related to the illness experience is crucial.

Case Example

Dying client (to the nurse): It's not the dying that bothers me as much as not knowing what is going to happen to me in the process.

Nurse: It sounds as though you can accept the fact that you are going to die, but you are concerned about what you will have to experience. Tell me more about what worries you.

By linking the emotional context with the content of the client's message, the nurse shows a desire to understand the situation from the client's perspective. Nurses need to be aware of the different physical and nonverbal cues clients give with their verbal messages. Noting facial expressions and nonverbal cues with "You look exhausted" or "You look worried" acknowledges the presence of these factors and normalizes them. Exercise 5-4 is designed to help you pick up another person's nonverbal cues.

As the nurse interacts with the client, there are opportunities to observe client strengths. Every client has healthy aspects of his or her personality and personal strengths that can be used to facilitate individual coping responses. Think about a client you have had or a person you know who has a serious illness. What personal strengths does this person have that could have a healing impact on the illness? Strengths can be courage, patience, fighting spirit, family, and so on.

Relying exclusively on client information without soliciting the perceptions of significant others can distort and limit history taking. If there is any reason to suspect the reliability of the client as a historian, significant others can supply information. Nursing judgment is also needed when family and client disagree about diagnosis, treatment goals, or ways to provide care. Comparing client and family data for congruence and differences is an important source of client data. The differences can be just as important as the agreement in developing the most appropriate nursing interventions. For example, if the client has one perception about self-care abilities and family members have a completely different perception, these differences become a nursing concern. Specific nursing diagnoses need to address the discrepancies in perceptions.

It is important to strike a balance between communicating with the client and with significant others accompanying the client. Sometimes health professionals treat clients who are elderly, adolescent, or physically handicapped as though they are mentally incapacitated in assessment interviews. Talking only with the adult members of a family instead of including the client in the dialogue or assuming the elderly or adolescent client has a limited understanding or interest devalues the person. This subtle and usually unintentional devaluing of the individual increases a sense of dehumanization and loneliness, a common occurrence in health care settings. On the other hand, family members are sometimes reluctant to challenge a client's perception of his or her physical or emotional condition in front of the client, yet both perspectives are needed for accurate assessment.

The last part of the assessment process in the orientation phase relates to determining the kind of help needed as well as who can best provide it. Assessment of the most appropriate source of help is an important but often overlooked part of the evaluation needed in the orientation phase.

Exercise 5-4 Interpreting Nonverbal Cues

Purpose: To identify and understand the role of nonverbal cues in the introductory, working, and termination phases of the therapeutic relationship.

Procedure:
A variety of photographs of nurse-client interactions will be provided, and each student will choose one. The student will examine the picture and creatively identify a phase it depicts, the tasks being accomplished by the nurse, and the response of the client.

Discussion:
Each student will share his or her picture and interpretation. Descriptions of each phase will be compiled on the board.

Communication Strategies. Initial contacts should be exploratory and somewhat tentative. Both the conversation and behaviors in the orientation phase are usually of a superficial nature. Keeping conversation to neutral topics rather than emotionally loaded subjects usually seems less invasive to the client in the beginning stages of the relationship. Most clients feel vulnerable in examining sensitive subjects before a trusting bond is established. Discussion of deep feelings and core issues will come later.

Knowledge of the client's developmental stage and current health situation may suggest possible topics for conversation. The acutely ill client will want short contacts that are to the point and related to providing comfort and care. Language and selection of topics should reflect the client's age and developmental level. For example, you would hold a different conversation with an adolescent client than you would with an elderly client. During the initial encounters with the nurse, the client begins to assess the nurse's trustworthiness (Ramos, 1992).

Communication is a two-way process. Kindness, competence, and a willingness to become involved are communicated through the nurse's words and actions. Does the nurse seem to know what he or she is doing? Is the nurse tactful and respectful of cultural differences? Data regarding the level of the nurse's interest and knowledge base are factored into the client's decision to engage actively in a therapeutic relationship.

Honesty and commitment are critical elements in trust. Consistency, dependability, and the honoring of commitments to the client foster the development of trust. When it is impossible for the nurse to honor a commitment, the client deserves a full explanation.

Trusting the nurse is particularly difficult for the seriously mentally ill, for whom the idea of having a caring relationship may be incomprehensible. Having this awareness helps the nurse depersonalize the experience of momentarily feeling overwhelmed by intense human emotions that many nurses experience and do not always easily understand. Most mentally ill clients respond better to shorter, frequent contacts until trust is established. Schizophrenic clients often enter and leave the space occupied by the nurse, almost circling around a space that is within visual distance of the nurse. With patience and tact, the nurse engages the client slowly, respecting the client's anxiety. Over time, brief meetings that involve an invitation and a statement as to when the nurse will return help reduce the client's anxiety, as indicated in the following dialogue.

Case Example

Nurse (with eye contact and enough interpersonal space for comfort): Good morning, Mrs. O'Connell. My name is Karen Quakenbush. I will be your nurse today.

(Patient looks briefly at the nurse and looks away, then gets up and moves away.)

Nurse: This may not be a good time to talk with you. Would you mind if I checked back later with you? *(The introduction coupled with an invitation for later communication respects the client's need for interpersonal space and allows the client to set the pace of the relationship.)*

Later, the nurse notices that Mrs. O'Connell is circling around the area the nurse is occupying but does not approach the nurse. The nurse can smile encouragingly and repeat short encounters with the client until the client is more willing to trust. *(Creating an interpersonal environment that places little demand on either party initially allows the needed trust to develop in the relationship.)*

Defining Goals. Often a client needs assistance in developing relevant health goals, but the level of assistance should always coincide with the client's capacity for self-help. Unless clients are physically or emotionally unable to participate in their care, they should be treated as active partners in developing personal goals.

Goals should have meaning to the client. Finding out the client's interests can influence the selection of environmental motivators and the development of specific nursing strategies. For example, modifying the exchange lists for a diabetic adolescent so that they include fast foods and substitutions that mimic normal adolescent eating habits may facilitate acceptance of unwelcome dietary restrictions imposed by the illness. The nurse conveys confidence in the client's capacity to solve his or her own problems by expecting the client to provide data, to make constructive suggestions, and to follow through with the agreed-on plan. Exercise 5-5 gives practice in establishing mutual goals with a client.

Working (Active Intervention) Phase

Once nurse and client together define the problem in the orientation phase, they move into the working phase.

Exercise 5-5 Establishing Mutual Goals

Purpose: To develop awareness of mutuality in treatment planning.

Procedure:

1. Read the following clinical situation and subsequent nursing goals.
2. Identify each goal as nurse-centered (N), client-centered (C), or mutual (M).

Mr. Singer, age 48 years, is a Caucasian, middle-class professional recovering from his second myocardial infarction. After his initial attack, Mr. Singer resumed his 10-hour workday, high-stress lifestyle, and usual high-calorie, high-cholesterol diet of favorite fast foods, alcohol, and coffee. He smokes two packs of cigarettes a day and exercises once a week by playing golf.

Mr. Singer is to be discharged in two days. He expresses impatience to return to work, but also indicates that he would like to "get his blood pressure down and maybe drop 10 pounds." The student nurse caring for Mr. Singer establishes the following treatment goals:

1. After three dietary teaching sessions, Mr. Singer will be able to identify five foods high in sodium content.
2. After discharge, Mr. Singer will nap for two hours each day.
3. During the dietary teaching session, Mr. Singer will list five foods high in calories and five foods low in calories.
4. Mr. Singer will exercise moderately for 10 minutes a day and will limit his weekly golf game to three holes.
5. Mr. Singer's diastolic blood pressure will be below 90 mm Hg at his one-month postdischarge examination.
6. Immediately after discharge, Mr. Singer will resume his executive work schedule.
7. Mr. Singer will remain symptom-free until discharge.

Discussion:

Discuss your answers. How could nurse or client goals be modified to become mutual treatment goals?

Characteristic of this phase is an atmosphere of trust and candor, which makes it easier for the client to discuss deeper, more difficult issues and to experiment with new roles and actions. In contrast with the orientation phase, in which roles are more individualistic, the working phase is characterized by interdependent role relationships; the client assumes more of a partnership with the nurse in problem solving and implementation.

The working phase is subdivided into two components: identification and exploitation. The *identification* component is parallel to the planning phase of the nursing process. Here, you and the client would mutually develop goals related to resolution of identified client health needs and decide on the type of assistance needed to achieve them. In the *exploitation* component, nurses help their clients seek out and use health care services and personal strengths in resolving the issues for which the client initially sought treatment. Corresponding to the implementation phase of the nursing process, in this phase, the nurse fosters the client's self-direction to whatever extent is possible in promoting his or her health and well-being. Peplau categorized the client role as dependent, interdependent, or independent, based on the amount of responsibility the client is willing or able to assume for his or her care.

The identification phase integrates mutuality with the client's autonomy as the nurse and client develop a working definition of the problem and brainstorm the best ways to meet treatment goals. The sorting-out process occurs more easily when nurses are relaxed and willing to understand views different from their own. Peplau (1997) suggests that a general rule of thumb in working with clients is to "struggle with the problem, not with the patient" (p. 164).

Clients need to feel they have played a major role in developing a plan and implementing it in ways that make sense to them. The role of the nurse is to provide enough structure and guidelines for the client to explore problem issues and develop realistic solutions, but no more than are needed (Ballou, 1998). You should avoid taking more responsibility for actions than the client or situation requires. Such an approach may be easier in the immediate situation, but important learning is lost. For example, it may seem more efficient to give a bath to a stroke victim than to watch the client struggle through the bathing process with the nurse providing coaching when the client falters. However, what happens when the client goes home if she has not learned to bathe herself?

The client's right to make important decisions, provided they do not violate self or others, is accepted by the nurse, even when it runs contrary to the nurse's thinking. This protects the client's right to autonomy, but it is not always easy to do when the nurse feels that the client is not acting in his or her own best interest. Consider what you would do as the community health nurse in the following situation.

Case Example

Mr. McEntee, 54 years old, is admitted for chest pain. His tests show increased occlusion of the cardiac vessels. All of the male members of his family died of coronary disease in their 50s. Three years ago he had coronary bypass surgery. Since the surgery, Mr. McEntee has conformed to a proper diet and exercised prudently. Although he was referred to the cardiac rehabilitation unit for aftercare, he has refused to go. A home visit shows that he is not adhering to his diet but that he goes to the gym daily to work out. The nurse questions his noncompliance and urges him to consider the implications.

Listening with heart as well as head, how would you try to understand Mr. McEntee's predicament? Why do you think he is acting in such a self-destructive way? What suggestions can you offer to the home care nurse to increase compliance?

Defining the Problem. Problem definition forms the basis for treatment. Defining the problem increases the probability of a satisfactory solution. The nurse acts as a sounding board, asking questions about parts of the communication that are not understood and helping the client describe the problem in specific and concrete terms.

The problem statement should be precise and concrete. "Mrs. Kane started to cry when talking about her son's accident" is much more helpful than stating, "Mrs. Kane is sad that her son was hurt in a motorcycle accident." The latter statement includes an inference about cause and effect that may or may not be true. The client's tears could relate to anger, disappointment, or hurt, and if so, responding to the client's needs on the basis of the inference would not be appropriate.

Clients usually find it easier to talk about factual data related to a problem rather than to express the feelings associated with the issue, or to talk about the feelings as though there were no factual data associated with the problem. Using open-ended questions and compound sentences to link situational facts and emotional effects allows for the most complete understanding. "It sounds as if you feel ____________ because of ____________" helps the nurse and client look at the strong interrelationship between the situational data and the emotional reactions to it. For many clients, events and feelings represent two separate and unconnected happenings. To experience the connection comes as a revelation.

Whenever the nurse fails to understand a part of the client's problem or expectations, the nurse should ask for clarification or for more specific information. The nurse might ask for concrete data to bring the client's needs into sharper focus, for example, "Describe for me what happened next" or, "Tell me something about your reaction to (your problem)." Time should be allowed between questions for the client to respond fully. Commonly, such questions are asked, but not enough time is allowed for the client to respond.

Pacing. The nurse needs to recognize the legitimacy of the client's need to proceed at a personally comfortable pace. Elderly adults will need a slower pace, and people in crisis will need a simple structured pace. Throughout the working phase, the nurse needs to be sensitive as to whether the client is still responding at a useful level. Looking at difficult problems and developing strategies to resolve those problems is not an easy process, especially when resolution will require significant behavioral changes. If the nurse is perceived as inquisitive rather than facilitative, communication breaks down. It is the responsibility of the nurse, not the client, to pace the interview in ways that offer support as well as challenge.

Use the client's behavioral responses as a guide for structuring deeper exploration.

Changes in client behaviors often are the best indicators of data collection that is proceeding beyond the client's tolerance level. Examples of warning signs that the pace needs adjustment include loss of eye contact, fidgeting, abrupt changes in subject, crying, inappropriate laughter, or asking to be left alone. At the same time, strong emotion should not necessarily be interpreted as reflecting a level of interaction stretching beyond the client's tolerance. Tears or an emotional outburst, or even a more prolonged negative exchange, may reflect honestly felt emotion. A well-placed comment such as, "It seems to make you sad when we talk about your daughter" acknowledges the feeling and may stimulate further discussion. Deciding whether or not to proceed is a clinical judgment that should be based on the client's response and overall body language. Sometimes just sitting with calm interest and an open posture is enough to help a client reduce the internal anxiety of expressing strong emotion. A simple statement such as, "It's all right to cry" or, "It's okay to feel angry; nobody would want this to happen" acknowledges the feeling component, gives the client permission to express it, and implicitly offers assistance in coping with difficult emotions.

Developing Realistic Goals. Goals develop from the nursing diagnosis. To be effective, goals should be achievable, behavioral, and realistic. The nurse assists the client in developing realistic short-term objectives to meet long-term treatment goals. Breaking a seemingly insoluble problem down into simpler chunks makes it more manageable. Deciding on a course of action for even a small part of the problem helps the client gain some control in the situation and usually reduces anxiety to a tolerable level. For example, a goal of eating three meals a day may seem overwhelming to a person suffering from nausea and loss of appetite associated with gastric cancer. A goal of having Jell-O or chicken soup and a glass of milk three times a day may sound more achievable, particularly if the client can choose the times. Packaging goals in terminology the client understands and accepts is more workable than having a goal the client considers beyond his or her capabilities.

Exercise 5-6 Selecting Alternative Strategies

Purpose: To help students develop a process for considering and prioritizing alternative options.

Procedure:

You have two exams within the next two weeks. Your car needs servicing badly. Because of all the work you have been doing, you have not had time to call your mother, and she is not happy. Your laundry is overflowing the hamper. Several of your friends are going to the beach for the weekend and have invited you to go along. How can you handle it all?

1. Give yourself five minutes to write down all the ideas that come to mind for handling these multiple responsibilities. Use single words or phrases to express your ideas. Do not eliminate any possibilities, even if they seem far-fetched.
2. In groups of three or four students, choose a scribe, and share the ideas you have written down.
3. Select the three most promising ideas.
4. Develop several small, concrete, achievable actions to implement these ideas.
5. Share the small-group findings with the class group.

Discussion:

1. In what ways were the solutions you chose similar or dissimilar to those of your peers?
2. Were any of your ideas or ways of achieving alternative solutions surprising to you or to others in your group?
3. What did you learn from doing this exercise that could help you and a client generate possible solutions to seemingly impossible situations?

Planning Alternative Solutions. All life situations have some element of choice. In even the most difficult nursing situations, there are some options, even if the choice is to die with dignity or to change one's attitude toward an illness or a family member. The nurse is in a unique position to enter a client's life and understand the depths of a dynamic life process in ways that help the client feel hope (Wang, 2000). After the nurse and client brainstorm all possible options and strategies to meet agreed-on health objectives, the planning needs to consider the perspectives of *all* stakeholders. For example, if a client wishes to go home rather than to a nursing home following hip surgery, how is this decision likely to affect other family members who will have to provide the necessary care? How does the client feel about his or her ability to provide self-care, and are these assumptions valid? Anticipating the needs of significant others affected by the client's illness or disability and planning how to handle them are important dimensions in the working phase.

During this phase of the relationship, nursing interventions should have a broader focus than simply correcting problem areas. Referral to community resources, enlisting family support, and integrating personal strengths can empower the client. Exercise 5-6 gives practice in developing and prioritizing alternative strategies when feeling overwhelmed by multiple stressors.

Implementing the Plan. Both nurse and client should monitor progress toward achievement of treatment goals. As the client begins to implement certain actions for coping more successfully with anxiety-provoking situations, you can offer anticipatory guidance and role rehearsal for the more difficult aspects of this process. Sometimes simply anticipating the worstcase scenario for a given action allows the client to see that the worst possibility is manageable. Feedback for the client regarding possible modifications when the situation warrants it is an equally important element of the process.

Implementation does not always mean the course will be smooth and uneventful, even when the plan is appropriate. Mistakes are to be expected. They do not have to destroy the work of this phase, but should be treated as new information requiring a modification in strategy. Developing alternative constructive coping mechanisms is as important to support as the actual plan. A useful comment might be, "It is important to keep in mind that you did a good job with this, and no one could have predicted the outcome." This statement removes the blame that so often accompanies failed efforts. Coping with unexpected responses can strengthen the client's problem-solving abilities by compelling the person to consider alternative options (i.e., a "Plan B") when the original plan does not bring about the desired results.

Most problems and health care needs have to be worked through slowly, with the client taking two steps forward and one step back. This slow progress is sometimes cause for discouragement. Like small children taking their first steps, the process is usually not a straight, linear progression. Offering the client reassurance based on the fact that the two small steps were taken and that those steps cannot be erased, even if the client is unable to achieve a short-term goal to complete satisfaction, is a source of valuable support. The more critical question is, "What is it about either the goal, the strategies used to meet the goal, or the appraisal of the need or problem that needs reworking?"

Sometimes the problem with implementation lies with the nurse's availability, but even in these cases there are ways to handle the situation that make a difference in how the client perceives the nurse's interest. Therapeutic responses should be clear and focused on the client's need, but should also respect the nurse's integrity. In the following example, both responses to the client's need take the same amount of time. Which is potentially more satisfying?

Case Example

Jenny Johnson, RN, is on her way to the staff lounge to take a much-needed break when Mr. Clemson stops her to discuss his concerns about the cardiac catheterization his son was scheduled for an hour ago. Jenny sighs, glances impatiently at her watch, and comments in a flat voice, "I'd be happy to talk with you about the procedure if you have any questions."

An alternative response, one that recognizes the legitimate needs of both client and nurse, might be as follows:

Jenny (in a warm voice and making direct eye contact): It's natural to be concerned, but this procedure usually takes at least two hours. I'll call the recovery room and find out if your son has arrived there yet. If he hasn't arrived, I'll leave a message for them to call me when he does arrive. I'll be off the unit for a short time now, but when I get back, I'd be happy to talk with you about the procedure if you have any questions.

In the second response, the nurse recognizes the legitimacy of the client's need as well as her own need and responds accordingly. Because the message is clear and congruent with her expression and action, it is more likely to comfort the client.

Challenging Resistant Behaviors. Sometimes in the working phase it is necessary to challenge behaviors that are getting in the way of goal achievement. Challenging resistant behaviors requires a special type of feedback because often the client is only partially aware of what is happening and of his or her role in the process (Garant, 1980). Because of this lack of awareness, these behaviors remain unavailable for direct exploration and negotiation. Before confronting a client, the nurse should anticipate possible outcomes. Sometimes asking open-ended questions may elicit self-awareness about a problem behavior in need of change, and the client may come to the same conclusion as the nurse about the need to modify behavior without a strong confrontation.

If this strategy does not work and you must challenge the meaning of the client's message, it is important to proceed with interpersonal precision, sensitivity, and accuracy. The nurse needs to appreciate the impact of the confrontation on the client's selfesteem.

Calling a client's attention to a contradiction in behavioral response is usually threatening. It should be accomplished in a tactful manner that welcomes, but does not necessarily demand, an immediate resolution. Constructive feedback involves drawing the client's attention to the existence of unacceptable behaviors or contradictory messages while respecting the fragility of the therapeutic alliance and the client's need to protect the integrity of the self-concept. To be effective, constructive confrontations should be attempted only when the following criteria have been met:

- The nurse has established a firm, trusting bond with the client.
- The timing and environmental circumstances are appropriate.
- The confrontation is delivered in a nonjudgmental and empathetic manner.
- Only those behaviors capable of being changed by the client are addressed.
- The nurse supports the client's right to self-determination.

Timing is everything. Enough time and interpersonal space should be given to allow the client an opportunity to reflect on the feelings surrounding the behaviors as well as on the thoughts and feelings aroused by the nurse's comments. More specific guidelines regarding constructive feedback are presented in subsequent chapters.

Case Example

Mary Kiernan is 5 feet 2 inches tall and weighs 260 pounds. She has attended weekly weight management sessions for the past six weeks. Although she lost 8 pounds the first week, 4 pounds in week two, and another 4 pounds in week three, her weight loss seems to have hit a plateau. Jane Tompkins, her primary nurse, notices that Mary seems to be able to stick to the diet until she gets to dessert, and then she cannot resist temptation. Mary is very discouraged about her lack of further progress.

Consider the effect of each response on the client.

Nurse: You're supposed to be on a 1200-calorie-a-day diet, but instead you're sneaking dessert. I think you need to face up to the fact that eating dessert while dieting is hypocritical.

Nurse: I can understand your discouragement, but you have done quite well in losing 16 pounds. It seems as though you can stick to the diet until you get to dessert. Do you think we need to talk a little more about what hooks you when you get to dessert? Maybe we need to find alternatives that would help you get over this hump.

The first statement is direct, valid, and concise, but it is likely to be disregarded or experienced as unfeeling by the client. In the second response, the nurse reframes a behavioral inconsistency as a temporary setback, a problem in need of a solution instead of a failure. By bringing in the observed strength of the progress achieved so far, the nurse confirms her faith in the client's resourcefulness. Both responses would probably require similar amounts of time and energy on the part of the nurse; however, the second response fits the goal of motivating the client to use inner resources. The external reinforcement of the nurse allows the client to continue progress toward her goal of losing 50 pounds over a six-month period.

Termination Phase

Unlike social relationships, therapeutic relationships have a predetermined ending (e.g., when the outcome criteria are achieved, the client is discharged, or the number of visits permitted by insurance is reached). The termination phase refers to the nursing interventions and behavioral responses occurring at the closure of a therapeutic relationship. Usually, the health-related goals and individual needs of the client dictate when it is time to summarize the major achievements in the relationship and discuss realistic plans for referral if necessary.

Termination, as the word implies, should be final. To provide the client with a hint that the relationship will continue is unfair. It keeps the client emotionally involved in a relationship that no longer has a health-related goal. Nurses need to be clear that good-bye means just that. This is a very difficult issue for nursing students, who either see no harm in telling the client they will continue to keep in contact or who feel they have used the client for their own learning needs and to leave is unfair. However, this perception underestimates the positive things that the client received from the relationship and denies the fact that good-byes, painful as they may be, are a part of life and certainly not new for the client or for the nursing student.

Just as the orientation phase is linked with the assessment phase, the termination phase of the nurse-client relationship shares characteristics with the evaluation phase. Termination is a significant issue in long-term settings such as skilled nursing facilities, bone marrow transplant units, rehabilitation hospitals, and state psychiatric facilities, in which long-term relationships can and do develop. Sometimes there is a tendency to shortchange the termination phase because it is more uncomfortable for both the nurse and the client than some of the other stages.

The process of termination will not be the same for every client. Different aspects of the relationship should be emphasized and, ideally, correlated with each client's individualized needs, temperament, and behavioral response. The nurse's behavioral response should match the level of other phases in depth and intensity. For very short-term relationships or for a superficial contact, a simple statement of the meaning of the relationship, factual reassurance based on client behaviors observed in the relational experience, and discussion of follow-up plans will suffice. The termination can take place during discharge planning. Always important is the assistance the nurse provides in helping a client decide the best options for him or her.

The importance of the relationship, no matter how brief, should not be underestimated. The client may be one of several persons the nurse has taken care of during that shift, but the relationship may represent the only interpersonal or professional contact available to a lonely and frightened person. Even if contact has been minimal, the nurse should endeavor to stop by the client's room to say good-bye. The dialogue in such cases can be simple and short: "Mr. Jones, I will be going off duty in a few minutes. I enjoyed working with you. Miss Smith, the evening nurse, will be taking care of you this evening." Anticipatory guidance in the form of simple instructions or reiteration of important skills may be appropriate, depending on the circumstances.

Care should be taken to recognize the variety of behaviors accompanying termination of a longer-term relationship (e.g., regression and a temporary return of maladaptive ways of coping). Clients react in a variety of ways to separation. Behaviors the nurse may encounter with termination include avoidance, minimizing of the importance of the relationship, temporary return of symptoms precipitating the need for nursing care, anger, demands, or additional reliance on the nurse. Sometimes this phase is perplexing for both nurse and client.

For the nurse, there is a sense of pride in watching someone grow and develop as a person. It is difficult to give this up or to experience loss of gains during the termination phase. For the client, there can be a fear of relapsing and losing ground with the new attitudes and competencies. All of these feelings are normal in the termination phase and are usually temporary. When the client is unable to express feelings about endings, the nurse may recognize them in the client's nonverbal behavior.

Case Example

A teenager who had spent many months on a bone marrow transplant unit had developed a real attachment to her primary nurse, who had stood by her during the frightening physical assaults to her body and appearance that were occasioned by the treatment. The client was unable to verbally acknowledge the meaning of the relationship with the nurse directly, despite having been given many opportunities to do so by the nurse. The client said she couldn't wait to leave this awful hospital and that she was glad she didn't have to see the nurses anymore. Yet this same client was found sobbing in her room the day she left, and she asked the nurse whether she could write to her. The relationship obviously had meaning for the client, but she was unable to express it verbally.

If the relationship has been rewarding, real work has been accomplished. Nurses need to be sufficiently aware of their own feelings so that they may use them constructively without imposing them on the client. It is appropriate for nurses to share some of the meaning the relationship held for them, as long as such sharing fits the needs of the interpersonal situation and is not excessive or too emotionally intense.

Appropriate self-disclosure in the termination phase might include thanking the client for sharing his or her experience with the nurse. Shared meanings enhance the human outcomes of the therapeutic relationship (Marck, 1990).

In a successful relationship, the client demonstrates the following outcomes:

- Adaptive progression toward health or wellbeing
- Satisfaction with role performance according to developmental level and constraints of the illness
- A self-reported or enacted value shift, indicating a deeper sense of personal integrity

Evaluation of outcomes should take into consideration all phases of the nursing process. Was the problem definition adequate and appropriate for the client? Were the interventions chosen adequate and appropriate to resolve the client's problem? Could the interventions be implemented effectively and efficiently to both the client's and the nurse's satisfaction?

Referral. Many clients will need a referral to a professional community-based resource other than a support group. When this occurs, nurses can play an important role in the referral process by thoroughly discussing with the client the reasons for the referral and helping to make the initial contact. The nurse should have the client's permission to transmit information to the referred resource. Often the nurse's summary of the relationship is helpful to the referral professional in planning future strategies. Summarizing goal achievement with the client and providing a copy of the summary information reinforces the client's sense of control and continuity of treatment. Peplau (1997) also suggests that nurses could contribute to the advancement of the profession by sharing their experiences with client reactions to the illness experience.

Gift Giving. Clients sometimes wish to give nurses gifts because they value the care nurses have given to them. In a nonprofessional relationship, it would be totally appropriate to exchange gifts; however, in a professional relationship, the issue of gift giving requires closer examination. Gift giving, especially during the termination phase, is an especially delicate matter that does not lend itself to absolute dictums, but instead invites reflection and professional judgment. In all cases, the nurse should reflect on questions such as these: What meaning does the gift have for the relationship, and in what ways might accepting it change the dynamics of the therapeutic alliance? Would giving or receiving a gift present issues for other clients or their families?

There is no one answer about whether gifts should or should not be exchanged. In fact, if the nurse handled every situation in the same fashion, the nurse would be denying the uniqueness of each nurse-client relationship. Each relationship has its own character and its own strengths and limitations, so what might be appropriate in one situation would be totally inappropriate in another. In general, however, nurses should not accept gifts of significant material value. Should this become an issue, the nurse could suggest making the gift to the health care agency or a charity. Exercise 5-7 is designed to help you think about the implications of gift giving in the nurse-client relationship.

Adaptations for Short-Term Relationships

Hagerty and Patusky (2003) argue that there is a need to reconceptualize the nurse-patient relationship to one of human relatedness, given the brevity of hospital stays in today's evolving health care arena. Health care consumers are increasingly expected to be active partners in their own health care (McGrath, 2005). Therapeutic relationships have to take place in minutes and hours rather than over days or weeks. Driven by the economics of managed care, nurses must help clients determine what they need and how to develop solutions that fit their situation much more quickly than previously. Although nurses can and should follow the phases of the relationship, developing a therapeutic relationship in short-term

Exercise 5-7 Gift-Giving Role-Play

Purpose: To help students develop therapeutic responses to clients who wish to give them gifts.

Procedure:
Review the following situations and answer the discussion questions.

Situation:
Mrs. Terrell, a hospice nurse, has taken care of Mr. Aitken during the last three months of his life. She has been very supportive of the family. Because of her intervention, Mr. Aitken and his son were able to resolve a long-standing and very bitter conflict before he died. The whole family, particularly his wife, is grateful to Mrs. Terrell for her special attention to Mr. Aitken.

Role-Play Directions for Mrs. Aitken
You are very grateful to Mrs. Terrell for all of her help over the past few months. Without her help, you do not know what you would have done. To show your appreciation, you would like her to have a $300 gift certificate at your favorite boutique. It is very important to you that Mrs. Terrell fully understand how meaningful her caring has been to you during this very difficult time.

Role-Play Directions for Mrs. Terrell
You have given the Aitken family high-quality care and you feel very good about it, particularly the role you played in helping Mr. Aitken and his son reconcile before Mr. Aitken's death. Respond as you think you might in this clinical situation, given the previous data.

Discussion:
1. Discuss the responses made in the role-playing situation.
2. Discuss the other possible responses and evaluate the possible consequences.
3. Would you react differently if a client gave you a gift of $200 or a hand-crocheted scarf? If so, why?
4. Are there gifts clients give a nurse that are intangible? How should these gifts be acknowledged?

care could be more accurately termed a working alliance with active support.

This therapeutic working alliance should focus quickly, with client and nurse working as partners on developing a shared understanding of the client's health problems. Based on this information, the work of the relationship turns to devising a mutually developed perspective about treatment goals that can be realistically achieved. Treatment outcomes will depend on the competence and motivation of the nurse and client respectively and the quality of the relationship itself (Egan, 2002). The same recommendations for self-awareness, empathy, therapeutic boundaries, active listening, competence, mutual respect, partnership, and level of involvement hold true as key elements of brief therapeutic relationships.

Orientation Phase: Establishing a Therapeutic Working Alliance. Introduce yourself and begin to develop rapport by expressing genuine interest in getting to know the client and what is important to him or her. Establishing a working alliance where time is an issue requires a "here and now" focus on problem identification and an emphasis on quickly understanding the context in which it arose. This emphasis on the here and now promotes hope, because small, short-term goals are achievable.

Begin your client assessment by asking the client the reason for seeking care. Eliciting the client's concerns and allowing the client to tell his or her story conveys respect and interest. Listen for what is left out, and pay attention to what the client's story elicits in you. Support and empathy will go a long way in building trust quickly. Dealing with the client's feelings with a statement such as, "Tell me more about . . ." (with a theme picked up from the client's choice of words, hesitancy, or nonverbal cues) keeps the conversation flowing. Nurses need to acknowledge client strengths, their efforts, and their willingness to actively participate in their care.

As with a longer-term relationship, your immediate objective is to get to know as much about the client as possible. Statements such as, "It's important for me to understand your feelings about your illness so we can work on them together" reinforces the idea that the nurse is concerned about the person, rather than focused on the disease or disorder. Because the time frame for a therapeutic relationship may be a few hours or days, nurses need to focus on what is absolutely essential, rather than what would be nice to know. Finding out how much the client already knows can save a lot of time. Clients who are computer savvy are often quite knowledgeable about health problems. They should be encouraged to ask questions, and in learning what they already know, nurses can correct misperceptions and add, rather than duplicate, information.

In contemporary health care, the client has to accept more responsibility for his or her health care than ever before. Planning will be smoother if the nurse and client choose problems that are of interest to the client, and that offer the best return on investment. Included in the planning should be the risks and cost/benefits for each targeted clinical outcome. Looking at the client's needs from a broader contextual perspective, one that takes into consideration which problems, if treated, would also help correct other health problems, has a double benefit in terms of client success and satisfaction. Engaging the client's family early in the treatment process is very helpful.

Working Phase. Brief relationships need to be solution-focused right from the beginning. Begin to work on small behavioral changes and related coping skills needed to meet client goals. Clients respond best to nurses who appear confident and empathetic. You need to convey a realistically hopeful attitude that the goals you develop with the client are likely to be achieved. Encourage expression of feelings and the development of concrete plans and strategies to meet mutually established treatment goals. An excellent way of helping clients discover the solutions that fit them best is by brainstorming. Brainstorming involves generating multiple ideas and suspending judgment until after all possibilities are exhausted. The next step is to look realistically at ideas that could work given the resources the client has available right now. Resistance can be worked through with empathetic reality testing.

Termination Phase. The termination phase in brief relationships is especially important because of the shortened time frame. Discharge planning is critical with shortened hospital stays. The nurse also needs to include what will happen after the hospitalization. The emphasis has to be on linkages between hospital and community care. Preventive care is also important. Inquiring about support systems and the client's knowledge of community resources provides a base for the types of information a client will need to ensure continuity of care.

Discharge planning should be thorough, with key points given in writing to the client. It also is important to check that the client understands the discharge instructions. Asking questions about the information provides the nurse with a better sense of what the client really understands rather than directly asking if the patient understands, or assuming that she does because she doesn't ask any questions. In the termination phase it is important to ensure that the client has sufficient sources of help in the community. Education about when to call the physician or nurse practitioner is also important, as is knowledge of medications. The nurse and client should mutually evaluate therapeutic outcomes.

SUMMARY

The nurse-client relationship represents a purposeful use of self in all professional relations with clients and other people involved with the client. Respect for the dignity of the client and self, mutuality, person-centered communication, and authenticity in conversation are process threads underlying all communication responses.

In contrast with social relationships, therapeutic relationships have specific boundaries, purposes, and behaviors. They are client-focused and are mutually defined by client and nurse. Effective relationships enhance the well-being of the client and the professional growth of the nurse. Each relationship has its own character, strengths, and limitations, and what may be appropriate in one nursing situation may be totally inappropriate in another.

The professional relationship goes through a developmental process characterized by four overlapping yet distinct stages: preinteraction, orientation, working (active intervention), and termination. The preinteraction phase is the only phase of the relationship the client is not part of. During the preinteraction phase, the nurse develops the appropriate physical and interpersonal environment for an optimal relationship, in collaboration with other health professionals and significant others in the client's life.

The orientation phase of the relationship defines the purpose, roles, and rules of the process and provides a framework for assessing client needs. The nurse builds a sense of trust through consistency of actions. Data collection forms the basis for developing relevant nursing diagnoses. The orientation phase ends with a therapeutic contract mutually defined by nurse and client.

Once the nursing diagnosis is established, the working or active intervention phase begins. Essentially, this is the problem-solving phase of the relationship, paralleling the planning and implementation phases of the nursing process. As the client begins to explore difficult problems and feelings, the nurse uses a variety of interpersonal strategies to help the client develop new insights and methods of coping and problem solving.

The final phase of the nurse-client relationship occurs when the essential work of the active intervention phase is finished. The ending should be thoroughly and compassionately defined early enough in the relationship that the client can process it appropriately. Primary tasks associated with the termination phase of the relationship include summarization and evaluation of completed activities and, when indicated, the making of concrete plans for followup.

Ethical Dilemma ▪ *What Would You Do?*

Kelly, age 20 years, has been admitted with a tentative medical diagnosis: rule out AIDS. John is a 21-year-old student nurse assigned to care for Kelly. He expresses concern to his instructor about the client's sexual orientation. The instructor notes that John spends the majority of his time with his only other assigned client, who is in for treatment of a minor heart irregularity. What conclusions might be drawn regarding the reason John spends so little time caring for Kelly? If you were John, what would be important to you in understanding and resolving your feelings?

REFERENCES

Anderson H: Postmodern collaborative and person-centered therapies: what would Carl Rogers say? *J Fam Ther* 23:339–360, 2001.

Ballou K: A concept analysis of autonomy, *J Prof Nurs* 14(2):102–110, 1998.

Benner P: *From novice to expert: excellence and power in clinical nursing practice*, Menlo Park, CA, 1984, AddisonWesley.

Bonnivier M: Management of self–destructive behaviors in an open outpatient setting, *J Psychosoc Nurs Ment Health Serv* 34(2):37–43, 1996.

Briant S, Freshwater D: Exploring mutuality within the nurse-patient relationship, *Br J Nurs* 7(4):204–206, 1998.

Carmack B: Balancing engagement and disengagement in caregiving. *Image* 29(2):139–144, 1997.

Carpenito LJ: Nurses, always there for you, *Nurs Forum* 35(2):3–4, 2000.

Chauhan G, Long A: Communication is the essence of nursing care, 2: ethical foundations, *Br J Nurs* 9(15):979–984, 2000.

http://www.cno.org/docs/prac/41033_Therapeutic.pdf.

Covington H: Caring presence: delineation of a concept for holistic nursing. *J Holist Nurs* 21(3):301–317, 2003.

D'Alessandro D, Dosa N: Empowering children and families with information technology, *Arch Pediatr Adolesc Med* 155(10):1131–1136, 2001.

Daniels L: Vulnerability as a key to authenticity, *Image J Nurs Sch* 30(2):191–193, 1998.

Deering CG: To speak or not to speak? Self-disclosure with clients, *Am J Nurs* 99(1 Pt 1):34–38, 1999.

Delbanco TL: Enriching the doctor-patient relationship by inviting the patient's perspective, *Ann Intern Med* 116:414–418, 1992.

Eckroth-Bucher M: Philosophical basis and practice of self-awareness in psychiatric nursing, *J Psychosoc Nurs Ment Health Serv* 39(2):32–39, 2001.

Egan G: *The skilled helper*, ed 7, Pacific Grove, CA, 2002, Brooks Cole Publishing.

Erlen JA, Jones M: The patient no one liked, *Orthop Nurs* 18(4):76–79, 1999.

Forchuk C: The orientation phase of the nurse-client relationship: testing Peplau's theory, *J Adv Nurs* 20:1–6, 1994a.

Forchuk C: Preconceptions in the nurse-client relationship, *J Psychiatr Ment Health Nurs* 1(3):145–149, 1994b.

Forchuk C: Development of nurse-client relationships: what helps? *J Am Psychiatr Nurses Assoc* 1:146–153, 1995.

Frankl V: *The doctor and the soul*, New York, 1955, Knopf.

Gallop R: Abuse of power in the nurse-client relationship, *Nurs Stand* 12(37):43–47, 1998.

Garant C: Stalls in the therapeutic process, *Am J Nurs* 80(21):662–669, 1980.

Godkin J: Healing presence, *J Holist Nurs* 19(1):5–21, 2001.

Hagerty B, Patusky K: Reconceptualizing the nurse-patient relationship, *J Nurs Scholarsh* 35(2):145–150, 2003.

Heinrich K: When a patient becomes too special, *Am J Nurs* 22(11):62–64, 1992.

Heery K: Straight talk about the patient interview, *Nursing* 30(6):66–67, 2000.

Henson RH: Analysis of the concept of mutuality, *Image J Nurs Sch* 29(1):77–81, 1997.

Katherine A: *Where to draw the line*, New York, 2000, Simon & Schuster.

Katz RL: *Empathy: its nature and uses*, London, 1963, Collier-Macmillan.

Kines M: The risks of caring too much, *Can Nurse* 95(8):27–30, 1999.

Lowry M: Self-awareness: is it crucial to clinical practice?: confessions of a self-aware-aholic, *Am J Nurs* 105(11): 72CCC–72DDD, 2005.

Marck P: Therapeutic reciprocity: a caring phenomenon, *Adv Nurs Sci* 13(1):49–59, 1990.

McGrath D: Healthy conversations: key to excellence in practice, *Holist Nurs Pract* 19(4):191–193, 2005.

McQueen A: Nurse-patient relationships and partnership in hospital care, *J Clin Nurs* 9(5):723–731, 2000.

Miller J: *The art of being a healthy presence*, Fort Wayne, Ind, 2001, Willowgreen Publications.

Morse J: Negotiating commitment and involvement in the nurse-patient relationship, *J Adv Nurs* 16:455–468, 1991.

Morse J: On comfort and comforting, *Am J Nurs* 100(9): 34–37, 2000.

Morse J, Bottorf J, Anderson G et al.: Beyond empathy: expanding expressions of caring, *J Adv Nurs* 17:809–821, 1992.

Myers S: Empathetic listening: reports on the experience of being heard, *Journal of Humanistic Psychology* 40(2): 148–174, 2000.

O'Kelly E: Countertransference in the nurse-patient relationship: a review of the literature, *J Adv Nurs* 28(2):391–397, 1998.

Olsen DP: Empathy as an ethical and philosophical basis for nursing, *Adv Nurs Sci* 14(1):62–75, 1991.

Oudshoorn A: Power and empowerment: critical concepts in the nurse-client relationship, *Contemp Nurse* 20(1):57–66, 2005.

Pearson A, Borbasi S, Walsh K: Practicing nursing therapeutically through acting as a skilled companion on the illness journey, *Adv Pract Nurs Q* 3(1):46–52, 1997.

Peplau HE: *Interpersonal relations in nursing*, New York, 1952, Putnam.

Peplau HE: Peplau's theory of interpersonal relations, *Nurs Sci Q* 10(4):162–167, 1997.

Ramos M: The nurse-patient relationship: theme and variations, *J Adv Nurs* 17:495–506, 1992.

Reynolds W: Peplau's theory in practice, *Nurs Sci Q* 10(4):168–170, 1997.

Rodgers BL, Cowles KV: A conceptual foundation for human suffering in nursing care and research, *J Adv Nurs* 25:1048–1053, 1997.

Rodwell C: An analysis of the concept of empowerment, *J Adv Nurs* 23(2):305–313, 1996.

Rogan F, Timmins F: Improving communication in day surgery settings, *Nurs Stand* 19(7):37–42, 2004.

Schoot T, Proot I, Meulen RT et al.: Actual interaction and client centeredness in home care, *Clin Nurs Res* 14(4):370–393, 2005.

Sheets V: Professional boundaries: staying in the lines, *Dimens Crit Care Nurs* 20(5):36–40, 2001.

Taylor B: Relieving pain through ordinariness in nursing: a phenomenologic account of a comforting nurse-patient encounter, *Adv Nurs Sci* 15(1):33–43, 1992.

Travelbee J: *Interpersonal aspects of nursing*, ed 2, Philadelphia, 1971, FA Davis.

Wang C: Knowing and approaching hope as human experience: implications for the medical-surgical nurse, *Medsurg Nurs* 9(4):189–192, 2000.

Williams A: A literature review on the concept of intimacy in nursing, *J Adv Nurs* 33(5):660–667, 2001.

Chapter 6

Bridges and Barriers in the Therapeutic Relationship

Kathleen Underman Boggs

OUTLINE

OBJECTIVES

At the end of the chapter, the reader will be able to:

1. Identify concepts that enhance development of therapeutic relationships: caring, empowerment, trust, empathy, mutuality, and confidentiality.
2. Describe nursing actions designed to promote trust, empowerment, empathy, mutuality, and confidentiality.
3. Describe barriers to the development of therapeutic relationships: anxiety, stereotyping, and lack of personal space.
4. Identify nursing actions that can be used to reduce anxiety and respect personal space and confidentiality.
5. Identify research-supported relationships between communication outcomes, such as client empowerment, and improvements in self-care.
6. Discuss how findings from a research study can be applied to clinical practice.

> *Being able to communicate was found to be one of the top three indicators of quality nursing care.*
>
> (Oermann, 1997)

Chapter 6 focuses on the components of the nurse-client relationship. The concepts and applications are integrated when they cannot logically be understood apart from one another. To establish a therapeutic relationship, the nurse must understand and apply the concepts of respect, caring, empowerment, trust, empathy, and mutuality, as well as confidentiality and veracity (Figure 6-1). Additional bridges fostering the relationship are the nurse's ability to put into practice the ethical aspects of respecting the client's autonomy and to treat the client in a just and beneficent manner. Appreciation of other concepts that may act as barriers to the relationship (e.g., anxiety, stereotyping, or violations of personal space or confidentiality) affects the quality of the relationship. Implementing actions that convey feelings of respect, caring, warmth, acceptance, and understanding to the client is an interpersonal skill that requires practice. Caring for others in a meaningful way improves with experience. Novice students may encounter interpersonal situations that leave them feeling helpless and inadequate. Feelings of sadness, anger, or embarrassment, although overwhelming, are common. Discussion of these feelings in peer groups, experiential learning activities, and theoretical applications helps students to grow. The self-awareness strategies identified in Chapter 4 and the use of educational groups described in Chapter 12 provide useful guidelines for working through these feelings.

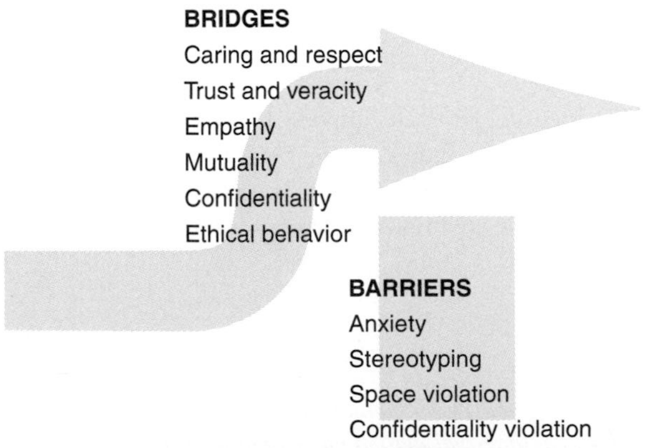

BRIDGES
Caring and respect
Trust and veracity
Empathy
Mutuality
Confidentiality
Ethical behavior

BARRIERS
Anxiety
Stereotyping
Space violation
Confidentiality violation

Figure 6-1 • Relationships can move in a positive or negative direction. Nursing actions can be bridges or barriers to a good nurse-client interaction.

BASIC CONCEPTS

Bridges to the Relationship

Respect

Conveying genuine respect for your client assists in building a professional relationship with him or her. As your mutual goal is to maximize the client's health status, you covey respect for his or her values and opinions. Asking clients what they prefer to be called and always addressing them as such is a correct initial step. Of course you avoid the sort of casual addresses portrayed in bad television shows, such as, "How are you feeling, honey?" or, "Mom, hold your baby" or, "How are we feeling today?" Hospitalized clients feel a loss of control in relation to interpersonal relationships with staff.

Barrier: Lack of Respect. In one study, clients felt devalued when they perceived that staff were avoiding talking with them or were unfriendly; they felt comforted when a little "chitchat" was exchanged (Williams & Irurita, 2004).

Caring

Caring is an intentional human action characterized by commitment and a sufficient level of knowledge and skill to allow the nurse to support the basic integrity of the person being cared for (Clarke, 1992). One person (the nurse) offers caring to another (the client) by means of the therapeutic relationship. The nurse's ability to care develops from a natural response to help those in need, from the knowledge that caring is a part of nursing ethics, and from respect for self and others. As a caring nurse, you will involve clients in their struggle for health and well-being rather than simply doing things for your clients.

Provision of a caring relationship that facilitates health and healing is identified as an essential feature of contemporary nursing practice in the Social Policy Statement of the American Nurses Association (ANA, 1995). In the professional literature, the focus of the caring relationship is clearly placed on meeting the client's needs. A formal model is even titled "patient-centered care." It involves understanding the client's perceived needs and expectations for health. This is a shift away from the old "I am the provider of treatment for this disease" kind of thinking (Lutz & Bowers, 2000). The behavior of "caring" is not an emotional feeling. Rather it is a chosen response to the client's need, the act of giving freely and willingly of oneself to another through warmth, compassion, concern, and interest. Nurses care for others during times of physical discomfort, emotional stress, and need for health maintenance. Caring has been identified as an ethical responsibility that guides a health care provider to advocate for the client (Branch, 2000).

Clients want us to understand why they are suffering. Platt (1995) noted that we tend to speak in a language of medicine that values facts and events. Clients, on the other hand, value associations and causes. To bridge this potential gap, health care providers need to convey to clients a sense that they truly care about the client's perspective. Caring has a positive influence on health status and healing. The applications section of this chapter describes how you communicate professional caring. In a caring relationship, clients can focus on accomplishing the goals of health care instead of worrying about whether care is forthcoming. The nurse gains from the caring relationship by experiencing the satisfaction of meeting the client's needs.

Families also need to experience a sense of caring from the nurse. Many families do not believe that the care provider has a clear understanding of the problems they are encountering while caring for their ill family member. This is especially true if the illness is not an easily observable defect or is a mental illness (Accordino, 1997).

Barrier: Lack of Caring. Although nursing has had a long-standing commitment to client-focused care, sometimes you may observe a situation in which you feel the nurse is meeting his or her own needs rather than the client's needs. At other times, a nurse can be so rushed to meet multiple demands that he or she forgets to focus on the client. Displaying an apathetic attitude is something student nurses are taught to avoid (Metz, 2000). Exercise 6-1 will help you focus on the concept of caring.

Empowerment

Empowerment is assisting the client to take charge of his or her own life (Reynolds, Scott, & Austin, 2000). The nurse using the interpersonal process provides the client with information, tools, and resources that help him or her build skills that can be used to reach the client's health goals. Empowerment is an important aim in every nurse-client relationship, and is addressed by nursing theories such as Orem's view of the client as an agent of self-care. Recent studies demonstrate that the more involved a client is in his or her own care, the better the health outcome is (Keller & Baker, 2000). At a personal level, empowered clients feel valued, adopt successful coping methods, and think positively. Empowerment has to do with people power: in helping our clients to take control of their lives, we identify and build on their existing strengths.

Barriers. Empowerment is purposeful. It encourages clients to assume responsibility for their own health. This is in direct contrast to the paternalistic attitude formerly found in medicine and characterized by the attitude of "I know what is best for you or I can do it better." One study in Australia showed that lack of information about giving care, managing medicines, or recognizing approaching crises was the major impediment to empowering family members to care for sick relatives (Wilkes, White, & O'Riordan, 2000). Failure to allow the client to assume personal responsibility, or failure to provide the client with appropriate resources or your ongoing support, undermines empowerment.

Exercise 6-1 Application of Caring

Purpose: To help students apply caring concepts to nursing.

Procedure:
Identify some aspect of caring that might be applied to nursing practice. Write each on the chalkboard or a transparency on the overhead projector so the entire group can see.

Discussion:
In a large group, discuss examples of how this form of caring could be implemented in a nurse-client situation.

Trust

Many writers, including Sheldon (2004), feel that establishing **trust** is the foundation in all relationships. The development of a sense of interpersonal trust, a sense of feeling safe, is the keystone in the nurse-client relationship (Pearson & Raeke, 2000). Trust provides a nonthreatening interpersonal climate in which the client feels comfortable revealing his or her needs to the nurse. The nurse is perceived as dependable. Establishment of this trust is crucial toward enabling you to make an accurate assessment of your client's needs.

Trust is also the key to establishing workable relationships (Bakir, 2000). For example, one study of Canadian nurses showed that trust in the employing agency was an important element in determining employee performance and commitment (Laschinger, 2000). According to Erikson (1963), trust is developed by experiencing consistency, sameness, and continuity during care by a familiar caregiver. Trust develops based on past experiences. In the nurse-client relationship, maintaining an open exchange of information contributes to trust. For the client, trust implies a willingness to place oneself in a position of vulnerability, relying on health providers to perform as expected. Trust appears as attitudes such as respect, honesty, consistency, faith, caring, and hope (Johns, 1996). Certain interpersonal strategies help promote a trusting relationship (Box 6-1).

Box 6-1 Techniques Designed to Promote Trust

- Convey respect.
- Consider the client's uniqueness.
- Show warmth and caring.
- Use the client's proper name.
- Use active listening.
- Give sufficient time to answer questions.
- Maintain confidentiality.
- Show congruence between verbal and nonverbal behaviors.
- Use a warm, friendly voice.
- Use appropriate eye contact.
- Smile.
- Be flexible.
- Provide for allowed preferences.
- Be honest and open.
- Give complete information.
- Provide consistency.
- Plan schedules.
- Follow through on commitments.
- Set limits.
- Control distractions.
- Use an attending posture: arms, legs, and body relaxed; leaning slightly forward.

Barrier: Mistrust. Mistrust has an impact not only on communication but also on healing process outcomes. Trust can be replaced with mistrust between nurse and client. Just as some agency managers treat employees as though they are not trustworthy (Johns, 1996), some nurses treat some clients as though they are misbehaving children. Such would be the case if a client fails to follow the treatment regimen and is labeled with the nursing

Exercise 6-2 Techniques that Promote Trust

Purpose: To identify techniques that promote the establishment of trust and to provide practice in using these skills.

Procedure:

1. Read the list of interpersonal techniques designed to promote trust.
2. Describe the relationship with your most recent client. Was there a trusting relationship? How do you know? Which techniques did you use? Which ones could you have used?

or

In triads, have one learner interview a second to obtain a health history, while the third observes and records trusting behaviors. Rotate so that everyone is an interviewer. Interviews should last five minutes each. At the end of 15 minutes, each observer shares findings with the corresponding interviewer.

Discussion:

Compare techniques.

diagnosis of "noncompliant." In other examples, the community health nurse who is inconsistent about keeping client appointments, or the pediatric nurse who indicates falsely that an injection will not hurt, are both jeopardizing client trust. It is hard to maintain trust when one person cannot depend on another. Energy that should be directed toward coping with health problems is rechanneled into assessing the nurse's commitment and trustworthiness. Having confidence in the nurse's skills, commitment, and caring allows the client to place full attention on the situation requiring resolution. Clients can also jeopardize the trust a nurse has in them. Sometimes clients "test" a nurse's trustworthiness by sending the nurse on unnecessary errands or talking endlessly on superficial topics. As long as nurses recognize testing behaviors and set clear limits on their roles and the client's role, it is possible to develop trust. Exercise 6-2 is designed to help students become more familiar with the concept of trust.

Empathy

Empathy is the ability to be sensitive to and communicate understanding of the client's feelings. It is a crucial characteristic of a helping relationship (May & Alligood, 2000; Reynolds et al., 2000). An empathetic nurse perceives and *understands* the client's emotions *accurately*. Empathy is the ability to put oneself into the client's position. Some nurses might term this as compassion, which has been identified by staff nurses as being crucial to the nurse-client relationship (Armstrong, Parsons, & Barker, 2000; May & Alligood, 2000). Communication skills are used to convey respect and empathy. Although expert nurses feel the emotions a client feels, they hold onto their objectivity, maintaining their own separate identities. As a nurse, you should try not to overidentify with or internalize the feelings of the client. If internalization occurs, objectivity is lost, along with the ability to help the client move through his or her feelings. It is important to recognize that the client's feelings belong to the client, not to you. Communicate your understanding of the meaning of a client's feelings by using both verbal and nonverbal communication behaviors. Validate the meaning of these feelings with the client.

Levels of Empathy. Attaining high levels of empathy is rewarding to both nurse and client. Carkhuff (1969) identified five levels of empathy. Use the information listed in Table 6-1 to understand the following case.

Table 6-1 Levels of Nursing Actions

Level	Category	Nursing Behavior
1	Accepting	Uses client's correct name Maintains eye contact Adopts open posture Responds to cues
2	Listening	Nods head Smiles Encourages responses Uses therapeutic silence
3	Clarifying	Asks open-ended questions Restates the problem Validates perceptions Acknowledges confusion
	Informing	Provides honest, complete answers Assesses client's knowledge level Summarizes
4–5	Analyzing	Identifies unknown emotions Interprets underlying meanings Confronts conflict

Level 1. *Unawareness of the client's message of feelings* is the lowest level of empathy. Because there is no evidence of active listening or understanding of the client's feelings, the nurse's response communicates significantly less than the client's does.

Case Example

Client (frantic): **Jamal [10 months old] has had a terrible cold for more than a week.**

Nurse (hurriedly, not looking at client): **Is he up-to-date on his immunizations?**

In this example, the nurse ignores the feeling tone of the client and changes the subject to obtain the desired information. The nurse's insensitivity may arise from boredom, lack of interest, bias, a heavy workload, or other reasons.

Level 2. *Superficial acknowledgment of the client's message* minimizes the client's feelings. The nurse shows awareness of superficial feelings but responds in a way that noticeably ignores the client's emotions.

Case Example

Client (frantic): Jamal [10 months old] has had a terrible cold for more than a week.

Nurse (with a casual glance): This is the time of year for colds. Everyone has one. He'll get over it.

In this example, the nurse responds to the content of the statement but not to the feeling tone of the client. The nurse minimizes the client's feelings.

Level 3. *Recognition of the client's message and some of the client's feelings* is somewhat helpful. In Level 3, the nurse responds to the meaning of the client's emotions. Verbal and nonverbal behaviors are congruent. The nurse's words reflect the client's concerns and feelings.

Case Example

Client (frantic): Jamal [10 months old] has had a terrible cold for more than a week.

Nurse (tone the same as the client's, making eye contact, leaning forward in chair): You're upset that Jamal has had this cold for more than a week.

Client (crying): Yeah. He's so little, and I want him to get better.

Nurse (breaking eye contact): He'll get better. The nurse practitioner will be in soon to examine him.

The nurse's first response shows a Level 3 empathy. The nurse accurately interprets the superficial feeling tone of client. Because the nurse seems to understand, the client feels free to provide more information. The nurse then reverts to a Level 2 response, however, and essentially ignores the client's tears. Level 3 responses are often a prelude to higher-level responses, which reflect the client's hidden emotions. Nurses who are unable to cope with deep feelings are unable to develop empathy beyond Levels 2 and 3.

Level 4. *Acknowledgment of the message and obvious feelings* demonstrates the nurse's willingness to understand and care about the client's concerns. Although there are still deep, hidden meanings of which the nurse is unaware, there is a forum for discussion. The nurse probes for information to expand the client's awareness and the nurse's understanding of the situation.

Case Example

Client (frantic): Jamal [10 months old] has had a terrible cold for more than a week.

Nurse (same voice tone as client, making eye contact, with attending, open posture): You are quite upset about this, aren't you?

Client (softly, spoken with tears): Yes. He's so little, and he just has to get better.

Nurse: You're afraid it might develop into something worse? (*Level 4*)

Client: Could he have pneumonia?

Nurse: I don't know. The nurse practitioner will examine him soon. How would you feel if he had pneumonia? (*Gathering data*)

Client: Oh, I couldn't stand to have him in the hospital away from me.

Nurse: You feel anxious about the possibility of hospitalization, in which the two of you would be separated, and what it might do to your close relationship. (*Level 4*)

Client: Yes, being separated would be awful.

In this example, the nurse begins responding on Level 3 and then moves to Level 4 responses. The nurse has not accurately perceived deeper feelings but gathers more data, which increases knowledge about the client and thus increases the probability of an accurate assessment of emotions.

Level 5. *Full therapeutic acknowledgment of the client's hidden message and meaning* adds significantly to the meanings behind the feelings. Because the nurse has a clearer, more objective view than the client, the nurse is able to state deep, hidden feelings unknown to the client.

Case Example

(Continued from previous example.)

Client: Oh, I couldn't stand to have him in the hospital away from me.

Nurse: What is it about the hospital separation from Jamal that makes you so anxious? (*Reflects hidden feelings, asks for more information*)

Client: It's just his being in the hospital.

Nurse (questions, still same feeling tone): Have you or anyone close to you been in the hospital?

Client: My brother, when he was young.

Nurse (seeking more information): And what was he there for?

Client: Pneumonia. He died there of complications!
Nurse: So now you're frightened that if Jamal has pneumonia and is hospitalized, he will die too, like your brother. (*Reflects deep feelings*)

Now that the nurse has full information, the interventions are more likely to address the client's individualized needs directly. The nurse then goes on to give information about pneumonia and provide reassurance that it is treatable. Armed with accurate data, the nurse can communicate the client's feelings to the physician so that the physician can discuss Jamal's diagnosis and treatment with the client to lessen the client's anxiety.

Barrier: Lack of Empathy. Failure to understand the needs of clients may lead the nurse to fail to provide essential client education. Or the nurse may fail to pro-

Exercise 6-3 Identifying Empathetic Responses

Purpose: To correctly identify levels of empathy for clinical situations.

Procedure:
Read the client statement, and then identify the nurse's response as to the correct empathy level (1, 2, 3, 4, or 5); place the number on the line to the left of the response.

1. *Client (on the verge of tears):* That doctor confused me so. He was in here for 10 minutes and I still don't know what's wrong with me.
Nurse:

_____ a. Doctors like that ought to give up medicine.

_____ b. You feel the doctor was confusing and didn't explain your medical problem.

_____ c. What time is it now?

_____ d. You're angry that the doctor was unable to adequately explain your medical condition.

_____ e. You feel exasperated about not knowing your current medical problem and helpless in knowing what you should do to take care of yourself.

2. *Client (in a hostile voice):* I'm sick of being poked at and stuck with needles. Go away and leave me alone.
Nurse:

_____ a. You're fed up with needles and wish to be left alone.

_____ b. Getting needles is part of being in the hospital.

_____ c. You're angry about having all these intrusive procedures and wish you didn't need them.

_____ d. Just remember to fill out your menu for tomorrow.

_____ e. With all these intrusive procedures, you feel vulnerable and defenseless, ready to go hide to get away from it all.

Exercise 6-4 Evaluating Mutuality

Purpose: To identify behaviors and feelings on the part of the nurse and the client that indicate mutuality.

Procedure:
Complete the following questions by answering yes or no after terminating with a client; then bring it to class. Discuss the answers. How were you able to attain mutuality, or why were you unable to attain it?

1. Was I satisfied with the relationship?
2. Did the client express satisfaction with the relationship?
3. Did the client share feelings with me?
4. Did I make decisions for the client?
5. Did the client feel allowed to make his or her own decisions?
6. Did the client accomplish his or her goals?
7. Did I accomplish my goals?

Discussion:
In large group, discuss mutuality.

vide needed emotional support. The literature indicates that major barriers to empathy exist in the clinical environment, including lack of time, lack of trust, lack of privacy, or lack of support from other professional colleagues (Reynolds et al., 2000). Several studies suggest that lack of empathy will result in less favorable health outcomes. Exercise 6-3 will help clarify information about empathetic responses.

Mutuality

Mutuality basically means that the nurse and the client agree on the client's health problems and the means for resolving them, and that both parties are committed to enhancing the client's well-being. This is characterized by mutual respect for the autonomy and value system of the other. In developing mutuality, the nurse maximizes the client's involvement in all phases of the nursing process. Mutuality is collaboration in problem solving.

Mutuality encompasses all phases of the nursing process and enriches nurse-client relationships. Evidence of mutuality is seen in the development of individualized client goals and nursing actions that meet a client's unique health needs. Exercise 6-4 gives practice in evaluating mutuality.

Nurses who respect differences between their own lifestyles and those of others have the capacity to attain mutuality in relationships. Such nurses involve clients in the decision-making process. They accept the decisions even if they do not agree with them. Effective use of values clarification as described in Chapter 3 assists clients in decision making. As discussed in this chapter, clients who clearly identify their own personal values are better able to solve problems effectively. Decisions then have meaning to the client, who thus has a higher probability of taking steps to achieve success. When a mutual relationship is terminated, both parties experience a sense of shared accomplishment and satisfaction.

Ethically-Based Professional Values of Veracity, Confidentiality, Autonomy, Justice, and Beneficence

As mentioned in Chapter 2, legal and ethical standards mandate specific nursing behaviors. These behaviors are based on professional nursing values that stem from the ethical principles described in Chapter 3. By adhering to these "rules," nurses build their therapeutic relationships with individual clients.

Veracity contributes to the establishment of a therapeutic relationship. When the client knows he or she can expect the truth from the nurse, the development of trust is promoted and helps build the relationship.

Confidentiality protects the client's right to decide who can have access to information about any aspect of health care or lifestyle. The client can feel reassured that the nurse generally will not divulge private information. Giving information is one way the client invests in the therapeutic relationship.

Information obtained through professional interviewing and history taking is used by the nurse and other health team members to arrive at an individualized client care plan. Relevant health-related data become a part of the client's permanent health record. Emphasis is placed on *pertinent* information. Recorded client data should be neither too sketchy nor too detailed. Information, especially confidential information, that does not contribute to the management of the client's care should not be included in the record. Data about the client or client's condition are not shared with the client's family or health professionals who are not directly involved in the client's care without the competent client's consent.

Confidentially and its legal and ethical limitations are discussed in Chapter 3. The nurse can explain that the client's record is kept where only members of the health team have access to it, and after discharge, is filed in medical records to help ensure the client's privacy. However, in this era of managed care, both nurses and their clients need to be aware that a number of agencies routinely audit records for both quality control and for financial payment requisites. Exercise 6-5 gives more information on confidentiality.

Barrier: Violations of Confidentiality. Confidentiality is breached if conversations are heard by other clients, visitors, or anyone else not involved in the direct care of the client. When conference rooms are unavailable for the sharing of sensitive information among client, nurse, and family, the nurse may close the door to the client's room. Perhaps an ambulatory roommate could be asked to leave the room if there is another place on the unit where clients are allowed to congregate.

The advent of computerized client information constitutes a new problem in the confidentiality issue. Once the information is entered into the computer, the nurse may not know under what circumstances it will be accessed. This is discussed in Chapter 23.

There are a few instances in which confidentiality is waived and clients are not allowed to restrict information to persons they approve or to those who have direct contact with their care. These are cases of suspicion of abuse of minors or elders, commission of a crime, or threat of harm to oneself or another person. Courts may also subpoena client records without the client's permission. Apart from these situations, the courts consider all communication between nurse and client as privileged communication.

Barriers to the Relationship

Many barriers described above affect the development of the nurse-client relationship. A few additional barriers

Exercise 6-5 Confidentiality and Setting

Purpose: To identify situations that are a breach of confidentiality and then to correct them.

Procedure:

Take one of the following situations, all of which depict a breach of confidentiality. In a group, do the following:

1. State how confidentiality has been broken.
2. Given the situation, what might be an appropriate response?

Situations:

1. You are eating lunch in the cafeteria with two fellow pediatric nurses who are discussing the behaviors of an abusive parent.
2. A nurse yells down the hall to you, "Your patient in 504 is ready to get off the bedpan."
3. On the postpartum unit, a nurse allows a husband to see his wife's chart.
4. You are riding in the elevator when two operating room nurses step on and comment, "It took four of us to tie him down for that IV."
5. You are on rounds. One physician, leaning over a client, suddenly remembers an order on another client and says, "Don't forget Mrs. Smith's enema. Give her a Fleet's enema this morning."

need your attention. Specifically, barriers in addition to the ones identified in the previous section include anxiety, stereotyping, and lack of personal space. Barriers inherent in the health care system are also commonly discussed in the professional literature. Under managed care, barriers often reflect cost-containment measures. Such barriers include lack of consistent assignment of nurse to client and increased use of temporary staff such as agency nurses or "floats." Lack of time can result from low staff-client ratios, but more often reflects the marked increase in early discharge or same-day (outpatient) surgeries. The primary care literature describes agency demand for minimal appointment time with clients. Primary care providers such as nurse practitioners are often constrained to focus just on the chief complaint to maximize the number of clients seen, leading to "the 15-minute office visit." Other system barriers include communication conflicts with other health professionals, conflicting values, poor physical arrangements, and lack of value placed on caring by for-profit agencies. These system barriers limit the nurse's ability to develop substantial rapport with clients. Adequate time is essential to develop therapeutic communication to achieve effective care responsive to client needs (Naish, 1996).

Anxiety

Anxiety is a vague, persistent feeling of impending doom. It is a universal feeling; no one fully escapes it. The impact on the self is always uncomfortable. It occurs when a threat (real or imagined) to one's self-concept is perceived. Anxiety is usually observed through the physical and behavioral manifestations of the attempt to relieve the anxious feelings. Although individuals experiencing anxiety may not know they are anxious, specific behaviors provide clues that anxiety is present. Similarly, although individuals may not be consciously aware of the factors that contribute to the anxiety-producing situation, others may be able to help them identify those factors, thus alleviating the anxiety. Exercise 6-6 identifies behaviors associated with anxiety. Four levels of anxiety are identified by Kreigh and Perko (1983). Expanding on this information, Table 6-2 shows how an individual's sensory perceptions, cognitive abilities, coping skills, and behaviors relate to the intensity and level of anxiety experienced.

A mild level of anxiety heightens one's awareness of the surrounding environment and fosters learning and decision making. Therefore, it may be desirable to allow a mild degree of anxiety when health teaching is needed or when problem solving is necessary. It is not prudent, however, to prolong even a mild state of anxiety.

However, higher levels of anxiety decreases perceptual ability. The anxious state is accompanied by verbal and nonverbal behaviors that inhibit effective individual functioning. For example, anxiety causes you to hold your breath, which can lead to even greater levels of anxiety

Exercise 6-6 Identifying Verbal and Nonverbal Behaviors Associated with Anxiety

Purpose: To broaden the learner's awareness of behavioral responses that indicate anxiety.

Procedure:

List as many anxious behaviors as you can think of. Each column has a few examples to start. Discuss the lists in a group, and add new behaviors to your list.

Verbal	Nonverbal
Quavering voice	Nail biting
Rapid speech	Foot tapping
Mumbling	Sweating
Defensive words	Pacing

Table 6-2 Levels of Anxiety with Degree of Sensory Perceptions, Cognitive and Coping Abilities, and Manifest Behaviors

Level of Anxiety	Sensory Perceptions	Cognitive/Coping Ability	Behavior
Mild	Heightened state of alertness; increased acuity of hearing, vision, smell, touch	Enhanced learning, problem solving; increased ability to respond and adapt to changing stimuli; enhanced functioning*	Walking, singing, eating, drinking, mild restlessness, active listening, attending, questioning
Moderate	Decreased sensory perceptions; with guidance, able to expand sensory fields	Loss of concentration; decreased cognitive ability; cannot identify factors contributing to the anxiety-producing situation; with directions can cope, reduce anxiety, and solve problems; inhibited functioning	Increased muscle tone, pulse, respirations; changes in voice tone and pitch, rapid speech, incomplete verbal responses; engrossed with detail
Severe	Greatly diminished perceptions; decreased sensitivity to pain	Limited thought processes; unable to solve problems even with guidance; cannot cope with stress without help; confused mental state; limited functioning	Purposeless, aimless behaviors; rapid pulse, respirations; high blood pressure; hyperventilation; inappropriate or incongruent verbal responses
Panic	No response to sensory perceptions	No cognitive or coping abilities; without intervention, death is imminent	Immobilization

*Functioning refers to the ability to perform activities of daily living for survival purposes.

(Puetz, 2005). Moderate to severe anxiety on the part of either nurse or client hinders the development of the therapeutic relationship. To accomplish goals and attain mutuality, higher levels of anxiety must be reduced. Once the presence of anxiety has been identified, the nurse needs to take appropriate action. Strategies to reduce anxiety are listed in Box 6-2.

Severe anxiety requires medical and psychiatric intervention to alleviate the stress. A prolonged panic state is incompatible with life. It is such an extreme level of anxiety that, without immediate medical and psychiatric assistance, suicide or homicide may ensue. Some of these interpersonal strategies used to reduce moderate anxiety also are used during severe anxiety and panic attacks as part of a team approach to client care.

Choosing from various strategies to reduce client anxiety can be difficult. Not all methods are appropriate or work equally well with all clients. If a nurse attempting to build trust pushes a client too fast into revealing what he or she is not yet ready to discuss, this can increase anxiety (Reynolds et al., 2000). Nurses need to accurately identify their client's level of anxiety, but they

Box 6-2 Nursing Strategies to Reduce Client Anxiety

- Active listening to show acceptance
- Honesty; answering all questions at the client's level of understanding
- Clearly explaining procedures, surgery, and policies, and giving appropriate reassurance based on data
- Acting in a calm, unhurried manner
- Speaking clearly, firmly (but not loudly)
- Giving information regarding lab tests, medications, treatments, and rationale for restrictions on activity
- Setting reasonable limits and providing structure
- Encouraging clients to explore reasons for the anxiety
- Encouraging self-affirmation through positive statements such as "I will," "I can"
- Using play therapy with dolls, puppets, and games
- Drawing for young clients
- Using therapeutic touch, giving warm baths, back rub
- Initiating recreational activities such as physical exercise, music, card games, board games, crafts, reading
- Teaching breathing and relaxation exercises
- Using guided imagery
- Practicing covert rehearsal

From Gerrard B, Boniface W, Love B: *Interpersonal skills for health professionals*, Reston, VA, 1980, Reston Publishing.

should also identify and reduce their own anxiety to help the client fully. Because anxiety can cloud one's perceptions, it interferes with relationships.

Stereotyping and Bias

Stereotyping is the process of attributing characteristics to a group of people as though all persons in the identified group possessed them. People may be stereotyped according to ethnic origin, culture, religion, social class, occupation, age, and other factors. Even health issues can be the stimulus for stereotyping individuals. For example, alcoholism, mental illness, and **sexually transmitted** diseases are fertile grounds for the development of stereotypes. Stereotypes have been shown to be consistent across cultures and somewhat across generations, although the value placed on a stereotype changes.

Stereotypes are learned during childhood and reinforced by life experiences. They may carry positive or negative connotations (e.g., all Jewish people are successful or not in business, or all Hispanics are honest or dishonest). Nurses may have personal biases based on conscious or often unconscious past learning. They may act on these unknowingly. Stereotypes negate empathy and erode the nurse-client relationship. Nurses must work to develop insight into their own expectations and prejudgments about people.

Stereotypes are never completely accurate: there are always variations within any group. All of us like to think that our way is the correct way and that everyone else thinks about life experiences just as we do. The reality is that there are many roads in life, and one road is not necessarily any better than another.

Emotions play a role in the value we place on negative stereotypes. Stereotypes based on strong emotions are called **prejudices**. Highly emotionally charged stereotypes are less amenable to change. In the extreme, this can result in discrimination. **Discrimination** is used to describe actions in which a person is denied a legit-

Exercise 6-7 Reducing Clinical Bias by Identifying Stereotypes

Purpose: To identify examples of nursing biases that need to be reduced. Practice in identifying professional stereotypes and in how to reduce them is one component of maintaining high-quality nursing care.

Procedure:

Each of the following scenarios indicates a stereotype. Identify the stereotype and how it might affect nursing care. As a nurse, what would you do to reduce the bias in the situation? Are there any individuals or groups of people for whom you would not want to provide care (e.g., homeless women with foul body odor and dirty nails)?

Situation A

Mrs. Daniels, an obstetric nurse who believes in birth control, comments about her client, "Mrs. Gonzales is pregnant again. You know, the one with six kids already! It makes me sick to see these people on welfare taking away from our tax dollars. I don't know how she can continue to do this."

Situation B

Mrs. Brown, a registered nurse on a medical unit, is upset with her 52-year-old female client. "If she rings that buzzer one more time, I'm going to disconnect it. Can't she understand that I have other clients who need my attention more than she does? She just lies in bed all day long. And she's so fat; she's never going to lose any weight that way."

Situation C

Mrs. Waters, a staff nurse in a nursing home, listens to the daughter of a 93-year-old resident, who says, "My mother, who is confused most of the time, receives very little attention from you nurses, while other clients who are lucid and clear-minded have more interaction with you. It's not fair! No wonder my mother is so far out in space. Nobody talks to her. Nobody ever comes in to say hello."

imate opportunity offered to others because of prejudice (Kavanaugh, 1991). Victims often suffer social isolation, distress, or difficulty finding employment (Crisp, Geider, Rix et al., 2000).

If nurses bring their biases with them to the clinical situation, they will distort their perception and prevent client change and growth. To reduce bias in clinical situations, nurses need first to recognize clients as unique individuals, both different from and similar to themselves. Acceptance of the other person needs to be total. This unconditional acceptance (described by Rogers in 1961) is an essential element in the helping relationship. It does not imply agreement or approval; acceptance occurs without judgment. The nurse who uses a nonjudgmental attitude with neutral responses conveys acceptance and develops meaningful client relationships. Mr. Fred Rogers, the children's television show host, ended his programs by telling his audience, "I like you just the way you are." How wonderful if we, as nurses, could convey this type of acceptance to our clients through our words and actions. Exercise 6-7 examines ways of reducing clinical bias.

Overinvolvement as a Boundary Violation

Objectivity is important if you are to provide competent, professional care (Sheldon, 2004). Sharing too much information about yourself or about your other clients can be a possible barrier if your client becomes unclear about his or her role in your relationship. A client may feel that if you are talking about other clients, you might also be talking to others about him or her. Vandegaer (2000) writes that the nurse making home health care visits might especially be likely to share irritations or job problems while in a client's home, especially if professional boundaries are blurred with social invitations to events such as family weddings and parties. She states that boundary violations are more common when the relationship is a long-term one. Many of us enjoy warm relationships with our clients, but if we are to remain effective, we need to be alert to the disadvantages of overinvolvement.

Violation of Personal Space

Personal space is an invisible boundary around an individual. The emotional personal space boundary provides a sense of comfort and protection. It is defined by past experiences, current circumstances, and our culture.

Proxemics is the study of an individual's use of space. Davis (1984) described optimal territorial space needed by most individuals living in western culture: 86 to 108 square feet of personal space. Other research has found that 60 square feet is the minimum needed for each client in multiple-occupancy rooms, and 80 square feet is the minimum for private rooms in hospitals and institutions. Critical care units offer even less square footage.

Among the many factors that affect the individual's need for personal distance are cultural dictates. In some cultures, people approach each other closely, whereas in others, more personal space is required. In most culures, men need more space than women do. People generally need less space in the morning. The elderly need more control over their space, whereas small children generally like to touch and be touched by others. Although the elderly appreciate human touch, they generally do not like it to be applied indiscriminately. Situational anxiety causes a need for more space. Persons with low self-esteem prefer more space as well as some control over who enters their space and in what manner. Usually people will tolerate a person standing close to them at their side more readily than directly in front of them. Direct eye contact causes a need for more space. Placing oneself at the same level (e.g., sitting while the client is sitting, or standing at eye level when the client is standing) allows the nurse more access to the client's personal space because such a stance is perceived as less threatening. Exercise 6-8 helps identify individual needs for personal space.

Hospitals are not home. Many of the diagnostic and treatment procedures that must be instituted in providing nursing care represent a direct intrusion into the personal space of the client. Commonly, procedures requiring tubes (e.g., nasal gastric intubation, administration of oxygen, catheterization, and intravenous initiation) restrict the mobility of the client and the client's sense of control over personal territory. When more than one health professional is involved in implementing the procedures, the impact of the intrusion on the client may be even stronger. In many instances, personal space requirements are an integral part of a person's self-image. When a person loses control over personal space, he or she may experience a loss of individuality, self-identity, and self-esteem. Maintain a social physical body distance of 4 feet when not actually giving care to avoid sending a message that may be interpreted as a desire for intimacy. Consider the issue of respect for

Exercise 6-8 Personal Space Differences

Purpose: To identify individual needs for personal space among different client populations.

Procedure:
Following is a list of factors affecting personal space. Each has a clinical example. Write another example (clinical or personal) for each factor.

1. Culture
   Mrs. Hopi, a Native American who is in the intensive care unit for a heart attack, is surrounded by her family and tribe members throughout her stay in the hospital. Would your family insist on being with you?
2. Sex
   Mr. Smith, a retired steel worker, greets his community health nurse with a smile and a gesture to enter his apartment. His ailing wife greets the nurse with outstretched arms and a kiss. If Mr. Smith greeted you this way, would your response be different?
3. Degree of acquaintance
   The nurse meets Mrs. Parker at the prenatal clinic for the first time. They maintain a distance of 5 feet during the initial interview. How far away would you sit?
4. Situational anxiety
   Mrs. Cook just returned from a brain scan, and she is quite anxious about the results. As the nurse attempts to comfort Mrs. Cook by placing her hand on Mrs. Cook's arm, Mrs. Cook snatches her hand away and retorts, "Just leave me alone."

Discussion:

1. What is your own preferred space distance? To what do you attribute this preference?
2. Under what circumstances do your needs for personal space change?

personal space in the clinical examples presented in Box 6-3.

When institutionalized clients are able to incorporate parts of their rooms into their personal space, it increases their self-esteem and helps them to maintain a sense of identity. This feeling of security is evidenced when a client asks, "Close my door, please." Freedom from worry about personal space allows the client to trust the nurse and fosters a therapeutic relationship. When invasions of personal space are necessary and occur while performing a procedure, the nurse can minimize their impact by explaining why a procedure is needed. Conversation with clients at such times reinforces their feelings that they are human beings worthy of respect and not just objects being worked on. Advocating for the client's personal space needs is an aspect of the nursing role. This is done by communicating client preferences to the members of the health team and including them in the client's care plan.

Home is not quite home when the home health nurse, infusion nurse, or other aides invade the client's personal space. Some modification of the nurse's "take charge" behavior is required when giving care in a client's home.

Nurses should be aware of their own space needs. Nurses who need more space themselves may feel uncomfortable entering a client's intimate space. Nursing actions that promote privacy and respect for the client's personal space will increase the nurse's sense of space.

Cultural Barriers

Cross-cultural communication is discussed extensively in Chapter 11. Cultural competence requires us to become aware of the arbitrary nature of our own cultural beliefs. True cultural competence is characterized by a willingness to try to understand and respond to our client's beliefs (Brody & Hunt, 2005).

Gender Differences?

The popular culture has recently given more attention to the notion that barriers exist when persons of the opposite gender try to communicate; however, no conclusive

Box 6-3 Clinical Examples of Personal Space Issues for Clients

- The nurse places the client on the bedpan without drawing the curtain on a postpartum unit. When the client protests, the nurse states, "Well, we're all girls here."
- The chief resident comes in with an entourage of residents and medical students. They draw the curtain and the chief resident, standing close to the client, informs the client that his cancer is terminal. The entourage moves on to the next client.
- Miss Jones has just been brought to the emergency room as a rape victim. Because of the circumstances, she is unable to change her clothes until she has been examined. It is an unusually busy night in the emergency room, and the policy is to practice triage and treat the most serious cases first. Because Miss Jones is not considered an emergency case, it will be some time before she is examined.
- Dr. Michaels has had an auto accident for which he is receiving emergency treatment by a multidisciplinary team. He is conscious, but no one calls him by name or seems to notice his wife standing outside the door.
- Barbara Burk has just been admitted to a psychiatric unit. The policy on the unit is to keep all valuables, razors, hand mirrors, and money locked up in the nurse's station. All clients must strip and shower under supervision soon after they arrive on the unit. It was not Barbara's choice to seek inpatient treatment, and she is very scared.
- Mr. Novack is admitted to the coronary care unit. He is hooked up to a cardioscope so his cardiac condition can be monitored continuously, and nasal oxygen is applied. The defibrillator is located close to his bed. His family is allowed to come in one at a time for five minutes once every hour as long as the visits do not interfere with nursing care or necessary treatment procedures.

Developing an Evidence-Based Practice

Jack S: *Engagement between mothers with children at-risk of developmental delays, public health nurses and family visitors in a blended home visiting program*, doctoral dissertation, McGill University, Toronto, 2004.

Though a hundred years of professional nursing has given us intuitive experience in building interpersonal relationships with clients and families, we are still developing a scientific basis for recommendations as to how to establish and maintain therapeutic relationships. This was a phenomenological (qualitative) study meant to identify and describe factors that influence these relationships. The working relationship between care providers making home visits and the mothers of infants at risk for developmental delays were observed.

Results: During a series of home visits, the 20 mothers who were interviewed identified a three-phase process:

1. Overcoming their vulnerability fears
2. Building trust
3. Seeking mutuality

Many factors affected the speed of development of the relationship, including visitor personality characteristics and the mothers' past experiences. Maintaining the relationship was influenced by the family perceptions about how valuable the visits were and the mother's ability to identify some short-term benefits from them.

Application to Your Clinical Practice: While this is a small study, findings do suggest that it is important to help the client recognize specific benefits that they have gained by maintaining their relationship with a visiting nurse. Do you think this evidence is strong enough to support Sheldon's statement (2004), quoted earlier in this chapter, that the need to establish trust is the foundation of the relationship? Does trust need to be established before mutuality?

research evidence exists showing that gender differences obstruct the therapeutic relationship. In fact, studies have been done that show little communication or primary outcome difference based on the gender of the care provider (van Dulmen & Bensing, 2000). Some physician studies report higher client satisfaction with female physicians, whereas others report higher satisfaction when both parties are of the same gender (Bernzweig, Takyama, Phibbs et al., 1997; Roter, Geller, Bernhardt et al., 1999). Although women have traditionally been considered to have more or better-developed communication skills, Colliver, Vu, Marcy, and others (1993) found in their study of medical students that male and female senior medical students performed equally well with respect to interpersonal and communication skills. In summary, although results are mixed, it appears that gender need not be a factor in developing therapeutic communication with clients.

APPLICATIONS

Many nursing actions recommended here are mandated by the American Nurses Association Code of Ethics for Nurses discussed in Chapter 2. The actions specified include confidentiality, autonomy, beneficence, veracity, and justice. Mutuality is addressed in the ANA position statement on human rights.

Steps in the Caring Process

Several articles identify four steps to help you communicate caring to your client (Clayton, 1991; Keller & Baker, 2000):

C = First *connect* with your client. *Offer your attention.* Here you introduce your purpose in developing a relationship with the client (i.e., meeting the client's health needs). Use the client's formal name, and avoid terms of endearment such as "sweetie." Show an intent to care.

A = The second step is to *appreciate* the client's situation. Although the health care environment is familiar to you, it is a strange and perhaps frightening situation for your client. Acknowledge his or her point of view and express concern.

R = The third step is to *respond* to what your client needs. What are his or her priorities? Expectations for health care?

E = The fourth step is to *empower* the client to problem solve with you. Here the client gains strength and confidence from the mutual experience while moving toward achievement of client outcomes.

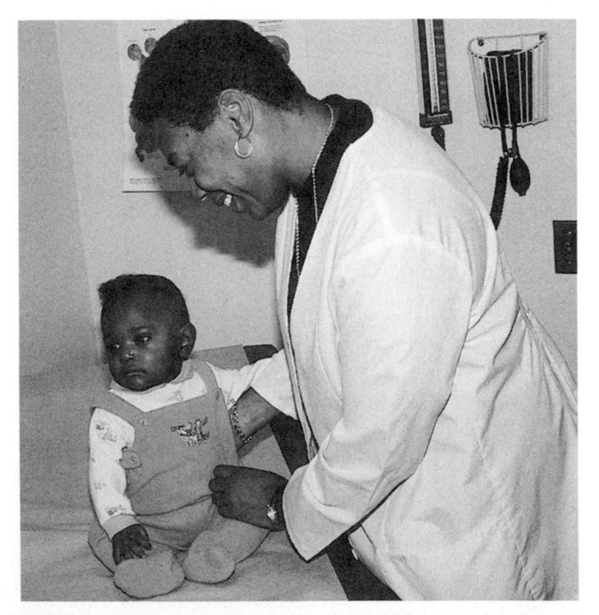

Infants lack verbal communication skills. The nurse's comforting touch and pleasant vocal tone help overcome this barrier. (Courtesy Adam Boggs.)

The ability to become a caring professional is influenced by your previous experiences. A person who has received caring is more likely to be able to offer it to others. Caring should not be confused with caretaking. Although caretaking is a part of caring, it may lack the necessary intentional giving of self. Self-awareness about feelings, attitudes, values, and skills is essential for developing an effective, caring relationship.

Strategies for Empowerment

Your method for empowering your clients should include the following key strategies (Skinner & Cradock, 2000; Spalding, 2000):

- *Accept* your client as he or she is by refraining from any negative judgments.
- *Explore the client's feelings* about his or her condition, discussing issues that may interfere with self-care.
- Form an alliance with the client, *mutually deciding* about his or her care.
- Reinforce the client's *autonomy*, for example, by allowing him or her to choose the content in your teaching plan.
- *Offer information* in an environment that enables him or her to use it.
- Make sure the client *actively participates* in the care plan.
- Clarify that the client holds the major *responsibility* for both the health care decisions he or she makes and their consequences.

We may never fully understand the decisions some clients make, but we support their right to do so.

Application of Empathy to Levels of Nursing Actions

Nursing actions that facilitate empathy are classified by Gazda (1987) into three major skills: (a) recognition and classification of requests; (b) attending behaviors; and (c) empathetic responses. Two types of requests are for information and action. These requests do not involve interpersonal concerns and are easier to manage. Another form of request is for understanding involvement, which entails the client's need for empathetic understanding. This type of request requires greater interpersonal skills. It can be misinterpreted as a request for action or information. The nurse may have to clarify whether the client needs only what he or she specifically asks for, or whether further exploration of the meaning of the need is necessary.

Attending behaviors facilitate empathy and include an attentive, open posture; responding to verbal and nonverbal cues through appropriate gestures and facial expressions; using eye contact; and allowing client self-expression. They also include offering time and attention, showing interest in the client's issues, offering helpful information, and clarifying problem areas. These responses encourage clients to participate in their own healing.

The third major skill is empathetic response. The nurse helps the client identify emotions that are not readily observable and connect them with the current situation. Using the actions listed in Table 6-1, the nurse uses attending behaviors and nursing actions to express empathy. Verbal prompts, such as, "Hmm," "Uh-huh," "I see," "Tell me more," and "Go on" facilitate expression of feelings. The nurse uses open-ended questions to validate perceptions. Using informing behaviors listed in Table 6-1 enlarges the database by providing new information. If the client's condition prevents use of familiar communication strategies to demonstrate empathy, the nurse can use alternative strategies. Use of techniques such as validation or touch may demonstrate empathy and help avoid frustration (Feil, 1996).

Reduction of Barriers in Nurse-Client Relationships

Recognition of barriers is the first step in eliminating them and thus enhancing the process of developing a therapeutic professional relationship. Practice with exercises in this chapter should help recognition of possible barriers. Findings from many studies, including the Keatinge et al. (2002) study of Australian nurses, emphasize the crucial importance of honesty, cultural sensitivity, and caring, especially in listening actively to suggestions and complaints from client and family. Refer to Box 6-4 for a summary of strategies to reduce barriers to the nurse-client relationship.

Box 6-4 Tips to Reduce Relationship Barriers

- Establish trust.
- Demonstrate caring and empathy.
- Empower the client.
- Recognize and reduce client anxiety.
- Maintain appropriate personal distance.
- Practice cultural sensitivity and work to be bilingual.
- Use therapeutic relationship-building activities such as active listening.
- Avoid medical jargon.

Respect for Personal Space

Before providing care, the nurse needs to assess the client's personal space needs. A comprehensive assessment includes cultural and developmental factors affecting the client's perceptions of space, how the client reacts to intrusions, how the client defends personal space, and nonverbal behaviors that may indicate loss of territory. All client populations require creative ways of handling personal space. To increase the client's sense of personal space, you can decrease close, direct eye contact. Instead, sit beside the client or position the chairs at angles for counseling or health teaching. Clients in intensive care units, where there are many intrusive procedures, benefit from decreased eye contact during certain times, such as when being bathed or during suction, wound care, and changing of dressings. At the same time, it is important for the nurse to talk gently with the client during such procedures and to elicit the client's feedback, if appropriate.

To minimize the loss of a sense of personal space and associated behaviors, the nurse demonstrates a high regard for the client's dignity and privacy. Closed doors for private rest and periods of uninterrupted relaxation are respected. Personal belongings are arranged and treated with care, particularly with very old and very young clients, for whom personal items may be highly significant as a link with a more familiar environment. Elderly clients can become profoundly disoriented in unfamiliar environments because their internal sensory skill in processing new information is often reduced. Encouraging persons in long-term facilities to bring pictures, clothing, and favorite mementos is an important nursing intervention with such clients.

Respect for Personal Space in Hospital Situations

Obviously, there is a discrepancy between the minimum amount of space an individual needs and the amount of space hospitals are able to provide in multiple-occupancy rooms. Therefore, the nurse must recognize individual needs for privacy and implement actions to increase the sense of personal space. Respect for the client's personal space can be accomplished by the following:

- Providing privacy when disturbing matters are to be discussed
- Explaining procedures before implementing them
- Entering another person's personal space with warning (e.g., knocking or calling the client's name) and, preferably, waiting for permission to enter
- Providing an identified space for personal belongings
- Encouraging the inclusion of personal and familiar objects on the client's nightstand
- Decreasing direct eye contact during hands-on care
- Minimizing bodily exposure during care
- Using only the necessary number of people during any procedure
- Using touch appropriately

Violations of Confidentiality

Discussing private information casually with others is an abuse of confidentiality. Nursing reports and interdisciplinary team case conferences are examples of acceptable forums for the discussion of privileged communication. An explicit norm of such conferences is that the information and feelings shared about a client are not discussed outside the conference except in the direct application of nursing care (Greve, 1990). To protect privacy, discussion of client care should preferably take place in a conference room with the door closed. This information includes change-of-shift reports, multidisciplinary conferences, one-on-one conversations with other health professionals about specific client care issues, and consultations with clients and their families. Newly implemented federal confidentiality regulations are discussed in Chapter 23.

Avoiding Cross-Cultural Dissonance

The ANA's statement on cultural diversity in nursing practice highlights the importance of recognizing intracultural variation and assessing each client as an individual (ANA, 1991). A nurse does not have to memorize a list of beliefs held by every culture to become culturally sensitive. Avoid barriers to communication that occur when a nurse generalizes a patient's beliefs based on his or her ethnic membership, rather than taking the time to learn the client's personal preferences (Brody & Hunt, 2005).

SUMMARY

This chapter focuses on essential concepts needed to establish and maintain a therapeutic relationship in nursing practice: caring, empowerment, trust, empathy, mutuality, and confidentiality. Respect for the client as a unique person is a basic component of each concept. Barriers affecting the development of the nurse-client relationship, such as anxiety, stereotyping, overfamiliarity, or intrusion into personal space, are described.

Caring is described as a commitment by the nurse that involves profound respect and concern for the unique humanity of every client and a willingness to confirm the client's personhood.

Empowerment is assisting the client to take charge of his or her own health.

Trust represents an individual's emotional reliance on the consistency and continuity of experience. The client perceives the nurse as trustworthy, a safe person with whom to share difficult feelings about health-related needs.

Empathy is the ability to perceive accurately another person's feelings and to convey their meaning to the client. Nursing behaviors that facilitate the development of empathy are accepting, listening, clarifying and informing, and analyzing. Each of these behaviors implicitly recognizes the client as a unique individual worthy of being listened to and respected.

Mutuality includes as much shared communication and collaboration in problem solving as the client is capable of providing. To foster mutuality within the relationship, nurses need to remain aware of their own feelings, attitudes, and beliefs.

A related concept is confidentiality: the nurse has an ethical responsibility, within limits, to respect the client's right to decide who can have access to his or her health information. The nurse needs to inform the client what types of information will be shared with other team members.

There are barriers as well as bridges in the establishment of a nurse-client relationship that affect the development of the relationship. Anxiety is a vague, persistent, and uncomfortable feeling of impending doom. A mild level of anxiety heightens one's awareness, but higher levels of anxiety decrease perceptual ability. The nurse needs to use anxiety- and stress-reduction strategies when clients demonstrate moderate anxiety levels.

Stereotypes are generalizations representing an unsubstantiated belief that all individuals of a particular

Ethical Dilemma ■ *What Would You Do?*

There are limits to your professional responsibility to maintain confidentiality. Any information that, if withheld, might endanger the life or physical and emotional safety of the client or others needs to be communicated to the health team or appropriate people immediately.

Consider the teen who confides his plan to shoot classmates. Can you breach confidentiality in this case? How about the 5-year-old child in whom you notice genital warts (HPV) on his anus, but who shows no other signs of sexual abuse?

social group, race, or religion share the same characteristics. No allowance is made for individual differences. Developing a nonjudgmental, neutral attitude toward a client helps the nurse reduce clinical bias in nursing practice.

Personal space, defined as an invisible boundary around an individual, is another conceptual variable worthy of attention in the nurse-client relationship. The emotional boundary needed for interpersonal comfort changes with different conditions. It is defined by past experiences and culture. Proxemics is the term given to the study of humans' use of space. To minimize a decreased sense of personal space, the nurse needs to demonstrate a high regard for the client's dignity and privacy.

REFERENCES

Accordino MP: Relationship enhancement as an intervention to facilitate rehabilitation of persons with severe mental illness, *J Appl Rehabil Counsel* 28(1):47–52, 1997.

American Nurses Association: *Cultural diversity in nursing practice* [position statement], Washington, DC, 1991, Author.

American Nurses Association: *Nursing's social policy statement*, Washington, DC, 1995, Author.

http://nursingworld.org, retrieved November, 2004.

Armstrong AE, Parsons S, Barker PJ: An inquiry into moral virtues, especially compassion, in psychiatric nurses, *J Psychiatr Ment Health Nurs* 7(4):297–306, 2000.

Bakir PH: Establishing mutual trust, *Schriftenr Ver Wasser Boden Lufthyg* 105:75–80, 2000.

Bernzweig J, Takyama JL, Phibbs C et al.: Gender differences in physician-patient communication, *Arch Pediatr Adolesc Med* 15(6):586–591, 1997.

Branch WT: The ethics of caring and medical education, *Acad Med* 75(2):127–132, 2000.

Brody H, Hunt LM: Moving beyond cultural stereotypes in end-of-life decision making, *Am Fam Physician* 71(3):429–430, 2005.

Carkhuff RR: *Helping and human relations*, vol 1, New York, 1969, Holt, Rinehart & Winston.

Clarke J: A view of the phenomenon of caring in nursing practice, *J Adv Nurs* 17:1283–1290, 1992.

Clayton G: Connecting: a catalyst for caring. In Chinn P, editor: *Anthology of caring*, New York, 1991, NLN.

Colliver JA, Vu NV, Marcy ML et al.: Effects of examinee gender, standardized patient gender and their interaction on standardized patients' ratings of examinees' interpersonal and communication skills, *Acad Med* 68(2):153–157, 1993.

Crisp AH, Geider MG, Rix S et al.: Stigmatization of people with mental illnesses, *Br J Psychiatry* 177:4–7, 2000.

Davis J: Don't fence me in, *Am J Nurs* 84:1141, 1984.

Erikson E: *Childhood and society*, ed 2, New York, 1963, Norton.

Feil N: Validation: techniques for communicating with confused old–old persons and improving their quality of life, *Top Geriatr Rehabil* 11(4):34–42, 1996.

Gazda GM: *Foundations of counseling and human services*, New York, 1987, McGraw-Hill.

Greve P: Keep quiet or speak up: issues in patient confidentiality, *Regist Nurse* 12:53, 1990.

Jack S: *Engagement between mothers with children at-risk of developmental delays, public health nurses and family visitors in a blended home visiting program*, doctoral dissertation, McGill University, Toronto, 2004.

Johns J: Trust: key to acculturation in corporatized health care environments, *Nurs Adm Q* 20(2):13–24, 1996.

Kavanaugh K: Values and beliefs. In Creasia J, Parker B, editors: *Conceptual foundations of professional nursing practice*, St Louis, 1991, Mosby.

Keller V, Baker L: Communicate with care, *RN* 63(1):32–33, 2000.

Kreigh H, Perko J: *Psychiatric and mental health nursing: a commitment to care and concern*, ed 2, Reston, VA, 1983, Reston Publishing.

Laschinger HK, Finegan J, Shamian J et al.: Organizational trust and empowerment in restructured healthcare: effects on staff nurse commitment, *J Nurs Adm* 30(9):413–425, 2000.

Lutz BJ, Bowers BJ: Patient-centered care, *Sch Inq Nurs Pract* 14(2):165–187, 2000.

May BA, Alligood MR: Basic empathy in older adults: conceptualization, measurement, and application, *Issues Ment Health Nurs* 21(4):375–386, 2000.

Metz D: Nurse urges care of patient, not customer [letter to editor], *Nebr Nurse* 33(4):4, 2000.

Naish J: The route to effective nurse-patient communication, *Nurs Times* 92(17):27–30, 1996.

Oermann MH: *Professional nursing practice: a conceptual approach*, Philadelphia, 2000, JB Lippincott.

Pearson SD, Raeke LH: Patients' trust in physicians, *J Gen Intern Med* 15(7):509–513, 2000.

Platt FW: *Conversation repair: case studies in doctor-patient communication*, Boston, 1995, Little, Brown.

Puetz BE: The winning job interview, *Am J Nurs* (Career Guide 2005 Supp):30–32, 2005.

Reynolds W, Scott PA, Austin W: Nursing empathy and perception of the moral, *J Adv Nurs* 32(1):235–242, 2000.

Rogers C: *On becoming a person*, Boston, 1961, Houghton-Mifflin.

Roter DL, Geller G, Bernhardt BA et al.: Effects of obstetrician gender on communication and patient satisfaction, *Obstet Gynecology* 93(5):635–641, 1999.

Sheldon LK: *Communication for nurses*, Thorofare, NJ, 2004, Slack.

Skinner TC, Cradock S: Empowerment: what about the evidence? *Practical Diabetes Int* 17(3):91–95, 2000.

Spalding N: The empowerment of clients through pre-operative education, *Br J Occup Ther* 63(4):148–154, 2000.

van Dulmen AM, Bensing JM: Gender differences in gynecologist communication, *Women Health* 30(3):49–61, 2000.

Vandegaer F: Issues in home care: environment, isolation and professional boundaries, *Adv Nurs* (October):25–26, 2000.

Wilkes L, White K, O'Riordan L: Empowerment through information, *Aust J Rural Health* 8(1):41–46, 2000.

Williams AM, Irurita VF: Therapeutic and non-therapeutic interpersonal interactions: the patient's perspective. *J Clin Nurs* 13(7):806–815, 2004.

Chapter 7

Role Relationship Patterns

Elizabeth Arnold and Kathleen Underman Boggs

OUTLINE

OBJECTIVES

At the end of the chapter, the reader will be able to:

1. Define role and role performance.
2. Describe the components of professional role socialization and stages of professional development.
3. Discuss the professional roles of the nurse.
4. Describe the nature of role performance as a nursing diagnosis.
5. Discuss the implications of role relationships for clients in health care.
6. Describe the nurse's role in client advocacy.

> *Helmer: Remember—before all else you are a wife and mother.*
>
> *Nora: I don't believe that anymore. I believe that before all else I am a human being, just as you are.*
>
> (Ibsen, 1879)

Chapter 7 explores the concept of role and role relationships from two perspectives: (a) as it relates to the professional nursing role; and (b) as it relates to significant role changes that many clients face as a result of illness or disability. Raudonis and Acton (1997) note that people in health care situations have special needs and that "the role of the nurse is to discover these needs, from the client's model of the world, and nurture the client towards optimal well-being" (p. 140). It is an awesome responsibility, and of particular importance as nursing moves into the community with less structured opportunities for human health care conversations.

Components of the professional nursing role include a specialized set of competencies and skills, professional involvement with clients marked by empathy and respect, and confidentiality.

BASIC CONCEPTS

Role is defined as the traditional pattern of behavior and self-expression performed by or expected of an individual by a given society. People have a large number of social and professional roles, some that they are born with (ascribed roles) and some that they acquire (acquired roles) during a lifetime. People can have several social roles simultaneously. For example, Marge is a professional nurse, a mother, a wife, a daughter, a lay minister in her church, and president of the parent-teacher association at her children's school. As the only girl in her family of origin and a nurse, her family anticipates certain caretaking behaviors of her that are not expected of her siblings. Multiple professional and social roles can create conflict when the expectations of one role interfere with the discharge of other important life roles or personal needs.

Roles and Role Relationships

Roles represent the social aspects of self-concept, with both performance and relationship dimensions affecting how people relate to one another. Social customs and expected professional standards of practice reinforce the performance aspect of role relationships. For example, consider the different but predictable professional role expectations of a lawyer, a physician, and a dentist. You would expect each of these professionals to have a very different set of skills and professional role competencies in helping you manage difficult life problems, based on their education and training. The same is true of professional nursing.

Behavioral standards for **role performance** differ based on cultural, gender, institutional, personal, and family expectations. Despite tremendous advances in equal opportunity, people still expect different role behaviors of men and women. For clients, significant changes in their behavioral ability to function in expected roles as a result of illness, disability, or other life changes can be devastating. Role relationships within the family and within the larger community are such an important dimension of the self that, in health care, they warrant their own special nursing diagnosis: *ineffective role performance*.

The relational aspect of roles is more complex and not as easily defined. Social customs impart different values to professional and social roles, which define a person's position, status, and influence within the community or group. Role relationships are recognizable through membership in a community or through differences in work responsibilities, cooperative activities, education, and social affiliations.

Some aspects of role relationships are reciprocal. Each person also plays a part in the implementation of specific role relationships characterized by the amount of effort and skill with which they discharge their role. The feedback they receive either reinforces or diminishes the status of the role. Two people having the same role can implement it differently, and responses to their implementation can vary significantly. Consider your own "role" as a nursing student and how it influences your relationships with clinical instructors, your clients, professional peers, your friends, and other significant people in your life. What do others expect of you, simply because you are a nursing student on your way to becoming a recognized health care provider?

Professional roles help direct therapeutic conversations. How nurses perceive their professional role and how they function as a nurse in that role have a sizeable effect on the success of interpersonal communication in the nurse-client relationship. Role relationships with a client can affect the quality of nursing care in the nurse-client relationship when the worth of the client as a person, for example, is judged on the basis of socioeconomic status, level of education, ethnicity, health state, or level of consciousness. They can affect effective treatment decision making when, for example, questioning a health care provider's professional judgment is not considered an appropriate behavior in the client's culture

Developing an Evidence-Based Practice

Foley BJ, Minick P, Kee C: Nursing advocacy during a military operation, *West J Nurs Res* 22(4):492-507, 2000.

This qualitative phenomenologic study was designed to explore the advocacy role experiences of military nurses and to provide a rich description of the common meanings of their advocacy practices. A purposive sample of 24 military nurses was interviewed and data analysis completed using a constant comparison methodology.

Results: Themes revealed one constitutive pattern associated with the concept of advocacy, namely safeguarding, with four related themes described as being the patient's voice, protecting, attending the whole person, and preserving the patient's personhood. A recommendation from this study is the need to coach nurses in how to relate to other members of the health team as the patient's advocate.

Application to Your Clinical Practice: As a profession, nurses need to develop research evidence and implement relevant study findings to advocate for the health and well-being of their clients. What themes do you associate with client advocacy in your clinical setting? Would these themes be the same or different in a community setting?

or when the family, not the client, is culturally expected to make important health care decisions.

APPLICATIONS

Professional Role Behaviors

Webster's Dictionary defines **profession** as a "calling requiring specialized knowledge and often long and intensive academic preparation." The criteria for identifying a discipline as professional originally developed by Flexner (1915) still hold true today (Box 7-1).

In contemporary nursing, Burnard (2004) has suggested that a very important defining characteristic of a profession is "a body of specific knowledge based on research" (p. 2). This emphasis on research will become increasingly important in modern health care, with its focus on evidence-based clinical practice and treatment outcomes.

In 1986, the American Association of Colleges of Nursing published examples of the essential values, attitudes, personal qualities, and professional behaviors associated with the profession of nursing. These examples, which carry moral, social, and competency expectations for the nurse's behavior, are outlined in Table 7-1.

Box 7-1 Flexner's Criteria of a Professional Role

- Members share a common identity, values, attitudes, and behaviors.
- A distinctive and substantial body of knowledge exists.
- Education is extensive, with both theory and practice components.
- Unique service contributions are made to society.
- There is acceptance of personal responsibility in discharging services to the public.
- There is governance and autonomy over policies governing activities of profession members.
- There is a code of ethics that members acknowledge and incorporate in their actions.

Nurses have a legal and moral obligation to maintain their competency and to work within the scope of their practice as defined in their state's Nurse Practice Act (see Chapter 2).

The professional nursing role should be clearly evident in every aspect of nursing care, but nowhere more fully than in the nurse-client relationship. Masters (2005) asserts that a professional nurse's *first* role responsibility is to the client. As a nurse, you are expected to act in a professional manner with clients, establishing realistic boundaries with them related to time, purpose of the interaction, and level of involvement (see Chapter 5).

Expected professional role behaviors should emphasize the following qualities:

- Ability to view clients as individual, holistic beings
- Respect for the basic human dignity of all clients, regardless of differences from oneself
- An attitude of cultural openness
- Sensitivity to individual clients' ability to access health care and adhere to prescribed regimens
- An understanding of the impact that illness and/or disability may have on clients
- Adherence to nursing standards of care
- Use of research evidence to improve nursing practice

(Masters, 2005)

Professional role behaviors in the nurse-client relationship include much more than simple caring; they require a sound knowledge base as well as specific technical and interpersonal competencies. On a daily basis, nurses must collect and process multiple, often indistinct pieces of behavioral data. They need to

Table 7-1 Values, Qualities, and Behaviors Associated with Professionalism in Nursing Practice

Essential Values*	Examples of Attitudes and Personal Qualities	Examples of Professional Behaviors
1. Aesthetics Qualities of objects, events, and persons that provide satisfaction	Appreciation Creativity Imagination Sensitivity	Adapts the environment so it is pleasing to the client. Creates a pleasant work environment for self and others. Presents self in a manner that promotes a positive image of nursing.
2. Altruism Concern for the welfare of others	Caring Commitment Compassion Generosity Perseverance	Gives full attention to the client when giving care. Assists other personnel in providing care when they are unable to do so. Expresses concern about social trends and issues that have implications for health care.
3. Equality Having the same rights, privileges or status	Acceptance Assertiveness Fairness Self-esteem Tolerance	Provides nursing care based on the individual's needs irrespective of personal characteristics.† Interacts with other providers in a nondiscriminatory manner. Expresses ideas about the improvement of access to nursing and health care.
4. Freedom Capacity to exercise choice	Confidence Hope Independence Openness Self-direction Self-discipline	Honors individual's right to refuse treatment. Supports the rights of other providers to suggest alternatives to the plan of care. Encourages open discussion of controversial issues in the profession.
5. Human dignity Inherent worth and uniqueness of an individual	Consideration Empathy Humaneness Kindness Respectfulness Trust	Safeguards the individual's right to privacy. Addresses individuals as they prefer to be addressed. Maintains confidentiality of clients and staff. Treats others with respect regardless of background.
6. Justice Upholding moral and legal principles	Courage Integrity Morality Objectivity	Acts as a health care advocate. Allocates resources fairly. Reports incompetent, unethical, and illegal practice objectively and factually.†
7. Truth Faithfulness to fact or reality	Accountability Honesty Inquisitiveness Rationality Reflectiveness	Documents nursing care accurately and honestly. Obtains sufficient data to make sound judgments before reporting infractions of organizational policies. Participates in professional efforts to protect the public from misinformation about nursing.

From American Association of College and University Education for Professional Nursing (1986). *Final report.* Washington, DC: American Association of Colleges of Nursing.

*The values are listed in alphabetic rather than priority order.

†From American Nurses Association: *Code for nurses*, Kansas City, MO, 1976, Author.

critically think through problems without getting lost in detail in very short periods of time and come up with workable solutions that clients want to implement. Through words and behaviors in relationship with other health care providers and agencies, nurses consistently serve as advocates for their clients and family members.

Today's nurse functions in a high-tech, managed health care environment in which the human caring aspects of nursing are easier to overlook. This provides unique challenges to the nurse-client relationship, such as shorter client contacts, decreased continuity, and lower levels of trust. Yet perhaps the nurse-client relationship and the caring communication that takes place within it will become *increasingly* important in helping clients feel cared for in a health care environment that sometimes neglects the psychosocial needs of clients in favor of cost-effectiveness and efficient use of time. Exercise 7-1 is designed to help you focus on your own self-development as a professional nurse.

Professional Nurse Role

Types of Professional Roles

Nurses currently are educationally prepared at the associate degree, baccalaureate, master's, and doctoral levels (Erickson & Ditomassi, 2005). Nurses function in different and sometimes overlapping roles, consistent with their educational preparation and clinical experiences (Box 7-2).

New professional roles emerging in the twenty-first century reflect the expanded advanced practice role of the nurse and include "entrepreneur, recruiter, editor, publisher, ethicist, labor relations expert, nurse anesthetist, lobbyist, [and] culture broker" (Roberson, 1992, p. 4). Because hospitals no longer are the primary settings for nursing practice, nurse practice roles take place in nontraditional as well as traditional health care settings. Nurses practice in the community; in prisons, schools, and homes; and with migrant workers in the field. They play an important role on health care teams working with the military, during disasters, in the justice system, with the homeless, and with medically disadvantaged client families. Increasingly nurses will be called upon to contribute to and present findings from evidence-based practice to inform policy makers, educators, and health care providers in a multidisciplinary health care environment. Exercise 7-2 is designed to help you look at the role responsibilities of different types of practicing nurses.

Exercise 7-1 Looking at My Development as a Professional Nurse

Purpose: To help students focus on their self-development as professional nurses.

Procedure:

Write the story of how you chose to become a nurse in a one- or two-page essay (may be done as a homework assignment). There are no right or wrong answers; this is simply your story. You may use the following as guides in developing your story.

1. What are your reasons for choosing nursing as a profession?
2. What factors influenced your decision (e.g., people, circumstances, or situations)?
3. What does being a nurse mean to you?
4. What fears do you have about your ability to function as a professional nurse?
5. How do you think being a nurse will affect your personal life?
6. What type of nursing do you want to pursue?

Discussion:

1. In what ways is your story similar to or different from those of your classmates?
2. As you wrote your story, were you surprised by any of the data or feelings?
3. Students can discuss some of the realistic difficulties encountered as nursing students, both professionally and personally, and ways to handle them. Through discussion, explore the following:
   a. The practices nursing students will need to follow to achieve their vision
   b. The types of supports nurses need to foster their ongoing professional development

Box 7-2 Professional Nursing Roles

Role	Role Responsibilities
Caregiver	Uses the nursing process to a. Provide complete or partial compensatory care for clients who cannot provide these self-care functions for themselves. b. Implement supportive/educative actions to promote optimum health. c. Reinforce the natural, developmental, and healing processes within a person to enhance well-being, comfort, function, and personal growth.
Teacher	Provides health teaching to individual clients and families. Develops and implements patient education programs to promote/maintain healthful practices and compliance with treatment recommendations. Guides individuals in their human journey toward wholeness and well-being through psycho-education.
Client advocate	Protects client's right to self-determination. Motivates individuals and families to become informed, active participants in their health care. Mediates between client and others in the health care environment. Acts as client's agent in coordinating effective health care services.
Manager	Coordinates staff and productivity. Delegates differentiated tasks to appropriate personnel. Facilitates communication within and among departments. Serves on committees to improve and maintain quality of care. Makes decisions and directs relevant changes to ensure quality care.
Evaluator	Sets quality assurance/care standards. Reviews records and monitors compliance with standards. Makes recommendations for improvement.
Researcher	Develops and implements research/grant proposals to broaden understanding of important issues in clinical practice and validate nursing theories as a basis for effective nursing practice.
Consultant	Provides specialized knowledge/advice to others on health care issues. Evaluates programs, curricula, and complex clinical data. Serves as expert witness in legal cases.
Case manager	Manages care for a caseload of clients. Coordinates cost-effective care options. Monitors client progress toward expected behavioral outcomes. Collaborates with other professionals to ensure quality care across health care settings.

Advanced practice nurses are registered nurses with a baccalaureate degree in nursing and a master's degree in a selected clinical specialty with relevant clinical experience. Certification and state licensing requirements vary according to state for practice in advanced practice roles. Box 7-3 identifies the four categories of advanced practice nursing in contemporary health care.

Regardless of the setting and specific application of professional nursing skills, different nursing role functions build on and reflect competence, critical thinking skills, and self-awareness. Interpersonal relationships provide the means by which these components of the professional nursing role interact with each other to provide quality nursing intervention. Exercise 7-3 helps you to explore the different specialty areas available for professional nurses.

New Professional Entry Roles in Nursing

In 2003, the American Association of Colleges of Nursing introduced two new types of professional roles in nursing in response to the nursing and nursing faculty shortages. The first, clinical nurse leader (CNL), prepares students for a generic master's-level leadership role, combining baccalaureate and master's preparation in an

Exercise 7-2 Professional Nursing Roles

Purpose: To help students explore different nursing roles.

Procedure:

Conduct an occupational interview with a practicing nurse about the different responsibilities involved in his or her job, the training and credentials required for the position, the client population encountered, the difficult and rewarding aspects of the job, and why the nurse chose a particular area or role in nursing. Write your findings in a short, descriptive summary. Questions you might ask are listed below, but you are also encouraged to create your own explorative questions.

- What made you decide to pursue nursing?
- What kinds of clients do you work with?
- What do you like best about your job?
- What would you do in an average workday?
- What is the most difficult aspect of your job?
- What kinds of preparation or credentials does your position require?
- What is of greatest value to you in your role as a professional nurse?

Discussion:

1. Were you surprised by any of your interviewee's answers? If so, in what ways?
2. What similarities and differences do you see in the results of your interview compared with those of your classmates?
3. In what ways can you use what you learned from doing this exercise in your future professional life?

Box 7-3 Advanced Practice Roles

Nurse practitioners (NPs) provide first-line health care services across the health-illness continuum in a variety of primary and acute care settings. They may practice either as an independent practitioner or in collaboration with a physician, depending on state laws. NPs can diagnose and treat common medical conditions and injuries, conduct physical exams and provide preventive care, and medically manage common chronic health problems in the community such as diabetes and high blood pressure. Acute care and specialty NPs (such as neonatal, pediatric, psychiatric, and geriatric NPs) use advanced clinical skills, diagnostic reasoning, and direct skilled management of specialized health care needs. Nurse practitioners can have prescriptive authority in most states, in conjunction with a statutorily mandated written agreement with a designated collaborating physician, approved by the State Board of Nursing.

Certified nurse-midwives provide a wide variety of first-line and clinical management of prenatal and gynecological care to normal healthy women. They perform uncomplicated delivery of babies in hospitals, private homes, and birthing centers, and continue with follow-up postpartum care. Certified nurse-midwives also have prescriptive authority under a mandated agreement with a designated collaborating physician, approved by the State Board of Nursing.

Clinical nurse specialists provide care in a range of specialty areas, such as cardiac, oncology, neonatal, pediatric, obstetric/gynecological, medical surgical, and psychiatric nursing. In some states, clinical specialists in psychiatric nursing can have limited prescriptive authority in accord with a statutorily mandated written agreement with a designated collaborating physician, approved by the State Board of Nursing. Clinical nurse specialists also perform indirect clinical nursing roles such as staff development, nursing education, administration, and informatics.

Certified registered nurse anesthetists administer anesthesia and conscious sedation in more than one-third of the hospitals in the United States.

Exercise 7-3 Exploring Advanced Practice Opportunities in Nursing

Purpose: To explore different specialty areas in nursing.

Procedure:

1. Select a specialty area about which you have an interest in learning more and obtain the American Nurses Association standards of practice for that specialty.
2. Interview a nurse in that specialty area.
3. Write a summary of your impressions of the practice of nursing in that specialty area, describing aspects that are especially important to you.

Discussion:

Students or student groups can present their summaries and discuss aspects of the specialty area that impress them the most. Do you see common threads across clinical specialties?

accelerated curriculum. The CNL "designs, implements, and evaluates client care by coordinating, delegating and supervising the care provided by the health care team, including licensed nurses, technicians, and other health professionals" (AACN, 2003, paragraph 2).

AACN also endorsed a second educational pathway leading to the doctor of nursing practice (DNP). This is envisioned as a terminal degree in advanced nursing practice for nurses who desire a clinical rather than research doctorate. The curriculum combines advanced nursing practice competencies with a solid foundation in clinical science, evidence-based practice methods, system leadership, information technology, health policy, and interdisciplinary collaboration (AACN, 2003). According to Mundinger (2005), the DNP degree will formalize an educational process leading to a doctoral degree designed to considerably expand and complement current master's specialty education and roles.

Role Socialization

Nursing students learn professional role behaviors through the process of professional role socialization. Role socialization is the process or set of activities a person uses to gain knowledge, skills, and behaviors in order to participate as a member of a particular group (Doheny, Cook, and Stopper, 1997). Cohen (1981) identified four steps in the professional socialization process (Box 7-4).

Box 7-4 Steps in the Socialization Process

1. Learn the technology of the profession: the facts, skills, and theory.
2. Internalize the professional culture.
3. Find a personally and professionally acceptable version of the role.
4. Integrate this professional role into all other life roles.

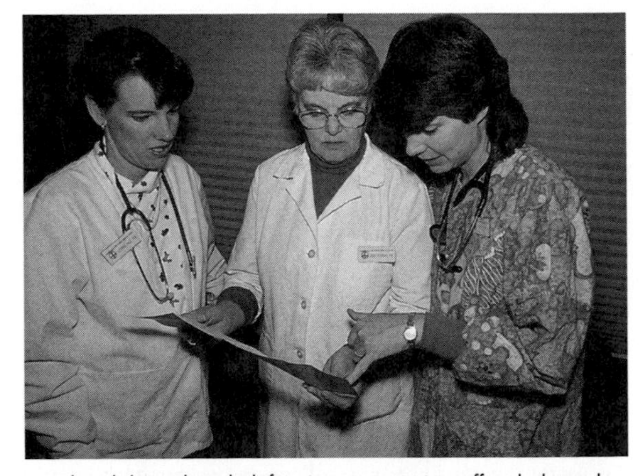

Nurses learn behavioral standards from instructors, nursing staff, and other students. (From Potter PA, Perry, AG: *Fundamentals of nursing,* ed 5, St Louis, 2001, Mosby.)

Initially, students focus on learning the "pure" form of nursing knowledge. In this first developmental stage, nursing students are dependent on the instructor to help them find the one "right answer" to health care problems. As they become more comfortable with foundational nursing knowledge, students begin to consider multiple options and to integrate professional judgment into clinical care planning. The second step in the socialization process involves internalizing the culture of professional nursing. The nursing faculty and unit preceptors serve as important socializing agents, helping students learn the values, traditions, norms, and competencies of the nursing profession (Neil, McCoy, Parry et al., 1998). As they watch their preceptors, other nurses, and their clinical faculty model desirable nursing behaviors, students begin to identify with them and to emulate these behaviors. They also are able to apply scientific knowledge to practice in a realistic manner and "to relate new material to their previous knowledge base" (Cohen, 1981, p. 18).

The last step in student socialization represents an internalization of professional norms and values, such that an individual integrates the nursing role with other life roles. With increasing clinical experience, nursing students become self-directed. They are able to tolerate ambiguity, create and work with alternative choices and diverse systems, and see the creative potential in all human beings, including themselves.

Professional Role Development as a Registered Nurse

Professional development as a nurse is a lifelong commitment. Formal means of professional development include continuing education, staff development, conference attendance, academic education, and research activities. However, many individuals also continue their professional growth through informal means such as consultation, professional reading, experiential learning, and self-directed activities.

Benner (1984, 2000) describes five developmental stages of increasing proficiency associated with the professional nursing role in clinical practice. The first developmental stage, referred to as the *novice* stage, occurs when the nurse first enters practice. With limited nursing experience, the novice nurse needs structure and tends to compare clinical findings to the textbook picture because he or she lacks the practice experience to do otherwise. Theoretical knowledge and confidence in the expertise of more practiced nurses also serve as guides to practice.

As the nurse progresses into stage 2, the *advanced beginner* stage, the nurse is better able to organize and prioritize clinical tasks and better able to assess and respond to the biological needs of clients. Although clinical analysis of health care situations is at a higher level than strict association with the textbook picture, the advanced beginner is only able to partially grasp the unique complexity of each client's situation.

Benner refers to stage 3 as the *competence* stage, typically occurring 1 to 2 years into nursing practice. Nurses in this stage are able to tailor nursing interventions to specific client needs. They begin to practice the "art" of nursing and participate in anticipatory planning. Performance is smoother and more coordinated, with increased evidence of diagnostic reasoning. The nurse views the clinical picture from a broader perspective and is more confident about his or her role in health care.

Stage 4, the *proficiency* stage, marks the transition from novice to expert. This stage occurs approximately 3 to 5 years into practice. Nurses in this stage are self-confident about their clinical skills. They are able to judge what things can wait and what things need immediate attention. They can recognize early warning signs of changes in a client's condition and they know what to do about it. Their psychosocial skills are well developed, and they are able to engage with the family of the client in a meaningful way.

Benner's *expert* stage of development, stage 5, is marked by a high level of clinical skill and the capacity to respond authentically and creatively to client needs and concerns. The expert nurse is able to sort through data and see the whole picture without getting lost in detail. Expert nurses can recognize the unexpected and work with it creatively. They demonstrate mastery of technology, sensitivity in interpersonal relationships, and specialized nursing skills in all aspects of their caregiving. Being an expert nurse is not an endpoint; nurses have the professional and ethical responsibility to continuously upgrade and refine their clinical skills through professional development and clinical skill training.

Expert or seasoned nurses often serve as mentors for their less-experienced colleagues. **Mentoring** is defined as a special type of professional relationship in which an experienced nurse or clinician (mentor) assumes a role responsibility for guiding the professional growth and advancement of a less-experienced person (protégé). A mentoring relationship can last over several months or years. Good mentors demonstrate role expertise and model the highest levels of personal professionalism. They share values and tips for success, providing support, structure, and challenges to the mentee or protégé. In many instances, they help facilitate contacts with significant people. Mentors are an invaluable resource for new nurses. Benefits to the mentor include satisfaction in seeing the achievements of the mentee and expansion of clinical excellence through others.

Role Stress

Nurses work daily with complex situations high in emotional intensity. The professional nursing role demands a commitment that sometimes exceeds the physical, emotional, and psychospiritual resources of an individual nurse. When this occurs, the nurse experiences **role stress**. Variables that lead to role stress include role pressures, role conflict, and role ambiguity.

Role pressures are external or internal circumstances, capable of change, that interfere with role performance. When role expectations are unclear, the workload is unreasonable, or several role demands occur simultaneously, professional as well as personal relationships suffer. Professional role pressures may be a result of perfectionism or of a confusion and uncertainty about the nature or validity of one's professional role. The individual nurse may experience simultaneous pressure from clients, the clients' relatives, nursing supervisors, and physicians, and can feel overwhelmed when each has different expectations of the nurse's role.

Role conflict occurs with competing demands between one or more role expectations. This can occur when a nurse feels torn between fulfilling the responsibilities of multiple life roles or when a nurse is asked to perform in ways that compromise client care (e.g., understaffing, being asked to perform a procedure that is beyond the scope of the nurse's practice or to supervise an unlicensed professional who lacks appropriate training for a treatment). Role conflict is usually present when you find yourself feeling resentful or uncomfortable with juggling all of your life responsibilities.

Role ambiguity occurs when roles are not defined clearly. The staff nurse who finds that most of her time is spent on paperwork and little on the direct nursing care originally specified in her job description may experience frustration, even though the work itself is easy. Exercise 7-4 offers an opportunity to explore multiple life roles and their impacts on one's life.

In addition to understanding how communication occurs within your workplace or agency system, you need to recognize your own response to conflicts you encounter (see Chapter 14). Especially within hospital systems, nurses recognize that constraints exist that may prevent them from going up against sources of power when they witness substandard care delivery to clients. Other situations involve unsatisfactory working conditions such as an unreasonable workload, a lack of support, or a feeling of futility about one's ability to make effective changes in the work environment. In a small study of 24 nurses, the majority perceived their

Exercise 7-4 Understanding Life Roles

Purpose: To expand students' awareness of the responsibilities, stressors, and rewards of different life roles.

Procedure:
1. Think of all the roles you assume in life.
2. Write a description of the specific responsibilities, stressors, and rewards related to each role.
3. Share some of your roles and their descriptions. (Share only what you feel comfortable revealing.)

Discussion:
As a group, discuss how these different aspects of life roles affect a person's overall functioning.
1. How can this help you to understand your clients better?
2. Discuss what would happen with these roles if you were incapacitated?
3. How might such a situation affect your coping ability?
4. How might it affect others?
5. What roles do you hold in common with other participants in this exercise?
6. What does the learning from this exercise suggest about possible role overload or conflict?
7. Identify one action you could take to reduce the strain of competing life roles.

work environment as more threatening than supportive. Phillips (1998) describes one response to such a situation as leaving by transferring to another unit or quitting your job. Obviously, removing yourself from the difficult situation helps you as an individual, but it does nothing to change the work problem.

Professional Self-Awareness

Self-awareness is a necessary antecedent to the full development of the professional role in nursing. Malloch and O'Grady (2003) assert that "knowing from the internal self what needs to be done and living those beliefs and values in the real world marks the leader's journey" (p. 101) in health care. Professional self-awareness related to the professional role promotes recognition of the need for continuing education, the acceptance of accountability for one's own actions, the capacity to be assertive with professional colleagues, and the capability of serving as a client advocate when the situation warrants it, even if it is uncomfortable to do so. In nurse-client relationships, professional self-awareness reflects on a balance between personal and professional use of self (see Chapter 5). Exercise 7-5 provides an awareness of personal strengths that can be important in developing a strong sense of professionalism.

Professional Communication in the Professional Nursing Role

Work Environment Communication

Effective communication among health care workers is essential for client health. A report from JCAHO noted that 24% of the sentinel events that lead to serious and deadly client outcomes could be attributed to lack of adequate staffing, interpersonal problems, or inadequate communication (Rosenstein and O'Daniel, 2005).

Networking

Networking is an essential component in building professional relationships and ultimately advancing your status within the profession. Your peers can be valuable sources of information. One of the authors of this book has used a book printed by her local nurse practitioner organization listing members' specialties to make nurse-to-nurse referrals.

When engaged in networking, you are making contacts with peers from as close as the nursing unit on the floor below to as far as a professional conference 500 miles away. By making contacts, nurses are communicating their expertise and sharing their ideas in a particular area of the profession while gathering information from their contacts. This give and take of information is often the

Exercise 7-5 Incorporating Personal Strengths in Role Development

Purpose: To help highlight the use of personal strengths as skills or assets in role development.

Procedure:

1. Pair up with another student.
2. Share a personal strength that you have observed about your assigned partner related to implementation of the professional nursing role, and describe the behavior that supports your assessment. (Examples might be persistence, sense of humor, balanced approach, energetic, thoughtful, caring, inquisitive, take charge, laid back, etc.)

Discussion:

1. Discuss how personal strengths can be used to enhance the professional role.
2. Compare and contrast what different students envisioned as personal strengths.
3. Did doing this exercise help you to learn something about the value of personal strengths?
4. Did anything surprise you about doing this exercise?
5. How can you use this information in your own role development?

bridge in networking with peers. For example, oncology nurses often exchange ideas about the best approaches to relieve side effects from chemotherapy and radiation therapy. Extensive networking among oncology nurses was the impetus for the formation of the Oncology Nursing Society. Networking is closely associated with coordination and collaboration activities, and is destined to become increasingly important in determining the future impact of advanced practice nursing.

Professional Rights

All health professionals, including nurses, have rights as well as significant responsibilities in interprofessional relationships with colleagues. Box 7-5 lists the American Nurses Association (2002) Bill of Rights for Registered Nurses. Rights carry with them corresponding responsibilities (see Box 7-6). Often, rightful acceptance of responsibilities fosters the automatic granting of rights by the other person. Think about your professional collegial relationships and your dual professional commitment to self and others. Think about the professional values identified in this book, and reexamine the components of professionalism. Each of those components is basically a professional responsibility.

Add your ideas for rights next to those responsibilities. Exchange ideas about professional rights and responsibilities with others.

Box 7-6 Chenevert's Rights in Nursing Practice

1. You have a right to be treated with respect.
2. You have a right to a reasonable workload.
3. You have the right to an equitable wage.
4. You have the right to determine your own reasonable priorities.
5. You have the right to ask for what you want, as long it does not interfere with the rights of others.
6. You have the right to refuse unreasonable requests without making excuses or feeling guilty.
7. You have the right to make mistakes and be responsible for them.
8. You have the right to give and receive information as a health professional.
9. You have the right to act in the best interest of the client as long as it is not in conflict with agency policy and respects the rights of others involved in the client's care.
10. You have the right to be human.

From Chenevert M: *Stat: special techniques in assertiveness training for women in the health professions*, ed 3, St Louis, 1988, Mosby.

Box 7-5 The American Nurses Association's Bill of Rights for Registered Nurses

- Nurses have the right to practice in a manner that fulfills their obligations to society and to those who receive nursing care.
- Nurses have the right to practice in environments that allow them to act in accordance with professional standards and legally authorized scopes of practice.
- Nurses have the right to a work environment that supports and facilitates ethical practice, in accordance with the Code of Ethics for Nurses and its interpretive statements.
- Nurses have the right to freely and openly advocate for themselves and their patients, without fear of retribution.
- Nurses have the right to fair compensation for their work, consistent with their knowledge, experience, and professional responsibilities.
- Nurses have the right to a work environment that is safe for themselves and their patients.
- Nurses have the right to negotiate the conditions of their employment, either as individuals or collectively, in all practice settings.

Reprinted with permission from American Nurses Association: *The Americal Nurse* 34(6), 2002, © 2002, American Nurses Association, Silver Springs, Md.

Professional Responsibilities

Nurses have a professional role responsibility to the individual, family, society, and the profession to do the following:

- Provide safe, competent nursing care according to accepted professional standards of care
- Act as an agent of change in the health care system
- Maintain the competence necessary for current nursing practice through continuing education
- Engage in scientific inquiry in evidence-based clinical practice
- Collaborate with other health professionals to ensure comprehensive care
- Educate and advocate for clients in the health care system

Diers (2004) suggests that the best source for nursing research comes from nursing practice itself. As a professional nurse, you will have opportunities to contribute to this body of knowledge if you look for them. Finally, multiprofessional health team collaboration is emerging as the most effective approach to resolving complex sociobiological health problems in the community.

Acting responsibly in nursing practice situations requires a willingness to go the extra step in establishing good working relations with professional colleagues, to try different interpersonal communication strategies, and to push on in the face of adversity. Most of the time, decisions are not either/or processes, but it is easy to lose sight of alternative options. Persistence and a good sense of humor are essential characteristics of honest interpersonal relationships with peers, reflecting a dual professional commitment to self and others.

Refusal of Assignment

Refusing an assignment is a serious matter, but there are times when the nurse must do just that to safeguard the client. The American Nurses Association (1995) takes the position that "nurses are accountable for judgments made and actions taken in the course of nursing practice. Neither physician's orders nor the employing agency's policies relieve the nurse of accountability for actions taken and judgments made" (review ANA position statement reference). This means that the nurse must have a clear knowledge of his or her professional duties, strengths, and limitations as an RN; skilled knowledge of medications, drug interactions, dosage, and side effects; and skill expectations for required clinical protocols and tasks. Before accepting an assignment, nurses must have the knowledge and skill to perform the tasks involved. The point of decision relates to taking a particular nursing action or delegating a nursing responsibility that would jeopardize the safety or health interests of the client. Personal factors also may be considered, for example, fatigue from working several shifts in a row (mandatory overtime) or, in the case of a pregnant nurse, when working with a client might present a medical danger to a developing fetus.

In making a decision to refuse an assignment, you need to use critical thinking skills to evaluate individual competence, explore other options for providing immediate care, and seek consultation as to alternate ways the client's care needs can be met. Once you have accepted an assignment, you need to make sure that the responsibility for the disputed care has been transferred to another qualified person if, in your professional judgment, you cannot safely provide it. *Under no circumstances may a nurse abandon a client.* Abandonment occurs when the nurse terminates a health relationship with a client without making reasonable arrangements with another person so that the client's nursing care can be continued.

Creating Work Environments to Support Professional Nursing Practice

Successful coping behaviors occur when a nurse believes he or she has some control to affect a situation. Change is most likely to occur when nurses recognize the need to work together among themselves and with their colleagues. In a study of what types of environmental support create satisfaction for professional nurses, Kramer and Schmalenberg (2002) uncovered the following factors chosen by the majority of the nurses surveyed:

- Working with other nurses who are clinically competent
- Good nurse-physician relationships and communication
- Nurse autonomy and accountability
- Supportive nurse manager-supervisor
- Control over nursing practice and practice environment
- Support for education (inservice, continuing education, etc.)
- Adequate nurse staffing
- Paramount concern for the patient

Magnet Recognition

In an effort to develop and support work environments that are favorable to nurses, and as a result of extensive research studies that explored factors of excellence within the hospital setting, the American Nurses Association, through the American Nurses Credentialing Center (ANCC), developed the Magnet Recognition Program in 1993. The factors chosen by nurses in the Kramer and Schmalenberg (2002) study are consistent with quality indicators for hospitals achieving **magnet status.** This national program recognizes quality patient care and nursing excellence in health care institutions and agencies, and identifies them as work environments that act as a "magnet" for professional nurses desiring to work there because of the institutions' excellence. To achieve magnet status, a hospital must fulfill a set of criteria designed to measure the strength and quality of their nursing. The ANCC identifies the following objectives of the Magnet Recognition Program (ANCC, 2006):

- Recognizing nursing services that use the Scope and Standards for Nurse Administrators (ANA, 2003) to build programs of nursing excellence for the delivery of nursing care of patients
- Promote quality in a milieu that supports professional nursing practice
- Provide a vehicle for the dissemination of successful nursing practices and strategies among health care organizations using the services of registered professional nurses
- Promote positive outcomes

A magnet hospital is characterized as one in which nurses have a high level of job satisfaction and staff nurse turnover that is lower than normal. Nurses in a magnet hospital are valued and have a strong voice in decision making about care delivery. They are encouraged and rewarded for involvement in shaping research-based nursing practice. Staffing ratios are viewed as appropriate, and the hospital demonstrates excellent treatment outcomes and client satisfaction. Communication among health professionals is open, and there is an appropriate mix of health care personnel to ensure quality care. Exercise 7-6 can help you think about how you would see yourself in the professional nursing role in the future.

Becoming Key Players in the Health Care Arena

Malloch and Porter-O'Grady (2005) suggest that we are living in an information-based societal infrastructure that is primarily relational and which functions horizontally in a global world without boundaries. Professional nursing requires an expanded set of skill competencies in the twenty-first century, as presented in Box 7-7.

Box 7-7 New vs. Old Skill Sets for Professional Nurses in the 21st Century

Knowledge Worker	Employee
Conceptual synthesis	Functional analysis
Competent integrated care	Manual dexterity
Mobile skill set	Fixed skill set
Outcome-based practice	Process, value-based practice
Interdisciplinary team performance	Individual practice

Modified from Mallach K, Porter-O'Grady T: A new vessel for leadership: new rules for a new age. In *The quantum leader: applications for the new world of work*, Sudbury, MA, 2005, Jones and Bartlett.

Exercise 7-6 Envisioning the Future

Purpose: To help students think about the nursing role they would like to aspire to in the future. Envisioning the future helps nurses to develop focused career goals.

Procedure:

1. Envision your career five years after graduation.
2. Write a detailed narrative of what you would be doing and what your career would be like as you might describe it to a classmate at your five-year reunion.
3. Have one student take the role of the storyteller, and the other the role of the classmate at the reunion. The person taking the role of the classmate should ask questions to clarify any aspects of the speaker's career vision that are not clear.
4. Reverse positions and repeat.

Discussion:

1. How difficult was it for you to think about what you want to do in the future?
2. What steps will you have to take in order to achieve your goal?
3. How will you go about finding out more about the career path you see yourself taking?

Making the role of the professional nurse visible in the twenty-first century is a task that nurses must undertake to strengthen the public's recognition of the nursing profession. Individual nurses and nursing organizations need to work together to strengthen the professional nursing role. In addition to defining our professional roles in ways that are understandable to us as professionals, nurses need to project a positive activist image of the professional nursing role within their communities. The nurse can achieve a place as key player in the current health care system by doing the following:

- Developing partnerships with clients, health care professionals, policy makers, and community agencies in the care of vulnerable populations
- Reflecting on and documenting what nurses do and the broad scope of services they provide for the public
- Participating as members of multidisciplinary groups with defined expertise as nurses to address significant health care issues from a nursing perspective
- Maintaining competence and acting in a professional manner
- Advocating for systems of care that provide adequate accessible health care for all people
- Developing and participating in multidisciplinary continuing education programs to ensure continued competence as a professional nurse
- Promoting the public and professional understanding of the professional nursing role
- Contributing to ethical discussions that support principled practices in clinical settings

Burkhardt and Nathaniel (2002) also suggest that all nurses can and should participate individually and collectively in the advancement of the profession through the sharing of nursing research and knowledge in practice.

Client Applications

Patient's Bill of Rights

In today's health care environment, clients need to take a more active role in their care and must be willing to assume more responsibility for their health, with the help and direction of their health care providers. As clients are considered an integral part of the treatment team, their participation needs to be one of equal partnership, with shared power and authority as joint decision makers in their health care. With a mutual participation model of health care delivery, the client's thoughts, concerns, and questions should be welcomed. Every decision related to the client's diagnosis and treatment should be a joint decision with the medical team based on combined input and shared responsibility for implementing the recommendations. This use of the client's self-knowledge and inner resources allows health care practitioners to be more effective supporters of the health care of their clients.

Concern for the quality of care provided to consumers of health care led to the development of the Patients' Bill of Rights sponsored by the American Hospital Association (AHA) in 1992. More recently, the AHA reframed this document as a "patient care partnership" between health care provider and health care consumer and outlined expectations, rights, and responsibilities of both client and provider as collaborative partners in facilitating quality health care. This second document emphasizes the client's responsibility to actively engage with the care provider in their health care. Another document adopted by the US Advisory Commission on Consumer Protection and Quality in the Health Care Industry in 1998 is also used. Together these documents provide a framework for protecting the client's rights in hospital settings. Components of these documents are identified in Box 7-8.

Client Role Relationships and Health Status

An important outcome of health status, identified in *Healthy People 2010*, is optimal quality of life. In 1959, Parsons, a well-known sociologist, defined health as "the state of optimum capacity of an individual for the effective performance of his roles and tasks" (p. 10). Quality of life and role relationships are interconnected. That role relationships and performance matter to people as essential elements of their well-being is evidenced in the emergence of symptoms of depression, feelings of emptiness, and even suicidal thoughts when a significant personal or professional role ceases to exist. Examples of lost role relationships include job loss, divorce, retirement, death of a significant person, and a chronic or debilitating illness. Nurses always need to be sensitive to the changes in role relationships that even a minor illness or injury produces.

From the client perspective, loss of or changes in normal roles, role relationships, and role performance are important dimensions of their emotional pain in health care situations. Major changes in role performance occur when unexpected life events such as illness or injury alter role function. Illness or trauma can change an individual's social role from one of independent self-sufficiency to one of vulnerability and varying degrees of dependency on others, a personal role change from

Box 7-8 Protecting the Client's Rights

All clients have the right to:	Described as:
1. High quality hospital care	Right to respectful, considerate, nondiscriminatory skilled care by qualified health care providers Right to know the identity of the caregiver and their educational status as student, resident, trainee
2. Clean, safe environment	Right to know if anything unexpected happens, plus any resulting changes in care Right to a fair, fast, and objective review of any complaints related to the hospital stay
3. Participation in treatment decisions	Right to have full knowledge of all treatment options, including risks, benefits, anticipated outcome, long-term effects on quality of life Right to consent to or refuse a treatment and to choose whether or not to participate in a research study Parents, designated legal representatives can represent the client if clients are unable to make their own treatment decisions
4. Full information disclosure	Right to accurate and understandable information about all aspects of care Right to assistance in making informed decisions, if needed because of language or mental or physical disability
5. Protection of client privacy	Right to protection of all personally identifiable medical information as specified in legal written notice of privacy practices Right to review and copy personal medical records and to request changes if the record is not accurate, relevant, or complete
6. Access to emergency services	Right to screening and stabilization emergency services in cases of emergency without prior authorization or financial penalty
7. Discharge planning and referral resources	Right to information about resources for follow-up care, and when possible, training or coordination of post-discharge activities with community-based caregivers

Modified from US Advisory Commission on Consumer Protection and Quality in the Health Care Industry (1998): www.consumer.gov/qualityhealth/rights.htm and American Hospital Association (AHA): The Patient Care Partnership: Understanding Expectations, Rights, and Responsibilities (brochure) (2003), available at www.aha.org/aha/ptcommunication/partnership/index.html.

independence to dependence. For example, when lack of physical stamina after a heart attack prevents a woman from fulfilling her customary caregiving roles in the home, she can experience a loss of self-confidence and personal value that can affect her rehabilitation (Arnold, 1997).

Most people do not assume the sick role voluntarily. At the hospital door, the client forsakes, either temporarily or permanently, recognized social roles in the family, work situation, and community. Regardless of how competent the person may be in other life roles, questions about role performance inevitably arise when illness strikes. Often, clients must learn new role behaviors that are unfamiliar and unsettling to previously held self-concepts. Illness or disability, whether actual or perceived, also strain family equilibrium and coping abilities. Role performance is considered such an important element of a person's self-concept that it warrants its own nursing diagnosis (North American Nursing Diagnosis Association, 1991).

Case Example

Dan was diagnosed with dementia in his mid-50s. He was a man of many talents who headed a large accounting firm prior to his illness. His wife had never worked outside of the home. Dan handled all of the finances, and his wife generally deferred to him for decisions. His son is in his first year of college on a 4-year scholarship, and there is one younger child in the home. The progression of the disease has been swift and incapacitating. Because of his age, Dan had not yet invested in

long-term care insurance. He is too young for Social Security and is functional enough not to qualify for disability retirement. His illness creates significant changes for his wife, who now must take over running the household finances. His son is not sure whether he should come home or continue his studies. The younger child is robbed of a normal childhood role because of his father's illness.

In its most extreme forms, this nursing diagnosis can reflect a client's lack of hope about ever having a positive social identity or receiving acceptance from others as a functional member of society. In an assessment interview, the nurse asks open-ended, focused questions about the client's family relationships, work, and social roles (Box 7-9). The questions you do ask should be asked in a conversational manner at a pace the client can tolerate.

The nurse may be the only person who has the expertise and willingness to facilitate, in an objective, compassionate manner, discussions of the implications of role changes stemming from altered health status for the client. With shortened hospital stays, this discussion of potential role changes ideally should be part of the discharge planning and/or follow-up in the community. Nurses working in long-term rehabilitation settings can help their clients look at personal strength skills they may still possess that could be used in a different way, for example, good communication skills, persistence, patience, and so on. Many times clients are not aware of transferable skills that can be put to good use when previous capabilities are no longer available to them. Exercise 7-7 can help you understand the nature of transferable skills.

Society is not kind to people with disabilities of any kind, and judgments are made about individuals returning to their former roles, even after successful rehabilitation (Wynne, Shields, & Sirkin, 1992). Preconceived notions of role disruption for an ill or disabled person occur more commonly when the illness is protracted, recurrent, or seriously role disruptive. Nurses need to help clients learn how to respond to subtle and not-so-subtle discriminatory actions associated with people's lack of understanding of the client's situation. An important nursing intervention related to fortifying role relationships in the nurse-client relationship involves the advocacy role.

Box 7-9 Questions the Nurse Might Ask in Assessing Role Relationships

Family

"What changes do you anticipate as a result of your illness (condition) in the way you function in your family?"

"Who do you see in your family as being most affected by your illness (condition)?"

"Who do you see in your family as being supportive of you?"

Work

"What are some of the concerns you have about your job at this time?"

"Who do you see in your work situation as being supportive of you?"

Social

"How has your illness affected the way people who are important to you treat you?"

"To whom do you turn for support?"

"If ________________ is not available to you, who else might provide social support for you?"

Advocacy Roles in the Nurse-Client Relationship

Although advocacy has always been considered a fundamental and integral part of the nursing role, never has it been more important in a health care era focused on including the client as a part of the health team and protecting the client's right to self-determination. The ANA (2001) specifically addresses the advocacy responsibilities of nurses in its Code of Ethics for Nurses, stating, "the nurse promotes, advocates for, and strives to protect the health, safety and rights of the patient."

"Patient advocacy is a fundamental role and ethical responsibility of every nurse" (Frederich, Strong, & von Gunten, 2002, p.155). **Advocacy** can be defined as a nurse using the skills of teacher, counselor, and leader to protect and support the client's rights (Taylor, Lillis, & LeMone, 1997). Client advocacy is a professional role requiring not only self-awareness but also a broad knowledge base about the client in the health care system. Nurses have historically acted in the interests of clients who cannot act for themselves (e.g., children and clients who are immobilized, unconscious, or mentally disabled). Furthermore, nurses have been instru-

Exercise 7-7 Transferable Skills

Purpose: To help students identify the unique skills that can be transferred to other situations.

Procedure:

1. Think of the one achievement of which you are most proud.
2. List the strengths or personal actions that went into this accomplishment. For example, "I was a good swim instructor" can be recast into personal strengths such as, "I was a good swim instructor because I was dependable, organized, patient, and persistent; I am able to relate easily to children; and I was compassionate with slow learners and able to inspire others."
3. Identify the physical, psychological, and psychosocial characteristics that contributed to the accomplishment (e.g., athletic ability, being raised in a large family, ethnic origin).
4. Share your achievement with your classmates.

Discussion:

1. How many different aspects of yourself were you able to identify as being a part of your accomplishment?
2. What physical, psychological, and psychosocial characteristics contributed to your achievement?
3. As you listened to the other students' reports, did you think of any other factors present in your situation?
4. Do you see any of these talents or strengths as "transferable skills" you might use in other situations?
5. What did you learn about yourself from this exercise?
6. How might you apply what you learned in this exercise to working therapeutically with clients?

mental in giving information to clients about their health problems and in educating clients to care for themselves.

Types of Advocacy

The different types of advocacy are presented in Box 7-10.

Anticipatory Guidance. Anticipatory guidance is a form of primary prevention. Helping the client foresee potential difficulties decreases his or her stress. For example, respite care is needed at regular intervals in families with severely ill members. Having no relief from caretaking activities fosters strained family relations and potential client abuse. This need should be anticipated for families of clients with sustained handicaps or chronic illness.

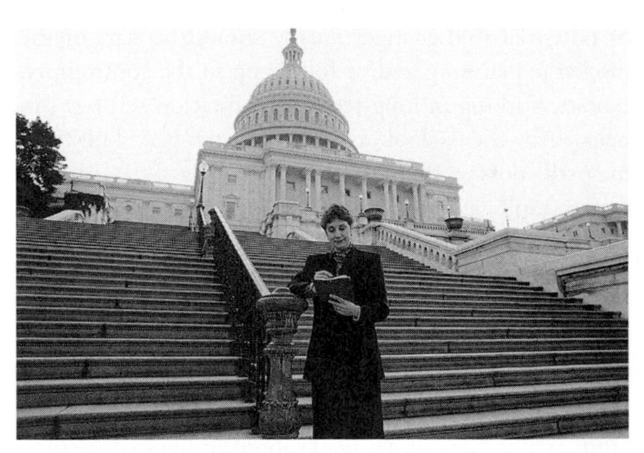

An important component of the nurse's role is advocacy for clients. (Courtesy University of Maryland School of Nursing.)

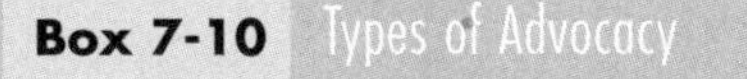

Box 7-10 Types of Advocacy

- Anticipatory guidance and primary prevention
- Role modeling
- Educational informing
- Providing support
- Collaboration and referral

Case Example

Tammy, the 15-year-old mother of Daniel, age 7 months, comes to your clinic. She was living with her mother, but her mom moved out of state. Tammy

works part-time at a fast food chain and has no other income. She wants to return to finish high school. Daniel is healthy but cannot roll over or sit up (developmental milestone delays), and his immunizations are not up-to-date. What kind of collaboration and referrals might you use to help?

Consider that the adolescent single parent with little financial support usually needs assistance with nutritional and economic resources (e.g., the Women, Infants, and Children [WIC] program for formula) and a referral to social services for follow-up. Providing information about ways to obtain public support services can help an adolescent mother meet her child's basic needs. Children with developmental disabilities benefit if the nurse explains motor development in infants to the parents. Each of these simple nursing actions acts to improve the client's or family member's capacity to cope and care.

Role Modeling. In the clinical setting, the nurse acts as a role model for appropriate behaviors. For example, you can model for a new mother by talking with her infant, smiling, and appropriately handling the infant. You could set limits in a kind but firm way with a misbehaving toddler. If you ask a child age-appropriate questions in the presence of his or her parents, you are modeling a useful interpersonal parenting behavior. This modeling often helps family members focus on minimizing stress and achieving simple, constructive goals in the clinical setting. With the frail, elderly client, you can model talking directly to the client instead of conversing only with the caregiver.

Educational Information. Your role as client advocate includes educational support and information. You are expected to inform clients about the nature of their health problems and the choices they have in seeking to modify their health care needs with nursing intervention. You can help your client gather information and learn health promotion behaviors.

Ongoing Support. An important part of your advocacy role is one of support, which you can offer when the informed client makes reasoned choices. In the advocacy role, nurses recognize clients' inherent right to make decisions for themselves and to take responsibility for their decisions. Nurses include the client as an equal partner in resolving health care needs and are respectful of client choices, even when the decisions reached are not what the nurse would recommend for the client.

Collaboration and Referral. Referral is another important component of client advocacy. Health-related problems are multidimensional and require the services of more than one health discipline. Often the nurse provides educational support as well as specific client data to other health professionals. Support may focus on the client's needs, nursing interventions, or information about the client's family. An interdisciplinary approach to client care in which all members of the health team pool their expertise to develop a workable care plan ensures comprehensive treatment.

Advocacy Process

As the client's advocate, you use an informational process, as presented in Box 7-11. Your base of power, in acting as an advocate, is your knowledge. You need to be aware of personal and professional ethics, values, and prejudices. For example, if a nurse thinks of elderly clients as helpless and equates aging with being taken care of, then the nurse will be likely to "take charge" of all client health activities for the elderly client, even those the client is still capable of performing with little or no assistance. In this situation, personal values have gotten in the way of individualized professional nursing values associated with client advocacy.

Understanding the System. To be successful as a client advocate, you need to know the environmental,

Box 7-11 Information Steps in Client Advocacy

- Knowledge of the personally held values of nurse and client
- Awareness of treatment and of professional and personal goals
- Information about professional nursing, environmental and interpersonal protocols, and the bureaucratic structure of the organizational work system
- Knowledge of potential power or recognition needs that could compromise the integrity of the client advocacy process
- Knowledge of how to mobilize community resources and referral processes

interpersonal, and bureaucratic system within which you work. It is important to understand how the communication flow filters through the different systems. Usually a combination of formal and informal communication with other staff is necessary for you to be effective.

Some of this knowledge can be gained by observing how communication is passed from person to person and by asking questions. Knowing how the various units are influenced by outside pressures (e.g., politics, financial constraints, consumer groups, and regulatory agencies) is as important as knowing who is in charge and who is influential in facilitating change. For example, one CEO of a health care organization writes about wanting to create a corporate cultural climate in which nurses feel empowered to advocate for client's viewpoints (Hofmann & Morris, 2000). He suggests putting nurses on agency committees, such as the ethics committee. Understanding the formal and informal power structure adds to the nurse's power base in effecting change on the client's behalf. With this knowledge base, the nurse is in a position to inform and assist the client in making the most of health care choices with the least amount of effort.

Steps in the Advocacy Process

Assess. Client advocacy is designed to help the client overcome feelings of helplessness and powerlessness in the hospital or health care treatment setting. Questions might center on the following: (a) What does the client believe is the most pressing problem? (b) What aspects of the problem might be a good place to start? (c) What supports (e.g., family, minister, rabbi, social services) are in place? (d) What health or social services is the client familiar with or resistant to considering? The client's powerlessness can be decreased when you provide anticipatory guidance, role-playing, modeling behaviors, education, and mobilization of community resources on the client's behalf.

Plan. When a problem situation is identified, you must act quickly to mobilize the necessary resources. Consultations are requested. The client or responsible family member is involved in the process of defining the problem and assuming as much responsibility as possible. Sometimes the nurse serves as dual advocate for the client and a family member. For example, in a child abuse situation, you need to act as an advocate of the child by taking the steps necessary to provide a protective and safe environment for the child. (By law, you are required to report suspected abuse.) You can be an advocate for the parents by referring them to appropriate community resources and helping them develop different methods for coping with situational stressors.

Implement. Another component of the advocacy role is to help the client become a self-advocate. More recently, this process has been referred to as empowerment (a model of which is found in Chapter 5). **Empowerment** requires a certain degree of assertiveness on the part of the nurse. Gibson (1991) describes the process as assisting individuals in asserting control over the factors affecting their lives. By maximizing clients' independence and minimizing their dependence, nurses are engaging in partnerships with their clients. If you have difficulty being assertive, then the client can hardly be expected to learn assertive interpersonal skills. You need to recognize when to speak for the client and when to encourage the client to speak up. In general, encouraging clients to take responsibility to speak on their own behalf is more effective.

Protect. As client advocate, you are seen as the client's protector. Client advocacy by nurses is becoming a legitimate role concept, used in the legal system in malpractice and negligence cases. A nurse who does nothing is generally held more liable than one who tries to do something within the scope of nursing practice and fails. The law is particularly interested in client advocacy as it relates to the presence of inadequate or improper medical care of the nurse's client. Therefore, nurses must not only be knowledgeable, but they must also be willing and able to assert their knowledge in situations involving poor medical management of a client.

Client advocacy acts as a connective link between ethics and the law. Providing appropriate information that allows a client to make an informed choice conforms to client's rights under the law, and supporting the client's right to make a decision that may or may not be compatible with the nurse's recommendation indicates an ethical commitment to ensure the client's self-determination. Exercise 7-8 provides a clinical situation in which the nurse's advocacy role is in conflict with traditional nursing and medical advice.

Evaluate. The effectiveness of your advocacy is a valuable resource, especially when usual means of providing information and care fail to meet the client's need.

Collaborate. Collaborate with colleagues to provide better outcomes for your client. **Collaboration** refers to an interactive process requiring that the involved individuals combine their expertise, skills, and resources to solve a problem or achieve a goal (Stichler, 1995). It includes comments from all parties and active integration of viewpoints of all participants (Coeling and Cukr, 2000). Thus, a broader database can be pooled to design a comprehensive care plan for the client.

Collaboration is an essential component of the professional nursing role in today's social world (Hales, Karshmer, Montes-Sandoval et al., 1998). Collaboration needs to occur with a broad spectrum of other health professionals, as well as among nurses. Never before has the potential for conflict been so great in the health care system. As society redefines every citizen's right to health, more and sicker clients are demanding higher-quality services, in spite of declining resources. Studies have

Exercise 7-8 Client Advocate Role-Play

Purpose: To understand the nurse advocacy role in difficult and conflict-filled clinical situations.

Procedure:

1. Read the following clinical situation and answer the questions in writing.
2. Have one student play the role of the client and another play the role of the nurse.
3. After the role-play, examine your written answers. See whether there are any changes you would like to make.
4. Finally, make up a situation and give it to your colleague with the same questions. Role-play the situation with your colleague, this time taking the role of the client.

Situation:

A 65-year-old man has been a client on the medical unit for 10 days, and you are assigned to care for him for the next four days. Diagnostic workup and tests reveal that he has cancer of the larynx. Surgery is indicated and has been scheduled. The doctor discusses his diagnosis and prognosis with him in your presence.

During the next two days, the client becomes increasingly withdrawn and introspective. Subsequently, he requests to speak with you and the physician. He states that he does not wish to have any surgery performed and no medication given, that he "has lived a good life" and would like you and the health team to accept his decision to die. He asks that no tube feedings or intravenous fluids be given. He asks that you cooperate and support his wishes.

Discussion:

1. What would your reaction be in this situation?
2. What does the statement "death with dignity" mean to you?
3. Do you think the client has the right to refuse treatment that may be life-sustaining?
4. What nursing care should you provide for this man as he continues to refuse food and fluids (keeping in mind that the client is an equal partner in his care)?
5. What conflicts does this situation pose for you? How would you see yourself dealing with them?
6. How can you, as a nurse, respect the integrity of a client's decision when it conflicts with promoting maximum client health functions?
7. Does the client's age influence your acceptance of his decision?
8. How will you support the client when faced with other health care professionals who disapprove of the client's decision?
9. What risks will you be taking in supporting the client?

Adapted from Uusral D: Values clarification in nursing: application to practice, *Am J Nurs* 78:2058-2063, 1978.

shown a significant relationship between excellent communication and collaboration, and improved client outcome or reduced client mortality (Coeling and Cukr, 2000; Rosenstein & O'Daniel 2005; Tschannen, 2004) (see Chapter 22 for more details about collaboration).

The concept of collaboration means working simultaneously in a new relationship with one another and with the client. This new relationship requires that nurses, physicians, other health professionals, and the client communicate effectively with one another and view one another as coming from different perspectives, but as having an important joint influence on client care. All members share responsibility to ensure different aspects of holistic, safe, effective, and compassionate care for clients.

Sharing information and ideas with other health care professionals leads to increased trust and mutual respect. With a nursing perspective, the nurse provides a holistic assessment of health care issues and important information about how likely the client is to accept medical treatment protocols. Because of the nature of their professional responsibilities, nurses are often in a better position to help clients explore different options and to plan creatively the most effective approach. A collegial relationship means not only that clients receive better care but also that the nurse finds the experience of collaboration personally and professionally affirming (Mauksch, 1981).

Coordinate. Coordination is closely related to collaboration, the difference being that with collaboration there may be more joint direct interaction with a client. In **coordination**, two or more people provide services to a client or program separately and inform each other of their activities. A careful assessment of the nature of the client's self-care requirements often reveals that he or she has a need beyond the scope of your professional practice or experience.

To make an appropriate referral, you need to identify the health care professional who can best serve the client's need and then contact that person. In making referrals, you need a good sense of personal or professional limitations and an adequate understanding of health, human services, and community resources. Your agency's social worker is usually the expert on whom you call. Having knowledge about referral sources helps match the client's needs and preferences with the best resource. Some referral source factors to be considered include compatibility with the client's expressed need, financial resources, accessibility (time as well as place), and ease of contact. Ease of contact and financial considerations sometimes are forgotten elements in coordination efforts, much to the detriment of the client's welfare (see Chapter 22 for a more detailed description of collaboration and coordination activities).

Interestingly, Welchman and Griener (2005) strongly view advocacy as both an individual and a collective professional responsibility, with the latter best served through professional associations. They note that "what actually seems to have happened is that nurses have been burdened with a responsibility that most professions assign, with good reason, to their professional associations" (p. 296), as the collective duties associated with advocacy have a much broader platform than most nurses can accomplish as individuals. These authors suggest a partnering of individual nurses willing to make a difference at the association level, as well as for their individual clients, and nursing associations willing to use their resources to bring about critical health care changes.

SUMMARY

How nurses perceive their professional role and how they function as a nurse in that role has a sizeable effect on the success of interpersonal communication in the nurse-client relationship. The professional nursing role should be evidenced in every aspect of nursing care, but nowhere more fully than in the nurse-client relationship. A professional nurse's *first* role responsibility is to the client. Because hospitals no longer are the primary settings for nursing practice, nurse practice roles take place in nontraditional as well as traditional health care settings. Advanced practice roles include the nurse practitioner, clinical nurse specialist, certified nurse-midwife, and nurse anesthetist. Two new roles, the clinical nurse leader and the doctor of nursing practice, were introduced in 2003.

Nurses learn professional role behaviors through the process of professional role socialization. Professional development as a nurse is a lifelong commitment. Benner's five developmental stages of increasing proficiency describe the nurse's progression from novice to expert. Mentorship and continuing education assist nurses in maintaining their competency and professional role development.

Because the professional nursing role demands such a strong commitment from nurses, the nurse can experience

Ethical Dilemma ■ *What Would You Do?*
Bishop and Scudder (1996) said that nurses have a professional obligation not only to provide efficient, effective, and attentive care but also to do so in the context of a caring relationship. What do you think they meant by this statement? What does this statement have to do with the nurse's role? Why is this an ethical issue?

role stress, experienced through role overload, role conflict, or role ambiguity. Good communication helps mitigate nursing stress and dissatisfaction, as does having a work environment that supports the professional development of nurses. Effective communication among health care providers also is essential for positive client health outcomes.

Advocacy is an important component of the professional nursing role. As client advocates, nurses assist clients in reworking role definitions lost through illness and assisting clients and families with the recovery process.

REFERENCES

American Association of Colleges of Nursing: *Values, qualities, and behaviors associated with professionalism in nursing practice*, Washington, DC, 1986, Author.

American Association of Colleges of Nursing: *Working paper on the role of the clinical nurse leader*, 2003; available online: http://www.aacn.nche.edu/Publications/WhitePapers/ClinicalNurseLeader.htm.

American Hospital Association: *A patient's bill of rights*, Chicago, 1992, Author.

American Nurses Association: *Code of ethics for nurses with interpretive statements*, Silver Spring, MD, 2001, American Nurses Publishing.

American Nurses Association: *Scope and Standards for nurse administrators*, ed 2, Washington, DC, 2003, American Nurses Association.

American Nurses Association: The right to accept or reject an assignment, *NursingWorld Reading Room* [website], 1995; available online: http://nursingworld.org/readroom/position/workplac/wkassign.htm

American Nurses Credentialing Center: *Magnet recognition program: recognizing excellence in nursing services: application manual*, Silver Spring, MD, 2004, Author.

American Nurses Credentialing Center: Objectives of the magnet recognition program, revised April 6, 2006. In *ANCC Magnet Recognition Program*, 2006; available online: http://www.nursingworld.org/ancc/magnet/index.html.

Arnold E: The stress connection: women and coronary heart disease, *Critical Care Nurs Clin North Am* 9(4):565–575, 1997.

Benner P: *From novice to expert: excellence and power in clinical nursing practice*, Menlo Park, CA, 1984, Addison-Wesley.

Benner P: *From novice to expert: excellence and power in clinical nursing practice*, comm ed, New York, 2000, Prentice Hall.

Bishop AH, Scudder, JR Jr: *Nursing ethics: therapeutic caring presence*, Boston, 1996, Jones and Bartlett.

Burkhardt M, Nathaniel A: *Ethics and issues in professional nursing*, ed 2, Clifton Park, NY, 2002, Delmar Thompson Learning.

Burnard P, Chapman C: *Professional ethical issues in nursing*, Philadelphia, 2004, Elsevier.

Coeling HV, Cukr PL: Communication styles that promote perceptions of collaboration, quality, and nurse satisfaction, *J Nurs Care Qual* 14(2):63–74, 2000.

Cohen H: *The nurse's quest for a professional identity*, Menlo Park, CA, 1981, Addison-Wesley.

Diers D: *Speaking of nursing: narratives of practice, research, policy, and the profession*, Sudbury, MA, 2004, Jones and Bartlett.

Doheny M, Cook C, Stopper M: *The discipline of nursing: an introduction*, ed 4, Stamford, CT, 1997, Appleton & Lange.

Erickson J, Ditomassi M: The clinical nurse leader: new in name only, *J Nurs Educ* 44(3):99–100, 2005.

Flexner A: Is social work a profession? In *Proceedings of the National Conference on Social Work*, New York, 1915.

Frederich ME, Strong R, von Gunten CF: Physician-nurse conflict: can nurses refuse to carry out doctor's orders, *J Palliat Med* 5(1):155–158, 2002.

Gibson CH: A concept analysis of empowerment, *J Adv Nurs* 16:354–361, 1991.

Grossman D: Enhancing your "cultural competence," *Am J Nurs* 94(7):58–62, 1994.

Hales A, Karshmer J, Montes-Sandoval L et al.: Preparing for prescriptive privileges: CNS-physician collaborative model, *Clin Nurse Spec* 12(2):73–82, 1998.

Ibsen H: *A doll's house*, 1879.

Kramer M, Schmalenberg C: Staff nurses identify essentials of magnetism. In McClure M, Hinshaw AS, editors, *Magnet hospitals revisited: attraction and retention of professional nurses*, Washington, DC, 2002, American Nurses Publication.

Malloch K, Porter-O'Grady T: *The quantum leader: applications for the new world of work*, Sudbury, MA, 2005, Jones and Bartlett.

Masters K: *Role development in professional nursing practice*, Sudbury, MA, 2005, Jones and Bartlett.

Mauksch I: Nurse-physician collaboration: a changing relationship, *J Nurs Adm* 6:35, 1981.

Mundinger M: Who's who in nursing: bringing clarity to the doctor of nursing practice: 2005, *Nurs Outlook* 53(4):173–176, 2005.

NANDA: *Nursing diagnoses: definitions and classifications 2003–2004,* Philadelphia, North American Nursing Diagnosis Association.

Neil K, McCoy A, Parry C et al.: The clinical experiences of novice students in nursing, *Nurs Educ* 23(4):16–21, 1998.

North American Nursing Diagnosis Association: *Classification of nursing diagnoses: proceedings of the ninth conference,* Philadelphia, 1991, JB Lippincott.

Parsons T: Definitions of health and illness in the light of American values and social structure. In Jaco E, editor, *Patients, physicians and illness,* Glencoe, NY, 1959, Free Press.

Phillips DE: Moral distress in nursing. In Friedman E, editor, *Choices and conflict,* Chicago, 1998, American Hospital Publishing.

Raudonis BN, Acton G: Theory-based nursing practice, *J Adv Nurs* 26(1):138–145, 1997.

Roberson M: Our diversity gives us strength: comment and opinion, *Am Nurse* 24(5):4, 1992.

Rosenstein AH, O'Daniel M: Disruptive behavior and clinical outcomes: perceptions of nurses and physicians, *Am J Nurs* 1:54–64, 2005.

Stichler JF: Professional interdependence: the art of collaboration, *Adv Pract Nurs Q* 1(1):53–61, 1995.

Taylor C, Lillis C, LeMone P: *Fundamentals of nursing: the art and science of nursing,* ed 3, Philadelphia, 1997, Lippincott-Raven.

Tschannen D: The effect of individual characteristics on perceptions of collaboration in the work environment, *Medsurg Nurs* 13(5):312–319, 2004.

Welchman J, Griener G: Patient advocacy and professional associations: individual and collective responsibilities, *Nurs Ethics* 12(3):296–304, 2005.

Wynne L, Shields C, Sirkin M: Illness, family theory and family therapy: conceptual issues, *Fam Process* 31:4–17, 1992.

Chapter 8

Life's Losses and Endings and the Nurse-Client Relationship

Elizabeth Arnold

OUTLINE

OBJECTIVES

At the end of the chapter, the reader will be able to:

1. Define loss and identify types of losses people face in a lifetime.
2. Describe the stages of death and dying.
3. Discuss the concept of palliative care.
4. Describe two theoretical frameworks used to describe the grieving process.
5. Define grief and describe common patterns of grieving.
6. Discuss the nurse's role in helping people deal with loss and grief.
7. Apply concepts of palliative care to nursing strategies in the care of the dying patient.

Chapter 8 examines how the nurse-client relationship functions in times of loss, with a particular focus on palliative care, grief and grieving, and nursing interventions at the end of life. Current research indicates that clients in the intensive care unit rank communication with professional caregivers as one of the most important skills at end of life, equal to or even superseding clinical skills (Curtis, 2004). Yet this important topic is not addressed in many nursing programs. As with other types of nurse-client relationships, self-awareness of your own personal feelings about loss, death, and grieving, combined with knowledge of the dying process, is important. These self-understandings can help you connect with clients and their families in a more authentic and empathetic manner.

BASIC CONCEPTS

Loss

Corless (2001) defines **loss** as "a generic term that signifies absence of an object, position, ability or attribute" (p. 352). It is a part of everyone's personal life journey. Many losses are sudden and unexpected; others are prolonged and can be experienced with relief as well as sorrow. Some are minor and easily resolved, while others are monumental, requiring significant time and emotional work to resolve. Although the concepts of loss and grieving are frequently associated with death and loss of relationship, loss is a much broader concept (Martin & Doka, 2000). Box 8-1 lists general assumptions about loss.

Feelings of loss can occur when giving up an old role for a new one—even if it is a positive move—or losing a place or object of special significance. People categorize loss according to its personal meaning to them. Each contains an element of saying good-bye to what was and beginning a new sense of self without the lost object, of building on the past while knowing you cannot return to it. Consider the following normal life events and reflect on the linking theme among all of them:

Box 8-1 General Assumptions About Loss

- The experience of loss is universal.
- Loss involves pain.
- Losses that are significant produce emotional upheaval.
- Loss requires change and adjustment to situations that are new, uncertain, and unchosen.
- Loss can impact many lives.

Adapted from Carson VB, Arnold EN: *Mental health nursing: the nurse-patient journey*, Philadelphia, 1996, Saunders, p. 662.

- A wife loses a 35-year-old marriage because her husband no longer finds her attractive.
- A cherished family pet dies.
- A wife watches as her husband disappears behind the wall of Alzheimer's disease.
- A middle-aged man loses his job of 24 years as a result of corporate downsizing.

The feelings associated with various losses differ only in the intensity with which they are encountered as a personal experience. As Mark Twain so poignantly expressed: "Nothing that grieves us can be called little; by the eternal laws of proportion a child's loss of a doll and a king's loss of a crown are events of the same size" (Mark

Exercise 8-1 The Meaning of Loss

Purpose: To consider personal meaning of losses.

Procedure:

Consider your answers to the following questions:

- What losses have I experienced in my life?
- How did I feel when I lost something or someone important to me?
- How was my behavior affected by my loss?
- What helped me the most in resolving my feelings of loss?
- How has my experience with loss prepared me to deal with further losses?
- How has my experience with loss prepared me to help others deal with loss?

Discussion:

1. In the larger group, discuss what gives a loss its meaning.
2. What common themes emerged from the group discussion about successful strategies in coping with loss?
3. How does the impact of necessary losses differ from that of unexpected, unnecessary losses?
4. How can you use in your clinical work what you have learned from doing this exercise?

Twain Quotes, 2002). While painful, losses offer unique opportunities for personal growth. Conversations about loss are not easy, as they reveal our vulnerability (Larson & Tobin, 2000). Other people want to hear that all is well and don't necessarily invite the grieving person to discuss their loss in any depth.

Case Example

"It's as if it just happened. The memories are so vivid—if I close my eyes, I can see the waiting room, hear the sounds of the hospital, see the strained faces of other visitors awaiting those precious few moments permitted for visiting an ill loved one. I recall sitting in the waiting room with my family gathered around. I can see the fear and dread in the eyes of my sisters and my dad, my husband and my children, my brothers-in-law, nieces, and nephews. We waited in silence—each of us knowing the outcome, but each praying privately that we were wrong. I can remember the expression on the doctor's face as he walked toward us. What I can't remember is what the doctor said, except for his final words: 'I am so sorry. We did everything we could to save your mother, but I am so sorry, we lost her.'"

To ignore or minimize end-of-life dialogue shortchanges clients in successfully coping with the final phase of life. It is important for nurses to understand their personal feelings about loss and death so that they can be fully present to dying clients and their families. Exercise 8-1 will assist you to examine the meaning of loss from a personal perspective.

Multiple Losses

Robinson and McKenna (1998) suggest that one loss can precipitate multiple losses. For example, the Alzheimer's disease victim doesn't lose only his memory. Accompanying his cognitive loss are profound psychological losses of role, communication, and independence. The nurse becomes a facilitator who can help the family strengthen its coping strategies in times of loss and grief by offering emotional support and providing useful direction and community referrals. Simply recognizing the multiple losses inherent in what seems to be a single loss is helpful to clients' families.

Multiple losses, whether stemming from one or many losses, are more complex and may take longer to resolve. The most helpful intervention is to focus on one relationship at a time, instead of trying to address the losses together. Putting into words the difference between a single loss and multiple losses often is reassuring to clients and families.

Death: The Final Loss

Death is the final chapter of the life cycle for all of us. As an event, death represents the physical ending of all that life holds: successes, failures, relationships, careers, laughter, and pain. Death may come suddenly without warning, or it can stalk a loved one, or us, over a long period of time. Death seeks the young and the old, the rich and the poor; it knows no favorites.

Silveira and Schneider (2004) suggest that "planning for the end of life is planning for the unknown" (p. 349). Death often is feared, even by those who believe in a spiritual afterlife. There is the fear of the unknown, the fear of losing everyone and everything, the fear of pain. Nurses are not immune from that fear. Nurses cling to life and struggle against death with the same intensity as the clients for whom they compassionately care, yet nurses are called on to rise above their feelings so that they can provide solace and support for the dying person and their loved ones. Nurses must achieve a balance between maintaining their own professional objectivity and psychological well-being and providing the empathy and support needed by their clients.

Everyone involved with the client—family, significant others, and health care providers—is confronted with the dying process. As Chenitz (1992), a nurse who died from AIDS, so eloquently stated, "Like many people with AIDS, I am not afraid of death. I am afraid of dying. The dying process and how that will be handled is of great concern to me. Everyone is going to die. Death is part of life. However, AIDS brings with it a terrible, painful, often humiliating dying process and that terrifies me" (p. 454). Chenitz's concerns are our concerns. How will we continue to provide compassion, assurance, and competence when we are faced with the dying person's pain, overwhelming losses, and feelings of sadness and anger?

Stages of Death and Dying

Nurses need to have a knowledge and understanding of the stages of death and dying so that they can be a support and not a hindrance to the client (Kellar, 1983). Kübler-Ross (1971) provides a framework for understanding the process of dying that is also applicable to the process of grieving. This framework includes five stages: denial, anger, bargaining, depression, and acceptance.

Denial. Commonly, when a client learns that his or her condition is terminal, the initial reaction is one of shock and disbelief. **Denial** is a temporary adaptive response to the traumatic news. Some clients use denial as a defense for long periods of time. The nurse needs to be sensitive to the client's need for denial and work at the client's pace of acceptance. Kübler-Ross characterizes this stage as the "No, not me" stage.

Anger. Increasingly the reality of death makes its way into client awareness, which leads to anger. The anger is focused on the fact that others have life and health, the very things that the client is losing. The client lashes out at family, friends, and staff members, angry that people are overly solicitous, and angry that people do not do enough. The client can be angry at life and angry with God. Kübler-Ross refers to anger as the "Why me?" stage.

Bargaining. After clients have vented their anger, they often enter a stage of bargaining with God. This stage is reminiscent of childhood days when children plead with their parents. Kübler-Ross states that the client in the bargaining stage characteristically says, "Yes, me, but..." or, "If you just let me live until my son's graduation, I can die in peace." During this phase, it is important to allow the client to proceed at his or her own pace of understanding. By supporting hope and avoiding challenges to the client's reality, the nurse actually facilitates the process of living while dying.

Depression. Once the client has resolved the bargaining stage, the client comes to the "Yes, me" stage. Depression at the end of life is often undertreated, because to confront it means acknowledging the enormity of the forthcoming loss. Nursing strategies in this stage include helping clients to accept their feelings as being normal responses and staying present as an empathetic, listening witness to their experience. This is often a time when people value spiritual help or legal assistance with advance directives, if they have not done so previously. Having the caregiver accessible becomes increasingly important.

Acceptance. According to Kübler-Ross, the acceptance stage brings peace. Clients are neither happy nor terribly sad. They accept the inevitable, hopefully having brought closure to important, unfinished business. There is nothing left to do but to be with the people they love and just wait. This time period can be difficult for family members, as the acceptance phase allows the dying client to experience a sense of detachment and gradual withdrawal from the external world. Nurses can be helpful in explaining the seeming detachment that accompanies the acceptance stage, and the active "presencing without demand" that family members can offer to their loved one during this final stage of dying. This witnessing is a valuable final gift.

Palliative Care

End-of-life care has increasingly become important for all clinical specialties to address, given the demographics of aging in this nation and an extended life span for many previously terminal illnesses. **Palliative care** is "a clinical approach designed to improve the quality of life for clients and families coping with a life threatening illness" (Davies & Higginson, 2004, p. 14). Over the past decade, individuals with serious life-threatening illnesses such as cancer and chronic obstructive pulmonary disease have achieved a significantly longer time span from time of diagnosis to death as a result of new technologies and the discovery of new medications. With appropriate care, a client's quality of life can be quite good until close to the end of life. Palliative care for these disorders begins at time of diagnosis, with the comfort part of holistic care gradually increasing and active treatment receding as treatment protocols fail to achieve previous results.

Quality palliative care requires a broad skill set, which includes careful management of physical symptoms and emotional support for the client and family as they embrace this part of every person's life journey. Glass, Cluxton and Rancour (2001) note that "the transition from life to death is as sacred as the transition experienced at birth" (p. 49). Nurses are often called upon to witness and to support this life transition.

By providing a sound early assessment and symptom management of the physical, psychosocial, and spiritual distress associated with a terminal illness and the dying process, a palliative approach provides immeasurable comfort to clients and families. Dying alone is a fear that many clients have. Supportive palliative care increases the client's sense of empowerment and dignity, and maximizes the family's ability to fully support the client.

The foundation for palliative, end-of-life care is to follow what clients actually want for themselves (Silveira & Schneider, 2004). For some clients, being able to voice their concerns about pain control and having access to family and staff at the time of death is extremely important. Even when a client is comatose, the nurse should talk with him or her about the care being given and encourage family members to stay connected through communication, reminding them that hearing is the last sense to go.

Communication is a critical component of high-quality care provided at the end of life (Boyle, Miller, Forbes-Thompson, 2005; Cherlin, Fried, Prigerson et al., 2005). With the awareness of death comes a concurrent awareness of potential loss of relationships, loss of purpose, and loss of control. As a life-threatening disease takes its toll, there is a general weakness such that one can no longer do what previously was possible, and with it can come a profound questioning or loss of self. As Millspaugh (2005) notes, "Anything that threatens one's existence may result in the loss of one's 'is-ness' or sense of purpose and may readily be experienced as spiritual suffering" (p. 921).

Recognizing the importance of palliative care, the AACN, with national funding, established the End-of-Life Nursing Education Consortium (ELNEC). The ELNEC project is a national education initiative to improve end-of-life care in the United States. The project provides undergraduate and graduate nursing faculty, continuing education providers, staff development educators, pediatric and oncology specialty nurses, and other nurses with training in end-of-life care so they can teach this essential information to nursing students and practicing nurses. To date, over 2571 nurses representing all 50 states have received ELNEC training and are sharing this new expertise in educational and clinical settings. Over the next few years, ELNEC trainers will touch the lives of millions of people facing the end of life (AACN, 2006).

Grief

Bereavement derives from a Latin term meaning "to be robbed" (Martin & Doka, 2000). Corless (2001) defines **grief** as "a person's emotional response to the event of loss" and the "state of mental and physical pain that is experienced when the loss of a significant object, person, or part of the self is realized" (p. 353). As such, it is an adaptive process with two major goals: healing oneself and recovering from the loss. The process of achieving these goals is often referred to as grief work.

Each person needs to grieve in his or her own way, but nurses can play an active role in supporting clients and families in this process. Jeffries (2005) notes, "A grieving person may need to be heard over and over again without receiving any advice, interpretations or words of wisdom" (p. xxiv). The grieving process can continue in some form and level of intensity for a long time. As people absorb a loss, common emotional behaviors can include sudden mood swings and recurring, wavelike, roller coaster–like feelings of sadness and loss. These wavelike feelings are more likely to occur when a person is alone, when something in the environment reminds the person of the loss, or during holiday or anniversary periods, when the feelings of loss are acute.

Case Example

"I would think I was doing okay, that I had a handle on my grief. Then without warning, a scent, a scene on television, an innocuous conversation would flip a switch in my mind, and I would be flooded with memories of my mother. My eyes would fill up with tears as my fragile composure dissolved. My grief lay right under the surface of my awareness and ambushed me at times and in places not of my choosing."

For some, the void can seem unending and the grief work feels unrelenting. C. S. Lewis (1963), writing of the death of his wife, stated, "No one ever told me that grief felt so like fear.... Part of every misery is...the fact that you don't merely suffer but have to keep on thinking about the fact that you suffer. I not only live each day in grief, but also live each day thinking about living each day in grief" (p. 3).

Theoretical Frameworks

Lindemann's Work on Grief. Lindemann (1944) pioneered the concept of grief work based on interviews with bereaved persons suffering a sudden tragic loss. From these interviews he identified patterns of grief, physical symptoms that accompany it, and emotional changes in people who had experienced significant losses. Box 8-2 lists Lindemann's four major observations about grief.

Box 8-2 Lindemann's Major Observations About Grief

- Acute grief is a definite syndrome with both psychological and physical symptoms.
- Grief may occur immediately after a crisis; it may be delayed; it may be exaggerated; or it may appear to be absent, which is considered pathological grief.
- Sometimes the typical pattern of grief is distorted.
- Distorted patterns of grief can be transformed into a normal grief reaction with appropriate clinical interventions.

Engel's Contributions. Engel (1964) built on the work of Lindemann in identifying the phases of grief work and psychological disturbances that commonly accompany unresolved grief. While helpful in understanding the grief process, not everyone follows the sequential pattern in an orderly manner. To some extent, the intensity of grieving depends on the relationship the person had with the deceased, other stressors occurring at the same time, and the level of social support at the time of loss. According to Engel, successful grieving involves three phases: (a) shock and disbelief, (b) developing awareness, and (c) restitution.

In the *shock and disbelief phase*, a newly bereaved person may feel alienated or detached from normal—"literally numb with shock; no tears, no feelings, just absolute numbness" (Lendrum & Syme, 1992, pp. 24–25). Sometimes a client may report seeing or hearing the lost person, or sensing his or her presence. These are not hallucinations brought about by a biological misfiring of neurotransmitters; they are normal temporary responses to extreme stress. Clients who have lost body parts through amputation sometimes physically feel sensations or pain in the missing limb. This initial disbelief and denial is an emotional buffer protecting one against a powerful assault to the integrity of the self. It does not mean that the client or family is delusional (Levin, 1998). Commenting that the symptoms, feelings, and sensations of unreality typically lose their intensity and become less frequent as time passes is a comfort to many people.

Case Example

Client: Sometimes when I'm driving home from work, I can actually hear Nancy talking to me. It's eerie. I know she's dead, but it feels so real. Am I going crazy?

Nurse: Mary, when people have suffered the loss of someone very significant to them, they often do think they hear or see them. It can be very frightening and disorienting, but it really is a very normal response to a powerful loss of someone special.

The client needs a high level of structured support coupled with empathetic listening to work through the emotional pain immediately following a loss. It is very important during this phase to help the client's family share the pain of their loss. Talking about a significant loss with someone who is caring and concerned allows a person to make better sense of it, and helps externalize his or her personal pain. Sometimes the nurse's empathic presence and acknowledgment of the person's grief is enough. Other times, the nurse will have to provide a tangible structure, such as a family meeting, to facilitate this discussion. This supportive intervention can enhance the feelings of closeness that families need to have in time of extreme need.

The *developing awareness (middle) phase* occurs when the unique void created by the loss begins to penetrate consciousness. The bereaved becomes increasingly aware of the anguish created by the loss and has painful feelings of sadness and emptiness. Strong emotional reactions (e.g., anger at the deceased, anger at persons deemed responsible for the loss, extreme helplessness, hopelessness, or guilt) are common. Other people experience this phase as an ongoing, low-level ache reminding the person of the void in his or her life. In her book *Living through Personal Crisis*, Stearns (1984) poignantly addresses the physical expressions of loss when she writes, "A wide range of marked physical changes can accompany an experience of loss. Not only through tears do we cry out our pangs of grief. Under the stress of what has been unrecoverably lost, our bodies have a dozen ways of weeping with us" (p. 16). A person may experience physical symptoms such as heart palpitations, nausea, dizziness, tightness in the throat or chest, a sense of fatigue or physical heaviness, or digestive problems. These are normal responses to fully feeling the void. This pain is part of the blueprint people use as they develop a new sense of self that incorporates the loss experience but does not depend on the lost person or object for its validity. Clients appreciate the nurse who can reassure them that this is a normal response.

Sadness and an overwhelming sense of loss can coincide with a sense of disorganization and loss of self-confidence without the other person. Nurses can offer support to surviving family members by normalizing these feelings and encouraging them to use resources they may not have thought of as they seek new sources of support. A progressive, supported return to normal activities is essential to the healing process.

Case Example

"Throughout the year following my mother's death, I was aware of a persistent feeling of heaviness—not physical heaviness, but emotional and spiritual. It was as if a dark cloud hung over my heart and soul. I was easily tired, with little energy to do anything but the most essential activities, and even those frequently received perfunctory attention. My usual pattern of 'sleeping like a log' was disrupted, and in its place I experienced uneasy rest that left me feeling as if I had never closed my eyes."

The *restitution phase* is characterized a reemergence of hope. The bereaved person experiences new energy for coping, a returning sense of well-being, and a renewed belief in self. Sleeping and eating habits begin to stabilize, and the person demonstrates increased interest in developing realistic goals for the future. Undertaking new relationships and new ways of being in a world without the person characterize this phase. It is not a complete detachment from the person lost, but rather an integrated one that allows for personal growth. Anniversaries and certain circumstances will trigger memories.

Patterns of Grieving

Anticipatory Grief. The grieving process can begin before the actual loss occurs. **Anticipatory grief** is an emotional response that occurs before the actual loss, for example, on learning of a terminal illness in a family member, a coming eviction, or a projected job loss. With anticipatory grief, the feelings of uncertainty and ambivalence in wishing it could be over while at the same time holding on to the person, dreading the finality of the projected loss, make the grieving process less straightforward. Feelings of helplessness, anger, and an inability to get on with one's life accompany the normal feelings of sadness associated with grief. It feels as though there is no way to complete the grieving process.

Case Example

Marge's husband, Albert, was diagnosed with Alzheimer's disease 5 years ago. Albert is now in a nursing home. He does not know who Marge is anymore. The doctor told Marge that his disease is progressing rapidly and that he most likely will die within the next few years. Marge just turned 60 and has been living with this disorder since she was 55. She doesn't know whether the "next few years" means 1 year, 5 years, or more. Although she misses Albert, she feels guilty because she would like a life of her own and has "other feelings, of wishing he would die so that she can get on with her life, and feeling cheated out of a life she deserves."

Grief Responses in Sudden or Traumatic Situations. Grief responses in sudden traumatic situations can be complicated by the emotional shock of the trauma situation. The safety and predictability of one's world is forever weakened. The bereaved responds to triggers reminiscent of the original trauma, and often reexperiences the details of the traumatic event. These flashbacks can often include regrets or guilt over things that the bereaved did or didn't do just prior to the traumatic loss that contributes to their emotional pain.

Case Example

Christine's fiancé was killed in an auto crash about a month before her wedding. Her fiancé had invited her to attend a movie that night, but Christine had pleaded that she was too tired, so he went alone. After the car crash, Christine blamed herself for not going out with him or suggesting that they stay home and watch movies there.

Places, smells, and noises can stimulate anxiety, and hyperarousal is a common finding. Some people manage their anxiety through avoidance of anything reminding them of the original trauma and are more reluctant to engage in future relationships.

Chronic Sorrow. A less-known form of grieving referred to as chronic sorrow is defined by Burke, Eakes, and Hainsworth (1999) as the "presence of pervasive grief found in people with chronic illness, their caregivers and the bereaved" (p. 374). Unlike complicated grief, and quite distinctive from clinical depression, chronic sorrow occurs as a low-level, nagging awareness of an ongoing loss of potential, for example, in a parent with a brain-damaged child or mental illness, or the spouse of an Alzheimer's victim. It is an incomplete loss, but a loss nevertheless. Many people fail to recognize the experience of an ongoing incomplete loss as a legitimate loss to be grieved (Lafond, 2002). A variant of chronic sorrow is "unattended sorrow," a term coined by Levine (2005) to describe how failure to resolve and tie up loose ends from previous losses can intensify the experience of a current, fresh loss.

Complicated Grieving. **Complicated grieving** is defined as an incapacitating form of grief, unusually long in duration and involving disorganized, depressed behaviors. Professional help is usually required when a person is trapped in complicated grief. A history of depression, substance abuse, death of a parent or sibling during childhood, prolonged conflict or dependency on the deceased person, or a succession of deaths within a short period of time can predispose a person to complicated grief. Chronic grief related to death is characterized by attempts to keep the deceased person alive by talking about him or her frequently, maintaining his or her personal things intact, and expecting that the deceased will reenter the mourner's life.

Lindemann (1944) described symptoms of complicated grieving, which he termed "morbid grief reactions":

- Overactivity or agitation without a keen sense of one's loss
- Acquisition of symptoms experienced during the last illness of the deceased
- Alteration in relationships with friends and relatives, progressing to complete social isolation
- Repression of feelings and an absence of emotional display despite the significant loss
- Lack of initiative or poor decision making, which leads to dysfunctional living patterns (e.g., poor grooming, not cooking or eating, not cleaning self or home)
- Deterioration into a state of depression marked by agitation, insomnia, feelings of worthlessness, bitter self-accusation, or the need for self-punishment (becoming dangerously suicidal)
- Extreme hostility toward persons held responsible for the loss

Delayed Grieving. A variation of complicated grief includes the absence of grief in situations where it would be expected. For example, young men and women faced with constant death in the current war in Iraq often don't or can't take the time to mourn the deaths of their war comrades in a timely manner. The life-and-death demands of the situation don't allow for it. However, the feelings don't just disappear; instead, they may reappear in unexpected ways later in life. Delayed grieving involves the postponement of grieving for weeks, months, or years. Subsequent losses can trigger an extreme reaction that seems out of proportion to the current loss or lasts much longer than would be expected.

Exercise 8-2 A Personal Loss Inventory

Purpose: To provide a close examination of one's history with loss.

Procedure:

Complete each sentence and reflect on your answers:
The first significant loss I can remember in my life was ___________.
The circumstances were ___________.
My age was ___________.
The feelings I had at the time were___________.
The thing I remember most about that experience was ___________.
I coped with the loss by ___________.
The most difficult death for me to face would be ___________.
I know my grief over a loss is resolved when ___________.

From Carson VB, Arnold EN: *Mental health nursing: the nurse-patient journey*, Philadelphia, 1996, WB Saunders, p. 666.

For example, nurses will encounter clients who share information such as, "I never recovered from my son's death" or, "I feel like my life ended when my husband died." The client is identifying that grief work was never completed. Grieving that is incomplete or never attempted at all hangs over the individual and family like a dark cloud, blocking out the sun and resulting in long-term problems such as depression. It is important for the nurse to address this issue, even if the client is seeking help for an unrelated issue. The nurse can suggest a resource like the Grief Recovery Helpline or a grief support group. Exercise 8-2 helps you explore your own personal loss inventory.

APPLICATIONS

Roles of Nurses Working with Dying Clients

Helping Clients Achieve a Good Death

Although death is a necessary and unavoidable part of every person's life, it is a very uncomfortable topic to talk about. Talking with clients and families about death and dying is a complex process, complicated by the reality that the precise timing of death is not known. There are often many conflicting human factors associated with the dying process, and there is a general stigma attached to even thinking about the dying process.

The Institute of Medicine (1997) describes a good death as "one that is free from unavoidable distress and suffering for patients, families and caregivers; in general accord with patients and families' wishes; and reasonably consistent with clinical, cultural, and ethical standards" (p. 4). In a study of what constitutes a good death from the perspective of families, clients, and professionals, Steinhauser, Clipp, McNeilly et al. (2000) identified six elements: pain and symptom relief, transparent decision making, preparation for what to expect, achieving a sense of completion, contributing to others, and receiving affirmation as a whole person. Ultimately, the client's values and wishes should be the primary focus of caregiving and decision making about treatment issues at the end of life. Other authors identify three factors associated with a client's ability to achieve a good death (Côté & Peplar, 2005; Griffin & Rabkin, 1998):

- Keeping a sense of control
- Maintaining hope
- Having a sense of meaning and purpose in life

In addition to knowing what to expect, having financial affairs in order for some and making funeral arrangements prior to the actual death for others contribute to a good death, as does the comfort of care providers in talking about death and preparing the client and the family (Silveira & Schneider, 2004). Nurses often are the key informants about changes in the client's condition. In this role, nurses need to respect fundamental differences in the level of information an individual may desire. Listen and watch for cues. Some people will want to know everything, whereas others will not want to have this level of information. The response of the client should determine the content and pace of sharing information. Exercise 8-3 provides you with the opportunity to think about what constitutes a good death.

Developing an Evidence-Based Practice

Beckstrand R, Callister L, Kirchhoff K: Providing a "good death": critical care nurses' suggestions for improving end-of-life care, *Am J Crit Care* 15(1):38-45, 2006.

This survey study was part of a larger national study designed to elicit critical care nurses' view (N = 861) of end-of-life care in intensive care units. The goal of this report, consistent with the Institute of Medicine's recommendation to strengthen the knowledge base on end-of-life care, was to elicit suggestions on ways to improve end-of-life care.

Results: Study results indicated a common commitment of study subjects to helping clients achieve a good death, one marked with dignity and peace. Ways to achieve this goal were described as managing pain and discomfort, eliciting and following the clients' wishes for end-of-life care, facilitating family presence at time of death, and communicating effectively with other members of the health care team. Barriers were identified as time constraints, staffing patterns, and treatment decisions that did not reflect the clients' needs or wishes.

Application to Your Clinical Practice: As people live longer and the trajectory between time of diagnosis and time of death lengthens, palliative care becomes increasingly important. How could you, as a nurse, effectively help clients to die with dignity in a hospital setting? In a home setting?

Care of the Family: Family Meetings and Family Interventions

Inclusion of the family is an important dimension of holistic end-of-life care. The family can be an important support to the client. Equally important, they will need

Exercise 8-3 What Makes for a Good Death

Purpose: To help students focus on defining the characteristics of a good death.

Procedure:

1. In pairs or small groups, think about, write down, and then share briefly examples of a "good" and a "not-so-good" death that you have witnessed in your personal life or clinical setting.
2. What were the elements that you thought contributed to its being a "good" or "not-so-good" death?

Discussion:

Were there any common themes found in the stories as to what constitutes a "good" death? How could you use the findings of this exercise in helping clients achieve a "good" death?

to be able to prepare for the death of their loved one in ways that have meaning to them. Most will need the support and coaching of the health care team to do so. Family members often have trouble talking to each other about the death and its impact on them. It is "normal" for the loss to have a different impact on each family member, because each has had a unique relationship with the lost person (Martin & Doka, 2000). Giving family members permission to have different types of feelings about the loss often is comforting.

Family members should be included in decision making and in preparing for every aspect of the client's death. Nurses can facilitate such preparation by proactively providing comfort and responding compassionately to the unvoiced needs of clients and families for information and support (Mok & Chiu, 2004). Flexibility in allowing family and/or significant others access to the client, while taking care that the visits are not taxing for the client, can be equally comforting for clients and involved family members. Thinking about preparations after the death can also be helpful and, in some cases, healing for the client to plan as well as for the family. Box 8-3 identifies family communication needs at the end of life.

Box 8-3 Family Communication Needs at End of Life

- Honest and complete answers to questions
- Updates about the client's condition and changes as they occur
- Understandable explanations
- Frequent opportunities to express concerns and feelings in a supportive, unhurried environment
- Information about what to expect—physical, emotional, spiritual—as death approaches
- Discussion of whom to call, legal issues, memorial or funeral planning
- Appreciation of the conflicts that families experience when the illness dictates that few options exist (are they prolonging life or prolonging the dying phase?)
- Short private times to communicate with the client

The health care team, of which the nurse is a key member, can provide significant support for family members. Proactive planned family meetings can help alleviate family anxiety about the dying process, reduce unnecessary conflict between family members, and assist family members with important decision-making processes.

A family meeting allows the nurse to learn about the client and family values and preferences regarding end-of-life care and to answer difficult questions in a supportive environment. Although the physician more commonly leads the discussion, this is not always the case; nurses often are part of the health team called upon to conduct the family conference. The discussion of the client's condition should be compassionate and understandable. Curtis (2004) recommends that there be a higher ratio of family member-to-health care provider speaking time and that there be follow-up communication using a consistent physician-nurse team approach. Helping clients and their families understand the importance of advance directives and do not resuscitate (DNR) orders for withdrawal or noninitiation of life-sustaining treatments is an important aspect of communication; it helps prevent later conflicts among family members when tensions arise near the time of death (Boyle et al., 2005).

Box 8-4 Talking with Families About Care Options at End of Life

If neither durable power of attorney nor written directive is in effect:

- Determine who should be approached to make the decisions about care options.
- Determine if any key members are absent. (Try to keep those who know the client best in the center of decision making.)
- Find a quiet place to meet where each family member can be seated comfortably.
- Sit down and establish rapport with each person present. Ask about the relationship each person has with the client and how each person feels about the client's current condition.
- Try to achieve a consensus about the patient's clinical situation, especially prognosis.
- Provide a professional observation about the client's status and expected quality of life—survival vs. quality of life. Ask what each person thinks the client would want.
- Should the family choose comfort measures only, assure the family of the attention to patient comfort and dignity that will occur.
- Seek verbal confirmation of understanding and agreement.
- Attention to the family's emotional responses is appropriate and appreciated.

Adapted from Lang F, Quill T: Making decisions with families at the end of life, *Am Fam Physician* 70(4):720, 2004.

Nurses use a combination of presence, compassion, and quiet assurance to help clients and their families develop a comfort in talking about how they would like the controllable parts of the dying process to go. Guidelines for talking with families about the type of end-of-life care they want for their loved one are presented in Box 8-4.

It is difficult for anyone to remain in a relationship with another whose pain will not go away. This is the challenge for nurses: to remain in relationships with our clients and their loved ones even though we feel inadequate to the task. Our ability to listen and assist those who are grieving to understand their own feelings and behaviors through the use of open-ended statements such as "And then…"; "Tell me more"; "You felt…"; "How did you do that?"; "Who was with you?"; and "How did you feel?" is sometimes all that is needed to encourage the grieving process. Nurses must be cognizant of the fact that grieving is not a yes-or-no process, nor is it cut-and-dried. "Yes, it is true that your loved one has died as a result of acquired immunodeficiency syndrome (AIDS)." "No, he will never come back." These are the only simple realities; beyond these, the grief process is complex. Yet Casarett, Kutner, and Abrahm (2001) assert that simply by sitting with a family and bearing witness to the family's expression of grief, health care providers provide important support.

Case Example

"I remember standing next to my mom's bed. We had gone to her room to pay our last respects. A young nurse stood near to me and reached out gently and touched my shoulder. Softly she said, 'I'll just stay here with you in case you need something.' When I looked at her I saw eyes brimming with tears and a profound sadness on her face. Her presence meant so much; I was grateful for her open expression of sorrow. It confirmed the pain we were all experiencing."

Nurses can offer assistance in other ways as well. Grief affects perceptions. Nurses can provide anticipatory guidance about what will happen in the dying process and about the process of grief, and they can act as a realistic sounding board in correcting misperceptions. Interventions that are helpful include the following:

- Informing the grieving person or family what to expect as far as the intensity and unpredictability of grief
- Affirming that the encompassing nature of grief can leave the grieving individual questioning his or her own mental stability
- Providing support and quiet, compassionate acceptance of the myriad of emotions that comprise the grief process

The following quote illustrates some of these characteristics of grief:

> Nurses have many opportunities to provide formal and informal teaching about a variety of strategies the client, whether individual or family, can use to help themselves. In the role of teacher, nurses can share simple but effective strategies that others can use to assist someone who is dealing with grief.

Box 8-5 lists suggestions the nurse can give to significant others involved with grieving individuals and families.

Box 8-5 Strategies for Supporting a Grieving Person

- Prepare meals.
- Provide transportation.
- Provide babysitting service.
- Help deal with financial issues.
- Clean home.
- Sit quietly with the grieving person.
- Encourage the person to talk about the deceased or the loss.
- Share a special memory about the deceased with the grieving person.
- Write down that memory so that the grieving person can reread it.
- Weeks and months after the funeral, call and ask how the grieving person is handling his or her grief.
- Avoid giving trite reassurances.
- Accept that your presence is worth more than 1000 words.

Self-Awareness: Reflecting on Personal Experiences with Grief

Nurses are confronted with their own grief as well as the grief of clients and their families and significant others. Unlike their clients, who live through one loss at a time, the nurse may experience several losses a week while caring for terminally ill clients and their families (Brunelli, 2005). It is important for nurses to examine their experiences with and feelings about grief and loss. How have we handled our grief experiences? Did we work our way through grief and not try to sidestep the pain of the loss? How would we cope if we were faced with what our client is facing? This examination is an ongoing one, stimulated by losses in the nurse's personal and professional life. Exercise 8-4 is designed to help you think about an important loss and how putting the feelings into words can be an important dimension of healing.

Using the Nursing Process in Working with Dying Clients

Working with dying clients and their families is a demanding task, but it can also be an emotionally enriching experience for the nurse. Not every nurse can be intimately involved with every dying client and family members. It is hoped that there is at least one nurse available to the client who is able to become involved in the client's pain, to withstand the client's anger, and to help the client in whatever way is needed in this experience of death. Exercise 8-5 is designed to help you think through some of the aspects of grieving.

Exercise 8-4 Words About Losing Someone Important

Purpose: To provide students with an opportunity to see how putting into words the meaning a person had for you could facilitate the grieving process.

Procedure:

1. Write a letter to someone who has died or is no longer in your life. Before writing the letter, reflect on the meaning this person had for you and the person you have become.
2. In the letter, tell the person what they meant to you and why it is that you miss them.
3. Tell the person what you remember most about your relationship.
4. Tell the person anything you wished you had said but didn't when the person was in your life.

With a partner, each student should share his or her story without interruption. When the student finishes his or her story, the listener can ask questions for further understanding.

Discussion:

1. What was it like to write a letter to someone who had meaning in your life and is no longer available to you?
2. Were there any common themes?
3. In what ways was each story unique?
4. How could you use this exercise in your care of clients who are grieving?

Exercise 8-5 A Questionnaire About Death

Purpose: To explore students' feelings about death.

Procedure:

Answer the following questions.

1. Who died in your first personal involvement with death?
   a. Grandparent or great-grandparent
   b. Parent
   c. Brother or sister
   d. Other family member
   e. Friend or acquaintance
   f. Stranger
   g. Public figure
   h. Animal
2. To the best of your memory, at what age were you first aware of death?
   a. Younger than 3 years
   b. 3 to 5 years
   c. 5 to 10 years
   d. 10 years or older
3. When you were a child, how was death talked about in your family?
   a. Openly
   b. With some sense of discomfort
   c. Only when necessary, and then with an attempt to exclude the children
   d. As though it were a taboo subject
   e. Do not recall any discussion
4. Which of the following most influenced your present attitudes toward death?
   a. Death of someone else
   b. Specific reading
   c. Religious upbringing
   d. Introspection and meditation
   e. Ritual (e.g., funerals)
   f. Television, radio, or motion pictures
   g. Longevity of my family
   h. My health or physical condition
   i. Other
5. How often do you think about your own death?
   a. Very frequently (at least once a day)
   b. Frequently
   c. Occasionally
   d. Rarely (no more than once a year)
   e. Very rarely or never
6. What does death mean to you?
   a. The end; the final process of life
   b. The beginning of a life after death; a transition; a new beginning
   c. A joining of the spirit with a universal cosmic consciousness
   d. A kind of endless sleep; rest and peace
   e. Termination of this life, but with survival of the spirit
   f. Do not know

Exercise 8-5 A Questionnaire About Death – *cont'd.*

7. If you had a choice, what kind of death would you prefer?
   a. Tragic, violent death
   b. Sudden, but not violent death
   c. Quiet, dignified death
   d. Death in the line of duty
   e. Death after a great achievement
   f. Suicide
   g. Homicide victim
   h. There is no "appropriate" kind of death
8. If it were possible, would you want to know the exact date on which you are going to die?
   a. Yes
   b. No
9. If your physician knew that you had a terminal disease and a limited time to live, would you want him or her to tell you?
   a. Yes
   b. No
   c. It would depend on the circumstances
10. What efforts do you believe ought to be made to keep a seriously ill person alive?
    a. All possible efforts should be made (e.g., transplantation, kidney dialysis)
    b. Efforts should be made that are reasonable for that person's age, physical condition, mental condition, and pain
    c. After reasonable care, a natural death should be permitted
    d. A senile person should not be kept alive by elaborate artificial methods
11. If or when you are married, would you prefer to outlive your spouse?
    a. Yes, I would prefer to die second and outlive my spouse
    b. No, I would rather die first and have my spouse outlive me
    c. Undecided or do not know
12. What effect has this questionnaire had on you?
    a. It has made me somewhat anxious or upset
    b. It has made me think about my own death
    c. It has reminded me how fragile and precious life is
    d. Other effects

It is this nurse who accepts the client's denial as long as the client needs to use this defense. It is this nurse who can say to the client, "I can see how angry you are, and I wish that I could make you better." It is this nurse who can assist the client to see that berating family members may not be the best method for dealing with his or her sense of powerlessness. It is this nurse who communicates a care plan to the rest of the staff so that everyone has an understanding of the client's changing needs. Finally, it is this nurse who helps family members deal with their own grief as they prepare to say goodbye. Morgan (2001) describes a basic social process between nurse and client in palliative care, which she labeled protective coping and adjustment. This process involves nursing interactions that *protect*, *maintain*, and *safeguard* the integrity of clients while at the same time helping them to determine and act upon actions that are in their own best interests.

In planning care for the dying client, the nurse applies the steps of the nursing process, bearing in mind the principles of end-of-life care presented in Box 8-6.

Box 8-6 Principles of End-of-Life Care

- Discussions of medical futility with patients and family will be more effective if they include concrete information about treatment, its likelihood of success, and the implications of the intervention and nonintervention decisions.
- Effective decision making at the end of life can be improved by the use of advance directives and surrogate decision makers.
- Ethnic and cultural traditions and practices influence the use of advance directives and health care decision-making surrogates.
- Taking the time to explore the client's perceptions about quality of life at the end of life is a core component of clinical assessment and is essential to ensuring optimal outcomes.
- The cost of failing to offer clients and families a full range of end-of-life care options, services, and settings is an incalculable toll in terms of quality of life and utilization of appropriate health care resources at the end of life.

Modified from Bookbinder M, Rutledge DN, Donaldson NE et al.: End-of-life care series: part I: principles, *Online Journal of Clinical Innovations* 4(4), 2001. Copyright 2001, Cinahl Information Systems. Reprinted by permission.

Assessment. There are a number of important areas for the nurse to assess when working with the dying client, including the client's feelings about death, cultural response to and spiritual beliefs regarding death, life experiences with death, developmental level, role within the family, and support system. All of these factors interact to shape the client's response to death.

The assessment of *feelings* has already been addressed in the discussion of the stage of death and dying. What was not covered was the manner in which clients express their feelings. Generally, clients hint about their underlying feelings and concerns. Thus, the nurse must be attuned not only to nonverbal clues that clients communicate but also to their use of symbolic language.

Clients may refer to their deaths as a great struggle, "a last train ride," or "the biggest fight of my life." The use of symbolic language with a sensitive listener usually means that the client is willing to talk about issues of loss, saying good-bye, and taking care of unfinished business. The nurse assesses a client's readiness to openly discuss death and, one hopes, responds in a way that says, "You can talk to me." Sometimes the nurse is the most convenient or the only person who allows the client this freedom.

In assessing the *family's feelings* related to their loved one's death, the nurse must be aware that the family's reaction is not always synchronous with that of the client. For instance, the client may be ready to openly grieve, but the family is still denying the reality of death. The nurse must also help the family to deal with their feelings so that they can provide empathetic and loving support to the client.

Culture plays an important role in how a dying person and family members cope with death. Nurses need to consider how grief is expressed by the client's culture. Nurses need to examine their own cultural biases so that they are not judgmental toward cultural beliefs and practices that are important to clients and their families. Cultural beliefs about death affect the nurse's role in a number of areas. For instance, culture may dictate such things as (a) the type of care that is given to provide comfort to the dying person; (b) the use of nonprofessional as well as professional caregivers; (c) the understanding of the causes of illness and death; (d) funeral or burial rites; and (e) definition of acceptable sick role behavior and grief responses.

Spiritual beliefs and religious practices regarding death are another crucial area for the nurse to assess. In assessing spiritual needs, the nurse needs to be attuned to clients' verbal and nonverbal behaviors indicative of their feelings and thoughts toward God. Clients may refer to God in a guarded, indirect way; they may joke about God; or they may openly plead with God. These clients are indicating their need to talk about and to God, and this need is as essential for the nurse to address as administering pain medication. Steinhauser, Voils, Clipp et al. (2006) suggest using the probe "Are you at peace?" as a useful way to ask the client about spiritual concerns without being intrusive. The dying process, grief, and death itself herald a spiritual crisis—a crisis of faith, hope, and meaning. The resolution of this crisis is an integral aspect of emerging from grief healed and whole and confronting death with peace and acceptance. In fact, it is not unusual for a client who has previously declined spiritual interventions to desire them as he or she moves into the final phase of life. Exercise 8-6 is helpful for nurses in examining the patterns and meaning in their own lives, and may be a useful strategy to assist clients to do the same.

Exercise 8-6 Blueprint for My Life Story

Purpose: To view life as a whole, integrated process.

Procedure:

This is a two-part exercise. First, make a single life line across a blank sheet of paper, beginning with your birth. Identify the significant events in your life, and insert on your worksheet the age that you were when the event or moment occurred. When you are finished, answer the following questions:

Childhood

1. What was your happiest time as a child?
2. What were your saddest times?
3. What did you hope to become when you grew up?
4. Who were your companions as a child?
5. How did you view your mother? Your father? Your grandparents?
6. How did you feel about your home? Your neighborhood?
7. As a child, who was your most important relationship with?
8. Were boys and girls treated alike in school? In the family?
9. Where was your favorite space?
10. Where did you live as a child?

Adolescence

1. What subjects did you like best in school?
2. How and when did you get your first job?
3. Who were your companions as an adolescent, and what did you do with them?
4. Who was your first girlfriend or boyfriend?
5. Who had the most significant influence on you as an adolescent? In what ways?
6. What was most important to you as an adolescent?

Adulthood

1. What was the best job you ever had? The worst?
2. If you could choose your career again, what would you choose?
3. If you could relive any part of your life, what would it be?
4. What parts of your life are you particularly proud of?
5. Look back over your life. When were you happiest? Saddest?
6. What have you learned about life from the process of living?
7. What was the most exciting part of your life?
8. Who has influenced your life most as an adult?
9. If you could make three wishes, what would they be?

Record your answers in whatever way seems most appropriate to you. Spend some time thinking about the events you have identified on your life line and the answers you have provided in the narrative. Reflect on your life as a whole, with you as the primary actor, producer, and director. Think about ways in which you could write the remaining chapters of your life so they have special meaning for you.

Discussion:

In the larger group, discuss your lifeline.

1. In what ways were you surprised or comforted by the events that emerged from your lifeline?
2. As you contrast your lifeline with those of your classmates, do common themes emerge?
3. How could you use common themes as the basis for discussion with clients?

Religious practices and rituals are important to clients in the final phase of life. The nurse needs to assess the importance of such rites and facilitate their performance. Although the nurse may not understand the exact meaning of the religious rite for the client, displaying reverence and respect toward the client's need for specific religious practices helps the client feel more comfortable. In addition, the nurse recognizes that facilitating these practices touches the client's inner core and helps him or her to move toward a peaceful death (Bryson, 2004).

Previous life experiences with death may affect clients' attitudes toward their own dying, either positively or negatively. For instance, if clients have experienced the death of a loved one or a friend who was able to face death with equanimity, they may not view death as something to be feared.

Developmental level is an influencing factor in a person's attitude toward death. The young child views death entirely differently from the elderly client, and this difference should influence nursing strategies. A child younger than 3 years has no clear concept of what death means. By 3 years of age, children begin to play at death as if it is a game, without any conception of the finality associated with the reality. Very young children react to the anguish and the grief of those around them but are confused as to why everyone is so sad. Preschoolers understand that death involves leaving, but they believe that it is gradual and temporary. Cartoons on television, which commonly depict characters dying and coming back to life, reinforce this belief.

Children between 6 and 9 years tend to personify death and view it as a person who causes people to die. The older school-age child, 10 to 12 years of age, understands that death is the cessation of bodily life. The adolescent may vacillate between a mature and a childlike attitude toward death. Regardless of the age of the child, questions should be answered directly and honestly at the child's level of comprehension. It is important to consider the question from the child's perspective. In answering questions, think about what the child *wants* to know, and what the child *needs* to know. Depending on the question, you may need to explore it further with the child to be sure you understand what is being asked.

Adults between 18 and 45 years of age are fully aware of the finality of death, but they tend to believe that only old people die. They are so involved with the tasks of generativity, family, and career that death is not a common thought. Between the ages of 45 and 65 years of age, adults have accepted their own mortality as a concept, but not as a reality that will happen to them. They have probably already experienced the death of their parents or some of their peers.

Adults older than 65 years are more in touch with their mortality, in part because of the aging process itself, and in part because of the increase in the number of deaths of close associates and family members of their generation. Concerns about dying and being a burden to family members become immediate (Carson & Arnold, 1996). Elderly clients often want to die. Often doing a life review focused on things the person is proud of and helping the client connect with important people or religious affiliations helps with unfinished business. Elderly people are afraid of dying alone, and for some, this may be a reality if they have outlived most of their contemporaries and have few friends. The nurse may be the only person willing to help them make this transition.

Family role is another area that the nurse needs to assess in relation to the dying client. Different roles within the family carry with them differing amounts of responsibility, some requiring significant personal and family functional adjustments when a family member dies.

The nurse also examines the client's *support system* and its availability as a resource. The presence or absence of a loving and supportive family is a determining factor in the client's ability to cope (Bauman, 2000). The family may need as much support as the client in coping with the dying process with their loved one. For instance, if a client is expressing anger and is particularly abusive to a spouse, the spouse may be confused and frightened. A situation like this would require some mediation on the part of the nurse, not only to help the client deal with his or her anger more appropriately but also to provide the spouse with an understanding of the client's behavior.

Analysis. Any or all of the following nursing diagnoses could be appropriate when working with the dying client and family members:

- Ineffective coping related to impending death
- Anticipatory grieving related to expected death
- Dysfunctional grieving related to expectant death
- Fear related to known and unknown factors of expected death
- Alteration in self-concept related to death
- Spiritual distress related to impending death

Planning. The care of dying clients and their families requires open and consistent communication among all members of the health team. Usually the nurse coordinates the planning and evaluation of care.

Ideally, one nurse is responsible for the primary care of the client, keeps the rest of the health team members informed of new issues, and seeks their input to plan and to evaluate care. This approach prevents fragmentary and inconsistent care and allows the client to be cared for totally.

Although goals for care are individualized to particular clients and their families, the following general goals provide a framework for developing more specificity:

- The client will vent anger in appropriate ways.
- The client will explore and evaluate his or her life experiences.
- The client will identify areas of concern over "unfinished business."
- The client will use religious practices appropriate to his or her beliefs.
- The client will verbalize a sense of personal order and meaning associated with the dying process.
- The client will spend private uninterrupted time with his or her family.

Intervention. In meeting these goals, most of the nurse's interventions will focus on communication. Lindemann (1944) studied dying persons and their families for 30 years and summarized three key components in providing care for them: (a) open, empathetic communication; (b) honesty; and (c) tolerance of emotional expression.

Evaluation. The evaluation of care of dying clients and their families is an ongoing and continuous process. In some cases, nurses may consider their interventions successful if the client dies in peace surrounded by loved ones. For some clients, though, this kind of death is not possible, and yet this does not mean that nursing interventions were ineffective. If a client persists in a state of denial until the end, this is the client's right. Although nurses may feel this is not the ideal way to depart from life, it is the client's needs that are paramount in directing care. In general, nursing care of the dying client is successful when the nurse is sensitive to the needs of the client and family and meets those needs in a loving and gentle way. For one client, such care will involve the nurse's quiet presence while the client cries and mourns; for another, it will involve the nurse's faithfulness in light of the client's angry behavior; for still another, it may be the nurse's willingness to pray with him or her for a peaceful death. Everyone experiences death differently, and it is the uniqueness of each person's experience that the nurse attempts to tap into and facilitate. Dobratz (2002) describes a human life pattern in dying patients that is "shaped by self-integration, inner cognition, creation of personal meanings, and connection to others and a higher being" (p. 139).

Talking About Death

It is always important to find out what the client or family already knows and is asking. For example, to a client who asks, "Am I going to die?" the nurse might respond, "What is your sense of it?"

Talking about death with clients is not something that comes easily to the nurse. Few schools of nursing

Box 8-7 Guidelines for Communicating with Terminally Ill Clients

- Avoid automatic responses. Each person and family is unique and deserves to be treated as such.
- Relate person to person. Show humor as well as sorrow.
- Use your mind, eyes, and ears to hear what is said as well as what is not said.
- Respect the individual's pattern of communication and ways of dealing with stress. Support the client's desire for control of his or her life.
- Humility and honesty are essential. Be willing to admit that you do not know the answer.
- Maintain a sense of calm. This will help the client's sense of control.
- Never force the client to talk. Respect the client's need for privacy and be sensitive to the client's readiness to talk.
- Let the client lead the discussion to the future. Be comfortable with focusing on the here and now. (This discussion is not a one-time event; openings for discussion should be encouraged as the client's condition worsens.)
- Be willing to allow the client to see some of your fears and vulnerabilities. It is much easier to open up to someone who is "human and vulnerable" than to someone who appears to have all the answers.
- Provide short, frequent times for family members to be with the dying client (without overtiring the client).

actually teach nurses how to converse with the dying client. In addition, nurses are subject to the same societal influences that the client is. These influences paint death as a topic to be avoided at all costs. Nurses often feel ill prepared to deal with the emotional turmoil generated by the task. Yet at the end of life, they need to be fully responsible for their own performance in caring for dying clients, while at the same time acting on behalf of clients who no longer are able to act for themselves (Olthuis, Dekkers, Leget et al., 2006). The dying person often has a very strong need to express these feelings, and nurses can be facilitators of this process if they allow themselves to be a healing presence. Box 8-7 provides guidelines for communicating with terminally ill clients.

Case Example

"A hospice social worker enters the bedroom of a man who lies dying, surrounded by anxious family members. She kneels beside his bed, takes his hand and asks, 'Would you like me to tell you what I see?' With his consent, she tells him she senses his struggle. She sees also that his disease is becoming larger than his ability to fight it. Her quiet honesty disarms all defenses, enabling the man and his family to take a step beyond their fear and begin facing the pain of their approaching losses. She continues to kneel there as emotion fills the room. That is healing presence" (Miller, 2001, p. 12).

In addition to communication, the nurse's interventions can focus on helping the client come to terms with unfinished business and spiritual needs. Both issues may become sources of anxiety if the client has not dealt with them previously. Providing spiritual care through the use of clergy and the nurse's own interventions—providing presence and touch and encouraging use of prayer and scripture reading—are all important in meeting identified spiritual needs. A compassionate intervention would be to provide the client and family with the privacy necessary to talk and comfort one another and to share thoughts and physical closeness not possible when frequent interruptions by nursing staff occur.

Care of clients in the final phase of life should *always* be guided by the values and preferences of the individual patient. Allowing clients to maintain control over whatever they can helps preserve independence (Steinhauser et al., 2000). Common symptoms during the last days of life include withdrawal from the external world physically with longer periods of sleeping or coma, hallucinations or illusions, loss of appetite and interest in food, changes in bowel and bladder function with diminished and concentrated urine, confusion, restlessness and agitation, significant noisy changes in breathing, and changes in skin temperature and color. Pain management is critical to providing effective end-of-life care. It is important to ask clients to rate their level of pain, with 1 being the lowest and 10 the highest. With children and clients who speak English as a second language, the Wong-Baker FACES Pain Rating Scale can be particularly helpful (see Figure 8-1). Opioids such as morphine and lorazepam (Ativan) can keep most clients comfortable.

End-of-Life Decision Making

Thelan (2005) defined **end-of-life decision making** as "the process that healthcare providers, patients and patients' families go through when considering what treatments will or will not be used to treat a life threatening illness" (p. 29). Ideally, end-of-life decisions related to life-limiting, incurable disease should be expressed in writing as an **advance directive**. This is a legal document that can be revoked or revised at any time by its author.

The enactment of the Patient Self-Determination Act in 1990 mandates that all individuals receiving medical care receive written information about advance directives

0
NO HURT
1
HURTS
LITTLE BIT
2
HURTS
LITTLE MORE
3
HURTS
EVEN MORE
4
HURTS
WHOLE LOT
5
HURTS
WORST

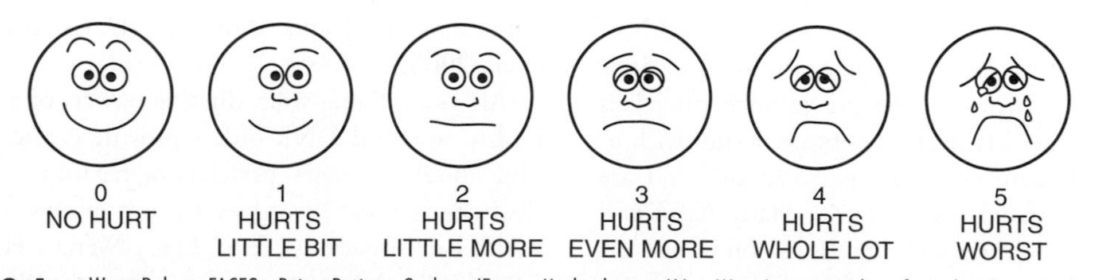

Figure 8-1 • Wong-Baker FACES Pain Rating Scale. (From Hockenberry MJ: *Wong's essentials of pediatric nursing*, ed 7, St Louis, 2005, Mosby, p.1301. Copyrighted by Mosby, Inc. Reprinted with permission.)

Box 8-8 Types of Advance Directives

Living Will	Documents the client's preferences for medical treatment should the client be unable or incompetent to state them. (Legal status of living wills varies from state to state.)
Medical Power of Attorney for Health	Legal document with designation of a proxy authorized to make health care decisions should the client be unable to do so.
Durable Power of Attorney	Legal document with designation of a proxy authorized to make financial decisions and to represent the client's interests, should the client be unable to do so. Durable power of attorney can be revoked in writing at any time, as long as the client is competent.
Do Not Resuscitate (DNR) Orders	Written directions about not resuscitating the client if the client's breathing or heartbeat stops.

and their right to accept or reject them. Examples of advance directives include a living will, DNR orders, and a durable power of attorney for health care, as identified in Box 8-8. Since life-threatening medical emergencies can occur at any time, all adults—even the healthiest—could benefit from having advance directives in place concerning care at the end of their life.

At the same time, nurses need to be aware of and respect cultural differences in making decisions about end-of-life care (LaVera, Crawley, Marshall et al., 2002). Searight and Gafford (2005) identify three factors that affect end-of-life decision making and are culturally at variance with the U.S. and western European models of health care: communication of bad news, locus of decision making, and attitudes toward advance directives and end-of-life care. Many ethnic groups do not wish to have direct disclosure of a terminal diagnosis and are hesitant to discuss advance directives. Many Asian and Native American cultures feel that discussion of end-of-life care compromises hope in the face of terminal illness and can precipitate unnecessary depression. In Hispanic, Chinese, and Pakistani communities, family members deliberately protect terminally ill clients from knowledge of their condition (Searight & Gafford, 2005).

Nurses need to accept the client's cultural values as a starting point for discussing end-of-life options in the nurse-client relationship. Stressing shared goals (e.g., relief of suffering) sometimes can help bridge the gap between cultures. A general inquiry about health care practices at end of life helps ensure cultural safety for clients and families (Cleary, 2005).

The ANA believes that nurses should play a primary role in helping their clients make the best choices for end-of-life care. They suggest the nurses can ask the following questions regarding the client's wishes about advance care directives (ANA, 1995):

- Do you have basic information about advance care directives, including living wills and durable powers of attorney?
- Do you wish to initiate an advance care directive?
- If you have already prepared an advance care directive, can you provide it now?
- Have you discussed your end-of-life choices with your family and/or designated surrogate and health care team? (ANA, 1991)

This discussion should take place in a compassionate, gentle manner, paced at the client or client family's pace and level of understanding. Unfortunately, even with an advance directive in place, family members sometimes want to override the wishes of a client who is no longer able to express his or her wishes. This can create an ethical conflict for the nurse, who often is called on to play a significant role in helping families sort out different agendas and agree on a course of action when the client is unable to do so. The nurse needs to appreciate that honoring the expressed wishes of the client is the ultimate decision. A comparative study of stress levels in families of terminally ill clients with or without advance directives demonstrated significantly less stress levels in families with advance directives (Davis, Burns, Rezac et al., 2005).

Although living wills, durable powers of attorney for health care, and DNR orders provide explicit information about a client's preferences regarding end-of-life treatments, these directives are not always followed in health care situations (Teno, Lynn, Wenger et al, 1997). Communicating with families about the client's status and meeting with them to address specific questions and goals of care should happen frequently when the client's health status begins to decline or show a change.

Bereavement and the Family System

Death, separation, and divorce inevitably alter the dynamics of a family system. Grieving families must not only mourn the loss, but must at the same time re-establish homeostasis within the family, often involving significant realignment of family roles. When the death is untimely, out of sequence (as in the case of a child's death), or complicated by stigma (as in the case of the death of an AIDS victim or drug addict), the challenge for the family is even greater.

Loss of a parent can be traumatic at any age, but it is particularly so for children and adolescents. Greeff and Human (2004) identified overall family hardiness, emotional and practical support provided by the family, support from extended family and friends, spiritual beliefs, and resilient personality traits such as optimism as helpful in assisting children to successfully grieve the loss of a parent. The emotional pain of a divorce can be as severe, if not worse, for a spouse or children because the person is still around but not available to the family as a unit. The American Association of Family Therapists suggests the following areas should be addressed (Weiss, 2000):

- What type of losses has the family experienced? What are the dates?
- How did they or their parents/grandparents historically handle situations involving loss?
- How has the family discussed bad news?
- How has the family expressed sadness in the past?
- Are outward expressions of emotions considered a weakness? Is there a gender distinction?
- How has the family managed loss? Have they put it in the past and moved on? Have those members who wished to talk about their loss been able to talk openly?
- Do family members take on specific roles in the bereavement process?
- Is there a gender-based difference in the ways that family members cope?
- How have children been included in the bereavement process?
- What types of rituals of mourning were used in their families of origin?

Helping Parents Communicate with Children. Losses are particularly difficult for children because they don't have the cognitive development and life experiences to process them completely. The nurse can play an important role in helping parents communicate unpleasant family changes to their children. Children do not have the same understandings as adults about critical issues such as death, mental illness in a parent, divorce, or incapacity of a primary caregiver. They often have fantasies about what happened. They worry about the implications of a changed set of circumstances, but usually do not voice their concerns unless there is a safe place and opportunity to do so. Nurses can encourage parents to set aside a specific time each day simply to hear the thoughts and reactions of their child about a sudden change in the health of a parent or a death of significant person in their lives.

Parents can help their children understand difficult situations by explaining in a concrete, direct way what has happened, using words the child can understand. Stating that a parent who has died has "gone to a better place" or "is happy now" is not helpful, because the child may believe that he or she was not able to make the parent happy enough to remain with the family. Often parents mistakenly believe that their children should be spared details, but this is not true. It is important that parents encourage questions and answer them truthfully.

Maintaining daily routines in the child's life following a tragedy is critical. Children need to know that they are safe and will be taken care of by the remaining adults in their life. If changes must be made, the child should have ample time to make the adjustment rather than have a sudden move thrust upon them without discussion. Children dealing with loss may need more physical contact and reassurance. If the parent is not able to provide the level of communication a child needs to cope with the emotional turmoil of a lost family member, the nurse can be instrumental in helping with appropriate referrals.

Each child grieves in his or her own way. There are some commonalities, however, and parents need to know—and expect—that their child will show regressive behavior, anger, fear, and crying in response to the loss of a significant person in their life. Normalizing the occurrence of these behaviors as an expected event can facilitate temporary acceptance. Children don't express their grief in the same way as adults. Because children may be sad one minute and then playing outside with friends the next, adults may not understand that their grief is intense and long-lasting. It is experienced in a less continuous manner, and children tend to handle it with activity rather than with words. It is essential to help children to express their feelings by proactively putting into words the frustration, sadness, and need to mourn the loss that most children feel.

A child's developmental level also affects how the child will respond to an incapacitating illness or death in the family. For example, 6-year-olds may act out by hitting the parent or by refusing to attend school, whereas adolescents may seem to take the critical event in stride, but will withdraw or show a sharp decline in school performance. Rask, Kaunonen, and Paunonen-Ilmoneum (2002) found that adolescents experienced a sense of loneliness, fears about death, and intrusive breakthrough feelings surrounding the loss of a loved one.

Nurses also may need to help families talk to their children about a child's terminal diagnosis. Most families are hesitant to talk about this with children. In fact, care providers share this discomfort in a society where only the elderly are expected to die. When children receive false information or reassurance about their condition, they don't know what to believe because their intuition and physical symptoms are in conflict with information received from the adults they trust. This discrepancy compounds their sense of isolation and experience of being different. Often children are aware they will die, but lack the words to express their concern. Nurses are in an ideal position to help children and their parents talk about what is happening.

SUMMARY

This chapter describes the experience of grief that accompanies life's losses. Although grief and loss are universal experiences, they profoundly affect us. It is essential for nurses to approach grief and loss both from a theoretical perspective, clearly understanding expected stages and behaviors, and an experiential perspective, understanding their own feelings and responses to loss and grief. The pioneer work of Kübler-Ross, Lindemann, and Engel deepens our understanding of death and dying and the grieving process. This combined perspective provides the nurse with a wisdom that allows him or her to help clients as they grapple with a variety oflosses.

Palliative care is a clinical approach designed to improve the quality of life for clients and families coping with a life-threatening illness, beginning with a terminal illness diagnosis. With appropriate palliative care, a client's quality of life can be quite good until close to the end of life.

The nurse is attuned to the issues of loss and grief and can best assist through compassionate presence and offering therapeutic suggestions to the client and family throughout the dying process. Talking with clients about advance directives is a professional responsibility of the nurse, and it reduces unnecessary conflict among family members at this critical time in a person's life. So often, losses and having to say good-bye leave us with regrets; we wish we could have said more, given more, and somehow been able to feel less pain. Part of the nurse's role, through compassionate communication, presence, and anticipatory guidance, is to diminish those regrets and ease the grief of loss. It is both a blessing and a challenge to the nurse to be able to share and participate in a client's deepest and most meaningful life experiences, including the experience of loss. End-of-life care provides nurses with a unique opportunity to make a meaningful and lasting contribution to the health and well-being of their clients and their families.

> **Ethical Dilemma ■ *What Would You Do?***
> Francis Dillon has been on a ventilator for the past three weeks. It appears as though there is little chance of recovery, yet his family is reluctant to take him off the ventilator. What do you see as the ethical issues, and how would you, as the nurse, address this problem from an ethical perspective?

REFERENCES

Advance directives and life-sustaining treatment: a legal primer, *Hematol Oncol Clin North Am* 16(6):1381–1396, 2002.

American Association of Colleges of Nursing: *End-of-Life Nursing Education Consortium (ELNEC) fact sheet, updated March 2006*, Washington, DC, 2006, Author; available online: http://www.aacn.nche.edu/ELNEC/about.htm.

American Nurses Association: ANA position statements: Nursing and the patient self determination acts, *ANA Nurs World*, 1991; available online: www.nursingworld.org/readroom/position/ethics/etsdet.html.

Bauman S: Family nursing: theory-anemic, nursing theory-deprived, *Nurs Sci Q* 13(4):286–291, 2000.

Boyle D, Miller P, Forbes-Thompson S: Communication and end-of-life care in the intensive care unit, *Crit Care Nurs Q* 28(4):302–316, 2005.

Brunelli T: A concept analysis: the grieving process for nurses, *Nurs Forum* 40(4):123–128, 2005.

Burke M, Eakes G, Hainsworth M: Milestones of chronic sorrow: perspectives of chronically ill and bereaved families, *J Fam Nurs* 5(4):374–389, 1999.

Bryson K: Spirituality, meaning, and transcendence, *Palliative Support Care* 2(3):321–328, 2004.

Carson VB, Arnold EN: *Mental health nursing: the nurse-patient journey*, Philadelphia, 1996, WB Saunders.

Casarett D, Kutner J, Abrahm J: Life after death: a practical approach to grief and bereavement, *Ann Intern Med* 134(3): 208–215, 2001.

Chenitz WC: Living with AIDS. In Flaskerud JH, Ungvarski PJ, editors, *HIV/AIDS: a guide to nursing care*, Philadelphia, 1992, WB Saunders.

Cherlin E, Fried T, Prigerson H et al.: Communication between physicians and family caregivers about care at the end of life: when do discussions occur and what is said? *J Palliat Med* 8(6):1176–1185, 2005.

Cleary A: Respecting each other, *J Palliat Med* 8(1):4–6, 2005.

Corless I: Bereavement. In Ferrell B, Coyle N, editors, *Textbook of palliative nursing*, New York, 2001, Oxford University Press.

Côté J, Peplar C: A focus for nursing intervention: realistic acceptance or helping illusions, *International Journal of Nursing Practice* 11:39–43, 2005.

Curtis JR: Communicating about end-of-life care with patients and families in the intensive care unit, *Crit Care Clin* 20:363–380, 2004.

Davies E, Higginson J, editors: *Palliative care: the solid facts*, Milan, 2004, European Office of the World Health Organization.

Davis B, Burns J, Rezac D et al.: Family stress and advance directives: a comparative study, *Am J Hosp Palliat Care* 7(4):219–229, 2005.

Dobratz M: The pattern of becoming: self in death and dying, *Nurs Sci Q* 15(2):137–142, 2002.

Engel G: Grief and grieving, *Am J Nurs* 64(7):93–96, 1964.

Glass E, Cluxton D, Rancour P: Principles of patient and family assessment. In Ferrell B, Coyle N, editors, *Textbook of palliative nursing*, New York, 2001, Oxford University Press.

Greeff A, Human B: Resilience in families in which a parent has died, *Am J Fam Ther* 32(1):27–42, 2004.

Griffin K, Rabkin J: Perceived control over illness, realistic acceptance and adjustment in people with AIDS, *J Soc Clin Psychol* 17:407–424, 1998.

Institute of Medicine: *Approaching death: improving care at the end of life*, Washington, DC, 1997, National Academy Press.

Jeffries J: *Helping grieving people: a handbook for care providers*, New York, 2005, Brunner-Routledge.

Kellar MH: What is it like to be dying? *Nursing* 13(9):65–67, 1983.

Kübler-Ross E: What is it like to be dying? *Am J Nurs* 71:54, 1971.

Lafond V: *Grieving mental illness: a guide for patients and their caregivers*, ed 2, Toronto, 2002, University of Toronto Press.

Lang F, Quill T: Making decisions with families at the end of life, *Am Fam Physician* 70(4):719–723, 2004.

Larson D, Tobin D: End-of-life conversations: evolving practice and theory, *JAMA* 284(12):1573–1578, 2000.

LaVera M, Crawley M, Marshall P et al.: Strategies for culturally effective end of life care, *Ann Intern Med* 136(9): 673–677, 2002.

Lendrum S, Syme G: *Gift of tears: a practice approach to loss and bereavement counseling*, London, 1992, Routledge.

Levin B: Grief counseling, *Am J Nurs* 98(5):69–72, 1998.

Levine S: *Unattended sorrow: recovering from loss and reviving the heart*, Emmaus, PA, 2005, Rodale.

Lewis CS: *A grief observed*, Greenwich, CT, 1963, Seabury Press.

Lindemann E: Symptomatology and management of acute grief, *Am J Psychiatry* 101:141, 1944.

Mark Twain Quotations, Newspaper Collections, & Related Resources; available online: www.twainquotes.com.

Martin T, Doka K: *Men don't cry…women do: transcending gender stereotypes of grief*, Philadelphia, 2000, Brunner-Mazel.

Miller J: *The art of being a healing presence*, Ft. Wayne, IN, 2001, Willowgreen Publishing.

Millspaugh D: Assessment and response to spiritual pain: part I, *J Palliat Med* 8(5):919–923, 2005.

Mok E, Chiu P: Nurse-patient relationships in palliative care, *J Adv Nurs* 48(5):475–483, 2004.

Morgan A: A grounded theory of nurse-client interactions in palliative care nursing, *J Clin Nurs* 10(4):583–584, 2001.

Olthuis G, Dekkers W, Leget C et al.: The caring relationship in hospice care: an analysis based on the ethics of the caring conversation, *Nurs Ethics* 13(1):29–40, 2006.

Rask K, Kaunonen M, Paunonen-Ilmoneum M: Adolescent coping with grief after the death of a loved one, *Int J Nurs Pract* 8(3):137–142, 2002.

Robinson D, McKenna H: Loss: an analysis of a concept of particular interest to nursing, *J Adv Nurs* 27:779–784, 1998.

Searight H, Gafford J: Cultural diversity at the end of life: issues and guidelines for family physicians, *Am Fam Physician* 71(3):515–522, 2005.

Silveira M, Schneider C: Common sense and compassion: planning for the end of life, *Clin Fam Pract* 6(2):349–368, 2004.

Stearns A: *Living through personal crisis,* Chicago, 1984, Thomas Moore Press.

Steinhauser KE, Clipp EC, McNeilly M et al.: In search of a good death: observations of patients, families, and providers, *Ann Intern Med* 132(10):825–832, 2000.

Steinhauser KE, Voils C, Clipp E et al.: "Are you at peace?: one item to probe spiritual concerns at the end of life, *Arch Intern Med* 166(1):101–105, 2006.

Teno J, Lynn J, Wenger N et al.: Do advance directives provide instructions that direct care? *J Am Geriatr Soc* 45:508–552, 1997.

Thelan M: End of life decision making in intensive care, *Crit Care Nurse* 25(6):28–37, 2005.

Weiss M: AAMFT's clinical update on bereavement and loss, *Clin Update* 2(6), 2000.

Part III
Therapeutic Communication

Chapter 9
Communication Styles

Kathleen Underman Boggs

OUTLINE

OBJECTIVES

At the end of the chapter, the reader will be able to:

1. Describe the component systems of communication.
2. Cite examples of body cues that convey nonverbal messages.
3. Identify cultural implications of communication.
4. Describe the effects of gender on the communication process.
5. Define interpersonal competence.
6. Identify five communication style factors that influence the nurse-client relationship.
7. Discuss how metacommunication messages may affect client responses.
8. Identify client interpretations of nurses' nonverbal communication strategies.
9. Discuss application of one or more research studies for evidence-based clinical practice.

To "communicate effectively with clients and their families" is one of the 16 competencies deemed very important for health providers in the twenty-first century.
(Pew Health Professions Commission, 1995)

Chapter 9 explores styles of communication as a basis for applying communication skills and strategies in the nurse-client relationship. Since effective communication has been shown to produce better health outcomes, greater client satisfaction, and increased client understanding, nurses should be interested in improving their communication styles. Style is defined in Norton's *Communicator Style* (1983) as the manner in which one communicates. Verbal style includes pitch, tone, and frequency. Nonverbal style includes speech accompanied by facial expression, gestures, body posture and movement, eye contact, closeness to or distance from the other person, and so on. These nonverbal behaviors are clues clients provide to help us make sense out of the clients' words. Sharpening observational skills to gather data needed for nursing assessments, diagnosis, and intervention is of special value to the nurse in planning care for clients. Knowledge of communication styles allows a more client-centered, goal-directed approach to resolving difficult health care issues. Both the client and the nurse enter their relationship with their own specific style of communication. Some individuals depend on a mostly verbal style to convey their meaning, whereas others rely on nonverbal strategies to send the message. Some communicators emphasize giving information; others have as a priority the conveying of interpersonal sensitivity.

BASIC CONCEPTS

Metacommunication

Communication is a combination of verbal and nonverbal behaviors integrated for the purpose of sharing information. Within the nurse-client relationship, any exchange of information between the two individuals also carries messages about how to interpret the communication.

Metacommunication is a broad term used to describe all of the factors that influence how the message is perceived (Figure 9-1). An example is the "play fighting" observed in animals and children. Bateson noted that for an organism to "play" at fighting, it must both appear to be fighting and simultaneously appear not to be actually fighting but merely simulating. This message about how to interpret what is going on is metacommunication (Mitchell, 1991). Metacommunicated messages may be hidden within verbalizations or be conveyed as nonverbal gestures and expressions. The following case example should clarify this concept.

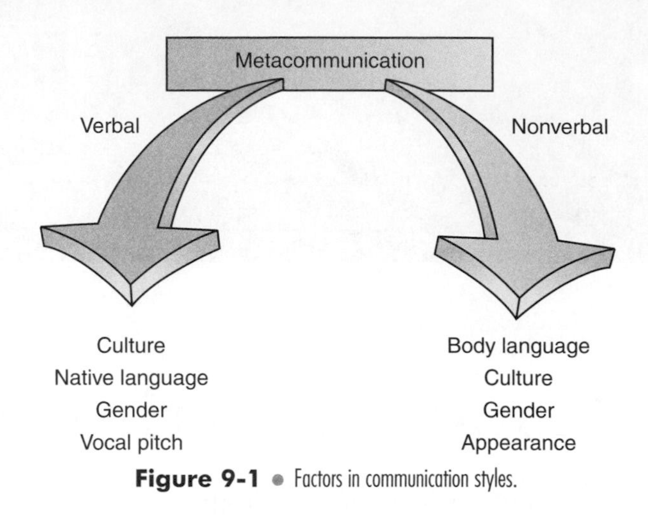

Figure 9-1 • Factors in communication styles.

Case Example

In their 1997 study, Patch, Hoang, and Stahelski found that there was greater compliance to requests when they were accompanied by a metacommunication message that demanded a response about the appropriateness of this request:

Student (smiling): We nursing students are trying to encourage community awareness in promoting environmental health and are looking for people to hand out fliers. Would you be willing?

(Metacommunication): I realize that this is a strange request, seeing that you do not know who I am, but I would really appreciate your help. I am a nice person.

Metacommunication in the nurse-client conversation conveys messages about how to interpret meaning through both verbal and nonverbal cues. For example, during their conversation, the nurse conveys a verbal message of caring to her Caucasian, middle-class client by making appropriate, encouraging responses, and a nonverbal message by maintaining direct eye contact; presenting a smooth face without frowning; and using a relaxed, fluid body posture without fidgeting.

In a professional relationship, verbal and nonverbal components of communication are intimately related. A student studying American Sign Language for the deaf was surprised that it was not sufficient merely to make the sign for "smile," but rather she had to actually show a smile at the same time. This congruence helped convey her message.

The nurse nonverbally communicates acceptance, interest, and respect for the client through eye contact, body posture, head nodding at pivotal points in the conversation, and frequent smiling. In studies, nurses' touching of clients has been reported to be perceived both positively as an expression of caring and negatively as a method of control (Mulaik, Megenity, Cannon et al., 1991). You need to help the client understand and assimilate the discrepancy so that content can be dealt with directly. For example, when you enter a room to ask Mr. Salsa if he is having any postoperative pain, he may say "No," but grimace and clutch his incision. If you comment on the incongruent message, he may admit he is having some discomfort. When nonverbal cues are incongruent with the verbal information, messages are likely to be misinterpreted.

Verbal Communication

Words are symbols used by people to think about ideas, share experiences with others, and validate the meaning of perceptions about the world and one's place in it. Without the use of spoken language, people would be severely limited in their ability to classify and order information in ways that can be understood. Choice of words is influenced by many factors (e.g., your age, race, socioeconomic group, educational background, and gender) and by the situation in which the communication is taking place.

The interpretation of the meaning of words may vary according to the individual's background and experiences. It is dangerous to assume that words have the same meaning for all persons who hear them. Language is useful only to the extent that it accurately reflects the experience it is designed to portray. Consider, for example, the difficulty an American has communicating with a person who speaks only Vietnamese, the dilemma of the young child with a limited vocabulary who is trying to tell you where it hurts, or the anguish of a man with Alzheimer's disease who is desperately attempting to communicate.

There are two levels of meaning in language: denotation and connotation. Both are affected by one's culture. **Denotation** refers to the generalized meaning assigned to a word; **connotation** points to a more personalized meaning of the word or phrase. For example, most people would agree that a dog is a four-legged creature, domesticated, with a characteristic vocalization referred to as a bark. This would be the denotative, or explicit, meaning of the word. When the word is used in a more personalized way, it reveals the connotative level of meaning. "What a dog" and "His bark is worse than his bite" are phrases some people use to describe personal characteristics of human beings, rather than a four-legged creature. Translating such phrases for individuals not familiar with their connotation requires explanation of their more personalized meaning. The nurse should be aware that many communications convey only a part of the intended meaning. We should never assume that the meaning of a message is the same for the sender and the receiver until mutual understanding is verified. For example, a 3-year-old child remarked to her mother, who was pregnant at the time, that the mother was getting fat. The mother, assuming the child was referring to changes associated with the pregnancy, launched into an elaborate explanation of why she was fat. "But, that's not what I meant, Mommy!" her daughter said. "I meant your legs are getting fat." Mother and child were talking to each other, but they were not communicating about the same issue. The best way we can be sure we are getting our message across is to ask for feedback (Telles, 1995).

English as a Second Language

Some people speaking English as a second language say the most difficult aspect is trying to translate expressions for which there is no equivalent English meaning. For others it is the many slang terms, or phrases that have double meanings. Many who learn English as an adult continue to think in their native language, translating words into a more familiar dialect before processing them in or out. Extra time needs to be allowed for information processing, especially when clients are experiencing emotional tension and are more likely to rely on their native language to assist them in sending and receiving information. Verification of message content is even more essential with clients from different cultural backgrounds to make sure that nuances of language do not get lost. When speaking with a client who uses English as a second language, allow time between messages. Use planned spaces of silence, which allow them time to understand your meaning and to prepare a response.

Slang and Jargon

Different age groups in the same culture may attribute different meanings to the same word. For example, an adult who says, "That's cool" might be referring to the temperature, whereas a teenager might convey his satisfaction by using the same phrase. In health care, the "food pyramid" is understood by nurses to represent the basic nutritional food groups needed for health; however, the term may have limited meaning for individuals not in the health professions.

Medical Jargon. Beginning nursing students often report confusion while learning all the Latin and medical terminology required for their new role. Remembering our own experiences, we can empathize with clients who are attempting to understand their own health care. Careful explanations help clients overcome this communication barrier. For successful communication, words used should have a similar meaning to both individuals in the interaction. An important part of the communication process is the search with the client for a common vocabulary so that the message sent is the same as the one received.

Case Example

Rutledge (2004) writes about an oncology nurse who developed a computer databank of cancer treatment terms. When admitting a new client, Mr. Hagler, she used her computer template to create for him an individualized terminology sheet with just the words that would be encountered by him during his course of five chemotherapy treatment cycles.

Pitch and Tone in Vocalization

The oral delivery of a verbal message, expressed through tone of voice and inflection, sighing, or crying, is referred to as paralanguage. It is important to understand this component of communication because it affects how the verbal message is likely to be interpreted. For example, the nurse might say, "I would like to hear more about what you are feeling" in a voice that sounds rushed, high-pitched, or harsh. The same statement might be made in a soft, unhurried voice that expresses genuine interest. In the first instance, the message is likely to be misinterpreted by the client, despite the good intentions of the nurse; the caring intent of the nurse's message is more apparent to the client in the second instance. Voice inflection (pitch and tone) suggests mood and either supports or contradicts the content of the verbal message. When the tone of voice does not fit the words, the message is less easily understood and is less likely to be believed. For example, expressing anger in a flat tone of voice as though the matter is of no consequence contradicts the meaning of the message and the intensity of the emotion the individual is feeling. Thus, it is very difficult for the person receiving the message to respond appropriately. A message conveyed in a firm, steady tone is more reassuring than one conveyed in a loud, abrasive, or uncertain manner.

Vocalization Variations. In some cultures, sounds are punctuated, whereas in other cultures sounds have a lyrical or singsong quality. Contrast, for example, the vocalization of some clients raised in an Eastern culture with that of clients from a Western culture. The vocal inflections are quite different. Nurses need to orient themselves to the characteristic voice tones associated with different cultures to avoid being distracted by them in the process of communication. The tone of voice used to express anger and other emotions varies according to culture and family. For example, it is sometimes difficult for an American nurse to tell when someone from another culture is angry because their vocalization of strong emotion may be more controlled. By contrast, loud, rapid vocalization may seem angrier than intended, when in reality they just convey culturally learned emotional intensity. Through repeated interaction with clients, the nurse learns to understand the message the client is trying to communicate. Chapter 11 discusses cultural communication in detail.

Nonverbal Communication

The majority of person-to-person communication is nonverbal. Think of the most interesting lecturer you ever had. Did this person lecture by making eye contact? Using hand gestures? Moving among the students? Learners generally are most interested in lectures whose nonverbal actions convey enthusiasm. The function of nonverbal communication is to give us cues about what is being communicated. Channels for nonverbal communication include touch, proxemics, body movements, posture, gestures, facial expression, and eye movements.

When the nonverbal cue is inconsistent with the verbal message, which do you believe? If you knock on your instructor's office door and seek help, do you believe her when she says she'd love to talk if you see her grimace and roll her eyes at her secretary? Can you think of a situation where you change the meaning of a verbal

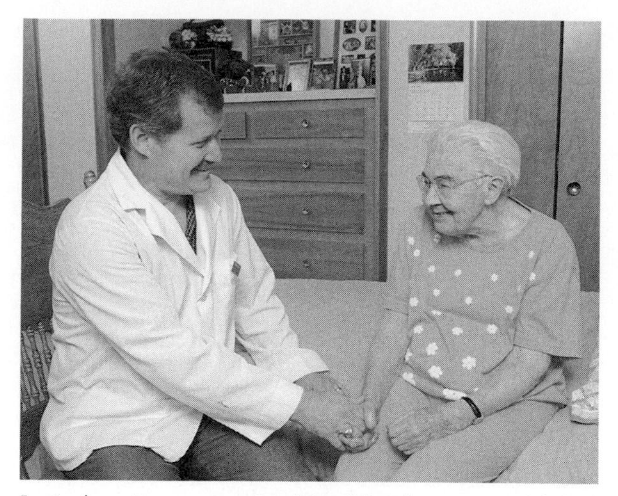

Emotional meanings are communicated through body language, particularly facial expression. (From deWit, SE: *Fundamental concepts and skills for nursing*, Philadelphia, 2001, Saunders.)

message by giving nonverbal "don't believe what I say" cues?

Physicians and nurses use nonverbal communication to build rapport with clients. Observing the client's nonverbal behavior may reveal vital information that will affect the nurse-client relationship. For example, a worried facial expression and lip biting may suggest an anxious client. Assessing the extent to which the client uses nonverbal cues to communicate emotions helps you communicate better. Assessment of nonverbal behaviors and their meanings must be verified with the client because body language, although suggestive, is imprecise. When communication is limited by the client's health state, the nurse should pay even closer attention to nonverbal cues. Pain, for example, can be assessed through facial expression even when the client is only partially conscious.

Touch

Touching a client is one of the most powerful ways a nurse has to communicate nonverbally. Within a professional relationship, touch can convey caring and reassurance. Touch is thought by some expert nurses to promote healing. Care must be taken, however, to abide by the client's cultural proscriptions about the use of touch. This varies across cultures. An example would be the proscription some Muslim men and Orthodox Jewish men follow against touching women outside of family members. They might be uncomfortable shaking the hand of a female health care provider. In another example, some Native Americans use touch in healing, so that casual touching may be taboo (Giger & Davidhizar, 1990). Of course, gender also influences the client's perception of the meaning of being touched.

In primary health care, the nurse's touch is an important component of assessment. The nurse uses touch to convey caring. Some nurses use **therapeutic touch** as part of a method of alternative health care. This healing touch involves a deliberate, specific skill designed to harness energy in order to promote healing. All nurses caring directly for clients use touch to assist. Their touching contact helps the client walk, roll over in bed, and so on. However, just as you are careful about invading the client's personal space, you must take care about when and where on the body clients are touched to avoid misinterpretation.

Many health care providers shake hands when they first meet their client in an ambulatory or community setting. In the American culture, a firm handshake signals equality. However, if your client was raised in some other cultures, he might be expecting a handshake to be soft rather than firm.

Case Example

While giving care to an unconscious woman, her nurse used soothing touch and conversation. She also encouraged the client's husband to do the same. When the woman later regained consciousness, she told the nurse that she recognized her voice! (Miller, 2004)

Proxemics

Proxemics is the use of body space, or the individual's perception of what is a proper distance to be maintained between the person's body or possessions and others. Use of space communicates messages. Clues to client behavior can be obtained by observing their possessions as you make a home visit or care for a client in a long-term facility. Some Asian cultures have elevated the serene use of living space to an art form (feng shui).

Although there is potential for misreading nonverbal cues, researchers have demonstrated that nonverbal behavior can be correctly used to make accurate inferences (Gifford, 1991). Each culture proscribes expectations for appropriate distance depending on the context of the communication. For example, the Nonverbal Expectancy Violations Model defines "proper" social distance for an interpersonal relationship as 1½ to 4 feet in western cultures. Canfield (2002) more specifically states that Americans feel crowded if someone stands closer than 3 feet. According to him, the interaction's purpose determines appropriate space, so that appropriate distance in space for intimate interaction would be zero distance, with increased space needed for personal distance, social distance, and public distance. In almost all cultures, zero distance is shunned except for loving or caring interaction. In giving physical care, nurses enter this "intimate" space. Care needs to be taken when you are at this closer distance, lest the client misinterpret your actions. Knowing the client's usual nonverbal pattern of communication is important in assessing the nature and meaning of changes in behavior. Violating the client's sense of space can be interpreted as threatening.

Generally, nonverbal manifestations of communication are considered useful for expressive and social communication and may be more reliable than their verbal counterparts. To be effective in your work, nonverbal behavior should be congruent with and reinforce the verbal message. For example, if a nurse smiles while telling the nurse-manager that his or her assignment is too much to handle, the seriousness of the message is negated.

Nonverbal Body Cues

Kinesics is an important component of nonverbal communication. Commonly referred to as **body language**, it is defined as involving the conscious or unconscious body positioning or actions of the communicator. Words direct the content of a message, whereas emotions accentuate and clarify the meaning of the words. Often the emotional component of a message can be indirectly interpreted by observing the client's body language, for example, bowing the head or slumping the body in despair after receiving bad news, or nodding the head while gazing down as if in subservience.

Posture, rhythm of movement, and gestures accompanying a verbal message are other nonverbal behaviors associated with the overall process of communication. Body stance may convey a message about the speaker. For example, speaking while directly facing a person conveys more confidence than turning one's body at an angle. A slumped, head-down posture and slow movements give an impression of lassitude or low self-esteem, whereas an erect posture and decisive movements suggest confidence and self-control. Rapid, diffuse, agitated body movements may indicate anxiety. Vigorous, directed actions might suggest confidence and purpose. More force with less focused direction in body movements may symbolize anger.

Facial Expression

Eye contact and facial expressions appear to be particularly important in signaling our feelings. We respond to the expressive qualities of another's face, often without even being aware of it. Research suggests that individuals who make direct eye contact while talking or listening create a sense of confidence and credibility, whereas downward glances or averted eyes signal submission, weakness, or shame. In addition to conveying confidence, maintaining direct eye contact communicates honesty (Puetz, 2005). Allowing your eyes to wander around during a conversation may convey disinterest or even dishonesty. Almost instinctively, individuals use facial expression as a barometer of another person's feelings, motivations, approachability, and mood.

Facial expression is important in conveying a message; it connects the words presented in the message and the internal dialogue of the speaker. Facial expression either reinforces or modifies the message the listener hears. When the verbal message is inconsistent with the nonverbal expression of the message, the nonverbal expressions assume prominence and generally are perceived as more trustworthy than the verbal content. The power of the facial expression supporting the verbal content far outweighs the power of the actual words.

Six common facial expressions (surprise, sadness, anger, happiness/joy, disgust/contempt, and fear) represent global, generalized interpretations of emotions common to all cultures (Canfield, 2002). Although facial expression is often a strong indicator of emotional response to a situation, there are exceptions. Some clients control their facial expressions to mask underlying emotion. In an assessment of facial expression, the nurse notes a *lack* of appropriate facial expression as well as evidence of strong emotion in the facial expression. Because the eyes and corners of the mouth are least susceptible to control, they may provide the most informative data to support or contradict the overall communication picture the client presents.

Case Example

A client smiles, but narrows his eyes and glares at the nurse. An appropriate comment for the nurse to make

might be, "I notice you are smiling when you say you would like to kill me for mentioning your fever to the doctor. It seems that you might be angry with me."

Clothing as a Nonverbal Message

Everyone is familiar with sayings like "dress for success." The business world has long noted the role clothing plays in conveying an image of a serious professional. Styles of nursing uniforms have evolved rapidly in the last decade. Is there one you associate with the image of a professional nurse?

Effects of Gender on Communication

Communication patterns are integrated into gender roles defined by an individual's culture. Gender differences in communication studies have been shown to be greatest in terms of use and interpretation of nonverbal cues (Hyde, 1990). This may reflect gender differences in intellectual style as well as culturally reinforced standards of acceptable role-related behaviors. Newer studies seem to question whether traditional ideas about male and female differences in communication are as prevalent as previously thought. And, of course, there are wide variations within the same gender. In our survey of the literature, results in several studies indicated some specific differences between men and women in their communication patterns. In some studies, gender differences occur in both the *content* and in the *process* of communication. However, recent literature tends to show little difference in communication according to gender, such as reports by Kindler, Szirt, Sommer et al. (2005) and Dunn (2004). A Swedish study even seemed to suggest that opinions about existence of gender differences not only are inaccurate but affect nurses' work performance, since they may be expected to live up to others' (biased) expectations (Larsson, 2005). Other studies show different styles may be more greatly associated with social status differences in the two communicators than a function of gender (Helweg-Larsen, Cunningham, Carrico et al., 2004).

What is factual and what is stereotype? More health care communication studies need to be done before we will really know. The following summarizes some traditional thinking about gender-related differences in communication content and process in both nonverbal and verbal communication. This is followed by a limited list with citations of actual results found in various research studies.

Women were traditionally said to tend to avoid conflict and to want to smooth over differences. They were said to demonstrate more effective use of nonverbal communication and to be better decoders of nonverbal meaning (Cotton-Huston, 1989; Keeley-Dyreson, Burgoon, & Bailey, 1991). Also they were said to disclose more personal information. Feminine communication was thought to be more person-centered, warmer, and more sincere (Reeder, 2005).

Study results do show that women tend to use more facial expressiveness, smile more often, maintain eye contact, touch more often, and nod more often (Hall, Irish, Roter et al., 1994; Helweg-Larsen et al., 2004). Women have been noted to be more constrained in use of gestures, perhaps since they have been taught at a young age to keep their arms, hands, and legs close to their bodies. Other results indicate that women have a greater range of vocal pitch and also tend to use different informal patterns of vocalization than men. Females use more tones signifying surprise, cheerfulness, and unexpectedness. Women tend to view conversation as a connection to others. When there are communication problems between parent and child, daughters tend to benefit more from social support (Landman-Peeters, Hartman, vanderPempe et al., 2005).

Traditionally, men in western cultures were thought to communicate in a more task-oriented, direct fashion, demonstrate greater aggressiveness, and boast about accomplishments. They also have been viewed as more likely to express their disagreement (Reeder, 2005; Sullivan, 2004).

Study results do show that men prefer a greater interpersonal distance between themselves and others and that they use gestures more often. Men are more likely to maintain eye contact in a negative encounter, though overall they maintain less direct eye contact. Studies have shown that men use less verbal communication than women do in interpersonal relationships (Juang & Tucker, 1991). Men are more likely to initiate an interaction, talk more, interrupt more freely, talk louder, disagree more, use hostile verbs, and talk more about issues (Sullivan, 2004). Men are also more likely to use conversation as a contest for status (Molella, 2001).

Gender Differences in Communication in Health Care Settings

Weisman and Teitelbaum (1989) suggest that more effective communication occurs when the provider of the care and the client are of the same gender, although this was not found to be true in other studies (Collier, Vu, & Marcy, 1993). Female physicians have been shown to spend more time during a client's health visit in positive talk, counseling, and emotionally focused communication (Roter, Hall, & Aoki, 2002). In the professional health care setting, women have been noted to use more active listening, using encouraging responses such as "Uh-huh," "Yeah," and "I see," and to use more supportive words (Bernzweig, Takayama, Phibbs et al., 1997; Hall et al., 1994). No gender differences in communication of pain were found by Decker and Perry (2003).

Cultural Variations in Communication

While there is clear evidence that effective communication is related to better client health outcomes, higher client satisfaction, and better compliance, there is less evidence showing how cultural competency directly affects health outcomes (Betancourt, 2004). However, there is anecdotal evidence that our communication is perceived through the filter of our client's cultural beliefs. For this reason, our health information is not always relevant to the client. Giger and Davidhizar, writing in early 1990, thought that many nurses lacked an understanding of communication principles and the techniques necessary to communicate effectively with clients from backgrounds other than their own. To communicate as a culturally competent professional, you need to develop an awareness of the values of a specific client's culture and adapt your style and skills to be compatible with that culture's norms. Chapter 11 deals in depth with intercultural communication concepts.

Most other nonverbal behaviors are culturally specific, learned unconsciously through observation. Sometimes a nonverbal gesture you find acceptable may be perceived as rude in another culture. For example, the nurse may mean to signal approval to her Brazilian client by putting thumb and index finger into a circle for "okay," but in Brazil this is considered an obscene gesture! Cultural taboos can inhibit nonverbal behaviors. For example, different cultures have distinct rules about eye contact. Some ethnic clients culturally tend to avoid eye contact when listening and use eye contact when speaking. The nurse who thinks the African-American or Appalachian client is inattentive to explanations because there is little eye contact during the conversation with the nurse may actually be experiencing a normal, culturally specific nonverbal behavior (Atkinson, Morten, & Sue, 1991).

Developing an Evidence-Based Practice

Kindler CH, Szirt L, Sommer D et al.: A quantitative analysis of anesthetist-patient communication during the pre-operative visit, *Anaesthesia* 60(1):53-59, 2005.

Kindler and colleagues conducted a quantitative analysis of communication between physicians and their client in Switzerland. Fifty-seven preoperative anesthesiologist-client discussions were videotaped and then analyzed for the purpose of identifying the structure and the content of communication that occurred during these interactions.

Results: Results showed that gender had no impact on the content of communication. On average, clients in this study asked six questions, as compared to an average of three questions asked in another study of primary care clients. Physician verbalizations dominated the conversations. Communication was facilitated when physicians asked open-ended questions or made affective comments.

Application to Your Clinical Practice: Effective communication affects client health outcome, satisfaction, and understanding. This study provides evidence that asking open-ended questions promotes communication. Could a similar study be done to examine interaction between nurses and clients?

APPLICATIONS

Knowing Your Own Communication Style

The style of communication used by the health provider can influence client behavior, especially regarding compliance with treatment. Exercises in prior chapters should give you basic skills used in the nurse-client relationship, but you bring your own communication style with you, as does your client. Because we differ widely in our personal communication styles, it is important to identify your style and understand how to modify it for certain clients. Personality characteristics influence your style.

For example, would you be described as more shy or assertive? One nurse might be characterized as "bubbly," whereas another is thought of as having a "quiet" manner. Similarly, clients have various styles. The communication styles of the nurse and client need to be compatible. Think about the potential for incompatibility in the following case.

Case Example

Nurse (in a firm tone): **Mr. Ruth, it is time to take your medicine.**

Mr. Ruth (complaining tone): **You are so bossy.**

Recognize how others perceive you. Consider all the nonverbal factors that affect a client's perception of you. Your gender, manner of dress, appearance, skin tone, hairstyle, age, role as a student, gestures, or confident mannerisms may make a difference. Exercise 9-1 may increase your awareness of gender bias.

The initial step in identifying your own style may be to compare your style with that of others. Ask yourself, "What makes a client perceive a nurse either as authoritarian or as accepting and caring?" The Exercise 9-2 video may help you to compare your style with that of others. The next step is to develop an awareness of alternative styles that you can comfortably assume if the occasion warrants. Next, it is important to figure out whether some other factors influence whether your style is appropriate for a particular client. How might their age, race, socioeconomic status, or gender affect their response to you?

Interpersonal Competence

Kasch (1984) proposes that nurse-client communication processes are based on the nurse's interpersonal competence. **Interpersonal competence** develops as the nurse comes to understand the complex cognitive, behavioral, and cultural factors that influence communication. This understanding, together with the use of a

Exercise 9-1 Gender Bias

Purpose: To create discussion about gender bias.

Procedure:
In small groups, read and discuss the following. The following comments are made about care delivery on a geriatric psychiatric unit by staff and students: "Male staff tend to be slightly more confident and to make quicker decisions. Women staff are better at the feeling things, like conveying warmth."

Discussion:
1. Were these comments made by male or female staff?
2. How accurate are they?
3. Can you truly generalize any attribute to *all* males and females?

Exercise 9-2 Self-Analysis of Video Recording

Purpose: To increase awareness of students' own style.

Procedure:
With a partner, role-play an interaction between nurse and client. Video record or use the video capacity of your cell phone to record a 1- to 2-minute interview with the camera focused on you. The topic of the interview could be "identifying health promotion behaviors" or something similar.

Discussion:
What posture did you use? What nonverbal messages did you communicate? How did you communicate them? Were your verbal and nonverbal messages congruent?

broad range of communication skills, helps the nurse interact with the client as he or she attempts to cope with the many demands placed on him or her by the environment. Good communication skills are associated with competency, as demonstrated in Smith's research (2005). Results identified communication skills as one of the attributes of those expert nurses who were perceived as having clinical credibility. In dealing with the client in the sociocultural context of the health care system, two kinds of abilities are required: social cognitive competency and message competency.

Social cognitive competency is the ability to interpret message content within interactions from the point of view of each of the participants. By embracing the client's perspective, you begin to understand how the client organizes information and formulates goals. This is especially important when your client's ability to communicate is impaired by mechanical barriers such as a ventilator. Clients who recovered from critical illnesses requiring ventilator support reported fear and distress during this experience (Happ, 2000).

Message competency refers to the ability to use language and nonverbal behaviors strategically in the intervention phase of the nursing process to achieve the goals of the interaction. Communication skills are used as a tool to influence the client to maximize his or her adaptation. When your instructor responds to your answer with a smile and affirmative head nod, saying, "Great answer," doesn't this make you feel successful?

Box 9-1 Behavioral Communication Styles in Nurse-Client Relationships

To Increase Involvement

Nurse demonstrates commitment:
- Responds to client as an individual
- Uses close physical distance
- Gives time to the client
- Establishes common ground
- Anticipates needs

Nurse shows perseverance:
- Gets to know client's family
- Follows through on promises and goals

Nurse acts as an advocate:
- Becomes involved
- Connects the client with the system
- Acts as a buffer or go-between
- Adapts or bends rules to meet client's needs

Client tests behavior (personal):
- Is nurse a "good person"?
- Tests for dependability
- Evaluates "likeability"
- Requests personal disclosures

Client tests behavior (professional):
- Is nurse a "good nurse"?
- Obtains information from other clients
- Looks for indicators of empathy
- Evaluates competency
- Tests for ability to keep a confidence

Client makes overtures:
- Acts like a "good patient"
- Is friendly, jokes
- Seeks time with nurse

Client makes decision to trust:
- Conversation content less social, more meaningful
- Relinquishes vigilance

To Decrease Involvement

Nurse depersonalizes the client:
- Refers to client by bed number or diagnosis
- Uses formal terms of address
- Has no time to talk

Nurse maintains superefficient attitude:
- Gives impression of business
- Interactions focus on physical care
- Ignores emotional behavior and cues that client wants to discuss difficult questions
- Does not provide meaningful information to client about condition

Nurse does not trust client:
- Suspects ulterior motives
- Keeps client "in the dark"

Client avoids therapeutic relationship:
- Does not selfdisclose
- Is late or absent from scheduled meetings or activities
- Focuses conversation on symptoms rather than feelings

Client does not trust the nurse:
- Becomes overly manipulative
- Is demanding

Client expresses discomfort nonverbally:
- Avoids direct eye contact
- Fidgets when conversation "gets personal"
- Refuses to talk
- Turns head or body away from nurse

Style Factors Influencing Relationships

The establishment of trust and respect in an interpersonal relationship with client and family is dependent on open, ongoing communication style (Winn, Cook, & Bonnel, 2004). Having knowledge of communication styles is not sufficient to guarantee successful application. You need to understand how the materials discussed in this chapter interrelate. Box 9-1 lists some communication styles that increase or decrease involvement in the nurse-client relationship.

Responsiveness of Participants

How responsive the participants are affects the depth and breadth of communication. Some clients are naturally more verbal than others. It is easier to have a therapeutic conversation with extroverted clients who want to communicate. The nurse will want to increase the responsiveness of less verbal clients, and there are many ways to enhance communication responsiveness. Verbal and nonverbal approval encourages clients to express themselves. Therapeutic skills and strategies that promote responsiveness include active listening, demonstration of empathy, and acknowledgment of the content and feelings of messages. Sometimes acknowledging the difficulty a client is having expressing certain feelings, praising efforts, and encouraging use of more than one route of communication helps. Such strategies demonstrate interpersonal sensitivity. A responsive care provider has been shown to improve compliance with the treatment regimen and to be preferred by clients themselves (Worchel, Prevatt, Miner et al., 1995).

Roles of Participants

Paying attention to the role relationship of the communicators may be just as important as deciphering the content and meaning of the message. The relationships between the roles of the sender and of the receiver influence how the communication is likely to be received and interpreted. The same constructive criticism made by a good friend and by one's immediate supervisor is likely to be interpreted differently, even though the content and style are quite similar. Many studies, including that of Giannantonio, Olian, and Carroll (1995), show that communication between subordinates and supervisors is far more likely to be influenced by power and style than by gender. When roles are unequal in terms of power, the more powerful individual tends to speak in a more dominant style (Simkins-Bullock & Wildman, 1991). This is discussed in Chapter 22.

Validation of Individual Worth

Styles that convey "caring" send a message of individual worth that sustains the relationship with the client. For example, in a study of physician providers, a "warm" communication style resulted in more information being shared by the client (Gerbert, Johnston, Bleecker et al., 1997). Another study of children with birth defects showed that parents want a provider to show caring, to give information, and to allow them time to talk about their own feelings (Strauss, Sharp, Lorch et al., 1995).

Confirming responses validate the intrinsic worth of the person. These are responses that affirm the right of the individual to be treated with respect. They also affirm the client's autonomy (i.e., his or her right, ultimately, to make his or her own decisions). For example, in a nurse-client relationship, the nurse acts deliberately to accept and confirm the humanity of the client.

Disconfirming responses, on the other hand, disregard the validity of feelings by either ignoring them or by imposing a value judgment. Such responses take the form of changing the topic, offering reassurance without supporting evidence, or presuming to know what a client means without verifying the message with the client. In a study of communication interactions between nurses and physicians, Garvin and Kennedy (1988) found that more experienced nurses used more confirming communication than did younger, less experienced nurses. These findings suggest that communication skills are learned. Try Exercise 9-3 for practice in using confirming skills.

Remember from Chapter 3 that the ethical principle of beneficence can be used to guide your care. If faced with an ethical dilemma situation such as the one at the end of this chapter, what would you do? Which ethical principle should guide your intervention? Are your actions legally defensible?

Context of the Message

Communication is always influenced by the environment in which it takes place. It does not occur in a vacuum, but is shaped by the situation in which the interaction occurs. Taking time to evaluate the physical setting and the time and space in which the contact takes place—as well as the psychological, social, and

Exercise 9-3 Confirming Responses

Purpose: To increase students' skills in using confirming communication.

Procedure:
Change these disconfirming, negative messages into positive, confirming, caring comments.
1. "Three of your 14 blood sugars this week were too high. What did you do wrong?"
2. "Your blood pressure is dangerously high. Are you eating salty foods again?"
3. "You gained five pounds this week. Can't you stick to a simple diet?"

Discussion:
Was it relatively easy to send a positive, confirming message?

cultural characteristics of each individual involved—gives you flexibility in choosing the most appropriate context.

Involvement in the Relationship

Relationships generally need to develop over time because communication changes with different phases of the relationship. In these days of managed care, nurses working with hospitalized clients have less time to develop a relationship, whereas community-based nurses may have greater opportunities. Reexamine the behaviors in Box 9-1 to decide which you could use to increase your clients' involvement. How would culture affect behaviors described in this box? To begin to explore ethical problems in your nursing relationships, consider the ethical dilemma provided.

Box 9-2 Suggestions to Improve Your Communication Style

- Adapt yourself to client's cultural values.
- Make eye contact.
- Display pleasant, animated facial expressions.
- Smile often.
- Maintain attentive, upright posture.
- Attend to proper proximity and increase space if client shows signs of discomfort such as gaze aversion, leg swinging, or rocking.
- Use touch with client if appropriate to the situation.
- Use humor, but avoid gender jokes.
- Attend to proper tone and pitch, avoiding being overly loud.
- Avoid using jargon.
- Use active listening and respond to client's cues.
- Verbalize respect for client and address the client formally.
- Use confirming, positive comments.

SUMMARY

Communication between nurse and client or nurse and another professional involves more than the verbalized information exchanged. Box 9-2 summarizes suggestions for improving your communication style. Professional communication, like personal communication, is subtly altered by changes in pitch of voice and use of accompanying facial expressions or gestures. This chapter explores factors related to effective styles of verbal and nonverbal communication. Cultural and gender differences associated with each of these three areas of communication are discussed. For professionals, maintaining congruence is important. Style factors affecting

Ethical Dilemma ■ *What Would You Do?*

Katy is due for her initial six-month employment evaluation from her supervisor, Mr. Singh. Katy knows she has made several client care mistakes and fears she may be terminated. Mr. Singh has on two occasions touched Katy inappropriately, with suggestive, nonverbal gestures. Mr. Singh intimates to Katy that if she divulges these incidents she will not receive a favorable evaluation and will not be recommended for continued employment.

What ethical principle is being violated in this situation? What would you do if you were in Katy's place? Identify behavior options and their possible outcomes.

the communication process include the responsiveness and role relationships of the participants, the types of responses and context of the relationships, and the level of involvement in the relationship. Confirming responses acknowledge the value of a person's communication, whereas disconfirming responses discount the validity of a person's feelings. More nonverbal strategies to facilitate nurse-client communication are discussed in later chapters.

REFERENCES

Atkinson D, Morten G, Sue D: Minority group counseling. In Samovar L, Porter R, editors, *Intercultural communication: a reader*, ed 4, Belmont, CA, 1991, Wadsworth.

Bernzweig J, Takayama J, Phibbs C et al.: Gender differences in physician–patient communication, *Arch Pediatr Adolesc Med* 151:586–591, 1997.

Betancourt JR: Cultural competence-marginal or mainstream movement? *N Engl J Med* 351(10):953–955, 2004.

Canfield A: *Proxemics*, unpublished document, ERIC Document Reproduction Service No. ED473237, 2002.

Collier JA, Vu NV, Marcy ML: Effects of examinee gender, standardized patient gender, and their interaction on standardized patients' ratings of examinees' interpersonal and communication skills, *Acad Med* 68(2):153–157, 1993.

Cotton-Huston A: Gender communication. In King S, editor, *Human communication as a field of study*, Albany, NY, 1989, State University of New York Press.

Decker SA, Perry AG: The development and testing of the PATCOA to assess pain in confused older adults, *Pain Manag Nurs* 4(2):77–86, 2003.

Dunn LJ: Nonverbal communication: information conveyed through the use of body language, 2004; retrieved 2/23/05 from http://clearinghouse.mwsc.edu/manuscripts/70.asp.

Garvin BJ, Kennedy CW: Confirming communication of nurses in interaction with physicians, *J Nurs Educ* 27:20–30, 1988.

Gerbert B, Johnston K, Bleecker T et al.: HIV risk assessment: a video doctor seeks patient disclosure, *MD Comput* 14(4):288–294, 1997.

Giannantonio C, Olian JD, Carroll SJ: An experimental study of gender and situational effects in a performance evaluation of a manager, *Psychol Rep* 76(3):1004–1006, 1995.

Gifford R: Mapping nonverbal behavior on the interpersonal circle, *J Pers Soc Psychol* 61(2):279–288, 1991.

Giger JN, Davidhizar R: Transcultural nursing assessment, *Int Nurs Rev* 37(1):199–202, 1990.

Hall JA, Irish JT, Roter D et al.: Gender in medical encounters: an analysis of physician and patient communication in a primary care setting, *Health Psychol* 13(5):384–392, 1994.

Happ MB: Interpretation of nonvocal behavior and the meaning of voicelessness in critical care, *Soc Sci Med* 50:1247–1255, 2000.

Helweg-Larsen M, Cunningham SJ, Carrico A et al.: To nod or not nod: an observational study of nonverbal communication and status in female and male college students, *Psychol Women Q* 28(4):358–362, 2004.

Hyde JS: Meta-analysis and the psychology of gender differences, *Signs* 16(1):55–73, 1990.

Juang S, Tucker CM: Factors in marital adjustment and their interrelationships, *J Multcult Counsel Dev* 19(1):22–41, 1991.

Kasch CC: Communication in the delivery of nursing care, *Adv Nurs Sci* 6:71–88, 1984.

Keeley-Dyreson M, Burgoon J, Bailey W: The effect of stress on decoding kinesic and vocalic communication, *Hum Comm Res* 17(4):584–585, 1991.

Kindler CH, Szirt L, Sommer D et al.: A quantitative analysis of anesthetist-patient communication during the preoperative visit, *Anaesthesia* 60(1):53–59, 2005.

Landman-Peeters KM, Hartman CA, vanderPempe G et al.: Gender differences in the relation between social support, problems in parent-offspring communication, and depression and anxiety, *Soc Sci Med* 60(11):2549–2555, 2005.

Larsson US: Conceptions of gender: a study of female and male head nurses, *J Nurs Manag* 13(2):179–182, 2005.

Miller N: When you can't cure, is caring enough? *Nursing* 34(8):32, 2004.

Mitchell RW: Bateson's concept of metacommunication in play, *New Ideas Psychol* 9(1):73–87, 1991.

Molella RC: *Working life,* 2001, http://www.mayo health.org (refer to section on gender communication differences).

Mulaik JS, Megenity J, Cannon R et al.: Patients' perceptions of nurses' use of touch, *West J Nurs Res* 13(3):306–323, 1991.

Norton R: *Communicator style: theory, applications, and measures,* Beverly Hills, CA, 1983, Sage Publications.

Patch M, Hoang VR, Stahelski AJ: The use of metacommunication in compliance, *J Soc Psychol* 137(1):88–94, 1997.

Pew Health Professions Commission: *Critical challenges (3rd report)*, Washington, DC, 1995, Author.

Puetz BE: The winning job interview, *Am J Nurs* (Career Guide 2005 Supp):30–32, 2005.

Reeder HM: Exploring male and female communication: three lessons on gender, *J Sch Health* 75(3):115–118, 2005.

Roter DL, Hall JA, Aoki Y: Physician gender effects in medical communication, *JAMA* 288(6):756–764, 2002.

Rutledge D: What strategies are nurses using to overcome barriers? *ONS News* 19(9):4, 2004.

Simkins-Bullock J, Wildman BG: An investigation into the relationships between gender and language, *Sex Roles* 24(3/4):149–160, 1991.

Smith CS: Identifying attributes of clinical credibility in registered nurses, *Nurs Adm Q* 29(2):188–191, 2005.

Strauss RP, Sharp MC, Lorch SC et al.: Physicians and the communication of bad news, *Pediatrics* 96(1):82–89, 1995.

Sullivan EJ: Communicating effectively. In *Becoming influential: a guide for nurses*, Upper Saddle River, NJ, 2004, Prentice Hall.

Telles M: Good communication skills are crucial for nurses, *Nurs News* 45(5):4, 9, 1995.

Weisman CS, Teitelbaum MA: Women and health care communications, *Patient Educ Couns* 13(2):183–199, 1989.

Winn P, Cook JB, Bonnel W: Improving communication among attending physicians, long term care facilities, residents, and residents' families, *J Am Med Dir Assoc* 5(2):114–122, 2004.

Worchel FF, Prevatt BC, Miner J et al.: Pediatricians' communication style: relationship to parents' perceptions and behaviors, *J Pediatr Psychol* 20(5):633–644, 1995.

Chapter 10

Developing Therapeutic Communication Skills in the Nurse-Client Relationship

Elizabeth Arnold

OUTLINE

OBJECTIVES

At the end of the chapter, the reader will be able to:

1. Define therapeutic communication.
2. Identify the purposes of therapeutic communication.
3. Describe the characteristics of therapeutic communication.
4. Apply active listening and therapeutic communication strategies and skills.
5. Compare and contrast the use of selected verbal strategies to facilitate therapeutic communication.

> *The fundamental fact of human existence is person with person.... That special event begins by one human turning to another, seeing him or her as this particular other being, and offering to communicate with the other in a mutual way, building from the individual world each person experiences to a world they share together.*
>
> (Stewart, 1986)

Chapter 10 describes the fundamental principles of therapeutic communication. **Therapeutic communication** is a specialized form of communication used in health care settings to support, educate, and empower people to effectively cope with difficult health-related issues. In addition to words that allow for the active interchange of ideas and transmission of feelings about health-related matters, therapeutic communication also includes a wide range of nonverbal behaviors and activities that embrace reading, art expression, touch, and writing.

Therapeutic communication can take place in a variety of clinical settings ranging from neonatal intensive care units to nursing homes—and even to telenursing in cyberspace (Sharpe, 2001). As health care delivery moves to a community focus, therapeutic communication increasingly takes place in nontraditional care settings (e.g., prisons, schools, churches, the client's home, and ambulatory care settings). Although the same principles apply, the nurse will need to modify communication strategies to meet shortened time frames and environmental constraints imposed by managed care (Cahill, 1998). The nurse needs to document important points of the client's behavior and responses in appropriate charting and reports.

BASIC CONCEPTS

Therapeutic Communication

Therapeutic communication, a term coined by Ruesch (1961), is defined as a purposeful form of conversation designed to help a client achieve identified health-related goals through participation in a focused relationship. Therapeutic conversations are similar to those used spontaneously in social communications, with several notable distinctions. Self-disclosure by the health care provider is limited to meeting the health-related goals of the relationship. In contrast to social conversations, therapeutic conversations have a serious purpose related to improving the health and well-being of the client. Therapeutic conversations in health care should be empathetic. They are designed to help clients learn about their illness and how to cope with it, to comfort dying persons, and to assure clients that someone is there to be with them and ease their suffering (Pearson, Borbasi, & Walsh, 1997). Therapeutic conversations help make illness bearable by reinforcing self-esteem and supporting the natural healing powers of a person (Peplau, 1960).

In health care situations, the communication is goal-directed, time-limited, and focused. Conversations between nurse and client have defined rules about the nature of the communication and its duration and purpose; the topics focus on specific health care needs. Effective therapeutic communication focuses on the present health situation. Referred to as immediacy, the nurse encourages the client to focus on health-related concerns in the here and now. The nurse uses concrete, culturally specific language that matches the client's use of language. Avoiding language that is too medical or global increases the chance of the message being understood and responded to appropriately (Figure 10-1).

Purpose of Therapeutic Communication

The purpose of therapeutic communication is to provide a safe place for the client to explore the meaning of the illness experience and to provide the information and emotional support that each client needs to achieve maximum health and well-being. In many ways, the nurse functions as a skilled companion, using communication as a primary tool to achieve health goals (Pearson et al., 1997).

Each therapeutic conversation is unique (Caughan & Long, 2000) because the people holding them are different. Therapeutic communication considers each client's perspective and strengths, readiness to learn, ways of relating to others, physical and emotional condition, and sociocultural norms as relevant factors in planning and

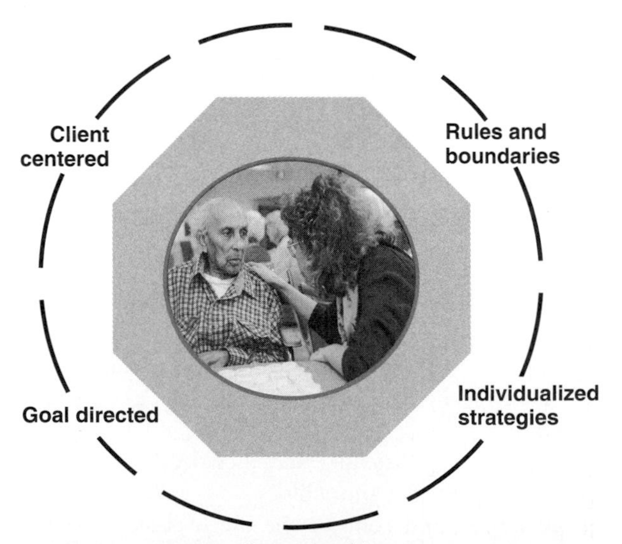

Figure 10-1 • Characteristics of therapeutic communication.

implementing communication strategies (SmithBattle, Drake, & Diekemper, 1997).

Talking aloud about complex problems allows clients and their families to hear themselves as they speak of difficult issues. The client is able to listen to his or her own feelings and thoughts and to receive thoughtful feedback from a health care professional. Much more than simply the transfer of information and ideas from one person to another, each therapeutic conversation helps clients realistically sort out priorities and actions they can take to better cope with their specific diagnoses and personal relationship needs. A therapeutic conversation tells the story of an illness, with both nurse and client taking different roles in telling it.

Active Listening

Effective therapeutic communication with clients begins with active listening (Bush, 2001). **Active listening** is defined as a dynamic, interactive process in which a nurse hears a client's message, decodes its meaning, and provides feedback to the client regarding the nurse's understanding of the message. The nurse should be sensitive not only to "what" is said but also to "how" it is said, and to what is left out of the message as well as to what is included.

Active listening means listening without making judgments or letting your own perceptions serve as a barrier to really hearing the client. It is a two-way, interactive process, with communication exchange expected between speaker and listener. Active listening involves aesthetic—as well as scientific, personal, and ethical—patterns of knowing in making interpretations. Gadow (1995) suggests, "In composing a narrative between nurse and patient, it does not matter who is author, because each is poet; it matters only that there are enough words between them to make a story" (p. 11). The goal of active listening is to fully understand what the other person is trying to communicate.

Active listening allows the health care provider to see a situation from the client's perspective and to convey that understanding in such a way that both parties understand its common meaning. Alderman (2000) refers to active listening as an art. Included in each participant's communicated message are important nonverbal instructions **(metacommunication)** about the interpretation of the message (see Chapter 9). Calero (2005) notes that if the verbal and the nonverbal messages are congruent, the message is credible. If the two are incongruent, the speaker will create doubt in the mind of the listener and the message will be questioned.

The listener notes the tone of voice, the pauses in the conversation, and his or her own intuitive feelings in receiving the message (Metcalf, 1998). If you notice nonverbal behaviors that seem to contradict words, or the client seems sad or distracted, you might want to call the client's attention to the discrepancy with a simple statement, such as, "I notice that you seem very quiet today. Is there something that I can help you with?"

The listener consciously uses both metacommunication and minimal verbal cues to encourage further communication. Referred to as *attending behaviors* (Box 10-1), these listening connections invite the client to communicate at a deeper level with the nurse. They convey both interest and a sincere desire to understand (Straka, 1997). Attending behaviors let the client know that you are focused on understanding their situation and that you are open to whatever the client has to say. Check in with your client periodically to make sure that what is being observed or heard is accurate. For example, you might say, "I'd just like to check in with you to make sure that I understand. Are you saying that...?"

Exercise 10-1 looks at the use of principles of active listening in familiar situations.

Barriers to Active Listening. Barriers to active listening can result from either nurse or client factors, such as the following:

1. *Preoccupation.* The nurse can become so involved with giving physical care or inner thoughts that listening to the client becomes secondary. Alternatively, the client may be too preoccupied with illness, pain, or worry to talk. Sometimes nurses listen only to the parts of the

Box 10-1 Effective Attending Behaviors in the Nurse-Client Relationship

- Full focus on the client and what he or she is saying
- Erect, open posture, with the upper torso slightly inclined toward the client
- Direct eye contact
- Minimal cues and nonverbal gestures, such as nodding, smiling
- Nonjudgmental facial expression mirroring the conversation
- Avoidance of premature or judgmental responses

Exercise 10-1 Active Listening

Purpose: To develop skill in active listening and an awareness of the elements involved.

Procedure:

1. Students break up into pairs. Each will take a turn reflecting on and describing an important experience they have had in their lives. The person who shares should describe the details, emotions, and outcomes of his or her experience. During the interaction, the listening partner should use listening responses such as clarification, paraphrasing, reflection, and focusing as well as attending cues, eye contact, and alert body posture to carry the conversation forward.
2. After the sharing partner finishes his or her story, the listening partner indicates understanding by (a) stating in his or her own words what the sharing partner said; and (b) summarizing perceptions of the sharing partner's feelings associated with the story and asking for validation. If the sharing partner agrees, then the listening partner can be sure he or she correctly utilized active listening skills.

Discussion:

In the large group, have pairs of students share their discoveries about active listening. As a class, discuss aspects of nursing behavior that will foster active listening in client interactions.

communication that interest them or to those that they assume are relevant. The nurse may be so absorbed in the content of a message that the nonverbal contradictions or qualifiers are not heard (Crowther, 1991).

2. *Personal insecurity.* If the client's need taps into a nurse's professional insecurity, a nurse's anxiety level can become high enough to obstruct receptive listening. For example, if a client is extremely critical of the nurse's performance, the nurse may have trouble listening fully to the client. Self-awareness is an essential characteristic of effective therapeutic communication (Rowe, 1999). Personal insecurity in the client also can present a barrier. Nurses should be aware that clients experiencing an illness or injury may feel embarrassed, fearful of criticism, or insecure about appearing vulnerable in health care situations. Normalizing feelings of insecurity and encouraging clients and families to tell their story in their own way is useful.
3. *Unusual speech patterns or behavioral mannerisms.* Thick accents, rapid or slow speech, a monotone voice, high-pitched laughter, or a tendency to ramble can make it more difficult to extract meaning from the client's words. Again, allow more time and help the client focus, without demanding that he or she interact in a certain way.
4. *Physical discomfort.* When the client experiences discomfort such as pain, hearing loss, being too hot or too cold, or feeling nauseated, it can halt communication and make listening more difficult.
5. *Psychological discomfort.* Communicating about emotionally charged material can increase anxiety so that the resulting client communication is vague, tangential, or so explosive that the meaning is difficult to capture or respond to constructively.
6. *Too much information.* Either given or received, a surplus of information reduces a person's ability to concentrate on the main points of a communication.

The issue is not whether barriers exist, but how to address them effectively. For example, the nurse might say to the client who rambles, "I'm feeling that time is limited here, so we need to stay on track. Tell me more about..." and return the focus to the topic under discussion.

Conditions That Influence Communication

Physical Factors

Regardless of the surroundings, your body posture gives a powerful message to the client, either inviting trust or conveying disinterest. Leaning forward slightly toward the client and nodding to signal that you are hearing the client's message convey the impression that what the client has to say is important to you. Moving a chair close to the client in a wheelchair enhances communication (Miller, 1990). Whether you are sitting or standing,

Box 10-2 Physical Behavioral Cues

Emblems: Gestures or body motions having a generalized verbal interpretation (e.g., handshaking, baby waving bye-bye, sign language).

Illustrators: Actions that accompany and exemplify the meaning of the verbal message. Illustrators are used to emphasize certain parts of the communication (e.g., smiling, a stern facial expression, pounding the fist on a table). Illustrators usually are not premeditated.

Affect displays: Facial presentation of emotional affect. Similar to the illustrators just discussed, the sender has more control over their display (e.g., a reproving look, an alert expression, a smile or a grin, a sneer). Affect displays seem to be more pervasive nonverbal expressions of the client's emotional state. They have a larger range of meaning and act to support or contradict the meaning of the verbal message. Sometimes the generalized affect is not related to a specific verbal message (e.g., a depressed client may have a retarded emotional affect throughout the relationship that has little to do with the communicated message).

Regulators: Nonverbal activities that adjust the course of the communication as the receiver gives important information to the sender about the impact of the message on the sender. Regulators include nodding, facial expressions, some hand movements, and looking at a watch.

Adaptors: Characteristic, repetitive, nonverbal actions that are client-specific and of long duration. They give the nurse information about the client's usual response to difficult emotional issues. Sample behaviors include a psychogenic tic, nervous foot tapping, blushing, and twirling the hair.

Physical characteristics: Nonverbal information about the client that can be gleaned from the outward appearance of the person (e.g., skin tone, descriptions of height and weight and relation to body shape, body odor, physical appearance [dirty hair, unshaven, teeth missing or decayed]).

Adapted from Blondis M, Jackson B: *Nonverbal communication with patients: back to the human touch*, ed 2, New York, 1982, Wiley, pp. 9-10.

your posture should be relaxed and, if possible, the upper part of your body should be inclined toward the client. Physical behavioral cues characteristically include the behaviors summarized in Box 10-2.

Clients need privacy for most health care conversations, and if you want the interaction to go well, you will need to make the setting as comfortable as possible. Sometimes a simple suggestion to the client, along with the rationale for it, greatly increases the client's comfort.

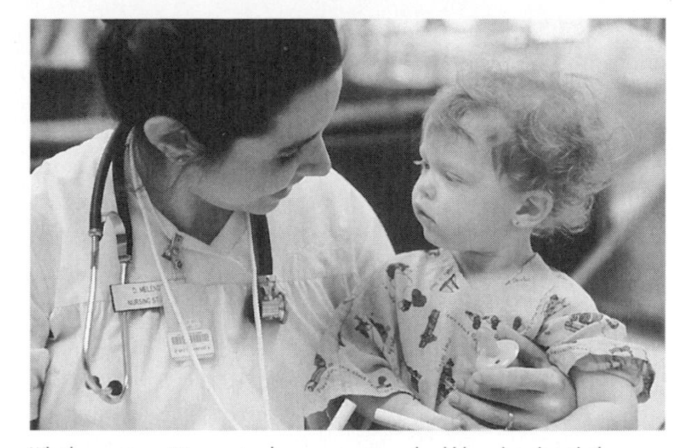

Whether you are sitting or standing, your posture should be relaxed, with the upper part of your body inclined slightly toward the client. (Courtesy University of Maryland School of Nursing.)

If the client is extremely anxious, or the conversation is likely to be complex or potentially anxiety-producing, it often is helpful to include someone the client trusts in the conversation. This person often is helpful in asking questions the client forgets to ask, and later can act as a resource when the client tries to recall the conversation.

Where the communication takes place in home care settings is more complex. Ask the family or client for a suitable quiet place. Freedom from interruption when discussing private matters enhances the impression that the nurse wants to give full attention to the client. Once a suitable place is determined, the nurse can ask for the family's cooperation in respecting the client's privacy.

The nurse also considers the amount of personal space a client requires for ease of conversation (Hall, 1959). Most therapeutic conversations take place within a social

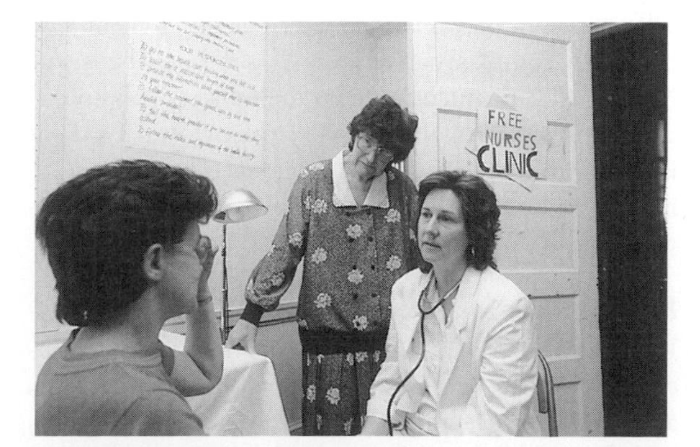

Most conversations take place within a social distance. (Courtesy University of Maryland School of Nursing.)

distance (3 to 4 feet is optimal); however, clients experiencing high levels of anxiety usually need more physical space for successful conversation, whereas clients experiencing a sudden physical injury or undergoing a painful procedure often appreciate having the nurse in close proximity to their head to talk them through the process and touch them. Some cultures require greater distance for comfort, whereas others do not. With experience, the nurse learns to gauge the amount of space the client needs. Nonverbal cues such as shifting position, rapid eye movements, and actually moving away slightly all suggest that the client may need more space (Knapp & Hall, 1997).

Timing

Timing is critical to the success of a therapeutic conversation. The nurse needs to assess, "Is this the right time to discuss the client's needs, and is there enough time to complete the discussion?" Cues from the client's behavior help the nurse determine emotional readiness and available energy. Sensitivity of the nurse to the presence of pain, variations in energy levels, and relationship needs of the client enhance communication. Planning for communication during periods when the client is more receptive to the idea and is able to participate is both time-efficient and respectful of the client's needs.

Clients do not always respond in the same way. Clients who show a distinct difference from their normal presentation in how they are interacting may be experiencing anxiety, pain, or anger. Here the nurse would reflect on previous conversations with the same client and make comparisons with other client observations in similar situations. For example, is the client's current way of expressing anger about the situation similar to or different from previous encounters? Is this a client who habitually complains about care, or is this new behavior? Making such distinctions helps the nurse ask additional questions and draw different conclusions. When a client is acting this way, the nurse might need extra time to inquire about the change in the client's behavior and its meaning in the present situation.

Personal Factors

Personal differences among clients related to socioeconomic status, previous life experience, education level, and occupational status influence the language, attitudes, and format of therapeutic communication, often unconsciously. Personal bias on the part of the nurse affects the ability to listen. Understanding the needs of a homeless client or the behaviors of a drug-addicted teenage mother may be difficult for a nurse who has never experienced the stresses associated with these lifestyles (Berne & Lerner, 1992). Although homosexuality is much more acceptable than it used to be, some nurses may find it more difficult to relate to clients with this lifestyle because of personal values and biases. Having a client of high social status or influence can affect communication because the nurse can feel intimidated.

Working with clients who refuse to comply or who have given up is a communication challenge for the nurse. When, despite health teaching, a client makes health choices that the nurse finds hard to accept, this too can influence communication. The alcoholic who persists in drinking and the HIV-positive mother who continues to become pregnant discourage the nurse's investment in communicating with these clients. Watching a client make choices that indicate the client has given up also makes therapeutic conversations difficult. For example, an 89-year-old woman with multiple health problems requiring nursing home care may be hard to motivate. Why should she live? Patience and understanding are key to success in helping this person make the right decisions for herself (Gorman & Devine, 1998). Self-awareness of personal prejudices and stereotypes that can interfere with communication allows nurses to communicate more effectively with their clients. It is always the nurse's responsibility to resolve personal value issues so that they don't sabotage the full acceptance needed for a therapeutic relationship.

Use of Language

Language helps clients connect different parts of their health stories and allows them to let others into their world. Weingarten (1992) noted that "every conversation creates an opportunity for connection and disconnection; reflection and haste; dialogue and monologue; understanding and misunderstanding; collaboration and instruction; no change and change" (p. 45).

Words can empower, comfort, challenge, and provide information to clients in distress. Language is the primary means by which people organize data about problems, explore different options, and validate with others the best solutions. For this reason, nurses should pay close attention to verbal expression and forms of language (Kettunen, Poskiparta, & Liimatainen, 2001) and *mirror them whenever possible*. Concentrating on issues

Box 10-3 Guidelines to Effective Verbal Expressions in the Nurse-Client Relationship

- Define unfamiliar terms and concepts.
- Match content and delivery with each client's developmental and educational level, experiential frame of reference, and learning readiness.
- Keep messages clear, concrete, honest, and succinct.
- Put ideas in a logical sequence of related material.
- Relate new ideas to familiar ones when presenting new information.
- Repeat key ideas.
- Reinforce key ideas with vocal emphasis and pauses.
- Keep language as simple as possible; use vocabulary familiar to the client.
- Focus only on essential elements; present one idea at a time.
- Use as many sensory communication channels as possible for key ideas.
- Make sure that nonverbal behaviors support verbal messages.
- Seek feedback to validate accurate reception of information.

of greatest importance is most likely to engage the client's attention. Messages that carry mental images of cultural significance to the client are more effective. Trust is stimulated by using conventional, everyday language; keeping the client's developmental and educational level in mind; and speaking in a general spirit of inquiry and concern for the client. Effective verbal messages address core issues in a clear, concise manner and take into account the principles listed in Box 10-3.

Don't overload the client with information. People can absorb only so much verbal information at one time. Introducing new ideas one at a time allows the client to process data more easily. Repeating key ideas and reinforcing information with concrete examples of concepts facilitates understanding and provides an additional opportunity for the client to ask important questions. At the same time, the nurse needs to be alert for nonverbal response cues from the client that support understanding or that reflect a need for further attention.

Developing an Evidence-Based Practice

McCabe C: Nurse-patient communication: an exploration of patients' experiences, *J Clin Nurs* 13:41-49, 2004.

This qualitative study was designed to elicit patient experiences of how nurses communicate. The study used a hermeneutic phenomenological methodology to analyze data from unstructured interviews. A purposive sample of eight patients in a general hospital was interviewed. The researcher used a reflective process of describing and interpreting themes and subthemes, and yielded four themes related to the patient's experience of how nurses communicated with them.

Results: Identified were lack of communication, attending, empathy, and friendly nurses. The lack of communication perceived by patients related to nurses making assumptions about their concerns and needs.

Application to Your Clinical Practice: As a profession, nurses need to develop patient-centered communication, which involves letting patients know the nurse recognizes their feelings. What steps could you take to ensure that your patients feel heard?

APPLICATIONS

Assessment Strategies

Building Rapport

Communication starts with building rapport in the beginning of a relationship or interview. Building rapport refers to establishing a trusting environment in which the client will feel comfortable sharing information about himself or herself. To the extent that a client feels safe, accepted, and validated by the nurse, the client will find it easier to access and share inner experiences in an authentic manner.

Building rapport starts with getting to know the client as a person (Crellin, 1998). After a brief introduction, use a broad opening statement, such as, "Tell me a little bit about what brought you to the clinic (hospital). I'd like to get an idea of what some of your issues and concerns are so that I can help you better." This type of message allows the client to tell his or her story without imposing the nurse's ideas. It invites the client to engage in a collaborative attempt to understand what is happening to the client that both nurse and client can recognize. The conversation becomes a shared reality about which both participants can dialogue.

It is important to allow each person to tell his or her story in a personal, authentic way (Platt & Gaspar, 2001). Roberts (1994) notes, "We cannot always control what happens to us in our lives, but we can control how we make meaning of it—by when, where, and how we tell the story and explain its significance" (p. 56). Nurses play an important role in helping clients and families tell their stories, including the ways in which gender, culture, and family norms have shaped their health experiences. Once the story is told, the nurse might say, "It probably would be of value for me to describe what we might do together today."

Although rapport building begins with the start of the relationship, it continues as a thread throughout the relationship. Building rapport requires the following:

- *Concentrating* on what is being said so that you can empathetically feed back to the client what you have heard
- *Listening* for key words and issues on which to comment and ask questions (to better understand what the client is truly saying and express empathy)
- *Objectivity* that allows you to experience clients as they are, not the way you'd like them to be
- *Staying* in the "here and now," focusing on the current issues and client concerns
- *Basic respect* for diversity, cultural, and gender differences between clients, as well as between nurse and client
- *Confident manner*, communicating caring and strength

Observation

The nurse needs to keep in mind that many clients suffer with problems of which they are not consciously aware or that they are unable to put into words. There are many different "channels" of nonverbal communication (e.g., facial expressions, vocal tones, gestures and body positions, body movements, touch, and personal space). Watch for nonverbal cues from the client that may signal how he or she is really feeling. Take special notice of whether cues such as the client's facial expression, body movements, posture, and breathing rate support or negate the meaning of the spoken message. For example, the client who verbally declares that he is ready for surgery and seems completely calm may be sending a very different message through the tense muscles the nurse accidentally touches. This is an obvious body language cue that the client may actually be nervous or upset, either consciously or unconsciously. Cues from the environment (e.g., a half-eaten lunch or noncompliance with treatment) can provide nonverbal evidence that a client is in distress. Although how a person really feels about a situation is often best evidenced through body language, nurses need to validate observations for complete accuracy. Lloyd and Weiten (2006) suggest that observing body language and other nonverbal cues when the nurse is speaking can also yield important information. For example, you might note if the client is drifting away and not paying attention, and you would want to comment on your observation, with a request for validation.

Facial expression, particularly around the eyes, is a major source of information when interpreted accurately. Often, a person's facial expression indicates whether the person is happy, sad, scared, confident, hostile, annoyed, or pleased. Ekman and Friesen (2003) describe

Table 10-1 Facial Expressions Associated with Different Emotions

Emotion Expressed	Facial Expression and Body Language
Anger, distress	Eyebrows down and together, forming "worry triangle"; cheeks stretched and flattened down; eyes without life in them; client may have difficulty looking at nurse
Anger, rage	Mouth and jaw firmly set; eyes narrow and alert; facial muscles taut; speech fast; lips curled under and tense; client usually looks directly at nurse with cold, hard stare
Guilt, shame	Head down, shoulders slumped; eyes down, avoiding direct eye contact; some twitching of facial muscles; face flushed; client may lick lips
Happiness, joy	Face smiling, laughing, "life" in the eyes; muscles relaxed, stretched upward and outward, nostrils flared; client looks directly at nurse
Contempt	Lips pursed, tense with corners turned up; jaw tense; eyes narrowed and focused
Interest	Forehead drawn upward; eyes wide open; smiling, mouth open; facial muscles relaxed
Fear	Muscles tense; head lowered; eye contact limited; mouth closed
Caring	Eyes soft; muscles relaxed; smiling

Data from Ekman P, Friesen W: *Unmasking the face*, Englewood Cliffs, NJ, 1975, Prentice Hall.

guidelines for interpreting facial expressions (Table 10-1) that may be useful in interpreting the nonverbal behaviors observed in nursing practice. At the same time, people do have control over their nonverbal behaviors, and they are influenced by the context in which they occur (Richmond & McCroskey, 2003). Culture also can influence facial expression, and the nurse should verify the meaning of a particular facial expression. Certain cultures (e.g., English, northern European) demonstrate less facial responsiveness than Latin cultures, especially with strangers, whereas some Asian cultures tend to cover negative emotions with a smile (Dowd, Giger, & Davidhizar, 1998).

Exercise 10-2 provides practice with observing and interpreting the meaning of nonverbal behaviors.

Asking Questions

Questions are an important form of communication in all phases of the nurse-client relationship, and they are a primary means of obtaining information from a client. The information needed and condition of the client help dictate the number and type of questions. Nurses need to ask enough questions so the client feels the nurse is listening, but not so many that the client feels he or she is being interrogated (Renwick, 1992). Questions fall into three categories: open-ended, closed-ended, and circular.

Open-Ended Questions. Telling the story of an illness rather than listing discrete facts helps individuals and families connect relevant elements (e.g., relationships, impact of the illness on self or others, environmental barriers, potential resources). Without this knowledge, nurses may not respond appropriately to a client's need. An **open-ended question** is similar to an essay question on a test. It is open to interpretation and cannot be answered by "yes," "no," or a one-word response. Such questions are designed to permit the client to express the problem or health need in his or her own words. Open-ended questions are used to elicit the client's thoughts and perspectives without influencing the direction of an acceptable response.

The wording is important, as is a friendly approach that respects the individual and gives the client as much control as possible in responding. A good starting question is, "Will you please tell me a little about yourself and why you came to the clinic today?"

Open-ended questions usually begin with "how," "what," "where," "when," "in what way," or "Can you tell me about…" The following are examples of open-ended questions:

"What are your plans after discharge?"
"Tell me about the accident."
"Where would you like to begin today?"
"What can I do to help you?"

Note that these questions are general, rather than specific, and open to a variety of answers. Follow up on all topics requiring further information using active listening responses and open-ended questions. Sometimes you will need to ask focused questions to elicit more details.

Exercise 10-2 Observing for Nonverbal Cues

Purpose: To develop skill in interpreting nonverbal cues.

Procedure:

1. Watch a dramatic movie (that you haven't seen before) with the sound off for 15 minutes.
2. As you watch the movie, write down the emotions you see expressed, the associated nonverbal behavior, and your interpretations of the meaning and the other person's response.

Discussion:

In a large group, share your observations and interpretations of the scenes watched. Discussion should focus on the variations in the interpretations of the nonverbal language. Discuss ways in which the nurse can use observations of nonverbal language with a client in a therapeutic manner to gain a better understanding of the client. Time permitting, the movie segment could be shown again, this time with the sound. Discuss any variations in the interpretations without sound versus with verbal dialogue. Discuss the importance of validation of nonverbal cues.

Exercise 10-3 Asking Open-Ended Questions

Purpose: To develop skill in the use of open-ended questions to facilitate information sharing.

Procedure:

1. Break up into pairs. Role-play a situation in which one student takes the role of the facilitator and the other the sharer. (If you are in the clinical area, you may want to choose a clinical situation.)
2. As a pair, select a topic. The facilitator begins asking open-ended questions.
3. Dialogue for 5 to 10 minutes on the topic.
4. In pairs, discuss perceptions of the dialogue and determine what questions were comfortable and open-ended. The student facilitator should reflect on the comfort level experienced with asking each question. The sharing student should reflect on the efficacy of the listening responses in helping to move the conversation toward his or her perspective.

Discussion:

As a class, each pair should contribute examples of open-ended questions that facilitated the sharing of information. Compile these examples on the board. Formulate a collaborative summation of what an open-ended question is and how it is used. Discuss how open-ended questions can be used sensitively with uncomfortable topics.

Although open-ended questions are desirable in most clinical situations, there are exceptions. Emergencies or other circumstances when information is needed quickly require the use of focused or closed-ended questions. For example, open-ended questions may not be appropriate to use with a woman in active labor or with a new admission to the emergency department. Exercise 10-3 provides an opportunity to practice the use of open-ended questions.

Focused Questions. A variation of the open-ended question is the focused question, which limits the response to a certain informational area but requires more than a "yes" or "no" response. The nurse uses focused questions to obtain data that are more specific. Sometimes people with limited verbal skills respond better to focused questions because they know how to respond. The following are examples of focused questions:

"Tell me more about the pain in your arm."

"You mentioned that you had the problem with your back before. How did this problem develop before?"

"Can you give me a specific example of what you mean by…?"

"What has been most difficult for you regarding…?"

"When would you say you began to feel the helpless feeling you describe?"

Closed-Ended Questions. **Closed-ended questions** resemble multiple-choice questions with limited answer options. The answer to a closed-ended question limits expression of the client's feelings, and it may take more questions to obtain the same information. They are useful in emergency situations, when the goal is to obtain information quickly and the client's emotional reactions are of secondary importance. Clients with limited social skills often can respond better initially to closed questions. Examples of closed-ended questions include the following:

"When was your last tetanus shot?"

"Does the pain radiate down your left shoulder and arm?"

"When was your last meal?"

"Have you had these symptoms before?"

Exercise 10-4 provides experience with assessing types of active listening responses.

Circular Questions. In contrast to linear questions, which explore the descriptive characteristics of a situation, **circular questions** focus on the interpersonal *context* in which an illness occurs. They are designed to identify family relationships and differences in the impact of an illness on individual family members. They serve to bring into view the interpersonal patterns and connections present in the current situation that are problematic or that could be potentially available to the client or family as resources. They are categorized as difference, behavioral effect, hypothetical, and triadic types. Examples of circular

Exercise 10-4 Differences in Active Listening Questions

Purpose: To help students identify differences in types of listening questions.

Procedure:

Examine the following questions. Mark those that are open-ended with an asterisk (*). Mark a focused question with a plus sign (+). Mark a closed-ended question with a minus sign (–).

Ms. Gai, did you have a productive therapy session?
How do you feel about it now that you've learned that you will be staying at your daughter's house?
What did the doctor say about your lower back pain?
Your tray will be here soon. Are you hungry?
And when you heard that, you felt...?
When the physician walked away, you felt rejected?
No one likes to be in pain; can I get you something for it?
In the past when your leg ached, what kinds of things helped?
What do you think about being transferred to a nursing home?
Tell me, what brought you to see the physician today?
Are you having that problem with arthritis in your hand again?
What would you like to discuss today while we take a walk?
How are you?
What happened to you after you fell down?
And then what did you think?
Do you feel like taking your medicine now or later?

questions are provided in Chapter 13. When asking circular questions, the nurse should maintain a neutral, accepting attitude toward the response, even when the answer is surprising or controversial.

Asking Follow-Up Questions. Many times, once the nurse has asked preliminary questions about a topic, whether open, focused, closed or circular, there is a need to follow up to get more information. Follow-up questions directly relate to the initial data and ask the client to expand on a particular topic, for example, "Now that you have told me about how you handle your diabetic diet in general, can you tell me about any modifications you have to make when you are ill or stressed?"

What the Nurse Listens For

It is essential to explore another's reality before one can be of any help. The words are important, but clients also bring attitudes, feelings, and values that must be recognized but are not always readily apparent to the client. For example, a client newly diagnosed with cancer may be aware of the diagnosis but may be much less clear about the accompanying fear, anger, uncertainty, and resentment that could affect treatment compliance. Box 10-4 presents what the nurse should listen for in assessment interviews.

Themes

The process of therapeutic communication involves much more than words. As Myers (2000) suggests, "any actual dialogue has an inner, subjectively experienced com-

Box 10-4 What the Nurse Listens For

- Content themes
- Communication patterns
- Discrepancies in content, body language, and vocalization
- Feelings, revealed in a person's voice, body movements, and facial expressions
- What is not being said as well as what is being said
- The client's preferred representational system (auditory, visual, tactile)
- The nurse's own inner responses
- The effect communication produces in others involved with the client

ponent" (p. 151). This subjective component refers to the **theme** or central idea (feeling) expressed through the communication. A theme is defined as the underlying feeling associated with concrete facts (e.g., feelings of powerlessness, fear, abandonment, and helplessness).

Listening for themes includes observing and understanding what the client is *not* saying as well as what the person actually reveals. For example, a client may tell you that he is not afraid of his surgery the next day. It is a simple in-and-out procedure, he says, and he plans to be back at work on Monday. At the same time, he is distressed that his girlfriend will not be able to go out with him the night before the operation "to get his mind off the surgery." Here the words create a mixed message. Identifying the underlying themes presented in a therapeutic conversation can relieve anxiety and provide direction for individualized nursing interventions.

Clients bring their life history to each health care situation, and the manner in which the change in health status affects each individual is unique and reflective of the patient's history as well as the current situation (Ramos, 1992). For example, the client may say to the nurse, "I'm worried about my surgery tomorrow." This is one way of framing the problem. If the same client presents his concern as, "I'm not sure I will make it through the surgery tomorrow," this changes the focus of the communication from a generalized worry to a more personal theme of survival. Alternatively, the client might say, "I don't know whether my husband should stay tomorrow for the surgery. It is going to be a long procedure, and he gets so worried." The theme (focus) expresses her concern about her relationship with her husband. In each of these communications, the client expresses a distinctive theme of concern about the up-

Exercise 10-5 Listening for Themes

Purpose: To help students identify underlying themes in messages.

Procedure:

1. Divide into groups of three to five students.
2. Take turns telling a short story about yourselves—about growing up, important people or events in your life, or significant accomplishments (e.g., getting your first job).
3. As each student presents a story, take mental notes of the important themes. Write them down so you will not be tempted to change them as you hear the other students. Notice nonverbal behaviors accompanying the verbal message. Are they consistent with the verbal message of the sharer?
4. When the story is completed, each of the other people in the group shares his or her observations with the sharer.
5. After all students have shared their observations, validate their accuracy with the sharer.

Discussion:

1. Were the underlying themes recorded by the group consistent with the sharer's understanding of his or her communication?
2. As others related their interpretations of significant words or phrases, did you change your mind about the nature of the underlying theme?
3. Were the interpretations of pertinent information relatively similar or significantly different?
4. If they were different, what implications do you think such differences have for nurse-client relationships in nursing practice?
5. What did you learn from doing this exercise?

Variation:

Students can break up into small groups and each create a clinical scenario in which two or more persons are dialoguing in relation to a situation or health problem. One person is in the helper role. Each group will dramatize their scenario to the larger group. Each student can listen for the emotional and informational themes and write a description of his or her impressions.

coming surgery. The nurse will want to assess differences in focus accurately and structure responses according to the client's emphasis.

Emotional objectivity in making sense of client themes is essential. Moving beyond the facts requires critical thinking skills and control of personal feelings and preferences. "Objectivity here refers to seeing what an experience is for another person, not how it fits or relates to other experiences, not what causes it, why it exists, or what purposes it serves. It is an attempt to see attitudes and concepts, beliefs and values of an individual as they are to him at the moment he expresses them—not what they were or will become" (Moustakas, 1974, p. 78). Exercise 10-5 provides practice in listening for themes.

Communication Patterns

Communication patterns offer another dimension in designing appropriate responses. Some clients exaggerate information, whereas others characteristically leave out highly relevant details. Some talk a lot, using dramatic language and multiple examples; others say very little. Evaluation of the client's present overall pattern of interaction with others includes strengths and limitations, family communication dynamics, and developmental and educational levels. Culture, role, ways of handling conflict, and ways of dealing with emotions reflect communication patterns. The nurse uses data about client communication patterns as the basis for understanding a client's response to health care and involvement in his or her care. For example, the nurse may give additional cues to the client who has difficulty with verbal expression. Mirroring the client's communication pattern (e.g., not being blunt with the client whose communication style lends itself to stories or metaphors) acknowledges that the nurse has heard and respects the client's communication pattern. Incorporating cultural understanding of communication style also is important (e.g., encouraging use of the client's own words as much as possible).

Intuitive Communication

Intuitive communication can occur as a personal listening response from within the nurse. Referred to as focusing, intuition represents a body-centered way of listening to feelings generated in the situation that carry meaning about the underlying issues and concerns (Klagsbrun, 2001). For example, the nurse may feel intuitively that something is not right with a client, even without objective evidence. When a nurse has no particular personal reason for reacting to the client with anger, fear, or sadness, this inner response may reflect a client's unexpressed feeling. Behavioral reactions that the nurse feels are out of proportion to the situation (e.g., complete calm before surgery, excessive anger, noncompliance or passive compliance with no questions asked, guarded verbalizations,

Table 10-2 Listening Responses

Listening Response	Example
Minimal cues and leads	Body actions: smiling, nodding, leaning forward Words: "mm," "uh huh," "oh really," "go on"
Clarification	"Could you describe what happened in sequence?" "I'm not sure I understand what you mean. Can you give me an example?"
Restatement	"Are you saying that . . . *(repeat client's words)*?" "You mean . . . *(repeat client's words)*."
Paraphrasing	*Client:* "I can't take this anymore. The chemo is worse than the cancer. I just want to die." *Nurse:* "It sounds as though you are saying you have had enough."
Reflection	"It sounds as though you feel guilty because you weren't home at the time of the accident." "You sound really frustrated because the treatment is taking longer than you thought it would."
Summarization	"Before moving on, I would like to go over with you what I think we've accomplished thus far."
Silence	Briefly disconnecting but continuing to use attending behaviors after an important idea, thought, or feeling
Touch	Gently rubbing a person's arm during a painful procedure

incongruent facial expressions or body language, or social withdrawal) can be danger signals. Nurses need to listen to their intuitive feelings, but it is also important to validate this intuitive knowledge with the client to fully understand the meaning of the behavior.

Therapeutic Listening Responses

Listening responses show the client that the nurse is fully present as a professional partner in helping the client understand a change in health status and the best ways to cope with it (Keller & Baker, 2000). Minimal verbal cues, clarification, restatement, paraphrasing, reflection, summarization, silence, and touch are examples of skilled listening responses the nurse can use to guide therapeutic interventions (Table 10-2).

Minimal Cues and Leads

Simple, encouraging leads can communicate interest. **Minimal cues** through body actions (e.g., smiling, nodding, and leaning forward) encourage clients to continue with their story. By not detracting from the client's message and by giving permission to tell the story as the client sees it, minimal cues promote client comfort in sharing intimate information. Short phrases such as, "Go on" or "And then?" or "Can you say more about…?" are also useful. Exercise 10-6 provides an opportunity to see the influence of minimal cues and leads on communication.

Clarification

Clarification seeks to understand the message of the client by asking for more information or for elaboration on a point. The strategy is most useful when parts of a client's communication are ambiguous or not easily understood. Failure to ask for clarification when part of the communication is poorly understood means that the nurse will act on incomplete or inaccurate information.

Clarification responses are expressed as a question or statement followed by a restatement or paraphrasing of part of the communicated message. "You stated earlier that you were concerned about your blood pressure. Tell me more about what concerns you." The tone of voice used with a clarification response should be neutral, not accusatory or demanding. Practice this response in Exercise 10-7.

Exercise 10-6 Minimal Cues and Leads

Purpose: To practice and evaluate the efficacy of minimal cues and leads.

Procedure:

1. Initiate a conversation with someone outside of class and attempt to tell the person about something with which you are familiar for 5 to 10 minutes.
2. Make note of all the cues that the person puts forth that either promote or inhibit conversation.
3. Now try this with another person and write down the different cues and leads you observe as you are speaking and your emotional response to them (e.g., what most encouraged you to continue speaking).

Discussion:

As a class, share your experience and observations. Different cues and responses will be compiled on the board. Discuss the impact of different cues and leads on your comfort and willingness to share about yourself. What cues and leads promoted communication? What cues and leads inhibited sharing?

Variation:

This exercise can be practiced with a clinical problem simulation in which one student takes the role of the professional helper and the other takes the role of client. Perform the same scenario with and without the use of minimum encouragers. What were the differences when encouragers were not used? Was the communication as lively? How did it feel to you when telling your story when this strategy was used by the helping person?

Exercise 10-7 Using Clarification

Purpose: To develop skill in the use of clarification.

Procedure:

1. Write a paragraph related to an experience you have had.
2. Place all the student paragraphs together, and then pick one (not your own).
3. Develop clarification questions you might ask about the selected paragraph.

Discussion:

Share with the class your chosen paragraph and the clarification questions you developed. Discuss how effective the questions are in clarifying information. Other students can suggest additional clarification questions.

Variation:

Have the student who creates the clarification questions ask these questions of the paragraph's author. Discuss in the larger group how effective the questions are in clarifying information.

Restatement

Restatement is an active listening strategy used to broaden a client's perspective or when the nurse needs to provide a sharper focus on a specific part of the communication. Restatement is like bracketing a phrase in a paragraph: it acts as a brief interruption designed to highlight a defined element of a message. Restatement is particularly effective when the client overgeneralizes or seems stuck in a repetitive line of thinking. To challenge the validity of the client's statement directly could be counterproductive. Repeating parts of the message in the form of a query serves a similar purpose without raising defenses, for example, "Let me see if I have this right…" (Coulehan, Platt, Egener et al., 2001). Restating a self-critical or irrational part of the message focuses the client's attention on the possibility of an inaccurate or global assertion. Restatement should be used sparingly and only as a point of emphasis. Otherwise it can sound stilted.

Paraphrasing

Paraphrasing is a response strategy designed to help the client elaborate more on the content of a verbal message. The nurse takes the original message and transforms it into his or her own words without losing the meaning. For the client, hearing his or her own words in a slightly different way provides a new means of hearing these

Exercise 10-8 Practicing Paraphrasing

Purpose: To practice paraphrasing as an active listening response.

Procedure:

Consider the following example, then write one appropriately rephrased sentence for each statement below.

Example: "I'm on a diet, but I seem to be gaining a lot of weight even though I usually try to stick to it faithfully."

Appropriate paraphrase: "You want to lose weight, but your diet isn't working?"

Inappropriate paraphrase: "You can't stick to your diet?"

1. "I need an operation, but can't take the time to have it until my business is doing better."
2. "The doctor just told me I have cancer, but I'm not sure what he means."

Exercise 10-9 Role-Play Practice with Paraphrasing and Reflection

Purpose: To practice use of paraphrasing and reflection as listening responses.

Procedure:

1. The class forms into groups of three students each. One student takes the role of client, one the role of helper, and one the role of observer.
2. The client shares with the helper a recent health problem he or she encountered and describes the details of the situation and the emotions experienced. The helper responds with the use of paraphrasing and reflection in a dialogue that lasts at least 5 minutes. The observer records the statements made by the helper. At the end of the dialogue, the client writes his or her perception of how the helper's statements affected the conversation, including what comments were most helpful. The helper writes a short summary of the listening responses he or she used, with comments on how successful they were.

Discussion:

1. Share your summary and discuss the differences in using the techniques from the helper, client, and observer perspectives.
2. Discuss how these differences related to influencing the flow of dialogue, helping the client feel heard, and the impact on the helper's understanding of the client from both the client and the helper positions.
3. Identify places in the dialogue where one form of questioning might be preferable to another.
4. How could you use this exercise to understand your client's concerns?
5. Were you surprised by any of the summaries?

concerns within a broader framework. The paraphrase statement is shorter and a little more specific than the client's initial statement so that the focus is on the core elements. Presented as a tentative statement—for example, "Let me see if I have this right," the paraphrase listening response invites but does not force a specific answer. Paraphrasing is particularly useful in the early stages of a relationship or when the client is raising a troublesome topic for the first time. It is also valuable in checking whether the nurse's translation of the client's words is an accurate interpretation of the message. Exercise 10-8 provides practice in paraphrasing. Exercise 10-9 is designed to help students role-play active listening responses.

Reflection

Reflection as a listening response focuses on the emotional overtones of a message. This listening response helps the client clarify important feelings and experience them with their appropriate intensity in relation to a particular situation or event. There are several ways to use reflection, including the following:

- Reflection on vocal tone: "I can feel the sense of anger and frustration in your voice."
- Linking feelings with the content message: "It sounds like you feel ___________ because _____________."
- Linking current feelings with past experiences: "It seems as if this experience reminds you of feelings you had with other health care experiences where you didn't feel understood."

Reflection as a listening response gives clients permission to *have* feelings and helps them to identify feelings they may not be aware of in new and unfamiliar circumstances. The nurse needs to know enough about the client to respond empathetically and accurately to the client's feeling. Reflective responses are most effective when they are used to accentuate or further develop the relation between content and feeling, and when the comment is expressed tentatively rather than as absolute fact.

Sometimes nursing students feel they are putting words into the client's mouth when they "choose" an emotion from their perception of the client's message. This would be true if you were choosing an emotion out of thin air, but not when the nurse empathetically considers the client's situation and does not go beyond the data the client presents. Reflection is different from interpretation in that it simply puts into words the feelings a

Exercise 10-10 Practicing the Use of Reflecting Responses

Purpose: To practice clarification, paraphrasing, and reflection as active listening responses.

Procedure:
This exercise may be done alone or in any size class group. Read the following situation:

Jamie, age 7 years, is dying of a chronic respiratory condition. His small stature and optimistic sense of humor have made him a favorite on the unit. Jamie's mom breaks down crying one day, saying to you, "I try to do good, to help out on the unit these last 4 weeks. Why is God punishing me this way? I can't take much more of this, staying here constantly, watching Jamie struggle for every breath. Only his intravenous fluids and oxygen keep him alive. Sometimes I think it would be better to stop them and let him die in peace."

1. Write appropriate nurse responses that reflect back to the mother your perception of the feelings underlying her statements.
2. Write other responses that reflect your perception of her feelings.
3. Combine the responses to attain an appropriate reflection of content and feeling. It may be easier to do this exercise for each sentence in the situation.

Discussion:
1. Was it more difficult to use reflection as a communication strategy? If so, why?
2. What did you personally learn from this exercise?

nurse senses or hears in the client's comments without either adding or subtracting from them. Exercise 10-10 gives practice in using reflecting responses.

Summarization

Summarization is an active listening skill used to review content and process. Summarization pulls several ideas and feelings together, either from one interaction or a series of interactions. Here the nurse reduces a lengthy interaction or discussion to a few succinct sentences. For example, the nurse might make a brief statement followed by the comment, "Tell me if my understanding of this agrees with yours." A summary statement is particularly useful before moving on to a different topic area. Exercise 10-11 gives practice in summarization.

Silence

Silence, used deliberately and judiciously, is a powerful listening response. The use of a pause can be very helpful during this type of interaction because it allows the client to think, while at the same time allowing the nurse to step back momentarily and process what he or she heard before responding. Too often a quick response addresses only a small part of the message or gives the client an insufficient opportunity to formulate an idea fully. A short silence to get in touch with the personal anxiety aroused by a client's response is appropriate before responding. On the other hand, long silences become uncomfortable. The silent pause should be just that, a brief disconnection followed by a verbal comment.

Another use of silence is to accentuate important points that you want the client to reflect on. By pausing briefly after presenting a key idea and before proceeding to the next topic, the nurse encourages the client to notice the most important elements of the communication.

When a client falls silent, it can mean that something has touched the client profoundly. Respecting the client's silence and sitting without breaking the mood can be important in sharing the meaning of the communication. Clients often marvel at the nurse's willingness to sit quietly and without awkwardness in their moments of silence. You can practice this skill in Exercise 10-12.

Touch

Touch, the first of our senses to develop, represents a person's first experience in communicating with another human being. Usually experienced as a nurturing, validating form of communication, touch remains a vital form of communication throughout life. Touch is a powerful listening response used when words would break a mood

Exercise 10-11 Practicing Summarization

Purpose: To provide practice in summarizing interactions.

Procedure:

1. Choose a partner for a pairs discussion.
2. For 10 minutes, discuss a medical ethics topic such as euthanasia, heroic life support for the terminally ill, or "Baby Doe" decisions to allow malformed babies to die if the parents desire.
3. After 10 minutes, both partners must stop talking until Participant A has summarized what Participant B has just said to Participant B's satisfaction, and vice versa.

Discussion:

After both partners have completed their summarizations, discuss the process of summarization, answering the following questions:

1. Did knowing you had to summarize the other person's point of view encourage you to listen more closely?
2. Did the act of summarizing help clarify any discussion points? Were any points of agreement found? What points of disagreement were found?
3. Did the exercise help you to understand the other person's point of view?
4. What should an effective summary contain? Is it hard to summarize a long conversation?
5. How did you determine which points to focus on in your summarization?

Exercise 10-12 Therapeutic Use of Silence

Purpose: To experience the effect of the use of silence as a listening response.

Procedure:

1. Two people act as Participants A and B.
2. Participant A plays the role of the nurse. Participant B is a healthy, ambulatory, 80-year-old female client in an extended-care facility who was placed there against her will by her family, who are moving to another state.
3. Participant B's role is to describe feelings (shock) at being institutionalized and to discuss the slow adjustment to new surroundings and new companions, describing both the positive and the negative aspects.
4. Participant A's objective is to make at least three deliberate efforts to use silence during the conversation (as a therapeutic device to encourage Participant B's consideration of life and problems).

Discussion:

After 10 minutes of role-playing, have a general discussion to share feelings about the effective use of silence.

or when verbalization would fail to convey the empathy or depth of feeling between nurse and client (Nelson, 1998; Straneva, 2000). A hand tenderly placed on a frightened mother's shoulder or a gentle squeeze of the hand can speak far more eloquently than words in times of deep emotion, whether sadness or joy. Clients in pain, those who feel repulsive to others because of altered appearance, lonely and dying clients, and those experiencing sensory deprivation or feeling confused respond positively to the nurse who is unafraid to enter their world

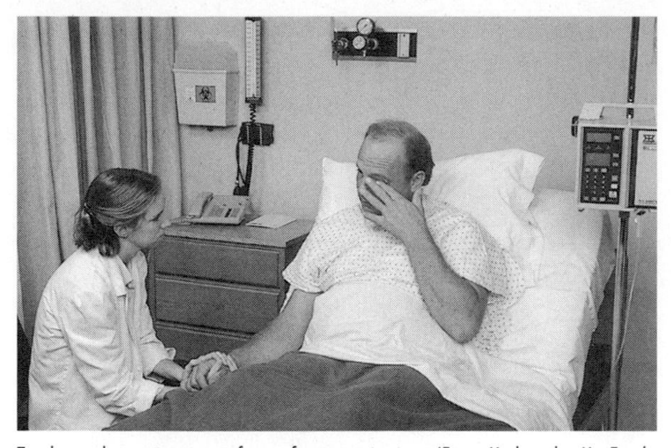

Touch can be an important form of communication. (From Harkreader H: *Fundamentals of nursing: caring and clinical judgment*, Philadelphia, 2000, WB Saunders.)

and touch them (Miller, 1990). Consider the use of touch with a brain-damaged client in the next example (Chesla, 1996).

Case Example

"I found out that if I held Sam's hand he would lie perfectly still and even drift off to sleep. When I sat with him, holding his hand, his blood pressure and heart rate would go down to normal and his intracranial pressure would stay below 10. When I tried to calm him with words, there was no response—he [had] a blood pressure of 160/90!" (Chesla, 1996, p. 202)

Touch can deepen the meaning of language. Expressive touch, when combined with words (e.g., in an arm placed around the shoulder or a touch on the hand), tends to enhance the feeling of comfort. Touch can be an important form of communication when words do not console or reassure. Holding a small child or placing your hand in another's during a painful procedure is as important a means of communication in the therapeutic relationship as knowing the right words to say. Touch is particularly useful as a form of communication with the elderly client who may be hard of hearing or have trouble seeing (Caris-Verhallen, Kerkstra, & Bensing, 1999).

Talton (1995) suggests, "For it to be a healing touch, however, you must touch with the intention of achieving a goal" (p. 61). She distinguishes task touch, delivered in the course of providing direct care to clients, from caring touch, which occurs as a form of communication (e.g., to reduce pain or offer comfort). Task touch—for example, gentle massage of a painful area—helps clients relax, whereas stroking the hand of a client with dementia helps reduce agitation.

People vary in their comfort with touch as a communication response. All cultures have norms about how people should touch each other and when touching is appropriate. In general, Latin cultures encourage touching, whereas many Asian cultures tend to prefer a more formal relationship. As in other aspects of the relationship, the nurse uses professional judgment about the strategy of touch and its possible interpretation by the client.

How individuals interpret the meaning of touch depends also on such factors as its duration, intensity, and the body part touched. Before reaching out to a client with touch, the nurse needs to assess the client's receptiveness to touch. Observation of the client will provide some indication, but the nurse may need to ask for validation. If the client is paranoid, out of touch with reality, verbally inappropriate, or mistrustful, touch is contraindicated as a listening response.

Healing touch is an energy-based form of therapeutic communication that, used judiciously, can deepen the nurse-client connection (Umbreit, 2000). Although this form of communication requires specialized training, it can be very beneficial to clients with pain or agitation.

Verbal Responses

People use word symbols to describe their reality, to reduce their anxiety or uncertainty, to collaborate or disagree with others, to develop relationships, and to express feelings and ideas. Nurses use a variety of verbal responses to teach, to encourage, to support, to provide information, to gather information, and to move a client in a certain direction toward goal achievement. Through verbal discussions, the nurse helps clients assess the healthy elements of their personality (their strengths) and to use those elements in coping with the current health problem. Active listening and verbal responses are inseparable from each other. Ideally, they support one another and provide a more complete picture. In making a verbal response, the nurse gives or changes the perspective on a health-related topic.

Most clients are not looking for brilliant answers from the nurse, but rather seek feedback and support that suggests a compassionate understanding of their particular dilemma. No matter what level of communication exists in the relationship, the same questions arise: "Who am I?"

"What is the meaning of my current experience?" "How can I cope with what is happening to me?" The same needs—"hear me," "touch me," "respond to me," "feel my pain and experience my joys with me"—are identifiable as basic underlying themes. Simple communication strategies to help clients feel understood include the following (Duldt, 1991):

- Allowing the client enough time to answer questions
- Informing the client of what the nurse is going to do and why
- Asking the client what his or her feelings are about what is happening

Verbal responses provide guidance and information to help clients assume responsibility for their health and well-being. With shorter time frames for actual client contact, nurses need to use verbal communication to connect with clients as partners from the first encounter in developing a mutually agreed-on focus for intervention based on client data, identifying and integrating client strengths to plan and implement treatment objectives, and using environmental supports and community resources to enhance treatment.

Verbal response strategies include mirroring, focusing, metaphors, humor, confirming responses, reframing, providing relevant feedback, and validation, all of which are designed to strengthen the coping abilities of the client, alone or in relationship with others. Although described individually for the purposes of this chapter, in real practice the nurse will integrate more than one, even in a single intervention. As with active listening responses, the nurse uses observation, validation, and patterns of knowing to gauge the effectiveness of verbal interventions. On the basis of the client's reaction, the nurse may have to use simpler language, use a different strategy, and adjust verbal response in whatever way is needed so that the client can fully understand the message. The way you say something is as important as the words you choose. Your voice should be firm, warm, moderate, and relaxed.

Mirroring Depth in Verbal Response

Regardless of content, the nurse's verbal responses should match the client's message in level of depth, meaning, and language (Johnson, 1980). The client needs to lead the way to any exploration of deeper feeling. If the client makes a serious statement, the nurse should not respond with a flip remark. Likewise, a superficial statement does not warrant an intense response. Responses that encourage a client to explore feelings about limitations or strengths at a slightly deeper but related level of conversation are likely to meet with more success.

Matching Response with Verbal Content

Verbal response should neither expand nor diminish the meaning of the client's remarks. Notice the differences in the nature of the following responses to a client:

Client: **I feel so discouraged. No matter how hard I try, I still can't walk without pain on the two parallel bars.**

Nurse: **You want to give up because you don't think you will be able to walk again.**

At this point, it is unclear that the client wants to give up, so the nurse's comment expands on the client's meaning without having sufficient data to support it. Although it is possible that this is what the client means, it is not the only possibility. The more important dilemma for the client may be whether his or her efforts have any purpose. The next response focuses only on the negative aspects of the client's communication and ignores the client's comment about his or her efforts.

Nurse: **So you think you won't be able to walk independently again.**

In the final response example below, the nurse addresses both parts of the client's message and makes the appropriate connection. The nurse's statement invites the client to validate the nurse's perception.

Nurse: **It sounds to me as if you don't feel your efforts are helping you regain control over your walking.**

Using Appropriate Vocabulary

The final match needed for successful communication is use of appropriate vocabulary. Using jargon or language that is beyond the client's educational level and experiential frame of reference generally means that little information will be retained. Unless the client is able to associate new ideas with familiar words and ideas, the nurse might as well be talking in a different language. More often than not, clients will not tell the nurse that they do not understand a verbal response for fear of either offending the nurse or revealing personal deficits. Talking down to a client or giving information that fails to take into account the client's previous experiences also tends to fall on deaf ears. Frequent validation with the client related to content can help reduce this problem.

Format is another factor to consider for full understanding. Some clients need a straightforward, concrete format; others respond favorably to more imaginative formats. Observation, really listening to the client's mode of expression, and cultural understanding of language nuances and meaning help the nurse select an appropriate format. Here is where the nurse uses artistry in choosing the most appropriate communication strategies for building and maintaining rapport.

Focusing

In past health care situations, the nurse often had extended time to talk with each client, but in today's health care delivery system, the nurse typically has a short time to gather relevant information and to assist clients in sorting through complex issues. Consequently, the nurse may have to help the client select the most pressing health care topic for discussion. To achieve this goal, the nurse might say the following to the client who is rambling about non–health-related matters:

"Mr. Solan, you have given me a lot to think about here, but I would like to hear more about how you are handling the surgery tomorrow. You mentioned that you were feeling afraid, and this is normal. I wonder if we could talk more about this."

Note that the nurse focuses on a topic raised by the client rather than a completely unrelated topic.

Sometimes the nurse helps the client focus on a single important thought or feeling with a simple statement such as, "This point seems worth looking at more closely." Although focusing is an extremely useful communication tool, the nurse should not force a client to focus on an issue that he or she is not yet willing to discuss. Rather, the goal is to open the door to the possibility of it being an issue worth exploring. You can always go back to a topic when the client is more receptive. For example, the nurse might say, "I can understand that this is a difficult topic for you, but I am here for you if you would like to discuss [identified topic] later."

Using Metaphors

Metaphor is a therapeutic communication strategy that portrays a nonthreatening mental picture that is similar to the dilemma a client is facing (Billings, 1991). A metaphor introduces a fresh perspective and provides the client with a foundation for learning new ways of functioning. Everyday metaphors such as "happy as a lark," "pain in the neck," "sharp as a tack," and "pillar of strength" demonstrate how a short phrase can convey a mental picture without needing fuller explanation.

A useful metaphor for understanding the basic therapeutic communication process is to consider how people play ball. The person who throws the ball (sender of a message) must aim the ball accurately so that the receiver can catch it easily. This means that the words used are to the point and fit the situation. The sender throws the ball with precision, aimed directly at the receiver. This means that the language used can be easily understood. The receiver deliberately stands in the proper position to catch it. This means that the nurse makes sure that the client is in a receptive position to hear the message. When the sender throws a fast ball (abstract vocabulary that the receiver has trouble understanding), a curve ball (manipulative or a message with a hidden agenda), or a slow ball (vague and tangential messages), the ball (message) catches the receiver off guard and misses the mark.

In *The Tale of the Velveteen Rabbit*, the author uses the metaphor of a young boy and his toy rabbit to help the reader understand the process of becoming real or authentic as essential to finding love. Nurses can also use short vignettes to get a point across. For example, with a noncompliant client who wants to be well doesn't take his or her medication, the nurse might say, "Now suppose that I wanted to lose weight. I go to the best dietitian, who tells me that I need to change my eating habits, eat low-fat foods, and exercise to lose weight. I thank her profusely but don't follow any of her advice. What chance do you think I would have of losing weight?"

Reframing Situations

Bandler and Grindler (1997) defined **reframing** as "changing the frame in which a person perceives events in order to change the meaning" (p. 1). It is not a distortion of reality, but rather a different, more positive interpretation. Meaning and behavioral responses are so interrelated that when the meaning changes, a person's responses and behaviors also change. The meaning of an event acts as a perceptual frame that guides subsequent action. For example, clients who look at a glass as half-empty and clients who see the same glass as half-full will approach the same situation differently.

Steps in the reframing process call for the nurse to discover a positive or useful element in the client's situation (Pesut, 1991). To illustrate, receiving a diagnosis of terminal illness is devastating, but once a person gets over the initial shock of the diagnosis, it can be reframed as a "gift" in that it gives the individual the opportunity to take advantage of the moment and to connect with significant people they might have taken for granted otherwise. Here, the nurse might ask a seriously ill client whether the illness has brought him closer to a family member or has caused him to contact a distant friend.

Reframing strategies emphasize client strengths. For example, the nurse might ask the client to identify coping strategies that have worked in the past and suggest that transferable skills such as persistence and creativity can be used in a different way in the current situation. The new frame must fit the current situation and be understandable to the client; otherwise, it will not work. This means that you should consider the reframing from several different perspectives and choose the one most likely to have the strongest impact.

Reframing a situation is helpful when blame is a component of a family's response to the client's illness. For example, the reason a person fails to take medication or continues to drink alcohol may have little to do with a desire to annoy or punish significant others. Helping a family to see these behaviors as symptoms of a medical illness for which they cannot assume responsibility helps the spouse or child reframe the situation as one they cannot control and leads to needed detachment.

Presenting Reality

Presenting reality to a client who is misinterpreting reality can be helpful as long as the client does not perceive that the nurse is arguing with or criticizing the client's perception of reality. A simple statement such as, "I know that you feel very strongly about ___________, but I don't see it that way" is a quiet way for the nurse to express his or her perceptions or the facts of a situation, thus introducing an alternate explanation for the client to consider. Another way of introducing reality is to validate the underlying feeling or to put into words an implied feeling, as seen in the following examples (note how the nurse does not challenge the client but addresses the feeling):

Client: **I can't talk to anyone around here. All you people seem to care about is the money, not the patient.**

Nurse: **It sounds like you are really feeling all alone right now.**

Using Humor

Humor is a powerful communication technique when used with deliberate intent for a specific therapeutic purpose. McGhee (1985) defines humor as "the mental experience of discovering and appreciating ludicrous or absurdly incongruous ideas, events, or situations" (p. 6).

The surprise element in humor can cut through an overly intense situation and put it in perspective. Once a person can appreciate the many absurdities and incongruities of life, the spirit lifts. Humor has the capacity to encourage a sense of intimacy, acceptance, and warmth, which can reduce emotional distance in the nurse-client relationship (Lynch & Anchor, 1991). Laughter increases β-endorphins, a neurotransmitter that creates natural highs and promotes healing (Cousins, 1976). A good joke creates a distraction, but it needs the proper context. Humor is most effective when rapport is well established and a level of trust exists between the nurse and client. A shared joke becomes a bond (and in some cases, almost a password) in well-established relationships (McGhee, 1998). When humor is used, it should focus on the idea, event, or situation, or something other than the client's humanity. Humor that ridicules is not funny.

Occasional use of humor is more effective than constant use. Constant use of humor can lead the client to minimize personal recognition of serious issues. It is up to the nurse to maintain the appropriate level of intensity and heightened interpersonal awareness in the relationship to help clients meet health goals. The following factors contribute to the successful use of humor:

- Knowledge of the client's response pattern
- An overly intense situation
- Timing
- Gearing to the client's developmental level

Before using humor, the nurse needs to collect enough data on the client to have a working knowledge of how a humorous remark or joke might be received. Some clients respond well to humor; others are insulted or perplexed by it. They may not see it as appropriate or culturally acceptable in a helping relationship. Because of their concrete thinking, small children cannot relate to humor as well as adults can. Adolescents respond enthusiastically to some types of humor and can be emotionally devastated by other humorous remarks, particularly if the comments directly relate to them as individuals.

Professional judgment in the use of humor is critical to its success. Humor is less effective when the client is tired or emotionally vulnerable. Instead, the client may need structure and calming support.

Confirming Responses

Confirming responses are statements designed to validate the client and enhance self-esteem. They respect and support the uniqueness of a client's experience. For example, the nurse might say to a mother reluctant to leave her small child, "I can see that it is hard for you to say goodnight to your little boy, knowing that he does not understand why you have to leave. Is there anything I can do to make it easier for you?" To the client who tells the nurse, "I know it is silly to worry about general anesthesia with one-day surgery. I don't know why I am so uptight about it," the nurse might say, "No, it is not silly; many people worry about anesthesia. Can you tell me more about what worries you?" With each confirming response, the nurse acknowledges the legitimacy of the client's feelings and invites the client to explore further the meaning of the message.

Disconfirming responses, in contrast, are those statements that contradict, minimize, or deny the client's feelings. They tend to lower the client's self-esteem and limit full disclosure (Heineken, 1982). Examples of disconfirming responses are provided in Table 10-3.

Giving Feedback

Feedback is a message sent from the receiver back to the sender in response to a message or observed behavior. Feedback reassures the client that the nurse is attending to the details provided by the client and is directing full attention to his or her problems. Accurate feedback can provide a broader, more constructive framework in which to view difficult problems. Verbal feedback provides, through words, the receiver's understanding of the sender's message and personal reaction to it. Nonverbal feedback registers the other's reaction to the sender's message through facial expressions such as those that show surprise, boredom, or hostility. Other nonverbal feedback can occur through behaviors such as leaving a situation or shutting down verbally. When you receive nonverbal messages suggesting uncertainty, concern, or inattention, you should use a listening response to fully appreciate what the client is having trouble understanding.

Table 10-3 Disconfirming Responses That Block Communication

Category of Response	Explanation of Category	Examples
False reassurance	Using pseudocomforting phrases in an attempt to offer reassurance	"It will be okay." "Everything will work out."
Giving advice	Making a decision for a client; offering personal opinions; telling a client what to do (using phrases such as "ought to," "should")	"If I were you, I would . . ." "I feel you should . . ."
False inferences	Making an unsubstantiated assumption about what a client means; interpreting the client's behavior without asking for validation; jumping to conclusions	"What you really mean is you don't like your physician." "Subconsciously, you are blaming your husband for the accident."
Moralizing	Expressing your own values about what is right and wrong, especially on a topic that concerns the client	"Abortion is wrong." "It is wrong to refuse to have the operation."
Value judgments	Conveying your approval or disapproval about the client's behavior or about what the client has said using words such as "good," "bad," or "nice"	"I'm glad you decided to . . ." "That really wasn't a nice way to behave." "She's a good patient."
Social responses	Polite, superficial comments that do not focus on what the client is feeling or trying to say; use of clichés	"Isn't that nice?" "Hospital rules, you know?" "Just do what the doctor says." "It's a beautiful day."

Helpful feedback is *descriptive* in nature. By simply describing one's reaction to a behavior and avoiding any evaluation of it, the receiver is free to use or discard the feedback. The following nursing responses demonstrate two types of feedback to a diabetic client:

Nurse: I can see that you are having trouble with understanding the importance of rotating sites for your injection. Why don't you tell me a little bit more about what you think about it, and then we can go over some ideas that I might have.

Nurse: You should have asked questions about rotating sites if you didn't understand it.

With the first response, the nurse makes an observation about the lack of understanding and asks for more information about the nature of the client's noncompliance. The client does not feel judged. The second response places all of the responsibility for noncompliance on the client. The nurse assumes that it is lack of understanding that precipitated the noncompliance, which may or may not be true. The client is likely to respond negatively, so that the nurse's response does not further the goal of compliance.

Effective feedback is *specific* rather than general. Telling a client he or she is shy or easily intimidated is less helpful than saying, "I noticed when the anesthesiologist was in here that you didn't ask her any of the questions you had about your anesthesia tomorrow. Let's look at what you might want to know and how you could get the information you need." With this response, the nurse provides precise information about an observed behavior and offers a solution. The client is more likely to respond with validation or correction, and the nurse can provide specific guidance.

Timing of feedback is crucial for effectiveness. Generally, feedback given as soon as possible after a behavior is observed is most effective. Other factors (e.g., a client's readiness to hear feedback, privacy, and the availability of support from others) need to receive consideration. Feedback should be appropriate to the needs of the situation and the client. For example, a very obese mother in the hospital was feeding her newborn infant 4 ounces of formula every four hours. She was concerned that her child vomited a considerable amount of the undigested formula after each feeding. Initially, the nursing student gave the mother instructions about feeding the infant no more than 2 ounces at each feeding in the first few days of life, but the mother's behavior persisted, and so did that of her infant. The nursing student then began to assess the mother's experience by asking questions and discovered that the mother's mother had fed her 4 ounces right from birth with no problem. As a new mother, this woman felt that she should follow her mother's guidelines. By considering the mother's past experience, the nurse was able to provide the educative support that allowed the client to see her infant as a unique human being and to feel comfortable and confident in feeding him a smaller amount of formula.

Avoid generalities and pick your battles wisely. Not all feedback is equally relevant. Nor is it always equally accepted. The benchmark for deciding whether or not feedback is appropriate is to ask, "Does the feedback advance the goals of the relationship?" and "Does it consider the individualized needs of the client?" If the answer to these questions is "no," the feedback may be accurate but inappropriate for the moment.

Usable feedback is perceived as interest and concern. In contrast, providing feedback about behaviors over which the client has little control only increases the client's feelings of low self-esteem and leads to frustration. For example, telling a cardiac client in the hospital with his second heart attack, "You should have known better than to go back to work so soon" is feedback the client already knows and cannot use in the present situation. Similarly, it is not useful to tell a 350-pound client, "You should lose some weight." Most obese clients are acutely aware of their weight problem.

Effective feedback is *clear*, *honest*, and *reflective*. Feedback supported with realistic examples is believable, whereas most clients will perceive feedback without documentation to support it as lacking in credibility. To illustrate from your nursing school experience, if you were told that you would have no trouble passing any of the exams in nursing school, you would wonder whether the statement was true. However, if your instructor said, "On the basis of past performance and the fact that your score on the entrance exams was high, I think you should have little problem with our tests as long as you study," you probably would have more confidence in the statement.

Assumptions stated as facts are difficult for the client to respond to. When the nurse tells the client, "I know what you mean," without asking the client whether the communication or situation has the same meaning for both, the nurse may be completely wrong. Feedback is relevant only when it addresses the topics under discussion and does not go beyond the data presented by the client. Switching the topic or focus of the conversation in the middle of a stream of thought tends to bring communication to a dead halt or to leave it at a superficial level.

Case Example

A nursing student had a client with pancreatic cancer who was in considerable pain, so that even shaving required effort almost beyond his endurance. It was one of the first days of spring, and the weather was bright and sunny. The client said to the nurse, "I wish I were dead; there is nothing to live for." The nurse responded, "It's such a beautiful day. At least that should have some meaning."

In this example, the nurse's answer reflected personal anxiety rather than the client's statement of anguish. With a complete switch in topic to one that had no connection with the ongoing subject, the nurse was ignoring the client's emotional needs and focusing on her own. In tense situations, it is not hard to make such a communication error. The nurse who recognizes his or her own discomfort as the basis for making such a switch might apologize to the client, acknowledge the nurse's own discomfort, and refocus the conversation back onto the client's needs.

Feedback sometimes can have a surprise twist leading to an unexpected conclusion, as shown in the following example.

Case Example

It was Jovan's third birthday. There was a party of adults (his mother and father; his grandparents; his great-uncle and great-aunt; and me, his aunt), because Jovan was the only child in the family. While we were sitting and chatting, Jovan was running around and playing. At a moment of complete silence, Jovan's great-uncle asked him solemnly: "Jovan, who do you love the best?" Jovan replied, "Nobody!" Then Jovan ran to me and whispered in my ear: "You are Nobody!" (Majanovic-Shane, 1996, p. 11)

Asking for Validation

Seeking validation is a special form of asking for feedback from a client based on the principle that meanings are in people, not in the words themselves. Clients differ in how they respond to a message, and these variations influence the ways they understand and use language. Validation is a way of checking out the accuracy of the message received by the nurse or of confirming that the client received the message sent by the nurse in the manner intended. Asking the client, "How do you feel about what I just said?" or, "I'm curious what your thoughts are about what I just told you" gives the client an opportunity and the interpersonal space to express his or her feelings.

If the client does not have any response, the nurse might follow up the inquiry with a simple statement suggesting that the client can respond later. For example, the nurse might say, "Many people do find they have reactions or questions about [the issue] after they have had a chance to think about it, and I would be glad to discuss them with you if you find you have some later on." Taking the time to ask for validation helps clients feel that the nurse genuinely cares about their feelings and fosters clients' sense of being full participants in their care (Heineken, 1998). Simply asking clients whether they understand what was said is not an adequate method of validating message content. Nurses need to rephrase or verbally reflect back to the clients their perceptions of what they hear and observe for complete accuracy.

Case Example

Mr. Brown (to nurse taking his blood pressure): I can't stand that medicine. It doesn't sit well. *(He grimaces and holds his stomach.)*

Nurse: Are you saying that your medication for lowering your blood pressure upsets your stomach?

Mr. Brown: No, I just don't like the taste of it.

Sometimes validation occurs in the client's behavior rather than through words.

Case Example

After a diabetes diet instruction class, Mr. Oxam questions the nurse as to whether the potato served him at lunch was an equivalent exchange for the toast he ate at breakfast. The nurse knows that the client has a basic understanding of the concepts related to food exchanges in diabetic diets. However, Mr. Oxam may need further information and practice to make concrete applications in his life.

Validation is a useful strategy to reinforce information and to ask clients about changes in their behavior that enhance compliance or reasons for noncompliance. In the following example, validation takes the form of tactful inquiry coupled with observational data.

Case Example

Jane Smith has been coming to the clinic to lose weight. At first she was quite successful, losing 2 pounds per week. This week, however, she has gained 3 pounds. The nurse validates the change with the client by simultaneously seeking additional information:

Nurse: Jane, over the past six weeks you have lost 2 pounds per week, but this week you gained 3 pounds. There seems to be a problem here. Let's discuss what might have happened and how we can get back on track with your goal of losing weight.

In using this strategy and form of query, the nurse describes the observed client behavior, remains nonjudgmental in asking for the client's perceptions of the behavioral change, and reaffirms the original treatment goal. Table 10-4 presents a summary of the different therapeutic interviewing skills presented in this chapter as they apply to the phases of the nurse-client relationship.

Anticipatory Guidance

Providing **anticipatory guidance** to clients likely to experience anxiety or vulnerability in an unfamiliar situation can significantly calm a client and allow more effective participation in his or her own health care. For example, a simple statement such as, "You've never had this procedure before. Let me explain how it works" can significantly allay a client's worry (Keller & Baker, 2000).

Table 10-4 Interviewing and Relationship Skills

Phase	Stage	Purpose	Skills
ORIENTATION PHASE			
	Rapport and structuring with the client	To build a working alliance	Basic listening and attending; information giving
INTERVENTION PHASE			
Assessment, engagement, and beginning active	Gathering information, defining the problem, identifying strengths	To determine how the client views the problems and what client strengths might be used in their resolution	Basic listening and attending; open-ended questions, verbal cues and leads
Planning, active	Determining outcomes: What needs to happen to reduce the self-care demand? Where does the client want to go?	To find out how the client would like to be: How would things be if the problems were solved?	Attending and basic listening; influencing; feedback
Implementation, active	Explaining alternatives and options	To work toward resolution of the client's self-care needs	Influencing; feedback balanced by attending and listening
TERMINATION PHASE			
Evaluation	Generalization and transfer of learning	To enable changes in thoughts, feelings, and behaviors; to evaluate the effectiveness of the changes in modifying the self-care need	Influencing; feedback; validation

Box 10-5 ABCs of a Cognitive Behavioral Approach

A refers to the **Activating event,** which creates an image in the person's mind.

B refers to the **Beliefs** surrounding the activating event. Beliefs can also include personal rules or demands a person makes on himself, and fixed attitudes.

C refers to the **Consequences**, which include a person's decision and behaviors representing the person's beliefs.

Cognitive Behavioral Strategies

Cognitive behavioral communication strategies are helpful in assisting resistant clients challenge self-defeating thoughts that threaten their productive involvement in their care. For whatever reason, people tend to make mental notes of their negative assumptions and focus on their mistakes or limitations rather than their successes. Cognitive-behavioral therapy (CBT) helps people look more objectively at their negative assumptions and to treat their inflexible thinking as hypotheses to be tested rather than as absolute fact. Once the nurse helps clients identify negative thoughts, clients are taught to challenge the validity of those thoughts and/or to replace them with a positive thought using an ABC approach (Box 10-5). The positive thought represents reality-based facts that contradict the negative thought or thinking pattern. By stopping or interrupting the negative thinking pattern and replacing it with positive thoughts, people can change both their mood and their behavior.

Case Example

Jack Norris is receiving an antidepressant medication for depression symptoms associated with his cancer diagnosis. He tells the nurse he wants to stop the medication because it feels like a "crutch" to him, and he doesn't want to depend on medication "to make him feel better." When the nurse queries him about his other medications, he says, "That's different, those are medications I need. My antidepressant is just to make me feel better."

Challenging and correcting thinking errors associated with faulty rigid attitudes that can shortchange a person's quality of life is a goal of CBT strategies. Applying the CBT model outlined in Box 10-5, the *activating event* (A) is Jack's prescription for diagnosed depressive symptoms. His *belief* (B) that using psychotropic medication is a sign of weakness and that he should be able to get along as well without it gets in the way of his being able to resolve his depressive symptoms, which in turn probably affects his efforts to cope with his cancer. The *consequence* (C) of going off the medication is a return of his depressive symptoms. In this case example, how would you help the client receive the help he needs for his emotional well-being?

When Face-to-Face Communication Is Not Possible

Ideally, all communication should involve face-to-face contact. When this is not possible, nurses should consider how their words might be interpreted. The number of behavioral cues decrease as communication becomes removed from direct interpersonal contact. Telephone calls represent a more distant way of communicating, whereas written communication is the most detached form of interpersonal contact. Even so, a written message is better than nothing when the interests of the relationship warrant it. A note can provide closure for the nurse and comfort for the client. There may be times, for instance, when a nurse must end with a client because of a sudden transfer without being able to say good-bye, or when a client dies on an off shift and the nurse would like to share thoughts with the family. Writing a note at least acknowledges the meaning of the relationship. When writing notes, consider the relevance of indirect communication cues such as the formality of the message, typed versus handwritten notes, and the nature of closing remarks.

With the sophistication of technology, nurses often are in contact with their clients solely by phone or computer technology. Sharpe (2001) notes that the electronic nurse-client relationship begins when the nurse comes online or begins speaking to the client on the phone. From that point forward, the nurse needs to follow defined standards of nursing care. Telephone communication is an important link for clients. Periodic informational telephone calls enhance family involvement in the long-term care of clients. Over time, some families lose interest or find it too painful to continue active commitment. Interest and support from the nurse reminds families that they are not simply nonessential, interchangeable parts in their loved one's life; their input is important.

Present-day technology has increasingly allowed people to use the Internet as a communications medium to share experiences with others having a disease condition, to consult with experts about symptoms and treatment, and to learn up-to-date information about their condition.

For example, it is often the nurse who places the call to the family when a client is near death or has died. When the connection is made, the nurse first clarifies that the person on the other end of the line is the correct significant other. Addressing the client's significant other by name centers the person. It is important to explain who you are and the reason for your call at the outset. Do not give details at this time (Buckman, 1992). Keep communication simple while providing clear directives as to the next step. In calling a client's responsible significant other, the nurse might use the following format: "Hello, is this Mr. Peters? My name is Judy Cooper, and I am a nurse at Bayley Hospital. Your son has been in an accident and was admitted to our emergency room. I know this must be a terrible shock to you, and I think it is important for you to come to the hospital as soon as possible. Are you familiar with the route to the hospital?"

Learning the details of a serious injury or the death of a relative with the direct support of hospital staff is more comforting than imagining things. Nursing personnel can interpret baffling medical data and provide practical advice regarding the next steps in caring for the client and the family. If the client has died, the nurse represents an anchor and calming presence in the face of an overwhelming crisis (Jacob, 1991). Having an opportunity to see the client in death and being able to say good-bye in person are important to families, because these opportunities allow natural closure to an important relationship.

Nurses should make every effort to deliver bad news in person. If the family directly asks whether the client has died, the nurse needs to answer truthfully. Other details are better discussed once the family has arrived on the unit. If the family wants details over the telephone, the nurse can respond with a simple statement, "As soon as you come in, we will be able to tell you everything that happened and we can answer your questions. Our experience is that being able to directly answer your questions in person is best." If the family member insists, the nurse can give only the most basic information and should conclude the brief explanation with the request that it would be better to discuss the events in person.

SUMMARY

This chapter discusses basic therapeutic communication strategies the nurse can use with clients across clinical settings. Application of communication strategies should fit the purposes of the relationship and the communication style of the nurse. The nurse uses clarification to obtain more information when data are incomplete. Restatement is appropriate when a particular part of the content is needed. Paraphrasing addresses the content or cognitive component of the communication. Reflection is a technique used more specifically to get at the underlying feelings or the affective part of the message. Silence gives the client additional opportunity to clarify thoughts and to process information. Touch is a nonverbal strategy that underscores verbal understanding or is used in place of verbal expression when words fail as a response to the depth of feeling expressed by the client. Summarization integrates the content and feeling parts of the message by rephrasing two or more parts of the message.

Open-ended questions give the nurse the most information because they allow clients to express ideas and feelings as they are experiencing them. By contrast, focused and closed-ended questions narrow the range of possible answers. They are most appropriate in emergency clinical situations, when precise information is needed quickly.

The nurse uses verbal communication strategies that fit the client's communication patterns in terms of level, meaning, and language. Other strategies include use of metaphors, reframing, humor, confirming responses,

> **Ethical Dilemma ▪ *What Would You Do?***
> You have had a wonderful relationship with a client and client family. They have revealed issues they had never talked about before and raised questions that extended beyond the health care situation that they did not have the time to finish. You are about to end your rotation. What do you see as your ethical responsibility to this client and family?

feedback, and validation. Feedback provides a client with needed information.

REFERENCES

Alderman C: The art of listening, *Nurs Stand* 14(20):18–19, 2000.

Bandler R, Grindler J: *Reframing*, Palo Alto, CA, 1997, Science and Behavior Books.

Berne M, Lerner HM: Communicating with addicted women in labor, *MCN Am J Matern Child Nurs* 17(1):22–26, 1992.

Billings C: Therapeutic use of metaphors, *Issues Ment Health Nurs* 12:1–8, 1991.

Buckman R: *How to break bad news: a guide for health care professionals*, Baltimore, 1992, Johns Hopkins University Press.

Bush K: Do you really listen to patients? *RN* 64(3):35–37, 2001.

Cahill J: Patient participation: a review of the literature, *J Clin Nurs* 7(2):119–128, 1998.

Calero H: *The power of nonverbal communication: how you act is more important than what you say*, Aberdeen, WA, 2005, Silver Lake Publishing.

Caris-Verhallen W, Kerkstra A, Bensing J: Nonverbal behaviour in nurse-elderly patient communication, *J Adv Nurs* 29(4):808–818, 1999.

Caughan G, Long A: Communication is the essence of nursing care: 2: ethical foundations, *Br J Nurs* 9(15):979–984, 2000.

Chesla C: Reconciling technologic and family care in critical-care nursing, *Image J Nurs Sch* 28(3):199–203, 1996.

Coulehan JL, Platt FW, Egener B et al.: Let me see if I have this right...: words that help build empathy, *Ann Intern Med* 135:221–227, 2001.

Cousins N: Anatomy of an illness, *N Engl J Med* 295(26): 1458–1463, 1976.

Crellin K: Eleven ways to build rapport, *Nursing* 98:48–49, 1998.

Crowther DJ: Metacommunications: a missed opportunity, *J Psychosoc Nurs Ment Health Serv* 29(4):13–16, 1991.

Dowd S, Giger J, Davidhizar R: Use of Giger and Davidhizar's transcultural assessment model by health professions, *Int Nurs Rev* 45(4):119–122, 1998.

Duldt B: I-thou in nursing: research supporting Duldt's theory, *Perspect Psychiatr Care* 27(3):5–12, 1991.

Ekman P, Friesen W: *Unmasking the face: a guide to recognizing emotions from facial expressions*, Englewood Cliffs, NJ, 2003, Prentice Hall.

Gadow S: *Relational ethics: mutual construction of practical knowledge between nurse and client,* paper presented to the conference "Philosophy in the Nurse's World: Practical Knowledge in Nursing," Institute for Philosophical Nursing Research, University of Alberta, Banff, Canada, 1995.

Gorman M, Devine J: What to do when your patient uses illicit drugs, *Am J Nurs* 98(3):54, 1998.

Hall E: *The silent language*, New York, 1959, Doubleday.

Heineken J: Disconfirmation in dysfunctional communication, *Nurs Res* 31(4):211–213, 1982.

Heineken J: Patient silence is not necessarily client satisfaction: communication problems in home care nursing, *Home Healthc Nurse* 16(2):115–120, 1998.

Jacob S: Support for family caregivers in the community, *Fam Community Health* 14(1):16–21, 1991.

Johnson M: Self-disclosure: a variable in the nurse-client relationship, *J Psychiatr Nurs* 18(1):17–20, 1980.

Keller V, Baker L: Communicate with care, *RN* 63(1):32–33, 2000.

Kettunen T, Poskiparta M, Liimatainen L: Empowering counseling—a case study: nurse-patient encounter in a hospital, *Health Educ Res* 16:227–238, 2001.

Klagsbrun J: Listening and focusing: holistic health care tools for nurses, *Nurs Clin North Am* 36(1):115–130, 2001.

Knapp ML, Hall JA: *Nonverbal communication in human interaction*, Orlando, FL, 1997, Holt Rinehart, and Winston.

Lloyd M, Weiten W: *Psychology applied to modern life: adjustment in the 21st century*, Belmont, CA, 2006, Thompson Higher Education.

Lynch T, Anchor K: Use of humor in medical psychotherapy. In Anchor K, editor, *Handbook of medical psychotherapy*, Lewiston, NY, 1991, Hogrefe & Huber.

Majanovic-Shane A: Metaphor: a propositional comment and an invitation to intimacy, 1996; available online: www.speakeasy.org/~anamshane/intima.pdf; paper presented at the Second Conference for Sociocultural Research, Geneva, Switzerland, Sept 1996.

McGhee M: Humor. In Snyder M, editor, *Independent nursing functions*, New York, 1985, Wiley.

McGhee P: Rx laughter, *RN* 61(7):50–53, 1998.

Metcalf C: Stoma care: exploring the value of effective listening, *Br J Nurs* 7(6):311–315, 1998.

Miller C: Understanding the psychosocial challenges of older adulthood, *Imprint* 37(4):67–69, 1990.

Moustakas C: *Finding yourself: finding others*, Englewood Cliffs, NJ, 1974, Prentice Hall.

Myers S: Empathetic listening: reports on the experience of being heard, *Journal of Humanistic Psychology* 40(2): 148–174, 2000.

Nelson J: Personal touch, *Nurs Stand* 12(36):18, 1998.

Pearson A, Borbasi S, Walsh K: Practicing nursing therapeutically through acting as a skilled companion on the illness journey, *Adv Pract Nurs Q* 3(1):46–52, 1997.

Peplau H: Talking with patients, *Am J Nurs* 60(7):964–966, 1960.

Pesut D: The art, science, and techniques of reframing in psychiatric mental health nursing, *Issues Ment Health Nurs* 12(1):9–18, 1991.

Platt FW, Gaspar DL: "Tell me about yourself"; the patient-centered interview, *Ann Intern Med* 134(11):1079–1085, 2001.

Ramos MC: The nurse-patient relationship: theme and variation, *J Adv Nurs* 17(4):196–206, 1992.

Renwick P: Teaching the use of interpersonal skills, *Nurs Stand* 7(9):31–34, 1992.

Richmond V, McCroskey J: *Nonverbal behavior in inter-personal relations*, Englewood Cliffs, NJ, 2003, Prentice Hall.

Roberts J: *Tales and transformations: stories in families and family therapy*, New York, 1994, Norton.

Rowe J: Self-awareness: improving nurse-client interactions, *Nurs Stand* 14(8):37–40, 1999.

Ruesch J: *Therapeutic communication*, New York, 1961, Norton.

Sharpe C: *Telenursing: nursing practice in cyberspace*, Westport, CT, 2001, Auburn House.

SmithBattle L, Drake MA, Diekemper M: The responsive use of self in community health nursing practice, *Adv Nurs Sci* 20(2):75–89, 1997.

Stewart J, editor: *Bridges not walls*, ed 4, New York, 1986, Random House.

Straka DA: Are you listening—have you heard? *Adv Pract Nurs Q* 3(2):80–81, 1997.

Straneva JA: Therapeutic touch: coming of age, *Holist Nurs Pract* 14(3):1–13, 2000.

Talton C: Touch—of all kinds—is therapeutic, *RN* 58(2):61–64, 1995.

Umbreit A: Healing touch: applications in the acute care setting, *AACN Clin Issues* 11(1):105–119, 2000.

Weingarten K: A consideration of intimate and non-intimate interactions in therapy, *Fam Process* 31:45–59, 1992.

Chapter 11

Intercultural Communication

Elizabeth Arnold

OUTLINE

OBJECTIVES

At the end of the chapter, the reader will be able to:

1. Define culture and describe related terminology.
2. Discuss the concept of intercultural communication.
3. Apply the nursing process to the care of the culturally diverse client.
4. Discuss characteristics of selected cultures as they relate to the nurse-client relationship.

> *If we are to achieve a richer culture, rich in contrasting values, we must recognize the whole gamut of human potentialities, and so weave a less arbitrary social fabric, one in which each diverse human gift will find a fitting place.*
>
> (Mead, 1988)

Chapter 11 focuses on cultural aspects of communication in health care. When health care providers do not recognize cultural differences, those differences can pose fundamental barriers that interfere with health care treatment access and compliance, as currently practiced in the United States (Louie, 2001). The health care system in the United States adheres to western values, which may be in serious conflict with the value standards held by clients from a nonwestern cultural system. These differences can result in unsafe health care (Searight & Gafford, 2005).

Today we live in a culturally heterogeneous society. The U.S. Census Bureau (2000) reported that 35% of the people in the United States identified themselves as non-white: those who identified as African American or Black made up 13% of the population; Hispanic, 13%; Asian/Pacific Islander, 4.5%; and American Indian/

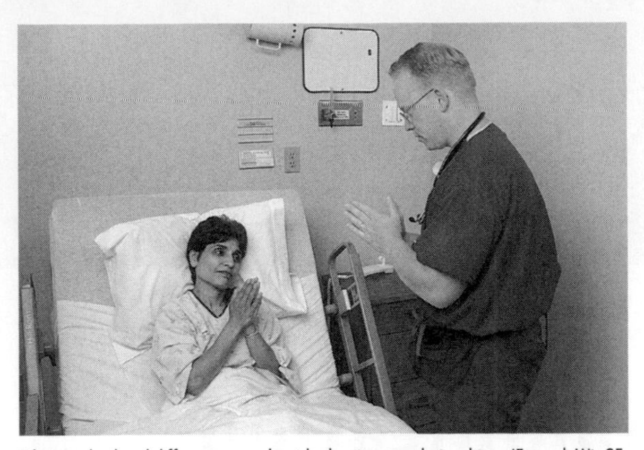

Ethnic and cultural differences need not be barriers to relationships. (From deWit SE: *Fundamental concepts and skills for nursing*, Philadelphia, 2001, Saunders.)

Alaskan native, 1.5%. A small but increasing number (2.5%) identified themselves as biethnic. Zoucha (2000) predicts that by mid-century, more than half of the U.S. population will be people currently classified as minorities. Canada reports a similar escalation in the number of immigrants, up 15% in the years preceding 1996, and three times the growth of the Canadian-born population (Canadian Nurses Association, 2000).

This demographic shift has significant implications for health and health care. Sutton (2000) notes, "People of diverse racial, ethnic, and cultural heritage suffer disproportionately from cardiovascular disease, diabetes, HIV/AIDS, and every form of cancer" (p. 58). Minority populations are often marginalized economically, occupationally, socially, and educationally, and these factors can adversely affect their access to early mainstream health care and compliance with treatment (James, 1997). Recognizing these disparities, *Healthy People 2010* identified "reducing health disparities" as an overarching goal of the nation's preventive health care agenda. To improve successful health care for every citizen, nurses must address cultural issues that are not always considered as part of a nursing intervention.

Learning about general cultural variations is essential to effectively communicating with ethnically diverse clients. Culture often plays a significant role in determining which illnesses and disorders are recognized as legitimate, which roles clients are expected to assume in their health care, and who becomes the culturally assigned expert in promoting, maintaining, and restoring health. Without a clear understanding of culturally acceptable behaviors during illness or disability, nurses may respond inappropriately.

BASIC CONCEPTS

Masters (2005) defines **culture** as a term used to explain "the norms of behavior and shared values among a particular group of people" (p. 157). These norms or standards of behavior develop from the customs, beliefs, and social institutions associated with different ethnic, racial, religious, and social groups (Office of Minority Health [OMH], 2001).

Cultural understandings become critical elements in effective provision of quality care. Our cultural beliefs influence feelings, attitudes, and behaviors; how we relate to others; our views of what is right and wrong; perceptions of health, illness, and death; appropriate rituals; and preferred methods of treatment. As Shweder (1991) notes, "When people live in the world differently, it may be that they live in different worlds" (p. 23). In trying to understand how individuals from another culture perceive themselves within the context of their environment, nurses need to suspend judgment, empathize, and try to understand the way that particular culture views the world. Culturally appropriate nursing interventions that consider the unique and individualized cultural history of an individual client and family and integrate this knowledge with the specific health needs and problem issues clients, families, and others present are more likely to be accepted.

Leininger's (1995) cultural nursing model provides a framework for understanding the cultural dimensions of nursing care (Figure 11-1). Culture is a community concept, grounding a person's life experience and connecting each individual with the larger community. Included in cultural expression are specific normative rules about daily living, role expectations, personal patterns of response, and child-rearing practices (Lipson, 1996). Culture provides the community with its strength and vitality, connecting each individual with the larger community. Family and cultural ties are a significant source of comfort and support to people in times of stress and illness. Lack of the social support that culture provides can foster a sense of alienation and helplessness.

Children learn the psychosocial aspects of their culture first from observing the behavior of their parents, and then from their experiences of peers, school, church,

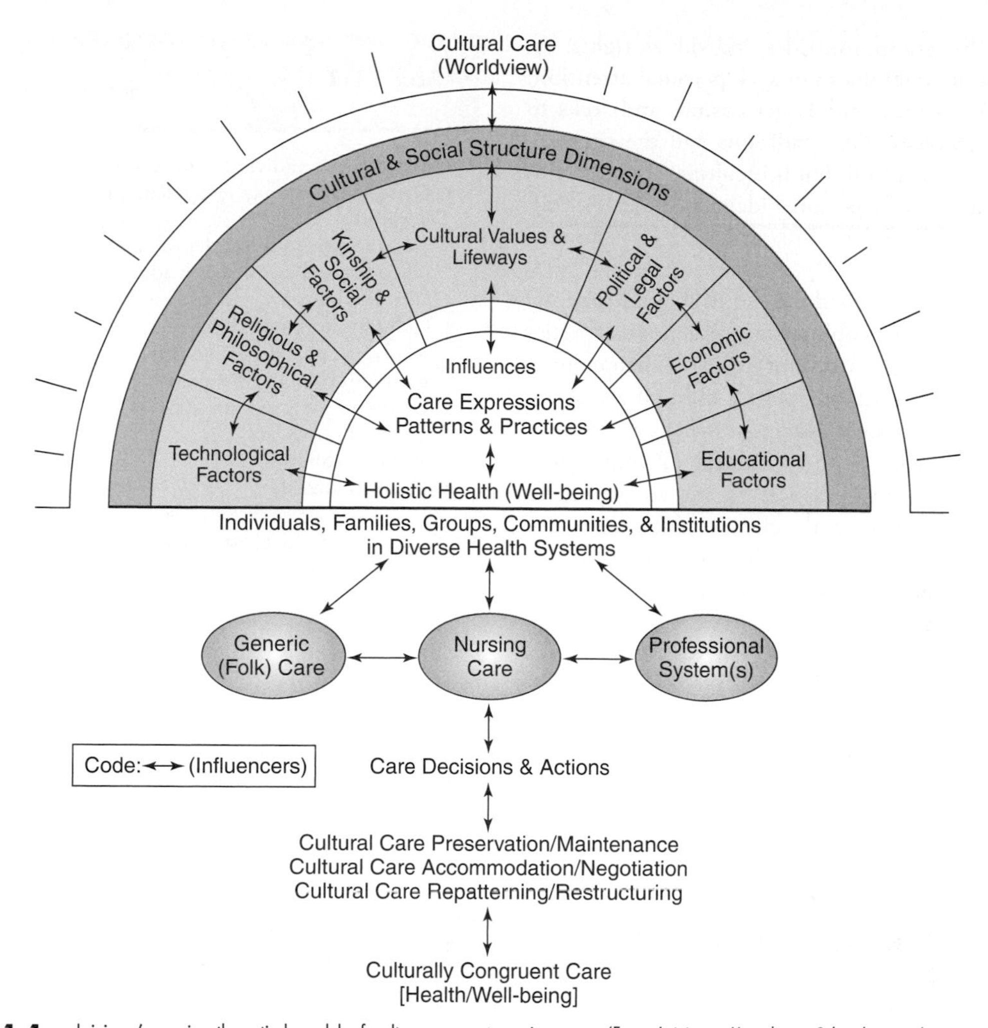

Figure 11-1 • Leininger's sunrise theoretical model of culture-congruent nursing care. (From Leininger M, editor: *Cultural care diversity and universality: a theory of nursing*, Sudbury, MA, 1991, Jones and Bartlett. Reprinted with permission.)

and the larger community. The latter may modify original perceptions, resulting in a counterculture for an individual. The psychosocial aspects of culture can create dilemmas for new immigrants who may have trouble integrating the beliefs of two ideologically different value systems.

The language of illness, its values, and its metaphors vary significantly from culture to culture. This is particularly true in western and eastern cultural beliefs about health and illness. Western culture, which dominates the health care system in North America, favors a more individualistic approach. Eastern cultures use a collectivistic social model. Davis (1999) points out that 70% of all cultures are supportive of a collectivistic societal model in which health care decisions are group decisions.

Case Example

Mohan is an Asian nursing student trying to cope with American society's cultural values of self-reliance and individualism. In contrast with his American student peers, Mohan seems nonaggressive and does not always act in his own best interest. He is guarded, by American standards, in what he reveals about himself, and it's hard to tell what he really needs or wants. Viewed from an Asian perspective, Mohan's behavior is not at all unusual. He comes from a collectivistic society in which

loyalty to the group overrides individual rights. In India, the individual does not seek personal attention; each person is part of the larger cosmos and seeks to blend harmoniously with traditions and the community. Achievements count, but it is culturally incorrect to view them as part of a personal identity (Kakar, 1991).

The ethical aspect of culture lies in the fundamental human beliefs, rights, obligations, and responsibilities that individuals hold as truth for people of their culture. Ludwick and Silva (2000) define cultural values as "enduring ideals or belief systems to which a person or society is committed" (p. 1). Ethical dilemmas arise when moral and health practices are not congruent. In both large and small ways, the client's value system may differ significantly from that of the nurse in health care situations. Respectful care, mandated in recently published cultural standards, requires the consideration of "the values, preferences, and expressed needs of the patient/consumer . . . provided in a manner compatible with their cultural health beliefs and practices and preferred language" (OMH, 2001, p. 5).

Culture affects all aspects of health care. Searight and Gafford (2005) identify the points of cultural diversity affecting health care (Box 11-1).

Box 11-1 Points of Cultural Diversity in Health Care

- Emphasis on individualism versus collectivism
- Definition of family (extended, nuclear, nonblood kinship)
- Common views of gender roles, child-rearing practices, and care of older adults
- Views of marriage and relationships
- Communication patterns (direct versus indirect; relative emphasis on nonverbal communication; meanings of nonverbal gestures)
- Common religious and spiritual-belief systems
- Views of physicians
- Views of suffering
- Views of afterlife

From Searight H, Gafford J: Cultural diversity at the end of life: issues and guidelines for family physicians, *Am Fam Physician* 71:3, 2005.

Exercise 11-1 is designed to help you appreciate the meaning of culture.

Cultural Competence

Cultural competence is defined as "a set of cultural behaviors and attitudes integrated into the practice methods of a system, agency, or its professionals, that enables them

Exercise 11-1 Meaning of Culture

Purpose: To help students appreciate the many dimensions of culture.

Procedure:

Often, the attitudes, feelings, and understandings people have about a culture are found in the words they associate with that culture.

1. Think about the word "culture" and write down all of the words and phrases that you can think of in response to the word. There are no right or wrong answers.
2. Assign a negative sign (−) to the words you perceive might have a negative value. Assign a positive sign (+) to the words you perceive might have a positive value. Do not assign any signs to words you perceive as being without a value.
3. Share your results with the other members of your class group.

Discussion:

1. Were you surprised at any of the words that popped into your mind?
2. What does your list tell you about your attitudes and feelings about culture?
3. In what ways were your words and phrases similar to or different from those of your classmates?
4. In what way did your answers reflect your own cultural background?
5. How could you use the information you gained from this exercise to provide culturally congruent care?

to work effectively in cross cultural situations" (Sutton, 2000, p. 58). Cultural competence in health care includes a substantive knowledge base of cultural values held by a particular cultural group *and* the ability to adapt individualized clinical nursing skills to fit the cultural context of each client in the nurse-client relationship. The American Academy of Nursing (1995) also includes issues of marginalization and vulnerability in society related to race, gender, and sexual orientation. Cultural competence in health care requires the nurse to understand and respond effectively to the rich values, beliefs, customs, and symbols of people of color that present themselves in all phases of health care delivery. It also requires culturally appropriate ways of speaking to clients and knowledge of culturally congruent ways to manage intercultural health care treatment (Smith, 1998).

Cultural competence starts with self-awareness. Everyone has a "cultural self," which provides an important context for understanding the personal self. To be culturally competent requires careful reflection on one's own values, attitudes, and perspectives, as well as knowledge of another's culture (Duffy, 2001; Leininger, 2000; Leonard & Plotnikoff, 2000). Exercise 11-2 provides an opportunity for you to reflect on your own cultural beliefs, values, and behaviors as a way of understanding the influence of culture in shaping your health care behaviors.

Cultural Terminology

Multiculturalism

Multiculturalism describes a heterogeneous society in which several diverse cultural worldviews can coexist with some general ("etic") characteristics shared by all cultural groups, and some ("emic") perspectives that are unique to a particular group. Leininger (2000) notes that the "emic perspective focuses on the local, indigenous, and insider's culture; the etic perspective focuses on the outsider's world and, especially, professional views" (p. 312).

Exercise 11-2 Cultural Self-Assessment

Purpose: To help students develop awareness of their own culture.

Procedure:

Think about your own culture and answer the following questions. Be as honest as you can; this will help you to be open and honest toward culturally diverse clients. There are no right or wrong answers.

1. Where did my family originate?
2. What do I attach importance to that could be considered a cultural value?
3. What do I believe about the gender roles of men and women? Are my beliefs different or consistent with those of my parents?
4. How much physical distance do I need in social interactions?
5. Who are the decision makers in my family, and whom do I look to for guidance in important matters?
6. What are my definitions of health and well-being?
7. If I needed health care, how would I respond to this need and what would be my expectations?
8. In a health care situation, what would be the role of my family?
9. In a health care situation, how important would religion be, and what would I need for spiritual comfort?

Discussion:

1. Share your observations with your classmates.
2. How difficult was it for you to really identify some of the behaviors and expectations that are part of your cultural self?
3. Were you surprised with any of your answers? If so, in what ways?
4. What did you learn about culture from hearing stories of other students? In what ways were their stories the same or different from your cultural story?
5. How can you use this exercise in communicating with culturally diverse clients?

Exercise 11-3 Recognizing Components of Group Culture

Purpose: To help students appreciate the multicultural components of everyday life.

Procedure:
1. Each student is to attend some type of group or community activity.
2. Observe as many behaviors, norms, rules, customs of dress, membership commonalities, roles, and so on as possible.
3. Write a descriptive summary of the group you observed that portrays an image of the group to others. Include what you have learned about the culture of this group and what you might be careful about in order to communicate effectively in this group.

Discussion:
1. Each student will share observations with the group and address the cultural components that are unique to this group.
2. Discuss how different cultural components impact on communication.
3. How should the nurse incorporate cultural awareness into communication?

Through an understanding of the contrasts between the emic and etic views of the same health care situation, the nurse is able to tailor communication in ways that respect these differences and enhance collaboration to find a common communication meeting ground. A multicultural perspective acknowledges the wide range of cultural groups as having equal value and very distinct characteristics that need to live with and understand each other (Pederson, 1991). In today's global social environment, with its rapidly changing demographics and increasingly interdependent world economy, the term *multiculturalism* fits most community definitions of culture. Exercise 11-3 examines the concept of multiculturalism through the lens of group study.

Acculturation

Acculturation is a term used to describe a socialization process in which a person from a different cultural group learns the cultural behavior norms of the dominant culture and begins to adopt its behaviors and language patterns. When people leave their country of origin, they leave behind a known social system, a familiar language, and cultural understandings that may have significantly less value in their new environment. Employment opportunities and housing options may be nonexistent or difficult to achieve for minority groups. For example, skilled physicians from other countries often have such strong hurdles to overcome to be similarly licensed in the United States that they choose different occupations to survive financially.

Successful acculturation requires an integrated sense of self that accepts the new culture while preserving significant cultural values as valid parts of the personal self. Socioeconomic status and education affect the level of acculturation, because those individuals with higher levels of either have more support options available to them.

Acculturation is a reciprocal socialization process in which both cultures influence each other to varying degrees through normal, ongoing exposure (Garrett & Herring, 2001). One of the best ways to learn about another culture is to spend time with people from that culture with an open mind and a sincere desire to understand their perspective.

Physical acculturation usually takes place before emotional acculturation. The concept of acculturation helps explain a significant portion of health and lifestyle behaviors. For example, cultural beliefs about etiology, ideal treatment, and prevention of illness may affect the utilization of health services.

A certain level of acculturation into the social structure of the majority group is essential for survival, even while respecting and accommodating important values from the original culture whenever possible. For example, the Vietnamese culture believes that a sick person will get well faster if the entire family is present to offer support (Davis, 2000). This practice conflicts with current protocols in many hospitals, which only allow two

Exercise 11-4 Family Culture Experiences

Purpose: To help students appreciate how culture is learned.

Procedure:

1. Identify and describe one family custom or tradition. It can relate to special family foods, a holiday custom, a child-rearing practice, or any other special tradition.
2. Describe the custom or tradition in detail.
3. Talk with a family member about how this family tradition originated in your family.
4. Discuss how this custom or tradition has changed over time.
5. Describe how this family tradition has affected your family functioning.

Discussion:

1. Share your family tradition with your classmates.
2. As a class, discuss how differences in family culture can influence health.
3. Discuss how knowledge of family customs can influence communication and health care promotion.

visitors at a time. With understanding and creativity, usually some adjustment can be made that recognizes and respects these cultural differences. Exercise 11-4 demonstrates how people learn cultural patterns.

Assimilation

A related concept is that of **assimilation**, a term used to describe a person's adoption of common behaviors, customs, values, and language of the dominant or mainstream culture, such that the political or ethnic identification with the original culture virtually disappears. The process of assimilation usually occurs over several generations, with each succeeding generation achieving greater integration with the dominant culture. For example, American-born, third-generation ethnic children may have little observable knowledge of their traditional culture and language or allegiance to their original heritage (Hernandez, 1995). At the same time, Bacallao and Smokowski (2005) suggest that we all carry vestiges of cultural traditions with us, without our awareness. Bicultural approaches that recognize a person as moving between the two cultures is likely to prove more effective.

Subculture

Subculture is defined as an ethnic, regional, economic, religious, or social group of people within the dominant culture who have adopted a cultural lifestyle different from that of the mainstream population. Dress, loyalty to a leader or cause, and distinctive differences in philosophy and behavior generally distinguish members of a subculture. Examples of subcultures in North America include the Amish, Jehovah's Witnesses, and the homeless. Jandt (2003) prefers the term "co-culture," which avoids the implication that one culture is superior to another.

Cultural Diversity

Cultural diversity is a term used to describe variations among cultural groups. Some physical and behavioral differences are obvious to most people. Interestingly, many people equate race and physical characteristics with ethnicity, despite the fact that culture is a social phenomenon, whereas race and physical characteristics are biological. Consider for example, people from Caribbean Islands and those from Africa both being called African Americans, despite the distinct difference in their heritage and resultant ethnic identities.

Spence (2001) also observed that with people from a different culture, "language, skin color, dress, and gestures, for example, are noticed and not passed over as they might be in encounters with people from one's own culture" (p. 102). Less obvious, but important, differences that involve spiritual, religious, political, social, or communal beliefs and values need further exploration. You also will need to consider a person's educational and socioeconomic background, length of residency in the United States, legal immigration status, age, gender, and whether the individual is exposed to people in the dominant culture or is living in an ethnic community. Cultural diversity can exist within the same community or a work group. Differences in cultural role expectations for the physician, social

Exercise 11-5 **Diversity in the Nursing Profession**

Purpose: To help students learn about the experience of nurses from a different ethnic group.

Procedure:

1. Each student will interview a registered nurse from an ethnic minority group different from their own ethnic origin.
2. The following questions should be asked:
   a. In what ways was your educational experience more difficult or easier as a minority student?
   b. What do you see as the barriers for minority nurses in our profession?
   c. What do you see as the opportunities for minority nurses in our profession?
   d. What do you view as the value of increasing diversity in the nursing profession for health care?
   e. What do you think we can do as a profession and personally to increase diversity in nursing?
3. Write a one- to two-page narrative report about your findings to be presented in a follow-up class.

Discussion:

1. What were the common themes that seemed to be present across narratives?
2. How do professional nurses view diversity, and how did doing this exercise influence your thinking about diversity?
3. Did you find any of the answers to the interview questions disturbing or surprising?
4. How could you use this exercise in becoming culturally competent?

worker, ward clerk, nurse, and physical therapist can affect decision making and task allocation in health care settings. Exercise 11-5 introduces you to the influence of culture on professional roles.

People tend to assume that common cultural values are shared among all members of a particular racial, ethnic, or religious group. In reality, significant differences usually exist. While recognition of diversity *between* cultures is a critical element in delivery of culturally competent care, the nurse must also recognize there can be significant diversity *within* a culture. Bromwich (1992) notes, for example, that artists, regardless of their ethnic heritage or gender, have more in common with other artists than they do with other members of their own cultural group.

In health care, cultural diversity in health priorities, meaning of the illness, treatment options, learning styles, power differentials, and decision making can become significant barriers to treatment if not recognized and respected. On the other hand, certain emotions are universal experiences; for example, Cochran (1998) observes that "tears have no color" (p. 53). Sadness over loss, illness, and difficult changes are universal experiences.

Cultural Relativism

Cultural relativism is a concept that proposes that each culture or ethnic group should be evaluated on the basis of its *own* values and norms of behavior, and not against the values and behavioral standards of another culture or ethnic group. This does not mean that all cultural practices are equally valid or appropriate, only that the nurse should respect the client's adherence to them as being appropriate to their culture. The concept of cultural relativism implies that sometimes cultural practices that seem bizarre to people outside the culture make perfect sense when they are evaluated within their own cultural context (Aroian & Faville, 2005).

Cultural relativism refers to the belief that cultures are neither inferior nor superior to one another, and that all cultures are equally worthy of respect. This concept allows nurses to care for clients with significantly different values without judging their behavior; allows them to transcend their own racial, ethnic, gender, cultural, and sociopolitical beliefs; and enables them to identify with people throughout the world and at all levels of human need.

Ethnicity

Ethnicity is defined as a personal awareness of certain symbolic elements that bind people together in a social context. The word "ethnic" derives from the Greek word *ethnos*, meaning "people." An **ethnic group** is a social grouping of people who share a common racial, geographic, religious, or historical culture. It is a sociopolitical construct that differs from race and the genetic characteristics of a population (Ford & Kelly, 2005). In contrast to culture, which does not always involve a conscious awareness of norms and symbols, ethnicity is a *chosen* awareness that reflects commitment to a cultural identity. In the United States, common ethnic groups include African-American, Native American, Hispanic, Asian, Indian, Jewish, Irish, Italian, Muslim, and Amish groups.

Holding a particular ethnic identity is not always a positive experience. The maltreatment of Native Americans, the enslavement of African Americans, the harassment and killing of six million Jews in World War II, the persecution of the Roma (Gypsies), the massacre of Croatians in Europe, the horror of the September 11, 2001, bombings in New York and Washington, D.C., and the brutal terrorism occurring concurrently with war create cultural and personal distrust of the "other" that spills over into health care.

Ethnicity is not the same as race, although people of color are sometimes treated as if the two were the same. Ethnicity is a social concept; race is a biological concept. Race refers to differences in external biological characteristics (e.g., color of the skin, facial features, and hair texture). People may share the same skin color but a vastly different ethnic experience.

Ethnocentrism

Ethnocentrism refers to a belief that one's own culture is superior to others. Lewis (2000) suggests that "ethnocentrism blinds us to the salient features of our own cultural makeup, while making us see other cultures as deviations from the correct" (p. 441). Taking pride in one's culture is appropriate, but when a person fails to respect the pride that people from a different culture take in their ethnic identity, it is easy to develop stereotypes; this can be highly destructive to a relationship. Duffy (2001) contends, "Stereotyping homogenizes a group of people based on unique characteristics" (p. 489). The problem with this way of thinking is that the identified characteristics may or may not be valid for either the group as a whole or individuals within it. Carried to an extreme, ethnocentrism fosters the belief that one culture has the right to impose the tenets of its culture onto another, leading to discrimination, property confiscation, violence, and terror. The deadly consequences of ethnocentrism were apparent in the Nazi persecution of the Jews during Hitler's regime in the name of the Aryan race, ongoing ethnic wars in the Middle East, and most recently in the September 11 bombings in the United States.

A variation of ethnocentrism (i.e., the belief that certain individuals or groups of people are inferior) happens on a smaller scale with the physically or mentally disabled, the urban poor, the homeless, persons with AIDS, and certain minority groups. Age, race, and disability discrimination are subtle forms of ethnocentrism that add to the feelings of devaluation and inferiority experienced even by members of a dominant culture. Canales and Howers (2001) suggest that understanding of diversity applies to anyone who is different, and that nurses need to broaden their conceptualization of cultural competence to include those who represent diversity for reasons other than cultural difference.

Case Example

"I knew a man who had lost the use of both eyes. He was called a 'blind man.' He could also be called an expert typist, a conscientious worker, a good student, a careful listener, and a man who wanted a job. But he couldn't get a job in the department store order room where employees sat and typed orders, which came over the phone. The personnel man was impatient to get the interview over. 'But you are a blind man,' he kept saying, and one could almost feel his silent assumption that somehow the incapability in one aspect made the man incapable in every other. So blinded by the label was the interviewer that he could not be persuaded to look beyond it." (Lee, quoted in Allport, 1982)

When the stereotyped label corresponds to undesirable personal traits in the eyes of the dominant culture—whether the deviation from the norm has a cultural, physical, or psychological origin—the person is at a distinct disadvantage because of the implied negative value judgments. Recognizing implied value judgments and taking the time to be sensitive to the subtle interpretations of value-laden ethnic terms in conversation can prevent misunderstanding and hurt feelings. Allport (1982) suggests using ethnic labels as adjectives rather than nouns. Thus the nurse would speak of the "person of color" rather than "the African American." This thoughtfulness seems particularly important when one considers that a person of color from Jamaica, for example, may

Exercise 11-6 Cultural Self-Assessment

Purpose: To help students examine stereotypes and their impact on communication and relationships.

Procedure:

The first part of this exercise should be written outside of class, anonymously, to encourage honest answers. The following list represents some of the groups in our society that carry familiar value-laden stereotypes:

African Americans	Homosexuals	People with sensory deficits
AIDS victims	Mentally ill persons	Teenage mothers
Asian Americans	Migrant workers	Homeless people
Elderly adults	Native Americans	
Hispanics	People on welfare	

1. Write down the first three words or phrases that come into your mind regarding each of these groups.
2. Make a grid to show stereotypes. Follow each cultural group with three columns listing positive, neutral, and negative connotations.
3. As a class group, take the collected words and phrases and decide whether they represent one or more culturally specific connotations. Place each word or phrase under the appropriate column for each group. Use an "X" to indicate repetitive words or phrases.

Discussion:

For each cultural group, consider the following:

1. Why do you think people believe that this cultural group possesses these characteristics?
2. What were the common themes of these groups? Did certain groups have more negative than positive responses? If so, how would you account for this?
3. In what ways did this exercise help you to think about your own cultural socialization process?
4. Did this exercise cause you to question any of your own assumptions about culturally different values?
5. From your view, what implications do these stereotypes hold for providing appropriate nursing care?
6. How can you use this exercise in your future care of culturally different populations?

Modified from Eliason M, Macy N: A classroom activity to introduce cultural diversity, *Nurse Educ* 17(3):32-35, 1992.

have no ancestral heritage from Africa, yet would be classified as African-American in our culture.

To provide quality care for clients from different cultures, the nurse must make a conscious effort to see each client as a unique individual with many complex characteristics, some of which happen to be different from those of the majority norm (Doswell & Erlen, 1998). Exercise 11-6 makes it easier to see the prevalence of stereotypes. Exposure to different cultures allows for a different perception of cultural differences and the universality of humanness.

Case Example

Mara has a stereotyped homogeneous view of Hispanic people. Her mother distrusts Hispanic people and has told her that Hispanic people are low-class and lack initiative. Without having had much exposure to Hispanic people, Mara's ideas reflect her mother's teaching and bear very little resemblance to reality. Her college roommate is Hispanic. As the roommates exchange experiences, they develop a shared history that is quite different from Mara's stereotype. Mara finds that her roommate is not so different from herself. Her roommate comes from a socioeconomic background similar to her own and is one of the best students in the class. Mara's knowledge of and attitude toward Hispanic people changes dramatically as a result of her firsthand experience with a person from a different culture.

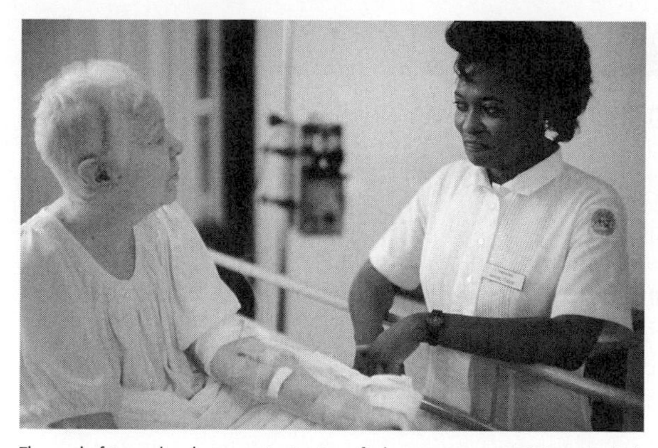

The goal of intercultural communication is to find a common ground through which people from different cultures can connect on many different levels with each other. (Courtesy University of Maryland School of Nursing.)

Intercultural Communication

Intercultural communication is defined as that which takes place between persons or groups from different cultures. Samovar, Porter, and McDaniel (2005) identify five components of culture relevant to the study of intercultural communication:

1. Perceptual elements
2. Patterns of cognition
3. Verbal behaviors
4. Nonverbal behaviors
5. The influence of context

Effectiveness as an intercultural communicator is dependent on two interactive experiences: developing a knowledge of other people and their cultures, and discovering more about yourself in the process of exposure to a different culture, which facilitates acceptance and appreciation of diversity in others (Jandt, 2003).

Different languages create and express different personal realities. The function of intercultural communication, regardless of the specific culture, is to direct actions, interpret the meaning of events and situations, connect past experiences with the present through imagination, and establish and maintain relationships with people (Nance, 1995).

Culture, expressed through language symbols, shapes the personalized meaning and experience of illness and health. It also influences methods of healing and the client's response to care (Purnell & Paulanka, 2005). People name objects, situations, events, qualities, and feelings in their own language symbols. Language helps people understand the motivations of others and makes their motivations known to others (Scott, 1991). People tell each other what is socially acceptable behavior and reinforce adaptive behavior. Effective intercultural communication helps people understand the implications of perceived differences in social behaviors.

Case Example

Benjamin Franklin's Comments on Native Americans

"Savages we call them, because their Manners differ from ours, which we think the Perfection of Civility; they think the same of theirs. Perhaps if we could examine the Manners of Different Nations with Impartiality, we should find no People so rude, as to be without any Rules of Politeness; nor any so polite, as not to have some Remains of Rudeness." (Benjamin Franklin, quoted in Jandt, 2003, p. 76)

Exercise 11-7 provides an opportunity to consider the implications of language barriers.

Linguistic rules about language structure and gender language use vary among cultures. Consider these two statements: "The family bears most of the responsibility for health care," and "The family has borne most of the responsibility for health care." This change from present to past tense results in a different form of the word (bears/has borne), which can confuse clients from other cultures. Some words in one culture have no translatable meaning in another culture. Thus nurses need to use precise language, be aware of linguistic language differences, and avoid slang and clichés with clients who display limited English skills. Watching word variations, asking the right questions, providing verbal cues, and allowing more time for clients with limited language skills to answer conveys interest and respect while also reducing anxiety.

Case Example

A nursing student from the Philippines said she was thoroughly confused by her instructor's slang expression, "I want to touch base with you." The student did not know how to respond because her literal translation of the sentence did not express its meaning to her. Had the instructor said, "I would like to talk with you," the student would have known how to respond.

Exercise 11-7 Understanding Language Barriers

Purpose: To help students understand the role of language barriers.

Procedure:

Situation 1
Lee Singh is a 24-year-old Korean patient who speaks no English. She was admitted to the maternity unit and has just delivered her first child, a 9-pound infant. It was a difficult labor because the infant was so big. The initial objectives of the health care providers are to help the client understand what is happening to her and to help her become comfortable with her baby.

Situation 2
Jose Perot is a 30-year-old Hispanic male who was admitted to the emergency department with multiple injuries after a car accident. His family has been notified, but the nurse is not sure they understand what has happened. They have just arrived in the emergency room.

1. Break up into groups of four or five students. Each group acts as a unit. The groups role-play Situation 1 and reverse roles for Situation 2.
2. The client group should completely substitute made-up words that only they understand for the words they would normally use to communicate in this situation. The made-up words should have the same meaning to all members of the client group.
3. The health provider group must figure out creative ways to understand and communicate with the client group.

Discussion:
1. In what ways was it different being the client and being the health provider group?
2. What was the hardest part of this exercise?
3. In what ways did this exercise help you understand the frustrations of being unable to communicate?

The concept of intercultural communication takes into account not only differences in words and dialects but also paralanguage differences such as voice volume, vocal tone, emphasis points and inflections, pronunciation, and national or regional accents. For example, in some cultures, a difference in vocal tone signals a distinct difference in the meaning of emotions such as sadness, anger, or sincerity. Intercultural communication also includes nonverbal differences in use of eye contact, flexibility of facial expression, gestures, use of touch, space needs for conversation, timing, and body posture (Purnell, 2000).

The goal of intercultural communication in the nurse-client relationship is to find a common ground through which people from different cultures can connect with each other on many different levels and in a meaningful way. Connections may be spontaneous or planned.

Case Example

"There weren't many Filipino nurses [in that hospital] and a lot of them were Caucasian and I remember this Black nurse...who was very, very nice. I think it was because she is not a Caucasian and she is able to feel with me. She probably sympathized with me who like her is from a different culture and had to move to Canada." (Pasco, Morse, & Olson, 2004, p. 243)

Culturally competent nurses integrate knowledge of their client's culture into all aspects of their communication, but particularly into their health teaching (Lester, 1998). More than simple language translation, the cultural meanings of illness, behaviors, and symptom expressions are important factors to consider, as are traditional approaches to treatments and family and decision-making styles. Sometimes the cultural differences are apparent, involving distinctive variations in diet and behavioral styles. A single gesture, for example, may have radically different meanings in different cultures. A thumbs-up gesture in America has a positive connotation, whereas in certain Middle Eastern cultures, it has an obscene meaning.

Although individual expression of culture and language differs significantly, basic human forms of interaction exist across culture and convey universal meaning. Nurses can sometimes transcend cultural differences with caring behaviors that are universally understood.

Case Example

A Chinese first-time mother, tense and afraid as she entered the transition phase of labor, spoke no English. Her husband spoke very little, and saw birthing as women's work. Callister (2001) relates, "The nurse could feel palpable tension that filled the room. The nurse could not speak Chinese either, but she tried to convey a sense of caring, touching the woman, speaking softly, modeling supportive behavior for her husband and helping her to relax as much as possible. The atmosphere in the room changed considerably with the calm competence and quiet demeanor of the nurse. Following the birth…the father conveyed to her how grateful he was that she spoke Chinese. She tactfully said, 'Thank you, but I don't speak Chinese.' He looked at her in amazement and said with conviction, 'You spoke Chinese.' The language of the heart transcends verbal communication." (p. 212)

Developing an Evidence-Based Practice

McElmurry B, Park C, Buseh A: The nurse-community health advocate team for urban immigrant primary health care, *J Nurs Scholarsh* 35(3):275-280, 2003.

This descriptive study was designed to describe an urban outreach health program for Latino immigrants, using a professional nurse and community advocate teamed together in providing health care delivery. Convenience samples of participants, staff, and other sources were used to describe the program and its effects in the Latino community.

Results: Findings indicated that pairing nurses with community health advocates greatly enhanced the project team's ability to provide preventive care in the Latino community. The combined resources provided culturally sensitive care to Latino immigrants and enabled them to seek and obtain appropriate health care.

Application to Your Clinical Practice: As professionals working in an increasingly multicultural society, nurses need to develop innovative ways to reach out to immigrants with limited knowledge and limited ways to access the health care system. What steps would you need to take as an individual nurse to encourage a stronger connection between culturally sensitive nursing care and the needs of immigrant populations?

APPLICATIONS

The first step in addressing a client's communication needs is developing self-awareness of your own cultural values and biases. The second step is developing a good understanding of the client's cultural values, health beliefs, and practices (Gravely, 2001). Later in the chapter, some generalizations about major cultural groups in North America are offered for discussion. This does not mean that everyone from a certain culture possesses the described characteristics. They are simply common patterns of beliefs and behaviors associated with a cultural group. Galanti (2004) presents the difference between stereotyping and providing common characteristics associated with a particular cultural group:

> The difference between a stereotype and generalization lies not in the content, but in the usage of the information. An example is the assumption that Mexicans have large families. If I meet Rosa, a Mexican woman, and I say to myself, 'Rosa is Mexican; she must have a large family,' I am stereotyping her. But if I think Mexicans often have large families and wonder whether Rosa does, I am making a generalization (p. 4).

Assessment

As with all clients, introduce yourself and ask how the client prefers to be addressed. Obviously it is important to pronounce your client's name correctly and to validate with the client that your pronunciation is accurate. Just the courtesy of trying to say a name correctly signals to the client that you are interested in knowing him or her as a person. If the client does not speak the same language, it is better to use the last name and title rather than the client's first name until rapport is established.

A general cultural assessment starts with the client's reality. By letting clients tell their stories and asking reflective questions to ensure understanding, the nurse learns to make sense of the cultural context of each client's health care need. Health care professionals sometimes mistakenly assume that illness is a single concept, but illness is a complex personal experience, strongly colored by cultural norms, values, social roles, and religious beliefs (Deetz & Stevenson, 1986). Some culture-specific behaviors in health care can appear to be dysfunctional or noncompliant when viewed by a person from a different culture; they often are quite appropriate from a transcultural perspective.

Case Example

Mrs. Campos had been in the United States for only a few years with her family and arrived carrying with her the same health problems she had been suffering for years in Mexico: nondescript abdominal pains, headaches, and a lack of energy. When she came to the United States, she was "found" by a plethora of social service workers and their agencies with money to spend on her health problems. They ushered her into the world of Western medicine as typically practiced in the United States; but far from providing the relief she hoped for, the system only seemed to increase her burden.

As she would undergo tests for one specific complaint, other problems would be diagnosed, until she boasted a medical history far more serious and complex than anything she had ever dreamed of in her village back in Mexico. Indeed, it was clear to her that her "new" health problems, for which expensive medicines, therapies, and even surgery were prescribed, were actually caused by living in the United States. Through all this, she was diagnosed as diabetic and would require insulin injections. She confided that she had never received a shot before coming to the United States and that she was told by Mexican friends that injections themselves would cause illness. Yet she had little choice but to submit to this foreign brand of medicine, unlike the more holistic and spiritual approaches she was accustomed to back home. (Anderson, 1998, p. 311)

If you were the nurse in this situation, how could you help Mrs. Campos feel more comfortable with the management of her health problems?

Table 11-1 Assessing Client Preferences When the Client Is from a Different Culture

Areas to Assess	Sample Assessment Approaches
Explanatory models of illness	"What do you think caused your health problem? Can you tell me a little about how your illness developed?"
Traditional healing processes	"Can you tell me something about how this problem is handled in your country? Are you currently using any medications or herbs to treat your illness? Are there any special cultural beliefs about your illness that might help me give you better care?"
Lifestyle	"What are some of the foods you like? How they are prepared? What do people do in your culture to stay healthy?"
Type of family support	"Can you tell me who in your family should be involved with your care? Who is the decision maker for health care decisions?"
Spiritual healing practices and rituals	"I am not really familiar with your spiritual practices, but I wonder if you could tell me what would be important to you so we can try to incorporate it into your care plan."
Cultural norms about cleanliness and modesty	"A number of our patients have special needs related to cleanliness and modesty of which we aren't always aware. I am wondering if this is true for you and if you could help me understand what you need to be comfortable."
Truth-telling and level of disclosure about serious or terminal illness	Ask the family about cultural ways of talking about serious illness. In some cultures, the family knows the diagnosis/prognosis, which is not told to the ill person (e.g., Hispanic, Asian).
Ritual and religious ceremonies at time of death	Ask the family about special rituals and religious ceremonies at time of death.

The way a client presents symptoms may reveal which aspects of the client's complaints are culturally acceptable and how the client's culture permits their expression. For example, in China, there is no specific term for depression. People with depressive symptoms present instead with multiple somatic symptoms because these symptom clusters are more acceptable in their culture. Being able to recognize the cultural meaning behind a health behavior gives the nurse an advantage in relating effectively and therapeutically with clients from different cultures. Table 11-1 presents topic questions the nurse can ask to better understand the cultural implications of an illness for a client.

Cultural Assessment Sequence

Nurses use a cultural assessment to understand the needs of clients from a different culture (Geissler, 1998; Rosenbaum, 1991). A cultural assessment consists of three progressive, interconnecting elements: a general assessment, a problem-specific assessment, and the culture-specific details needed to correctly analyze the meaning of behaviors and incorporate that into the treatment plan. This structure represents a logical organization of data and is easy for the client to follow. Exercise 11-8 provides practice with cultural assessment.

The *general* assessment component provides the nurse with an initial appraisal of cultural care issues that potentially could affect the treatment process. Common areas of cultural variation include client responses to pain, need for privacy/body exposure, eating preferences and style, consciousness of space and time, isolation and quiet, number of people involved in decision making, hygiene practices, religious and healing rituals, eye contact, and touch (Guarnaccia, 1998). Although most clients from a different culture will not spontaneously volunteer information about their cultural practices in health care, they usually are quite willing to share this information when asked by an interested health care provider. The general assessment also offers an opportunity for nurse and client to appreciate the commonalities across cultures. For example, the need to meet basic physiologic and safety needs and the need for the love and protection of the family are universal health care needs that transcend specific cultural beliefs.

The *problem-specific* stage of a cultural assessment allows the nurse to more fully understand each client's unique health care situation from a cultural perspective. Using a specific cultural assessment allows the nurse to place a particular client problem or need within its unique cultural context and to understand it. Here the nurse gathers data related to the condition or problem for which the client is seeking treatment.

Case Example

Wilma Martinez is a 67-year-old immigrant from El Salvador who moved to the United States to live with her daughter. Mrs. Martinez speaks only Spanish. Through her daughter's translations, the patient appears

Exercise 11-8 Cultural Assessment

Purpose: To help students identify cultural assessment data.

Procedure:

1. Select a specific ethnic culture and, using Leininger's model, interview someone from that culture. Information about different cultures can be found in the literature and on the Internet, or you may use your own personal experience with the ethnic culture you are describing.
2. Write a short report on that culture, including a discussion of values, traditions, health care beliefs, nutrition, and death rituals.
3. Share your written report with your classmates.

Discussion:

1. Discuss each ethnic culture and the common characteristics of the cultural group.
2. What important values did you uncover?
3. Discuss how the cultural values of a particular ethnic group have an impact on health care.
4. Discuss how the nurse can best meet the needs of culturally diverse clients while respecting their cultural identity.

to comprehend details of her illness and treatment. When asked if she understands what the doctor is saying, she invariably nods affirmatively. During a clinic visit, when Mrs. Martinez's daughter is not present, the physician arranges for a trained medical interpreter to be present. Later, the interpreter explains that Mrs. Martinez could not understand why the staff were insistent that she, rather than her daughter, make decisions. Mrs. Martinez stated, "In my country, the family decides." Assuming that her daughter would make the decisions for her, she saw no reason to sign the forms. She worried that signing forms would cause legal problems because of her immigration status. (Crawley, Marshall, Lo et al., 2002, p. 675)

In the above case example, cultural ways of negotiating the health care system were not easily understood by either the health care provider or the client.

The final phase of the cultural assessment integrates general and specific understandings into a comprehensive care plan that has meaning to the client. For example, if a restricted diet is a major part of the treatment protocol, every attempt is made to incorporate specific cultural foods into the food plan.

Diagnosis

NANDA (2005) identifies three nursing diagnoses that address cultural issues: impaired verbal communication related to cultural differences, impaired social interaction related to sociocultural dissonance, and noncompliance related to an individual's value system or beliefs about health and cultural influences. Used with culturally diverse clients, each diagnosis implies a negative clinical judgment of the client as being impaired or flawed, rather than simply different (Geissler, 1991). For example, the third diagnosis judges the client to be noncompliant, with the problem to be resolved in favor of the client's acceptance of North American medical standards. To comply with western medical protocols would place the client in conflict with personal cultural values. Thus the nursing diagnosis, while providing words about the client's difficulty, may not be usable as a valid descriptor. Knowing the cultural implications of the client's behavioral response, should the nurse still assume that the client is noncompliant and try to change the client's behavior? If you as a professional nurse wanted to make these diagnoses culturally congruent, how would you change their wording?

Planning

Language Barriers

Culture and communication are really separable from each other (Hecht, Ronald, Jackson et al., 2003). Clients from different cultures often identify language barriers as the most frustrating aspect of cultural diversity. They feel helpless, even desperate, when they cannot express their thoughts and feelings to someone who must be able to understand their meaning in order to help them. Acknowledging language difficulties and trying to find creative ways to share experiences are important for the client's acceptance of the nurse. Below are key concepts you should keep in mind in working with clients experiencing language barriers:

- Limitations in English proficiency should not be construed as a limitation of intellectual functioning.
- People can be highly literate in their language of origin, but functionally illiterate in English. This can create significant problems with effective health teaching.
- People tend to think in their native language, translating back and forth from English to their native language. This creates a delay in response that needs to be taken into account when speaking and responding.
- People always conduct an interior monologue about a message, often accompanied by visual imagery that reflects their cultural beliefs and experiences. This interpretative analysis may completely change the meaning of the original message, with neither party having awareness of the difference in interpretation.
- All written information should be given in the person's native language whenever possible. This enhances understanding and compliance.

Strategies the nurse can use when there are language barriers include using pictures and developing "flash cards" with commonly used hospital terms (e.g., pain, medicine, bathroom, can't sleep, hungry, hot, cold, and doctor) with the words in the client's language written beside them (Thompson, Thompson, & House, 1990). It also helps to learn a few key words related to the specific client's health care needs in the client's language and teach the client some simple English words to express health care needs.

Defining Role Relations

Cultural customs may require role relationships to be more formal, with well-defined boundaries and clearly verbalized expectations. For example, Asian clients respond best to a formal relationship. They favor an indirect communication style characterized by polite phrases and marked deference. Typically, the client waits for the information to be offered by the nurse as the authority figure. This behavior does not mean that the Asian client is timid, passive, or unwilling to participate in the treatment process. It simply is a cultural characteristic that needs to be acknowledged, respected, and accounted for in developing an individualized plan of care for a client exhibiting such culturally determined behavior. On the other hand, Hispanic clients need a more personal, informal, interpersonal format to feel comfortable. They respond best to a health professional who is open, warm, and willing to respond to personal questions (Pagani-Tousignant, 1992).

In some minority cultures, there is an unspoken tendency to view health professionals as authority figures, treating them with deference and respect but disregarding their advice. This value is so strong that a client often will not question the nurse or in any way indicate mistrust of this authority figure's counsel. Such clients simply will not follow the nurse's recommendations or will withdraw from treatment. Careful attention to the flow of the ethnic client or family's concerns helps to prevent this situation. Other factors related to role relations that nurses need to keep in mind include the following:

- Cultural distinctions between male and female roles are very strong in certain cultures, and this can affect decision making in health care (e.g., in Hispanic and Asian cultures, males are more likely to be the decision makers).
- Age and position in the family are relevant (e.g., decisions may be deferred to elders, and there may be role expectations of the eldest male, of females, and of children within the family).
- Religious and folk beliefs can influence the role of a child born with a disability.

Level of Family Involvement

Different ethnic groups define family differently. Some make little distinction between nuclear family and extended family as the basic family unit. Some cultures (e.g., Native American) include godparents, or even the community as a whole, in the family unit. Level of family involvement is another issue. For example, the degree of family involvement among Asian, Hispanic, and African-American cultures is apt to be much greater than the norm for the majority culture in the United States. Within these cultures, the extended family is the basic social unit. Health problems affecting one family member have direct implications for all other members of the family. Moreover, there also is a sex-linked hierarchy: the oldest male is the final authority on family matters in Asian and Hispanic cultures. For this reason, the nurse might address the husband first, even if another adult family member is the actual client. Identifying and including from the outset all decision makers and those who will be taking an active part in the care of the client recognizes the communal nature of family involvement in health care. For the Native American client, this may include many members of an immediate tribe or its spokesperson.

Time Orientation

Orientation to time and to time pressures differs in certain cultures, depending on whether the culture is past-, present-, or future-oriented. Our western health care culture's value of efficiency also often conflicts with time orientations in other cultures (e.g., in the Native American client). In North America, "time is money," and people are very concerned about such things as exact time frames for appointments and taking medications. Present-oriented time, however, does not consider the commitment to a future appointment as important as attending to what is happening in the moment. Giger and Davidhizar (1991) note, "A common belief shared by some African Americans and Mexican Americans is that time is flexible and events will begin when they arrive" (p. 105). Some flexibility with time schedules for nursing care procedures should be factored into the care plan for the culturally diverse client with a different sense of time. Even when cultures seem relatively similar in outlook, this may not always be the case. Lewis (2000) contrasts the difference in time orientation of a clock-conscious German person with that of his Italian counterpart in the next case example.

Case Example

Germans and Swiss love clock-regulated time, for it appears to them as a remarkably efficient, impartial, and very precise way of organizing life—especially in business. For Italians, on the other hand, time considerations will usually be subjected to human feelings.

"Why are you so angry because I came at 9:30?" an Italian asks his German colleague. "Because it says 9 a.m. in my diary," says the German. "Then why don't you write 9:30 and then we'll both be happy?" is a logical Italian response. The business we have to do and our close relations are so important that it is irrelevant at what time we meet. The meeting is what counts. (Lewis, 2000, p. 55)

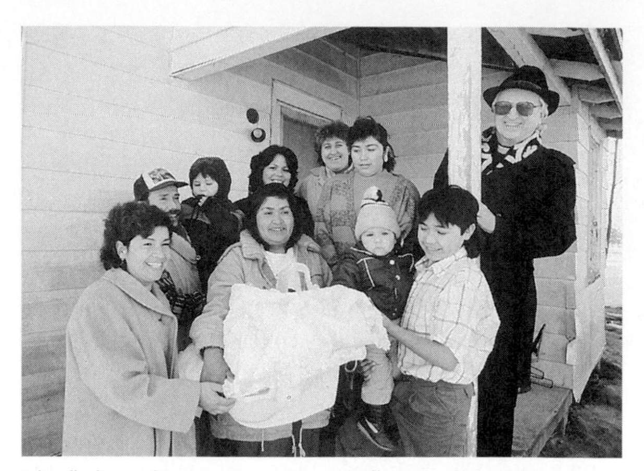

Culturally diverse clients experience the nurse's efforts to understand their culture as empowering. (Courtesy University of Maryland School of Nursing.)

Intervention

Interventions with clients from another culture rely on the same communication strategies discussed throughout this text. Culturally competent nurses also integrate the cultural knowledge base, skills, and attitudes needed to provide culturally sensitive health care to diverse cultural groups. Culturally appropriate nursing interventions should include the following:

- Respect for the client's belief in folk and natural traditional remedies
- Combining cultural folk treatments with standard medical practices to whatever extent is possible
- Familiarity with formal and informal sources of health care in the cultural community, including churches, *Shamans*, medicine men/women, *curanderos*, and other faith healers
- Respect for family position and gender distinctions when relating to family members about health care concerns
- Continuous use of active listening strategies and frequent validation with the client regarding the cultural appropriateness of your conclusions
- Remembering that the client is a person first, and a cultural person second

Empowering Clients

Culturally diverse clients experience the nurse's attempt to put their presenting problem into a cultural context as empowering. Clients belonging to ethnically disadvantaged groups are more likely to respond to health care providers who confirm their current dilemmas as set within social circumstances, values, and cultural experiences. Framing interventions within a culturally sensitive format that the client recognizes as familiar and valid, and openly discussing differences in backgrounds, norms, and health practices increases client understanding and compliance. Cultural sensitivity requires the nurse to pay attention to the client's nonverbal communication. Respectful use of touch, conversational distance, and tone of voice are essential components of therapeutic communication (Schim, Doorenbos, & Borse, 2005).

Case Example

An Oregon girl in an intercultural communication class asked a young man from Saudi Arabia how he would nonverbally signal that he liked her. His response was to smooth back his hair, which to her was just a common nervous gesture signifying nothing. She repeated her question three times. He smoothed his hair three times. Then realizing that she was not recognizing this movement as his reply to her question, he automatically ducked his head and stuck out his tongue slightly in embarrassment. This behavior was noticed by the girl, and she expressed astonishment that he would show liking for someone by sticking out his tongue. (Bennett, 1998, p. 180)

With clients demonstrating limited English proficiency, speak slowly and clearly; use simple words; and avoid slang, technical jargon, and complex sentences. Even if the client uses English most of the time, it is not unusual for the client or family member for whom English is a second language to revert to their native language in times of stress (Thompson et al., 1990). Although the client uses American words and phrases to communicate, they are translated into and processed in the client's native language. Sometimes it is difficult for the nurse to appreciate this double cognitive processing because the responses are in English, and the nurse is aware only that the client seems to be taking more time than usual. Tong, Huang, and McIntyre (2006) identify communication strategies that can be modified to meet the needs of culturally diverse clients in health care situations:

- Give the appearance of being patient and unhurried when teaching the client.
- Be aware of facial expressions indicating bewilderment, frustration, or being overwhelmed.
- Use the English-as-a-second-language style of phrasing—speak words slowly, with distinct separation of words and accentuation of important terms.
- Repeat explanations of important information in another way if the client does not seem to understand the original explanation.
- Use gestures, pantomime, body language, and visual cues to enhance understanding.
- Acknowledge effort and express belief in the client's ability to grasp the material.

The U.S. Department of Health and Human Services (2001) states, "Integral to provision of culturally competent health care services is familiarity with and respect of the traditional healing systems and beliefs of diverse cultural groups" (p. 52). This means that, whenever possible, nurses should incorporate traditional healing rituals and health practices into the treatment mix.

Using Culturally Based Teaching

Cultural differences affect a nurse's teaching and coaching functions. A useful teaching sequence for culturally diverse clients can be remembered with the mnemonic *LEARN: L*isten, *E*xplain, *A*cknowledge, *R*ecommend, and *N*egotiate (Campinha-Bacote, 1992). With this process, the nurse listens carefully to the client's perspective on his or her health problem, including cause, expectations for treatment, and information about family and others who traditionally are involved in the client's care. Once the nurse has a clear understanding of the client's perception of the problem, the nurse can explain his or her understanding of it using simple, concrete terminology, and then ask for validation that this perspective is correct.

After this discussion, the nurse can acknowledge the differences and similarities between perceptions. The information serves as a basis for planning interventions, with the nurse making specific recommendations to the client and negotiating a mutually acceptable treatment approach (Campinha-Bacote, 1991, 1992).

Throughout the negotiation process to determine goals and the means to achieve them, the nurse is respectful of the client's right to hold different cultural views. If family members traditionally are involved in decision making, they should be made an integral part of the relationship at each step in the process. The same information given to the client is shared with the family.

Specific teaching strategies can enhance culturally based recommendations. For example, incorporating storytelling as a teaching strategy is likely to facilitate success with the Native American client who is used to learning in this manner (Hodge, Pasqua, & Marquez, 2002). Providing a maternity client with booklets about breast-feeding written in her native language is a small yet meaningful gesture. The offering is tangible evidence of the nurse's acknowledgment of cultural differences. Box 11-2 provides general guidelines for teaching culturally diverse clients.

Box 11-2 General Communication Guidelines for Teaching Culturally Diverse Clients

- Use the same sequence and repeat phrases, expanding on the same basic questions.
- Speak slowly and clearly, and use concrete language the client can understand. Make the sentence structure as simple as possible.
- Encourage the client by smiling and by listening. Provide cues such as pictures and gestures.
- Avoid the use of technical language, and choose words that incorporate cultural terms whenever possible.
- Allow enough time, and do not assume that simply because the client nods or smiles that the communication is understood.
- Identify barriers to compliance, such as social values, environment, and language.
- Help the client develop realistic, culturally relevant goals.
- Incorporate culturally specific teaching formats (e.g., use an oral or storytelling format with clients who have oral teaching traditions).
- Close with cultural sensitivity: "I've really learned a lot today about [restate highlights]. Thanks for sharing with me."

Box 11-3 Guidelines for Using Interpreters in Health Care

- Whenever possible, the translator should not be a family member.
- Orient the translator to the goals of the clinical interview and expected confidentiality.
- Look directly at the client when either you or the client is speaking.
- Ask the translator to clarify anything that isn't understood by either the nurse or the client.
- After each completed statement, pause for translation.

Use of Interpreters

For clients who cannot communicate because of language differences, federal law *mandates* the use of a trained interpreter according to standards established by the Joint Commission on Accreditation of Hospitals and criteria published under Title VI of the Civil Rights Act. When an interpreter is not available, other means may be necessary. It is possible to use a family member who speaks both the native language and English, or it is possible to communicate in a more limited way. Having someone who can communicate with the client and who can understand the subtle nuances of the culture act as an intermediary often bridges the language gap (Newhill, 1990). Interpreters should be chosen with care, keeping in mind differences in dialects as well as differences in the sex and social status of the interpreter and the client if these are likely to be an issue. Children in the family should not be placed in the role of interpreter. Box 11-3 provides guidelines for the use of interpreters in health care interviews.

Applications to Special Populations

Schim et al. (2005) make the observation that "even when a *provider* and patient share the same ethnic or racial heritage, other aspects of diversity remain to be addressed" (p. 355), as there may be more differences among individuals within a culture than between cultural groups.

Culturally responsive approaches for health teaching and partnering with culturally diverse clients require an understanding of mainstream cultural values while simultaneously remembering that nurses "must be humanly responsive to the needs of people as human beings, not simply as cultural beings" (Kikuchi, 2005, p. 307). Knowledge of characteristic behaviors and values held by different cultures can help people communicate more effectively. At the same time, it is critical to keep in mind that culture is not a genetic trait; rather, it is a social concept related to a *shared* life experience of having specific values, communication patterns and symbols, family customs, political systems, and ethnic identity that influence health care, food choices, and occupational choices. Engebretson (2003) suggests that often it is only when people are directly exposed to another culture that their own beliefs are illuminated.

African-American Clients. African Americans account for 13 percent of the population of the United States, making them the largest minority group in the nation. For many African Americans, their ethnic cultural identity traces back to slavery and deprivation. The vestiges of this heritage are evidenced in a seriously disproportionate level of poverty, with its attendant social and health problems, and a visible need for further efforts to ensure equal access to care for this group. A smaller group emigrated voluntarily from countries such as Haiti and Jamaica.

Although African Americans are represented in every socioeconomic group, a significant percentage (approximately one-third) live in poverty (Spector, 2004). Clustered in crowded urban areas, lower-income African-American clients statistically are less likely to use regular preventive health services. They tend not to trust the formal health care system because of subtle and overt discrimination that has been a part of their lives for as long as they can remember. African Americans tend to rely on informal helping networks in the community, particularly those associated with their churches, until a problem becomes a crisis. Purnell and Paulanka (2005) advise that using the extended family system, particularly grandmothers, in providing support and health teaching is particularly useful when working with African-American clients in the community.

Establishing trust is a critical element for success with African-American clients, who are more willing to participate in treatment when they feel respected and are treated as treatment partners in their health care. Allowing these clients to have as much control over their health care as possible helps reinforce personal strengths and enhance their self-concept. This is a useful strategy with any client who feels oppressed and stigmatized by the health care system. Understanding the reasons behind a client's hostility and mistrust of the health care provider allows the nurse to be more patient and proactive.

Health Care Concerns. Health care concerns of African Americans cover a variety of social and physical diseases. The rate of AIDS, homicide, and drug abuse—social diseases associated more with poverty and substandard living conditions than with ethnicity—are significantly higher for African Americans than for Caucasian Americans. African Americans are also subject to higher rates of hypertension, adolescent pregnancy, diabetes, heart disease, and stroke. African-American males have a significantly greater chance of developing cancer and of dying from it (Spector, 2004).

Family. The family is the "primary and most important tradition in the African American community" (Hecht et al. 2003, p. 2). Loyalty to the extended family is a dominant value, and family members rely on each other for emotional and financial support (Littlejohn-Blake_& Darling, 1993; Sterritt & Pokorny, 1998). It is not uncommon for an entire entourage of family visitors to camp out in the hospital waiting room when one member has a serious illness.

Many low-income African-American children grow up in extended families because one or both parents cannot assume child care responsibilities and grandparents take on the role of primary caregiver. Littlejohn-Blake and Darling (1993) identify the taking in of family members and friends who need financial and/or emotional support as a resource strength of African-American families.

Religion. The church plays a central role in African-American culture. For centuries, it served as the primary social, economic, and community life center. African-American political leaders (e.g., Jesse Jackson, Ralph Abernathy, and the late Dr. Martin Luther King, Jr.) were also church leaders. Incorporating spirituality in the care plans for this population is important.

Many African Americans are Christian with strong fundamental beliefs. Prayer and the "laying on of hands" may be very important to your African-American client (Purnell & Paulanka, 2005). Because of the central meaning of the church in African-American life, incorporating the appropriate clergy in treatment plans is a useful strategy. Likewise, readings from the Bible and gospel hymns are sources of support during hospitalization.

A growing number of African Americans are practicing Muslims, a strict fundamentalist religion that emphasizes ethnic identity through dress and actions. The Muslim religion calls for dietary restrictions such as not eating pork or pork products, or "soul foods" such as greens and lentils. A Muslim client may refuse to take insulin if it has a pork base. Another less common religion practiced by some African Americans is voodoo, which consists of ritualistic ceremonies and is sometimes thought to create illness or emotional disturbance.

Case Example

Ms. Jones is a 56-year-old African American who was brought by her family to the psychiatric emergency service of a large city hospital. She claimed that her husband's lover had poisoned her. After a psychiatric examination, Ms. Jones was given the diagnosis of delusional disorder, jealous type. She was admitted to the inpatient psychiatric unit and started on a neuroleptic medication. However, the diagnostician failed to conduct a cultural assessment, which would have revealed that Ms. Jones felt she was experiencing voodoo illness. A more culturally relevant treatment would have included consultation with a folk healer (Campinha-Bacote, 1992).

Hispanic-American Clients. Hispanic Americans account for 13% of the population, and are projected to become the largest minority group in the United States by 2005 (U.S. Census Bureau, 2001). They represent a wide range of cultures and usually identify themselves as Hispanic Americans or Latinos. Mexican Americans sometimes refer to themselves as Chicanos. Typically, Hispanic clients identify their country of origin (e.g., Puerto Rico, Colombia, or San Salvador) in their self-description. They are very proud of their unique heritages and demonstrate distinct cultural differences. Much of the current growth in the Hispanic population of the United States consists of first-generation, new immigrants and older persons with lower socioeconomic status and limited health care resources. It is not uncommon to find Latinos living together in multiple family and ethnic communities.

Latino clients living in rural areas rely on *curanderos* (local folk healers and herb doctors) for most of their medical advice. The *curandero* uses a combination of healing practices, medicines, and herbs to cure illness. Specific dietary practices are included as treatment. It is important to determine whether the client ascribes to the hot and cold theory of treating illness. For example, many Hispanic clients view arthritis as a "cold" disease that should be treated with "hot" foods such as cornmeal, garlic, alcohol, coffee, onions, and chili peppers. "Hot" diseases such as constipation, diarrhea, and ulcers would be treated with "cold" medication, such as bicarbonate of soda and milk of magnesia (Cowell, 1988).

Health Care Concerns. Health care concerns of particular relevance to the Hispanic population are teenage drug abuse, adolescent pregnancy, lack of preventive care and prenatal health care, and a higher incidence of HIV infections in women and children than in the Caucasian population. Heart disease and cancer are the most common causes of death in the Latino population. Faith in God is closely linked with the Hispanic population's understanding of health care problems (Zapata & Shippee-Rice, 1999). Although not a universal belief among more highly educated people, Latino immigrants believe that illness can be the result of a great fright (*susto*) or falling out of favor with God. Latino women may be reluctant to express their private concerns in front of their children, even adult children. They often experience difficulty accessing health care services due to a variety of factors that extend beyond language barriers. Many are illegal immigrants and/or have low incomes and limited health insurance. A proactive prevention approach tailored to the health care needs of this minority population is essential to reducing the disparities in health and well-being found in the population (Chavez, Hubbell, & Mishra, 1999).

Hispanic clients typically use the formal health care system only as a short-term problem-solving strategy for health problems. They like to keep their problems within the family, so talking with a stranger, even if he or she is a health care provider, can be difficult. In a health care situation, the Hispanic client needs to develop *confianza* (trust) in the health care provider and often will ask personal questions to establish the bonding necessary for disclosure. This practice is not based on a desire to invade the nurse's privacy, but rather is the normal way the Hispanic client establishes an acceptable context for conversation (Pederson, 1988). Consequently, when asked, the nurse might provide simple information about marital status, number of children, or other nonintrusive data as a way of establishing trust.

Family. *Familismo* is a strong value in the Hispanic community (Juarez, Ferrell, & Boreman, 1998). The family is the center of the Hispanic client's life and serves as a primary source of emotional support. Hispanic clients are "family members first, and individuals second" (Pagani-Tousignant, 1992, p. 10). Family units tend to live in close proximity with each other and to depend on each other in crisis situations. Close friends are considered a part of the family unit. In the Hispanic (Latino) culture, cooperation is more important than competition, and competitive situations are avoided whenever possible. All major decisions are made by the family as a group rather than by the individual client, and the entire family is involved in the health care of a single family member. Latino families have strong cultural values and beliefs about the sanctity of life. Babies often sleep in the same room as the parents until the age of 2 years, and it is not unusual for children to sleep in the same bed as the parents as a regular practice in their country of origin.

Gender roles are relatively rigid, although this is changing. Latino women are socialized to serve their husbands and children without question (thus the concept of *la sufrida*, or the long-suffering woman) (Pagani-Tousignant, 1992). The nurse needs to be sensitive to the role of gender-specific cultural beliefs in treatment situations. The family must be included in all health care planning to serve both as a focus of care and as a resource to the patient.

Communication Patterns. Spanish is the primary language spoken in all Latin American countries except Brazil (Portuguese) and Haiti (French). Hispanic people tend to trust feelings more than facts. They are an extroverted people, able to tolerate close interpersonal contact, connect through touch, and be appreciative of people who recognize that their speech comes from the heart. On the other hand, physical touch and overfamiliarity are not acceptable to the Hispanic client early in a relationship (de Paula, Lagana, & Gonzalez-Ramirez, 1996). They first have to trust that the health care provider is truly interested in them. Hispanic people are sensitive and may be easily hurt, but they also easily react in a positive way if treated with respect and friendliness.

There are strict rules governing social relationships (*respecto*), in which higher status is given to older individuals and to males over females. This distinction can prove critical in communicating health information for purposes of informed consent.

Hispanic clients look for a warmth and friendliness (*personalismo*) in their health care providers, so it is important to ask about their well-being and to take extra time with finding out what they need. Hispanic clients usually are not assertive in health care interactions, preferring to express their reservations about treatment through noncompliance or silence.

Religion. Latino clients are usually deeply religious; the predominant religion is Catholicism. They view illness and suffering with a fatalistic acceptance having religious overtones (*si Dios quiere* [if God wishes]). The relationship between God and the individual is a close, intimate one, so much so that people can experience visions of God or the saints. In many western cultures, such behaviors might be incorrectly labeled as hallucinations.

Asian-American Clients. The third most common minority group in the United States is Asian Americans. Currently they make up 3.6% of the population, with an increase to 8.7% projected by 2050 (U.S. Census Bureau, 2001). Pagani-Tousignant (1992) notes that the cultural community of Asians and Pacific Islanders comprises more than 32 ethnic groups, with the most well-known being Chinese, Japanese, Indian, Korean, and Vietnamese. However, even within the same geographic grouping, significant cultural differences exist. For example, the Vietnamese and Hmong are both Indochinese, but the Hmong have no written language and have limited work skills, whereas many Vietnamese are highly literate people with sophisticated work skills.

Asian culture values hard work, education, and going with the flow of events. Its members have a deep respect for a harmonious coexistence with nature. The Asian culture supports the idea of people communicating and functioning under a set of prescribed rules and obligations that may seem foreign to people from more spontaneous cultures. In most Asian countries, there is an emphasis on politeness and correct behavior. The correct cultural behavior is to put others first and not to create problems. This can lead to vagueness in communication that is not always understandable to cultures that use a more direct communication style. Traditionally, the Asian client exercises significant emotional restraint in communication. Interpersonal conflicts are not directly addressed, and challenging an expert is not allowed (Chen, 2001). Jokes and humor are usually not appreciated because "the Confucian and Buddhist preoccupation with truth, sincerity, kindliness and politeness automatically eliminates humour techniques such as sarcasm, satire, exaggeration and parody" (Lewis, 2000, pp. 20-21).

Health care providers are considered experts. Asian clients are polite and submissive to avoid giving offense; they tend to nod and smile in agreement, even when they strongly disagree. The nurse needs to understand that the nodding does not always signify agreement, only that the listener is being attentive. It may be hard to tell what Asian clients are truly thinking or feeling because, typically, their facial expressions are not as flexible and their words are not as revealing as those of people in the dominant culture. A direct confrontation typically would not be a good communication strategy to use with an Asian client (Xu, Davidhizar, & Giger, 2004).

Health Care Concerns. Health is based on the ayurvedic principle, which requires harmony and balance between *yin* and *yang*, the two energy forces required for health (Louie, 2001). A blockage of *qi*, defined as the energy circulating in a person's body, creates an imbalance between *yin* (negative energy force) and *yang* (positive energy force) that results in illness (Chen, 2001). In this ancient representation, *yin* is the female force, containing all the elements that represent darkness, cold, and weakness. *Yang* represents the male elements of strength, brightness, and warmth. The Asian client seeks health care for symptom relief but does not view preventive health care as a priority (Lipson, Dibble, & Minarik, 1996).

Acupressure and herbal medicines are among the medical practices used by Asian clients to reestablish the balance between *yin* and *yang*. In some Asian countries, healers use a process of "coining," in which a coin is heated and vigorously rubbed on the body to draw illness out of the body. The resulting welts can mistakenly be attributed to child abuse if this practice is not understood. Traditional healers, such as Buddhist monks, acupuncturists, and herbalists, also may be consulted when someone is ill. The influence of eastern health practices and alternative medicine are increasingly incorporated into the health care of all Americans.

Health care concerns specifically relevant to this population include a higher-than-normal incidence of tuberculosis, hepatitis B, and some forms of cancer (U.S. Department of Health and Human Services, 2000). There is shame and stigma still attached to mental illness; they do not admit to mental problems, and are likely to describe depressive symptoms as sadness or physical symptoms (Kleinman, 1980). People with mental health issues do not seek early treatment because of shame and the lack of culturally appropriate mental health services (Louie, 2001).

Asian clients are stoic when in pain. The nurse can underestimate or neglect the Asian client's suffering. Asking the client about pain and suggesting possible feelings are helpful interventions. The Asian client also appreciates a clinician who is willing to provide advice in a matter-of-fact, concise manner.

Family members take an active role in deciding whether a diagnosis should be disclosed to a client, and they frequently are the recipients of this information before the client is told of the diagnosis, prognosis, and treatment options. Traditional Chinese culture does not allow clients to discuss the full severity of an illness; this creates challenges for mutual decision making based on full disclosure that is characteristic of western health care.

Case Example

A young Vietnamese woman gave birth to a healthy boy. During labor, the mother was smiling and said nothing. Seemingly, the labor process caused her no stress. The father remained at the hospital during the labor but assumed a passive role, entering the delivery room only to translate some instructions to his wife. On the postpartum unit, the client refused to take her medications with the ice water offered to her. She seemed reluctant to get out of bed other than to use the bathroom, and she refused to eat. Despite a smiling, polite posture during most of her postpartum course, she became visibly upset when the nurse brought her baby to her and made pleasing remarks about the infant (Hollingsworth, Brown, & Brooten, 1980).

To the casual observer, the client's behavior was perplexing; however, if the nurse viewed the same behaviors from a transcultural perspective, they made complete sense. Her composure during her labor and her politeness during postpartum were cultural responses dictated by the cultural need to remain stoic. In Vietnam, the newborn is bathed and clothed before the father has contact with it. This custom explains her husband's behavior in exiting the delivery room quickly and not spending initial time with his newborn infant.

The client's postpartum behavior has cultural meaning. The Vietnamese view childbirth as disturbing the balance between *yin* and *yang* (hot and cold) in the body. Only the body part to be examined can be exposed, and only in private. The client's refusal of medications was related to a fear of disturbing the balance between *yin* and *yang* in her body. Likewise, her poor eating pattern can be explained by this humoral imbalance. Only certain foods, such as chicken, rice, and pork, are thought to be "warm" foods. Postpartum women do not traditionally eat salads. Vietnamese women traditionally avoid early ambulation because of a belief that too much movement will prevent their distended internal organs from resuming their prepregnancy state. Finally, the nurse's enthusiasm in recognizing her new infant was unacceptable to the new mother because of a cultural belief that should a spirit overhear the comments and find the child desirable, the spirit might attempt to steal it away.

Family. The family is a powerful force in maintaining the religious and social values in Asian cultures. "Good health" is described as having harmonious family relationships and a balanced life (Harrison, Kagawa-Singer, Foerster et al., 2005). The weight of tradition and the community spirit strongly regulates individual behavior. Asian families traditionally live in multigenerational households, with extended family providing important social support (Jacobson, 1994). Individual privacy is uncommon. The Asian culture places family before individual welfare. The centrality of the family unit means that the individual may have to sacrifice his or her individuality if needed for the good of the family. The need to avoid "loss of face" by acting in a manner that brings shame to the individual is paramount, because loss of face brings shame to the whole family, including ancestors.

The family may consist of father, mother, and children; nuclear family, grandparents, and other relatives living together; or a broken family in which some family members are in the United States, and other nuclear family members are still living in their country of origin (Gelles, 1995). There is family pressure on younger members to do well academically, and the behavior of individual members is always considered within the context of its impact on the family as a whole. Family members are obligated to assume a great deal of responsibility for each other, including ongoing financial assistance. Older children are responsible for the well-being of younger children.

Traditional gender roles are strong. The husband or father acts as the primary authority figure, the decision maker in the household, and the family spokesperson in crisis situations. In contrast with many other societies, the elders in an Asian community are highly respected and well taken care of by younger members of the family

(Pagani-Tousignant, 1992). The wisdom of the elders helps guide younger family members on many life issues, including major health decisions (Davis, 2000). In more conservative Asian cultures, this includes even the choice of marriage partners.

Communication Patterns. Interpersonal communication takes place through prescribed roles and obligations, taking into account family roles, age, and position in the family. The Asian client views the health care provider as an authority figure, and in this culture a person must show complete respect for authority figures. It is almost impossible for the Asian client to argue or disagree with the nurse. Consequently, the nurse has to ask open-ended questions and clarify issues consistently in every interaction. If the nurse uses questions that require a yes or no answer, the answer may reflect the client's polite deference rather than an honest response. Explaining treatment as problem solving, asking the client how things are done in his or her culture, and working with the client to develop a culturally congruent solution usually is most effective (McLaughlin & Braun, 1998).

Asian men may have a difficult time disclosing personal information to a female nurse unless the nurse explains why the data are necessary for care, because in serious matters women are not considered as knowledgeable as men. Asian clients may be reluctant to be examined by a person of the opposite sex, particularly if the examination or treatment involves the genital area. Many Asians consider the head the repository of the soul, so that touching the head is seen as damaging to the equilibrium of the soul. For this reason, it is useful to explain the reason for touching the head before doing so (Santopietro, 1981).

Religion. Religion plays an important role in Asian society, and religious beliefs are tightly interwoven into virtually every aspect of daily life. Referred to as "Eastern religions," the major religious groups in Asian culture are Hindus, Buddhists, Sikhs, and Muslims.

According to Michaels (2003), Hinduism is not a homogeneous religion, but rather should be viewed as a living faith, a philosophical way of life with diverse doctrines, religious symbols, and moral and social norms. Being a Hindu provides a living membership in a communal society, and helps determine how individuals orient themselves within their culture. Approximately 80% of the people living in India are Hindus. Hinduism represents a pragmatic philosophy of life that specifically articulates harmony with the natural rhythms of life and the "right" or "correct" principles of social interaction and behavior. The *veda* refers to knowledge passed through many generations from ancient sages, which combined with Sanskrit literature provides the "codes of ritual, social and ethical behavior, called *dharma*, which that literature reveals" (Flood, 1996, p. 11). Hindus are vegetarians because it is against their religion to kill living creatures. Sikhism is a reformed variation of Hinduism in which women have more rights in domestic and community life.

Islam is a major world religion that is often identified with Asian culture, but in reality is found throughout the world. Followers of the religion are called Muslim. It is a monotheistic religion, with Allah identified as their higher power or God. Muhammad is his prophet.

Islam is the world's fastest growing religion, found predominantly in Southeast Asia. Islam is divided into four main groups: Sunni, Shi'a, Ismaili, and Ahmadiyya. People practicing this religion adhere to the Koran as the holy teaching of Muhammad. Faith, prayer, giving alms, and making a yearly pilgrimage to Mecca are requirements of the religion.

There can be no physical contact between a Muslim woman and a man who is not her husband. Physical modesty is of high value to the Muslim client, and the Muslim family may request that only female staff care for their female family members. Physical contact, eye contact, touch, and hugs between members of the opposite sex who are not family are avoided. Following the birth of a baby, women go into seclusion and don't shower for 10 days after the baby's birth (McKennis, 1999).

The Muslim religion is a way of life in which an individual submits entirely to Allah and follows Allah's basic rules about everything from personal relationships to business matters, including personal matters such as dress and hygiene. Islam has some strong tenets that affect health care, an important one being that God is the ultimate healer. Devout Muslims believe death is a part of Allah's plan, so to fight the dying process with treatment is wrong. Muslims believe that the dying person should not die alone. A close relative should be present, praying for God's blessing or reading the Koran. Once the person actually dies, it is important to perform the following: turn the body toward Mecca; close the person's mouth and eyes and cover the face; straighten the legs and arms; announce the death to relatives and friends; bathe the body (with men bathing men and women bathing women); and cover the body with white cotton (Servodido & Morse, 2001).

Buddhism represents a philosophical approach to life, which identifies fate, *Inn and Ko* as the primary factors impacting health and illness. Buddhists believe that *In* (cause) and *Ko* (effect) are variables that interact with fate and can influence people to be righteous and experience less stress and guilt, thereby promoting better health (Chen, 2001).

Native American Clients. Although Native Americans represent the smallest of the major ethnic groups in the United States, there are more than 500 federally recognized tribes and more than 100 tribes or bands that are state-recognized not recognized by the federal government. As an ethnic minority, Native Americans are among the least educated and poorest, with a much higher than normal incidence of social and health problems (Hodge & Fredericks, 1999). Terms to describe North American native people include Native Americans, First or Original Americans, Alaskan Natives, Aleuts, Eskimos, Metis (mixed blood), or Amerindians. Additionally, native people identify themselves as members of a specific tribe (Garrett & Herring, 2001).

Health Care Concerns. Native Americans suffer from much higher rates of mortality from chronic diseases such as tuberculosis, alcoholism, diabetes, and pneumonia. Domestic violence, often associated with alcoholism, is a significant health concern. Pain assessment is very important, because the Native American client tends to display a stoic response to pain (Cesario, 2001). Homicide and suicide rates are significantly higher than those for the general population (Meisenhelder, Bell, & Chandler, 2000). Health concerns of particular relevance to the Native American population are unintentional injuries (of which 75% are alcohol-related), cirrhosis, alcoholism, and obesity.

Family. The family is highly valued by the Native American, and the fundamental unit of society is the multigenerational family that lives together in close proximity. When two individuals marry, the marriage contract implicitly includes attachment and obligation to a much larger kinship system (Red Horse, 1997). Both men and women feel a responsibility to promote tribal values and traditions through their crafts and traditional ceremonies; however, women are identified as the standard bearers of the culture. A Cheyenne proverb graphically states, "A nation is not conquered until the hearts of its women are on the ground. Then it is done, no matter how brave its warriors nor how strong their weapons" (Crow Dog & Erdoes, 1990, p. 3). Cheshire (2001) notes, "It is the women—the mothers, grandmothers and aunties—that keep Indian nations alive" (p. 1534). Gender roles are less rigid than in other cultures, and family boundaries are extended to include people who are not blood-related. The nurse may need to include these people in care planning, because they can be a very important social support to the Native American client (Long & Curry, 1998). Because the family matriarch is often the primary decision maker, her approval and support may be required for compliance with a treatment plan (Cesario, 2001). Tribal identity is maintained through regular powwows and other ceremonial events.

Communication Patterns. Spector (2004) points out that nurses need to understand the value of nonverbal communication in therapeutic conversations with Native American clients. You will need to listen carefully with the Native American client, who is likely to speak in a low tone. Taking time to listen to the client and the family is critical, because Native Americans are likely to interpret a fast approach to their concerns as lack of interest. As an ethnic group, Native Americans are much more comfortable with long periods of silence than other groups. Native Americans are private people who respect the privacy of others and prefer to talk about the facts rather than emotions about them. Asking questions of each person individually is preferable. Direct eye contact is considered disrespectful, and Native American clients respond best to health professionals who stick to the point and do not engage in small talk. Learning for the Native American client is a passive process. Their learning style is observational and oral, so the use of charts, written instructions, and pamphlets is usually not well-received.

Case Example

When the nurse is performing a newborn bath demonstration, the Native American mother is likely to watch from a distance, avoid eye contact with the demonstrator, ask few or no questions, and decline a return demonstration. This learning style should not be seen as indifference or lack of understanding. Being an experiential learner, the Native American woman is likely to assimilate the information provided and simply give the newborn a bath when it is needed. (Cesario, 2001, p. 17)

Missed and late appointments and lack of compliance with treatment create frustration in the professional nurse, especially in today's managed care environment. For Native Americans, being on time or taking medication with meals (when three meals are taken on one day and two meals are eaten on another day) have little relevance (Cesario, 2001; Kavanagh, Absalom, Beil et al., 1999). Native Americans live in the present and view time on a continuum that has relevance only to what needs to be accomplished. They have little appreciation of scheduled time commitments, which in their mind do not necessarily relate to what needs to be achieved. Understanding this cultural belief and looking for the reason why the client is late from the Native American client's perspective can enhance communication (Cesario, 2001). Calling the client before making a home visit or to remind the client of an appointment is useful.

Religion. Native American health care beliefs and practices integrate religion with medical care, and spirituality plays a significant role in the maintenance and restoration of health in the Native American culture (Cesario, 2001; Meisenhelder et al., 2000). The religious beliefs of Native Americans are strongly linked with nature and the earth. There is a sense of sacredness in everyday living between "grandmother earth" and "grandfather sky" that tends to render the outside world extraneous (Kavanagh et al., 1999, p. 25).

Because the Native American way of life is so intimately connected to the plants, animals, waters, and spirits, illness is viewed as a punishment from God for some real or imagined imbalance with nature. Native Americans believe illness to be divine intervention to help the individual correct evil ways. In some cases, recovery is likely to occur only after the client is cleansed of the "evil spirits." Native Americans view death as a natural process, but they fear the power of dead spirits and use numerous tribal rituals to ward them off.

Spiritual ceremonies and prayers form an important part of traditional healing activities (Upvall, 1997). Because person and nature are one and the same, most healing practices are strongly embedded in religious beliefs. Native Americans may seek medical help from their tribal elders and *Shamans* (highly respected spiritual medicine men and women) who use spiritual healing practices and herbs to cure the ill member of the tribe (Pagani-Tousignant, 1992). For the Native American client, spiritual and herbal tokens or medicine bags placed at the bedside or in an infant's crib are essential to the healing process and should not be disturbed (Cesario, 2001).

Culture of Poverty. There are enough differences between the worldview of the dominant culture and the cultural worldview of those who fall below the poverty line to warrant special consideration of their needs in the nurse-client relationship. The culture of poverty is characterized by acute deprivation. The poor generally are disadvantaged educationally. They do not have the same access to the health care system and preventive health care because of cost and availability. The poor who seek health care are often subjected to long waits and sometimes experience rude treatment by health professionals who do not seem to want to help.

Exercise 11-9 Applying Cultural Sensitivity to Nursing Care

Purpose: To familiarize yourself with culture-specific elements of nursing care for several populations.

Procedure:

This can be done in small, even-numbered groups rather than as an individual exercise.

1. Each student creates a clinical scenario based on a client from a cultural group. Be creative, and write a situation in which ethnicity or cultural factors are present in the client's nursing needs.
2. Trade scenarios with another student, and write how you would incorporate cultural need and strategies into that student's care plan.
3. Each student presents the final case scenario with the care plan he or she developed.

Discussion:

Discuss in groups additional ways to incorporate cultural principles into nursing care.

Consequently, health-seeking behaviors among the poor and homeless tend to be crisis-oriented. The nurse needs to use a crisis-oriented approach for greatest impact.

Health Care Strategies. In our society, being poor often means being powerless. Many poor people feel that they have virtually no control over meeting their basic needs. Things that most of us take for granted, such as food, housing, clothing, the chance for a decent job, and the opportunity for education, are not available or sufficient for their needs. Often they have experienced violence rather than social justice as the means of providing their fundamental needs. Consequently, the idea that they can exercise choice in their lives and make a difference in their health care is not part of their worldview. They look to and expect others to take responsibility and to make things better. Poor people often do not take the initiative simply because their life experiences tell them they cannot trust that their own efforts will produce any change. This is a very difficult but important cultural concept for nurses to incorporate into their relationships with people of poverty. The nurse must take a proactive, persistent, and patient-oriented approach to understanding and working with this population (Minick, Kee, Borkat et al., 1998). Communication strategies that acknowledge, support, and empower the poor to take small steps to independence are most effective. Exercise 11-9 provides practice with a practical application of cultural sensitivity.

Evaluation

Evaluation of goals achieved in a transcultural nurse-client relationship should include answers to such questions as the following: Were the learning activities culturally specific and sufficient to produce the desired outcome? Is the client satisfied with the outcome? What cultural modifications are needed to provide the client with the content and process the client needs to achieve the objectives? In addition, the nurse needs to reflect on any potential biases that may have gotten in the way of providing culturally congruent care.

Ethical Considerations

Respect for human dignity is a major concern of ethical treatment. This means that the nurse pays strict attention to personal biases and stereotypes in interacting with clients from a different culture so as not to color the assessment or implementation of nursing interventions. It means treating each client as "culturally unique," with a set of assumptions and values regarding the disease process and its treatment, and acting in a nonjudgmental manner that respects the client's cultural integrity (Haddad, 2001). Ethics become particularly important in client situations requiring informed consent, health care decision making, involvement of family and significant others, treatment choices, and birth and death.

SUMMARY

This chapter explores the intercultural communication that takes place when the nurse and client are from different cultures. Culture is defined as a common collectivity of beliefs, values, shared understandings, and patterns of behavior of a designated group of people. Culture needs to be viewed as a human structure with many variations in meaning.

Multiculturalism describes a heterogeneous society in which diverse cultural worldviews can coexist with some general (etic) characteristics shared by all cultural groups and some (emic) perspectives that are unique to a particular group. Related terms include cultural diversity, cultural relativism, subculture, ethnicity, ethnocentrism, and ethnography. Each of these concepts broadens the definition of culture. Intercultural communication is defined as a communication in which the sender of a message is a member of one culture and the receiver of the message is from a different culture. Different languages create and express different personal realities.

A cultural assessment is defined as a systematic appraisal of beliefs, values, and practices conducted to determine the context of client needs and to tailor nursing interventions. It is composed of three progressive,

Ethical Dilemma ■ ***What Would You Do?***

Antonia Martinez is admitted to the hospital and needs immediate surgery. She speaks limited English, and her family is not with her. She is frightened by the prospect of surgery and wants to wait until her family can be with her to help her make the decision about surgery. As a nurse, you feel there is no decision to be made: she must have the surgery, and you need to get her consent form signed now. What would you do?

interconnecting elements: a general assessment; a problem-specific assessment; and the cultural details needed for successful implementation.

Knowledge and acceptance of the client's right to seek and support alternative health care practices dictated by culture can make a major difference in compliance and successful outcome. Health care professionals sometimes mistakenly assume that illness is a single concept, but illness is a personal experience, strongly colored by cultural norms, values, social roles, and religious beliefs. Interventions that take into consideration the specialized needs of the culturally diverse client follow the mnemonic *LEARN: L*isten, *E*xplain, *A*cknowledge, *R*ecommend, and *N*egotiate.

Some basic thoughts about the traditional characteristics of the largest minority groups (African-American, Hispanic, Asian, Native American) living in the United States relating to communication preferences, perceptions about illness, family, health, and religious values are included in the chapter. The culture of poverty is discussed.

REFERENCES

Allport G: The language of prejudice. In Eschholz P, Rosa A, Clark V, editors, *Language awareness*, ed 3, New York, 1982, St. Martin Press.

American Academy of Nursing: *Diversity, marginalization, and culturally competent health care: issues in knowledge development*, Washington, DC, 1995, Author.

Anderson W: Immigration and ethnicity: implications for holistic nursing, *J Holist Nurs* 16(3):301–319, 1998.

Aroian K, Faville K: Reconciling cultural relativism for a clinical paradigm: what's a nurse to do? *J Prof Nurs* 21(6):330, 2005.

Bacallao M, Smokowski P: "Entre dos mundos" (between two worlds): bicultural skills with Latino immigrant families, *J Prim Prev* 26(6):485–509, 2005.

Bennett M: *Basic concepts of intercultural communication: selected readings*, Yarmouth, MA, 1998, Intercultural Press.

Bromwich D: *Politics by other means: higher education and group thinking*, New Haven, CT, 1992, Yale University Press.

Callister L: Culturally competent care of women and newborns: knowledge, attitude, and skills, *J Obstet Gynecol Neonatal Nurs* 30(2):209–215, 2001.

Campinha–Bacote J: Community mental health services: a culturally specific mode, *Arch Psychiatr Nurs* 5(4):229–235, 1991.

Campinha-Bacote J: Voodoo illness, *Perspect Psychiatr Care* 28(1):11–16, 1992.

Canadian Nurses Association: Cultural diversity—changes and challenges, *Nursing Now: Issues and Trends in Canadian Nursing* 7:1–4, 2000.

Canales M, Howers H: Expanding conceptualizations of culturally competent care, *J Adv Nurs* 36(1):102–111, 2001.

Cesario S: Care of the Native American woman: strategies for practice, education and research, *J Obstet Gynecol Neonatal Nurs* 30(1):13–19, 2001.

Chavez LR, Hubbell FA, Mishra SI: Ethnography and breast cancer control among Latinas and Anglo women in southern California. In Hahn RA, editor, *Anthropology in public health*, New York, 1999, Oxford University Press.

Chen YC: Chinese values, health and nursing, *J Adv Nurs* 36(2):270–273, 2001.

Cheshire T: Cultural transmission in urban American Indian families, *Am Behav Sci* 44(9):1528–1535, 2001.

Cochran M: Tears have no color, *Am J Nurs* 98(6):53, 1998.

Cowell D: *Proceedings from the meeting of the National Institutes of Health: cultural implications of health care*, Washington, DC, 1988, National Institutes of Health.

Crawley L, Marshall P, Lo B et al.: (2002) Strategies for culturally effective end-of-life care, *Ann Intern Med* 136(9): 673–679, 2002.

Crow Dog M, Erdoes R: *Lakota woman*, New York, 1990, Grove Weidenfeld.

Davis AJ: Global influence of American nursing: some ethical issues, *Nurs Ethics* 6(2):118–125, 1999.

Davis R: The convergence of health and family in the Vietnamese culture, *J Fam Nurs* 6(2):136–156, 2000.

De Paula T, Lagana K, Gonzalez-Ramirez L: Mexican Americans. In Lipson JG, Dibble SL, Minarik PA, editors, *Culture and nursing care*, San Francisco, 1996, UCSF Nursing Press.

Deetz S, Stevenson S: *Managing interpersonal communication*, New York, 1986, Harper & Row.

Doswell W, Erlen J: Multicultural issues and ethical concerns in the delivery of revising care interventions, *Nurs Clin North Am* 33(2):353–361, 1998.

Duffy M: A critique of cultural education in nursing, *J Adv Nurs* 36(4):487–495, 2001.

Engebretson J: Cultural constructions of health and illness: recent cultural changes toward a holistic approach, *J Holistic Nurs* 21(3):203–227, 2003.

Flood G: *An introduction to Hinduism*, Cambridge, England, 1996, Cambridge University Press.

Ford M, Kelly P: Conceptualizing and categorizing race and ethnicity in health services research, *Health Serv Res* 40(5, pt 2):1658–1675, 2005.

Galanti GA: *Caring for patients from different cultures*, ed 3, Philadelphia, 2004, University of Pennsylvania Press.

Garrett M, Herring R: Honoring the power of relations: counseling Native adults, *Journal of Humanistic Counseling, Education and Development* 40(20):139–140, 2001.

Geissler EM: Nursing diagnoses of culturally diverse patients, *Int Nurs Rev* 38(5):150–152, 1991.

Geissler EM: *Cultural assessment,* St Louis, 1998, Mosby.

Gelles R: *Contemporary families,* Thousand Oaks, CA, 1995, Sage.

Giger J, Davidhizar R: *Transcultural nursing: assessment and intervention,* St Louis, 1991, Mosby.

Gravely S: When your patient speaks Spanish–and you don't, *RN* 64(5):64–67, 2001.

Guarnaccia P: Multicultural experiences of family caregiving: a study of African American, European American, and Hispanic American families, *New Dir Ment Health Serv* 77:45–61, 1998.

Haddad A: Ethics in action, *RN* 64(3):21–22, 24, 2001.

Harrison G, Kagawa-Singer M, Foerster S et al.: Seizing the moment, *Cancer* 15(104–112 supp):2962–2968, 2005.

Hecht M, Ronald L, Jackson L et al.: *African American communication: identity and cultural interpretation,* Mahwah, NJ, 2003, Lawrence Erlbaum Associates.

Hernandez D: *Children of immigrants,* Washington, DC, 1995, National Academy Press.

Hodge F, Fredericks L: American Indian and Alaska Native population in the United States: an overview. In Huff R, Kline M, editors, *Promoting health in multicultural populations,* Thousand Oaks, CA, 1999, Sage Publications.

Hodge FS, Pasqua A, Marquez C et al.: Utilizing traditional storytelling to promote wellness in American Indian communities, *J Transcult Nurs* 13(1):6–11, 2002.

Hollingsworth AO, Brown LP, Brooten DA: The refugees and childbearing: what to expect, *RN* 43:45–48, 1980.

Jacobson SF: Native American health, *Annu Rev Nurs Res* 12:193–213, 1994.

James DC: Coping with a new society: the unique psychosocial problems of immigrant youth, *J Sch Health* 67(3):98–102, 1997.

Jandt F: *An introduction to intercultural communication: identities in a global community,* Thousand Oaks, CA, 2003, Sage Publications.

Juarez G, Ferrell B, Boreman T: Influence of culture on cancer pain management in Hispanic patients, *Cancer Pract* 6:262–269, 1998.

Kakar S: Western science, eastern minds, *Wilson Q* 15(1): 109–116, 1991.

Kavanagh K, Absalom K, Beil W et al.: Connecting and becoming culturally competent: a Lakota example, *Adv Nurs Sci* 21(3):9–31, 1999.

Kikuchi J: Cultural theories of nursing responsive to human needs and values, *J Nurs Scholarsh* 37(4):302–307, 2005.

Kleinman A: *Patients and healers in the context of culture,* Berkeley, CA, 1980, University of California Press.

Leininger M: *Transcultural nursing: concepts, theories, research and practice,* ed 2, Hillard, OH, 1995, McGraw-Hill.

Leininger M: Founder's focus: Transcultural nursing is discovery of self and the world of others, *J Transcult Nurs* 11(4):312–313, 2000.

Leonard B, Plotnikoff G: Awareness: the heart of cultural competence, *AACN Clin Issues* 11(1):51–59, 2000.

Lester N: Culture competence: a nursing dialogue, *Am J Nurs* 98(8):26–33, 1998.

Lewis R: *When cultures collide: managing successfully across cultures,* London, 2000, Nicholas Brealey Publishing.

Lipson JG: Culturally competent nursing care. In Lipson JG, Dibble SL, Minarik PA, editors, *Culture and nursing care,* San Francisco, 1996, UCSF Nursing Press.

Lipson J, Dibble S, Minarik P: *Culture and nursing care: A pocket guide,* San Francisco, 1996, UCSF Nursing Press.

Littlejohn-Blake SM, Darling CA: Understanding the strengths of African-American families, *J Black Stud* 23(4):460–471, 1993.

Long C, Curry M: Living in two worlds: Native American women and prenatal care, *Health Care Women Int* 19(3): 205–215, 1998.

Louie K: White paper on the health status of Asian-Americans and Pacific Islanders and recommendations for research, *Nurs Outlook* 49:173–178, 2001.

Ludwick R, Silva M: Nursing around the world: cultural values and ethical conflicts, *Online J Issues Nurs* [serial online] 2000; available online: http://www.nursingworld.org/ojin/ethicol/ethics_4.htm.

Masters K: *Role development in professional nursing practice,* Sudbury, MA, 2005, Jones and Bartlett.

McKennis A: Caring for the Islamic patient, *AORN J* 69(6):1185–1206, 1999.

McLaughlin L, Braun K: Asian and Pacific Islander cultural values: considerations for health care decision-making, *Health Soc Work* 23(2):116–126, 1998.

Mead M: *Sex and temperament in three primitive societies,* New York, 1988, William Morrow & Co.

Meisenhelder M, Bell J, Chandler E: Faith, prayer, and health outcomes in elderly Native Americans, *Clin Nurs Res* 9(2):191–204, 2000.

Michaels A: *Hinduism: past and present,* Princeton, NJ, 2003, Princeton University Press.

Minick P, Kee C, Borkat L et al.: Nurses' perceptions of people who are homeless, *West J Nurs Res* 20(3):356–369, 1998.

Nance TA: Intercultural communication: finding common ground, *J Obstet Gynecol Neonatal Nurs* 24(3):249–255, 1995.

Newhill C: The role of culture in the development of paranoid symptomatology, *Am J Orthopsychiatry* 60(2):176–185, 1990.

North American Nursing Diagnosis Association: *Nursing diagnoses: definitions and classification, 2005–2006*, Philadelphia, 2005, NANDA International.

Office of Minority Health, U.S. Department of Health and Human Services: (2001). www.omhrc.gov.

Pagani-Tousignant C: *Breaking the rules: counseling ethnic minorities*, Minneapolis, MN, 1992, The Johnson Institute.

Pasco A, Morse J, Olson J: The cross-cultural relationships between nurses and Filipino Canadian patients, *J Nurs Scholarsh* 36(3):239–246, 2004.

Pederson P: *A handbook for developing multicultural awareness*, Alexandria, VA, 1988, American Association for Counseling and Development.

Pederson P: Introduction to the special issue on multiculturalism as a fourth force in counseling, *J Counsel Dev* 70:4, 1991.

Purnell L: A description of the Purnell model for cultural competence, *J Transcult Nurs* 11(1):40–46, 2000.

Purnell L, Paulanka B: *Guide to culturally competent care*, Philadelphia, 2005, FA Davis.

Red Horse J: Traditional American Indian family systems, *Families, Systems & Health* 15(3):243–250, 1997.

Rosenbaum J: A cultural assessment guide: learning cultural sensitivity, *Can Nurse* 87(4):32–33, 1991.

Samovar L, Porter R, McDaniel E: *Intercultural communication: a reader*, ed 11, Belmont, CA, 2005, Wadsworth.

Santopietro M: How to get through to a refugee patient, *RN* 44:43–48, 1981.

Saylor C: The circle of health, *J Holist Nurs* 22(2):98–115, 2004.

Schim S, Doorenbos A, Borse N: Cultural competence among Ontario and Michigan healthcare providers, *J Nurs Scholarsh* 371(4):354–360, 2005.

Scott JK: Alice Modig and the talking circles, *Can Nurse* 87(6):25–26, 1991.

Searight H, Gafford J: Cultural diversity at the end of life: issues and guidelines for family physicians, *Am Fam Physician* 71:3, 2005.

Searight HR, Gafford J: Effect of culture on end-of-life decision making, *AAHPM Bull*, Winter 2005, 6(4):1–4; available online: www.aahpm.org/education/05winterconvertarticle.pdf.

Servodido C, Morse E: End of life issues, *Nurs Spectr* 11(8DC):20–23, 2001.

Shweder RA: *Thinking through cultures*, Cambridge, MA, 1991, Harvard University Press.

Smith L: Concept analysis: cultural competence, *J Cult Divers* 5(1):4–10, 1998.

Spector R: *Cultural diversity in health and illness*, ed 6, Upper Saddle River, NJ, 2004, Pearson Prentice Hall.

Spence D: Prejudice, paradox, and possibility: nursing people from cultures other than one's own, *J Transcult Nurs* 12(2): 100–106, 2001.

Sterritt P, Pokorny M: African American caregiving for a relative with Alzheimer's disease, *Geriatr Nurs* 19(3):127–128, 133–134, 1998.

Sutton M: Cultural competence, *Fam Pract Manag* 7(9): 58–62, 2000.

Thompson WL, Thompson TL, House RM: Taking care of culturally different and non–English speaking patients, *Int J Psychiatry Med* 20(3):235–245, 1990.

Tong V, Huang C, McIntyre T: Promoting a positive cross-cultural identity: reaching immigrant students, *Reclaiming Children and Youth* 14(4):203–208, 2006.

U.S. Census Bureau: United States Department of Commerce, 2001; accessed 3/21/01: http://www.census.gov.

U.S. Department of Health and Human Services: *Healthy people 2010: national health promotion and disease prevention objectives*, Washington, DC, 2000, Author.

U.S. Department of Health and Human Services: *National standards for cultural and linguistically appropriate services in health care. final report*, Washington, DC, 2001, Author.

Upvall MJ: Nursing perspectives of American Indian healing strategies, *J Multicult Nurs Health* 3(1):29–34, 1997.

Xu Y, Davidhizar R, Giger J: What if your nursing student is from an Asian culture, *J Cult Divers* 12(1):5–12, 2004.

Zapata J, Shippee-Rice R: The use of folk healing and healers by six Latinos living in New England, *J Transcult Nurs* 10(2):136–142, 1999.

Zoucha R: The keys to culturally sensitive care, *Am J Nurs* 100(2):24GG–24II, 2000.

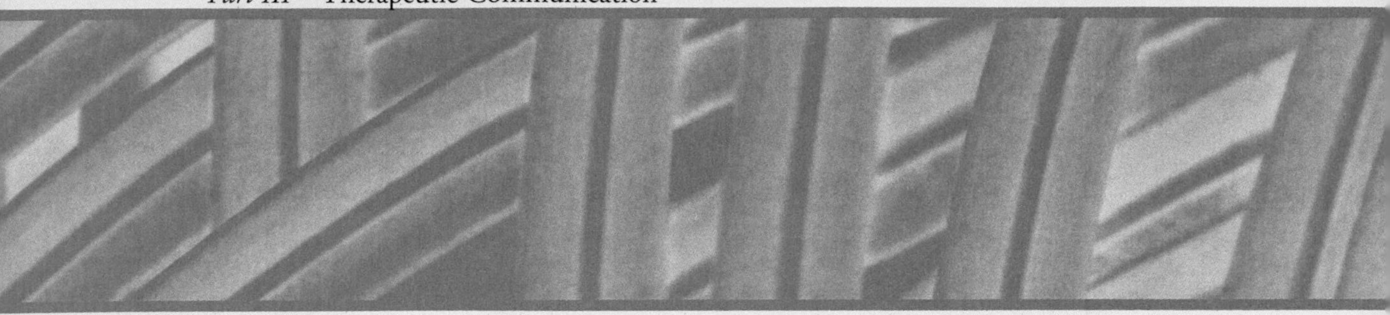

Chapter 12

Communicating in Groups

Elizabeth Arnold

OUTLINE

OBJECTIVES

At the end of the chapter, the reader will be able to:

1. Define group communication.
2. Identify the differences between primary and secondary groups.
3. Discuss factors that influence group dynamics.
4. Identify the stages of group development.
5. Apply group concepts in clinical settings.
6. Contrast different types of groups in heath care settings.

He knew intuitively how to be understanding and acceptant . . . This kind of ability shows up so commonly in groups that it has led me to believe that an ability to be healing or therapeutic is far more common in human life than we might suppose. Often it needs only the permission granted by a freely flowing group experience to become evident.

(Rogers, 1972)

Chapter 12 focuses on group communication in health care settings. At its most basic level, group communication is an integral form of communication in family, social, and work relationships and strongly influences a person's physical, emotional, and social development through the modeling and feedback a person receives in these relationships (Hawkins, 1998).

Group communication skills are an important dimension of professional growth in professional nursing. In work settings, groups represent an effective mechanism for discussing staff issues, effecting change, and establishing new work policies. Interdisciplinary health professionals work as a group to provide consistent and collaborative interactions for effective health care delivery (McGinley, Baus, Gyza et al., 1996).

Nurses use group formats to provide information and emotional support for clients and their families in a variety of health care settings ranging from preventive care to rehabilitation (Zahniser & Coursey, 1995). Therapy groups help people with behavior issues and low self-esteem learn more effective coping skills and achieve personal growth. Community health agencies provide important knowledge about lifestyle changes needed to promote health and well-being and to prevent illness. Support groups foster creative problem solving and provide community-based opportunities for people with serious health care problems to interact with others experiencing the same kinds of problems (Agapetus, 1996). As managed care limits interactions with health care professionals, support groups become increasingly important as a tool for people to share information about a specific illness, coping strategies, and resources (Yalom & Yalom, 1990).

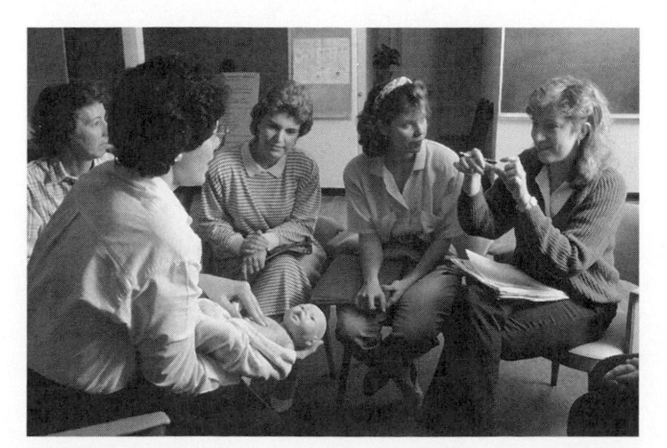

Groups offer a special forum for learning and emotional support. (Courtesy University of Maryland School of Nursing.)

BASIC CONCEPTS

A **group** is defined as (a) a gathering of two or more individuals (b) who share a common purpose and (c) meet over a substantial time period (d) in face-to-face interaction (e) to achieve an identifiable goal. A group is not simply a collection of individuals but rather a deliberate assembly of people who elect to be together because of a common cause, activity, purpose, or goal.

Every group has a unique collective personality. Groups develop a culture or personality, reflecting each group's unique behaviors. Relationships among members are interdependent, so that each member's behavior influences the behavior of other group members. Group cultures develop through shared images, values, and meanings that over time become the stories, myths, and metaphors about the group and how it functions.

Primary and Secondary Groups

Groups are categorized as primary or secondary groups. **Primary groups** are more spontaneous and linked to the values of an individual. Characterized by an informal structure and social process, group membership is either automatic (e.g., in a family) or is freely chosen because of a common interest (e.g., in scouting, religious, or civic groups). Primary groups are an important part of a person's self-concept, revealed in self-descriptions such as, "I am Jamie's mother."

Secondary groups are not spontaneous. They differ from primary groups in structure and purpose; they have a planned, time-limited association; a prescribed structure; a designated leader; and a specific, identified purpose. When the group achieves its goals, the group disbands. Examples include focus groups, therapy groups, discipline-specific work groups, interdisciplinary health care teams, and educational groups. People join secondary groups for one of three reasons: to meet personally established goals, to develop more effective coping skills, or because it is required by the larger community system to which the individual belongs. Exercise 12-1 presents a picture of the role groups play in a person's life.

Concepts Related to Group Dynamics

Group dynamics is a term used to describe the communication processes and behaviors occurring during the life of the group. They represent a complex blend of

Exercise 12-1 Role of Group Communication

Purpose: To help students gain an appreciation of the role group communication plays in their lives.

Procedure:

1. Write down all the groups in which you have been a participant (e.g., family; scouts; sports teams; community, religious, work, and social groups).
2. Describe the influence membership in each of these groups had on the development of your self-concept.
3. Identify the ways in which membership in different groups was of value in your life.
4. Identify the primary reason you joined each group. If you have discontinued membership, specify the reason.

Discussion:

1. How similar or dissimilar were your answers from those of your classmates?
2. What factors account for differences in the quantity and quality of your group memberships?
3. How similar were the ways in which membership enhanced your self-esteem?
4. If your answers were dissimilar, what makes membership in groups such a complex experience?
5. Could different people get different things out of very similar group experiences?
6. What implications does this exercise have for your nursing practice?

individual and group characteristics that combine with each other to achieve a group purpose. Group dynamics are an important influence on the success of goal achievement and member satisfaction (Figure 12-1).

Individual Characteristics

Commitment. Successful groups consist of members who are motivated to fulfill their responsibilities as group members. Members attend meetings through choice and feel

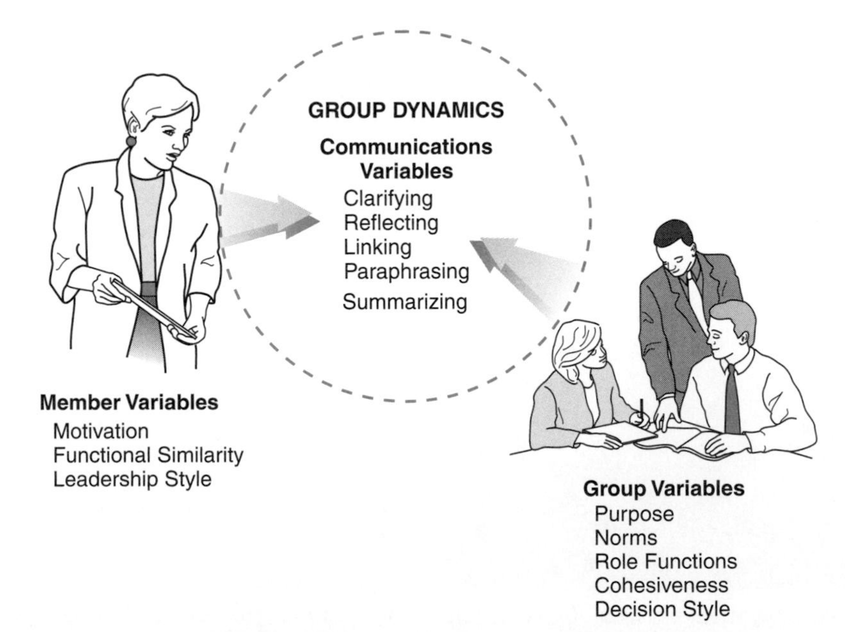

Figure 12-1 • Factors affecting group dynamics.

Exercise 12-2 Member Commitment

Purpose: To help students understand the connection of personal commitment to group dynamics.

Procedure:

1. In small groups of three to five students, think of a group to which you belonged that you would characterize as being successful.
2. What did you do in this group that contributed to its success?
3. What made this group easier to commit to than other groups to which you belonged? Be as specific as you can be about the factors that enhanced your commitment.
4. Have one student act as scribe and write down the factors that increased commitment to share with the rest of the class.

Discussion:

1. What are the common individual themes that emerged from the discussion?
2. Discuss the relationship of commitment to success.
3. Did commitment emerge as a major factor related to goal achievement?
4. Did commitment emerge as a major factor related to personal satisfaction?
5. What factors emerged as important variables in personal commitment?
6. How could you use what you learned in this exercise in client groups?

a sense of responsibility for the well-being of other group members. They achieve personal satisfaction from contributing to the group goal, which acts as reinforcement for further engagement. By contrast, lack of commitment results in group apathy, and rarely is the group task accomplished. The leader can increase group commitment by preparing members for the group before starting the group, allowing time to process possible resistance, and making group participation a matter of interest and benefit to

Exercise 12-3 Group Self-Disclosure: The Impact of Universality

Purpose: To provide students with the experience of universality and insight.

Procedure:

1. Break into groups of four to six people.
2. One person should act as a scribe.
3. Identify three things all members of your group have in common other than that you are in the same class and you are human (e.g., have siblings, have parents in the military, like sports or art).
4. Identify two things that are unique to each person in your group (e.g., only child, never moved from the area, born in another country, collect stamps).
5. Each person should elaborate on both the common and different experiences.

Discussion:

1. What was the effect of finding common ground with other group members?
2. In what ways did finding out about the uniqueness of each person's experience add to the discussion?
3. Did anything in either the discussion of commonalities or differences in experience stimulate further group discussion?
4. How could you use what you have learned in this exercise in your clinical practice?

individual members. Member commitment is discussed in Exercise 12-2.

Functional Similarity. Yalom (2005) describes **functional similarity** as meaning that group members have enough common intellectual, emotional, and experiential characteristics to interact with each other and to carry out the group objectives (Exercise 12-3). Some real-life examples illustrate the concept. Medication groups require a certain level of cognition because their goal is to provide education related to taking medication. The Alzheimer's disease victim, lacking the cognitive ability to acquire new information, generally does not benefit from such groups. A highly educated older adult placed in a group of young adults with limited verbal and educational skills is a misfit. In these cases, the different member becomes a group casualty. In another group, with clients who have similar issues, the outcome might be quite different.

The Ugly Duckling, a children's fairy tale of a baby swan trying to gain acceptance in a group of ducks, presents the dilemma of being different. It is difficult to be "one of a kind" and to capture a sense of belonging. Final acceptance and a sense of community comes when the swan recognizes and is recognized by the larger group as a part of the group membership. Careful selection of group members, based on their capacity to derive benefit from the group and to add to the discussion, is a critical individual variable in successful groups.

Functional similarity should not be confused with similarity of interpersonal communication style. Whereas it is important that group members speak enough of a common language to understand each other, differences in interpersonal styles help clients learn a broader range of behavioral responses. Having different ways of looking at things helps ensure a more lively discussion and a more productive outcome.

Group Variables

Purpose. The purpose of the group directly relates to the reason for the group's existence. It provides direction for membership decisions, development of group norms, and type of communication required to meet group goals. For example, if a group's purpose relates to medication compliance, the interventions would be educational. In contrast, a therapy group would relate to improved interpersonal functioning, with strategies designed to increase interpersonal insight into behavior. Common group purposes are presented in Table 12-1.

Table 12-1 Identifying Group Purpose

Group	Purpose
Therapy	Reality testing, encouraging personal growth, inspiring hope, strengthening personal resources, developing interpersonal skills
Support	Giving and receiving practical information and advice, supporting coping skills, promoting self-esteem, enhancing problem-solving skills, encouraging client autonomy, strengthening hope and resiliency
Activity	Getting people in touch with their bodies, releasing energy, enhancing self-esteem, encouraging cooperation, stimulating spontaneous interaction, supporting creativity
Education	Learning new knowledge, promoting skill development, providing support and feedback, supporting development of competency, promoting discussion of important health-related issues

Norms. **Group norms** are the behavioral standards expected of group members. Norms facilitate goal achievement because they provide the needed predictability for effective group functioning. For example, think of how a class group would operate if there were no behavioral standards. Suppose your instructor did not set a class agenda or provide expectations for student behavior. How satisfied would you be if students as well as the instructor did not hold you accountable for behaviors so that all might learn? What would it be like if you did not know what behaviors were needed to achieve a grade of *A* versus a *C*? Groups develop unspoken rules that shape the behaviors that a group will and will not tolerate. These norms reflect the values of its members. Some norms are universal standards, and others are specific to a particular group's dynamics.

Universal norms are behavioral standards held by most groups to be essential to the success of group life. Examples include confidentiality, regular attendance, and a willingness to share with others. Unless group members can trust that personal information revealed in the group will not be shared outside the group setting (confidentiality), the necessary trust will not develop. As with individual therapeutic relationships, some information about behaviors of individual clients may need to be shared with the health care team. If this is the case, members should understand beforehand what information will be shared and with whom.

Because the value of most groups depends on members sharing with each other, this is a prerequisite for group interaction. Regular attendance at group meetings is also critical to goal achievement. Without a commitment of attendance from each member, a group becomes an unstable means of promoting dialogue and action. Thus, repeated unexcused absences are not acceptable regardless of the reason; this is a universal norm.

Group-specific norms emerge from the combined expectations, values, and needs of group members. Although group members initially look to their leader to model important norms, other members will assume more active roles in defining and modifying behavioral standards as group trust evolves. Examples include the degree of individual risk taking, decision making, tolerance of humor and anger, focus on task or process, and level of leader control. For instance, some groups are characterized by blunt provocations designed to strip away a person's defenses and force members to confront their feelings. In other groups, confrontations are presented with tact and sensitivity. Once formed, norms are difficult to change, even when circumstances no longer warrant their existence. Exercise 12-4 will help you develop a deeper understanding of group norms.

Cohesiveness. **Cohesiveness** refers to the value a group holds for its members and their investment in being a part of the group (Yalom, 2005). Cohesiveness enhances commitment because people are willing to work harder to achieve individual and group goals when they value other group members and want to be a part of the group. Cohesiveness can develop from the appeal other group members personally hold for the individual, the significance of the group task, or the values and goals held by the group. Cohesiveness parallels the sense of mutuality and rapport that develops in successful one-to-one therapeutic relationships (Budman, Soldz, Demby et al., 1989).

Norms that encourage open expression of feelings, acceptance, and mutual support enhance cohesiveness, as does feeling valued by others. This, in turn, stimulates self-disclosure and a willingness to take interpersonal risks.

Caring for each other is strong outcome evidence of cohesiveness. The sense of human interdependency

Exercise 12-4 Identifying Norms

Purpose: To help identify norms operating in groups.

Procedure:

1. Divide a piece of paper into three columns.
2. In the first column, write the norms you think exist in your class or work group. In the second column, write the norms you think exist in your family. Examples of norms might be as follows: no one gets angry, decisions are made by consensus, assertive behaviors are valued, missed sessions and lateness are not tolerated.
3. Share your norms with the group, first related to the school or work group and then to the family. Place this information in the third column.

Discussion:

1. Were there many similarities between the norms you think exist in your school or work group and those that others in the same group had on their list?
2. Were there any "universal" norms on either of your lists?
3. Were you surprised either by some of the norms you wrote down when you thought about it or by those of your classmates?
4. Did you or other members in the group feel a need to refine or discuss the meaning of the norms on your list?
5. How difficult was it to determine implicit norms operating in the group?

Box 12-1 Communication Principles to Facilitate Cohesiveness

- Group tasks are within the membership's range of ability and expertise.
- Comments and responses are nonevaluative; they are focused on behaviors rather than on personal characteristics.
- The leader points out group accomplishments and acknowledges member contributions.
- The leader is empathetic and teaches members how to give feedback.
- The leader sanctions creative tension as necessary for goal achievement.

and community that develops within a group helps people who feel alienated to reconnect with others socially (Dallam & Manderino, 1997). Communication principles that enhance the development of cohesiveness are listed in Box 12-1. Research suggests that cohesive groups experience more personal satisfaction with goal achievement, and that members of such groups are more likely to join other group relationships (Brilhart & Galanes, 1997).

Group Think. Cohesiveness carried to an extreme results in **group think**, a term used to describe a group dynamic in which loyalty to the group and approval by other group members becomes so important that members are afraid to express conflicting ideas and opinions for fear of being excluded from the group. The group exerts pressure on members to act as one voice. Critical thinking and realistic appraisal of issues get lost (Janis, 1971; Rosenblum, 1982). The characteristics of group think are outlined in Figure 12-2.

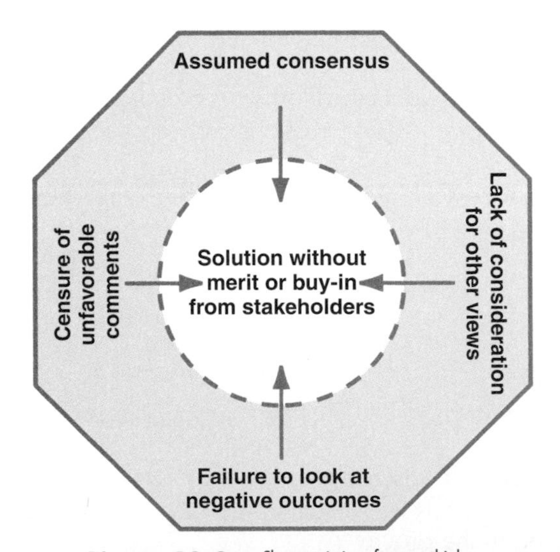

Figure 12-2 • Characteristics of group think.

Group Role Positions. People in groups assume roles that influence their communication and the responses of others. A person's role position in the group corresponds with the status, power, and internal image that other members in the group have of the member. Group members usually have trouble breaking away from roles they have been cast in despite their best efforts. For example, people will look to the "helper" group member for advice, even when that person lacks expertise or needs the group's help himself or herself. Other times, group members "project" a role position onto a particular group member that represents a hidden agenda or unresolved issue for the group as a whole (Gans & Alonso, 1998). For example, a monopolizer in a group is difficult to tolerate. Group members may resent the monopolization, but this person may actually serve a useful purpose for the group by diverting attention away from other members' equally critical issues. If the group as a whole seems to scapegoat, ignore, defer to, or consistently idealize one of its members, this group phenomenon can signify a group projection. Exercise 12-5 considers group role position expectation.

Some group members, because of the force of their personalities, emerge as dominant forces in a group. Groups often give power to the group members who best clarify the needs of the other group members or who move the group toward goal achievement. These are not always the group members making the most statements. A person can make few but very meaningful comments. What seems important is the ability to reflect and deliver the dominant thinking of a group in a concise, direct manner.

Case Example

Al is a powerful leader in a job search support group. Although he makes few comments, he has an excellent understanding of and sensitivity to the needs of individual members. When these are violated, Al speaks up and the group listens. His observations are always on target, and because he has the respect of the other group members, his opinions are influential in shaping the behaviors of other group members.

Exercise 12-5 **Headbands: Group Role Expectations**

Purpose: To experience the pressures of role expectations on group performance.

Procedure:

1. Break the group up into a smaller unit of six to eight members. In a large group, a small group performs while the remaining members observe.
2. Make up mailing labels or headbands that can be attached to or tied around the heads of the participants. Each headband is lettered with directions on how the other members should respond to the role. Examples:
   - Comedian: laugh at me
   - Expert: ask my advice
   - Important person: defer to me
   - Stupid: sneer at me
   - Insignificant: ignore me
   - Loser: pity me
   - Boss: obey me
   - Helpless: support me
3. Place a headband on each member in such a way that the member cannot read his or her own label, but the other members can see it easily.
4. Provide a topic for discussion (e.g., why the members chose nursing, the women's movement) and instruct each member to interact with the others in a way that is natural for him or her. Do not role-play, but be yourself. React to each member who speaks by following the instructions on the speaker's headband. You are not to tell each other what the headbands say, but simply to react to them.
5. After about 20 minutes, the facilitator halts the activity and directs each member to guess what his or her headband says, and then to take it off and read it.

Discussion:

Initiate a discussion, including any members who observed the activity. Possible questions include the following:

1. What were some of the problems of trying to "be yourself" under conditions of group role pressure?
2. How did it feel to be consistently misinterpreted by the group—to have them laugh when you were trying to be serious or ignore you when you were trying to make a point?
3. Did you find yourself changing your behavior in reaction to the group treatment of you—withdrawing when they ignored you, acting confident when they treated you with respect, giving orders when they deferred to you?

Modified from Pfeiffer J, Jones J: *A handbook of structured experiences for human relations training*, vol VI, La Jolla, CA, 1977, University Associate Publishers.

Role Functions. Role functions differ from the positional roles group members assume. Benne and Sheats (1948) described role functions as the behaviors members use to move toward goal achievement (**task functions**) and ensure personal satisfaction (**maintenance functions**). A healthy balance between task and maintenance functions increases group productivity. When task functions predominate to the exclusion of maintenance functions, member satisfaction decreases and there is less investment in the goal. Alternatively, groups in which maintenance functions override task functions do not always reach their goals and eventually will cease to exist. Group life flourishes, but little is accomplished. Members do not confront controversial issues, and the creative tension needed for successful group growth does not occur.

Within the group, a person may assume several different roles, although most people tend to gravitate toward one. Task and maintenance role functions found in most successful small groups are listed in Box 12-2. Exercise 12-6 gives practice in identifying task and maintenance functions.

Benne and Sheats (1948) also identified nonfunctional role functions in a group. Self-roles are roles a person uses to meet self-needs at the expense of other members' needs, group values, and goal achievement. Self-roles, identified in Table 12-2, detract from the group's work and compromise goal achievement by taking time away from group issues and creating discomfort among group members.

Box 12-2 Task and Maintenance Functions in Group Relations

Task Functions: Behaviors Relevant to the Attainment of Group Goals

- Initiating: Identifies tasks or goals; defines group problem; suggests relevant strategies for solving problem
- Seeking information or opinion: Requests facts from other members; asks other members for opinions; seeks suggestions or ideas for task accomplishment
- Giving information or opinion: Offers facts to other members; provides useful information about group concerns
- Clarifying, elaborating: Interprets ideas or suggestions placed before group; paraphrases key ideas; defines terms; adds information
- Summarizing: Pulls related ideas together; restates key ideas; offers a group solution or suggestion for other members to accept or reject
- Consensus taking: Checks to see whether group has reached a conclusion; asks group to test a possible decision

Maintenance Functions: Behaviors That Help the Group Maintain Harmonious Working Relationships

- Harmonizing: Attempts to reconcile disagreements; helps members reduce conflict and explore differences in a constructive manner
- Gatekeeping: Helps keep communication channels open; points out commonalties in remarks; suggests approaches that permit greater sharing
- Encouraging: Indicates by words and body language unconditional acceptance of others; agrees with contributions of other group members; is warm, friendly, and responsive to other group members
- Compromising: Admits mistakes; offers a concession when appropriate; modifies position in the interest of group cohesion
- Setting standards: Calls for the group to reassess or confirm implicit and explicit group norms when appropriate

Note: Every group needs both types of functions and needs to work out a satisfactory balance of task and maintenance activity.

Modified from Rogers C: The process of the basic encounter group. In Diedrich R, Dye, HA, editors, *Group procedures: purposes, processes and outcomes*, Boston, 1972, Houghton Mifflin.

Leadership. **Leadership** is defined as "interpersonal influence, exercised in situations and directed through the communication process, toward the attainment of a specified goal or goals" (Tannenbaum, Wechsler, & Massarik, 1988). Two basic assumptions support the function of group leadership: group leaders have a significant influence on group process; and most problems in groups can be avoided or reworked productively if the leader is aware of and responsive to the needs of individual group members, including the needs of the leader.

Effective leadership requires adequate preparation, professional leadership attitudes and behavior, responsible selection of members, and use of a responsible scientific rationale for determining a specific group approach.

Table 12-2 Nonfunctional Self-Roles

Role	Characteristics
Aggressor	Criticizes or blames others, personally attacks other members, uses sarcasm and hostility in interactions
Blocker	Instantly rejects ideas or argues an idea to death, cites tangential ideas and opinions, obstructs decision making
Joker	Disrupts work of the group by constantly joking and refusing to take group task seriously
Avoider	Whispers to others, daydreams, doodles, acts indifferent and passive
Self-confessor	Uses the group to express personal views and feelings unrelated to group task
Recognition seeker	Seeks attention by excessive talking, trying to gain leader's favor, expressing extreme ideas, or demonstrating peculiar behavior

Modified from Benne KD, Sheats P: Functional roles of group members, *J Soc Issues* 4(2):41-49, 1948.

Exercise 12-6 Task Functions Versus Maintenance Functions

Purpose: To help students identify task functions versus maintenance functions.

Procedure:

1. Break up into groups of eight students each.
2. Choose a topic to discuss (e.g., how you would restructure the nursing program; nursing and the women's movement; the value of a group experience; nursing as a profession).
3. Two students should volunteer to be the observers.
4. The students discuss the topics for 30 minutes; observers use the initial of each student and the grid below to mark with a tick (/) the number of times each student uses a task or maintenance function.
5. After completion of the group interaction, each observer shares his or her observations with the other group members.

Task Functions

Initiating ____

Information seeking ____

Clarifying ____

Consensus taking ____

Testing ____

Summarizing ____

Maintenance Functions

Encouraging ____

Expressing ____

Group feeling ____

Harmonizing ____

Compromising ____

Gatekeeping ____

Setting standards ____

Discussion:

1. Was there an adequate balance between task and maintenance activity?
2. What roles did different members assume?
3. Were the two observers in agreement as to members' assumptions of task versus maintenance functions? If there were discrepancies, what do you think contributed to their occurrence?
4. What did you learn from this exercise?

Personal characteristics needed by the group leader to be effective include a commitment to the group purpose; self-awareness of personal biases, values, and interpersonal limitations; and an open attitude toward group members. Beginning practitioners with knowledge of group dynamics can lead discussions, educational sessions, and some types of activity groups. Additional training and supervision are needed to lead a psychotherapy group effectively. Educational group leaders need to have expertise on the topic for discussion. Characteristics of effective and ineffective groups are presented in Table 12-3.

Table 12-3 Characteristics of Effective and Ineffective Groups

Effective Groups	Ineffective Groups
Goals are clearly identified and collaboratively developed.	Goals are vague or imposed on the group without discussion.
Open, goal-directed communication of feelings and ideas is encouraged.	Communication is guarded; feelings are not always given attention.
Power is equally shared and rotates among members, depending on ability and group needs.	Power resides in the leader or is delegated with little regard to member needs. It is not shared.
Decision making is flexible and adapted to group needs.	Decision making occurs with little or no consultation. Consensus is expected rather than negotiated based on data.
Controversy is viewed as healthy because it builds member involvement and creates stronger solutions.	Controversy and open conflict are not tolerated.
There is a healthy balance between task and maintenance role functioning.	There is a one-sided focus on task or maintenance role functions to the exclusion of the complementary function.
Individual contributions are acknowledged and respected. Diversity is encouraged.	Individual resources are not used. Conformity, the "company man," is rewarded. Diversity is not respected.
Interpersonal effectiveness, innovation, and problem-solving adequacy are evident.	Problem-solving abilities, morale, and interpersonal effectiveness are low and undervalued.

Effective leaders are good listeners. They are competent and able to convey warmth and understanding. Effective leaders adapt their leadership style to fit the changing needs of the group. Effective group leaders are committed to group goals and to supporting the integrity of group members as equal partners in meeting these goals. Effective group leaders have a clear understanding of their skills and limitations. Such knowledge allows the nurse to choose to explore new roles or to use previously untapped skills.

The *designated leader* in most health care settings is a health professional with training in group dynamics and process. *Emergent leaders* are informal leaders who emerge from the group membership and are recognized

Exercise 12-7 Clarifying Personal Leadership Role Preferences

Purpose: To help students focus on how they personally experience the leadership role.

Procedure:
Answer the following questions briefly:
1. What do you enjoy most about the leadership role?
2. What do you like least about the leadership role?
3. What skills do you bring to the leadership role?
4. What are the differences in your functioning as a group member and as a group leader?

Discussion:
1. What types of transferable skills did you find you bring to the leadership role? For example, are you an oldest child? Did you organize a play group? Did you teach swimming to mentally handicapped children in high school? Are you a member of a large family?
2. Were some of the uncomfortable feelings "universal" for a majority of the group?
3. What skills would you need to develop in order to feel comfortable as a group leader?
4. What did you learn about yourself from doing this exercise?

by other group members as powerful and often having equal status with the designated leader. Ideally, group leadership is a shared function of all group members, with many emergent leaders and each member contributing to the overall functioning of the group (Brilhart & Galanes, 1997). Exercise 12-7 is designed to help you develop an understanding of the leadership role.

Decision Making. Group decision making often yields a better product than individual solutions for three reasons. First, the knowledge, skills, and resources of all participants are available to influence the solution; group members build on one another's ideas. Second, because so many different perspectives are available in group thinking, it is more likely that positive and negative consequences of each solution will be considered. Third, if the decision is to be implemented by a group rather than an individual, including those affected by the solution in the decision-making process ensures ownership and greater likelihood of compliance. Each decision-making approach will have different consequences for the group.

The steps in group decision making follow a defined sequence. First, the group considers the nature of the problem and the amount of time and level of resources available to resolve it. Then the group brainstorms all possible solutions. Initially, the group gives equal weight to all proposed solutions, the only stipulation being that the solution must relate to the problem under discussion. Once the group generates sufficient ideas, group members begin to analyze potential alternatives and narrow their selection to the most promising ones. Group members consider the consequences of the refined alternatives and the impact on all of the people (stakeholders) who will be affected by the solution. The actual selection of the most promising solution is the outcome of the decision-making process. Further refinements occur as the solution gets implemented.

Developing an Evidence-Based Practice

Erwin P, Purves D, Johannes K: Involvement and outcomes in short-term interpersonal cognitive problem solving groups, *Counsell Psychol Q* 18(1):41-46, 2005.

This quantitative study was designed to explore the extent to which involvement in a short-term interpersonal cognitive problem solving group could predict improvement in interpersonal cognitive problem-solving skills. A convenience sample of 31 children were assigned to either an experimental (N = 16) or control (N = 15) group. All study participants were given a pre- and post-test for interpersonal cognitive problem-solving skills.

Results: Findings indicated significantly greater improvement in these skills with study participants in the experimental group compared to the control group. (N= 761) regarding barriers and facilitators to their utilizing research in clinical practice. Reported barriers included time constraints, lack of awareness about availability of research literature, insufficient authority and/or lack of support to make changes based on research findings, and lack of knowledge needed for critique of research studies. Facilitators included availability of time, access and support for review and implementation of research findings, and support of colleagues.

Application to Your Clinical Practice: Study findings suggest a significant relationship between group learning and positive outcomes for problem-solving skills. What kinds of problems do you see in your clinical experience that might lend themselves to short-term group intervention?

Concepts Related to Group Process

Group process refers to the structural development of the group, or its life cycle. Groups follow progressive stages of development that parallel the developmental stages of individual relationships. Each phase of group development has its own set of tasks that build and expand on the work of previous phases. Phases overlap, and the group can return to an earlier stage of development as it faces crises or as membership changes. Tuckman's (1965) theory of small group development provides an uncomplicated theoretical framework for examining group process at different stages in the life of the group. He described five stages: forming, storming, norming, performing, and adjourning.

Group process also describes the order in which topics are brought up and how the group responds to them both verbally and nonverbally. For example, expecting a newly formed group to move directly into problem resolution without first going through the necessary introductory stages of building trust can cause needless frustration and conflict. Having knowledge of group process helps the leader to recognize the conflict emerging in the storming phase of group development as a normal and necessary stage rather than as resistance on the part of individual members. Viewed in this way, the interventions are likely to be compassionate and productive.

APPLICATIONS

Comparison Between Group and Individual Communication

Group communication shares many of the characteristics of individual communication. The acceptance, respect, and understanding needed in individual relationships are essential components of effective group communication. Similar communication strategies of using open-ended questions, reflecting, paraphrasing, asking for clarification, linking, and summarizing are also important in group communication. Minimal cues in the form of eye contact with speakers and other group members, leaning forward, nodding, and smiling encourage sharing in groups. Allowing for pauses when it looks as though people are thinking is particularly important in groups. Usually it is anxiety-provoking but worthwhile to wait. Pauses serve a similar purpose of bracketing information and allowing think time. The group leader can use a variety of listening responses to respond to a client's statements, each of which can elicit a different focus.

Case Example

Group member: I hate my work. No matter how hard I try, I can't please my boss. I'd quit tomorrow if I could.

Leader: I'm not sure I quite understand your situation; could you tell me more about it? (*Asking for clarification*)

Leader: From what you say, it sounds as though you are feeling desperate. (*Reflecting*)

Leader: You're so unhappy with what is going on at work that you are thinking of quitting. (*Paraphrasing*)

As in individual relationships, the nurse links ideas with feelings and periodically summarizes member contributions, but there is an important distinction. Instead of simply linking ideas with feelings, the leader also links together common themes from two or more members.

Case Example

Carrie: I feel like giving up. I've tried to do everything right, and I still can't seem to get good grades in my classes.

Leader: I wonder if the discouragement you are feeling is similar to Mary's disenchantment with her job and Bill's desire to throw in the towel on his marriage.

Periodically, the leader summarizes or asks members to summarize the group's activities with an observational statement about the group dynamics for that session. For example, the nurse might say, "Today it seems as though we covered a lot of ground in finding useful strategies to reduce stress." Alternatively, the nurse might invite group members to respond: "We're almost out of time; I wonder if any of you have any final comments you'd like to make."

Although there are similarities, there are also important differences between individual and group communication strategies. Group communication is more complex because each member brings to the group a different set of perspectives, perception of reality, communication style, and personal agenda. Many people find it more difficult to express themselves in a group initially, and the leader may need to help them feel more comfortable. Because the focus is on group interaction rather than the I-thou communication of an individual therapeutic relationship, the leader might ask other group members for their reaction rather than give a personal response.

Case Example

Martha: I was upset with last week's meeting because I didn't feel we made any progress. Everyone complained, but no one had a solution.

Leader: I wonder if other people feel as Martha does. Would anyone like to respond to what Martha just said?

Box 12-3 Suggestions for Giving Feedback

- Be specific and direct.
- Support comments with evidence.
- Separate the issue from the person.
- "Sandwich" negative messages between positive ones.
- Pose the situation as a mutual problem.
- Mitigate or soften negative messages to avoid overload.
- Deliver feedback close to occurrence.
- Manner of delivery:
  - Assertive, dynamic
  - Trustworthy, fair, and credible
  - Relaxed and responsive
  - Preserve public image of recipient

From Haslett B, Ogilvie J: Feedback processes in task groups. In Cathcart R, Samovar L, editors, *Small group communication: a reader*, ed 5, Dubuque, IA, 1988, William C. Brown, p. 397.

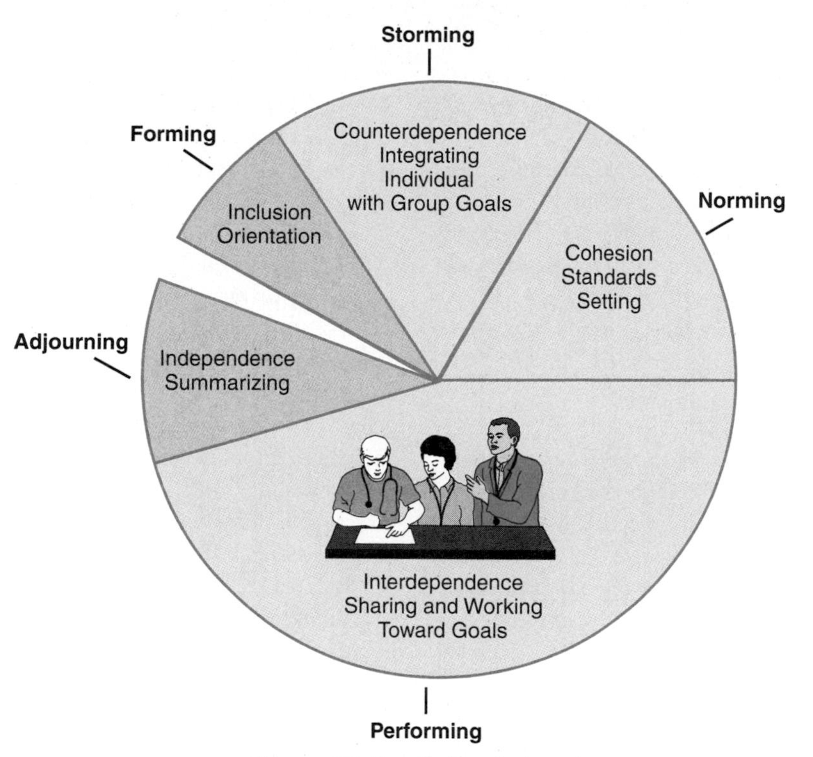

Figure 12-3 • The life cycle of groups.

A summary of suggestions for group communication feedback is presented in Box 12-3.

Leader Tasks in the Life Cycle of a Group

Figure 12-3 depicts the life cycle of groups. Descriptions of the tasks follow.

Before the Group Begins: Assessment and Planning

Before the group begins, the group leader considers the most effective structural framework for the group, given its purpose and goals. Foremost is the question, "What is the purpose of this group?" A well-defined group purpose gives direction to member selection and the establishment of group goals. Purpose dictates the group structure and format. A group's purpose can be educational, therapeutic, supportive, or designed to work on a particular problem or issue. For example, a medication group would have an educational purpose. A group for parents with critically ill children would have a supportive design, and a therapy group would have a therapeutic expectation. Exploration of personal experience would be limited and related to the topic under discussion in an education group. In a therapy group, such probing would be encouraged.

Defining the Goals of the Group

Group goals reflect the purpose of the group but differ in that they provide information about the therapeutic outcome a group hopes to attain through its efforts. For example, a group goal might be that the "group members will demonstrate knowledge of the actions and side effects of their medications." Group goals need to be achievable, measurable, and within the capabilities of group membership. Identifying a group goal helps the leader determine the time frame and type of membership needed to achieve the group objectives. Evidence of goal achievement justifies the existence of the group and increases client satisfaction.

Matching Client Needs with Group Goals

Matching group goals with client needs is essential. The leader needs to ask, "How will being in this group enhance a client's health and well-being?" When there is a good match and clients have the capacity to contribute to the group, members develop commitment and perceive the group as having value. When this is not the case, the group experience can be destructive. For example, clients with serious verbal difficulties, significant memory deficits, or limited tolerance for cooperative behaviors do best in group situations specially geared to meet their needs. Placing such a client in a therapy group in which group participation requires high-level cognitive processing would be inappropriate. "Patient mix difficult for the group" was the most commonly mentioned perceived barrier to nurse-conducted groups in a study completed by Van Servellen, Poster, Ryan et al. (1991).

Types of Group Membership

The leader needs to decide whether the group will have a closed or an open membership and whether the group goals are better achieved with a homogeneous or heterogeneous membership. **Closed groups** have a defined membership with an expectation of regular attendance and time commitment, usually at least 12 sessions. Group members may be added, but their inclusion depends on a fit with group-defined criteria. Most psychotherapy groups fall into this category. **Open groups** do not have a defined membership other than that imposed by the purpose and goals of the group. Anyone can attend. Individuals come and go depending on their needs, so that one week the group might consist of 2 or 3 members and the next week 15 members. Of necessity, norms are much looser. Most community support groups have open membership.

Another way of determining group membership is using homogeneous versus heterogeneous membership. **Homogeneous groups** have a common denominator pertaining to all members of the group, such as a diagnosis (e.g., breast cancer support group) or a personal characteristic (e.g., gender or age). Research indicates that such groups benefit clients who are coping with issues of exclusive importance to a particular group (e.g., a women's group focused on women's issues) (Prehn & Thomas, 1990). Psychotic clients and individuals with a specific diagnostic behavioral focus, such as eating disorders or drug addiction, Alcoholics Anonymous, ostomy clubs, Compassionate Friends, Alzheimer's disease family support groups, and gender-specific consciousness-raising groups are familiar examples of homogeneous groups.

Heterogeneous groups may represent a wide diversity of human experience and problems, consisting of members who vary in age, gender, and psychodynamics. Most psychotherapy and insight-oriented personal growth groups have a heterogeneous membership (Bertcher & Maple, 1985). Educational groups held on inpatient units (e.g., medication groups) typically are heterogeneous related to factors such as educational background, age, and gender.

Creating the Appropriate Environment

Complete privacy and freedom from interruptions are key considerations in selecting an appropriate site for group activity. The group should be conducted in a quiet, open space, apart from the mainstream of activity. The room should be neither too hot nor too cold and large enough to accommodate all participants comfortably. Holding meetings in the same room each time fosters continuity and trust. A sign on the door indicating the group is in session prevents unwelcome intrusions.

Seats should be comfortable and arranged in a circle so that each member has face-to-face contact with other members and clear access to the facial expressions and nonverbal cues that accompany member communication. Being able to see and respond to several individuals at one time is essential to effective group communication (see Figure 12-1).

The number of sessions, time of day, and frequency of meetings depend on the type of group and the group goals. For example, a work group might meet twice a month, whereas a therapy group might meet weekly. Support groups meet as often as once a week or as infrequently as once a month. An educational group might meet for one to eight sessions and then disband.

Although the length of a group session may vary, most groups meet for 60 to 90 minutes on a regular basis with established, agreed-on meeting times. Having a time that is convenient and does not conflict with the members' other obligations enhances group participation. Groups that begin and end on time help create an atmosphere of trust and predictability.

Determining Appropriate Group Size

The purpose and goals of the group will influence the number of members needed. In general, therapy and personal growth groups consist of six to eight members. With this number of people there is sufficient time and space to express feelings and get feedback. The group is large enough to contain a diversity of opinions and ideas, yet small enough to permit intimate connection with all of the other members. Generally, therapy groups should not have fewer than five members. With less than this number, interaction tends to be more limited, and if one or more members are absent, the group interaction can become intense and uncomfortable for the remaining members. Educational groups are traditionally larger than therapy groups. Twelve to 20 members is common, but because the focus is on relating to the presentation of a speaker, the level of interaction is not as important as it is in a therapy group.

Conducting a Pre-Group Interview

If the group has a therapeutic purpose, the leader may want to meet with the prospective members before the first meeting. The purpose of this interview is to explain the goals of the group, assess the client's suitability for placement in the group, describe the type of commitment needed, and structure an opportunity for the client to ask questions. The description of the group and of its members is kept short and simple. The nurse asks potential clients what they hope to obtain from the group experience and the kinds of issues they wish to explore. Using this approach, the nurse has a better idea of client expectations and is better able to correct misperceptions. The leader allows ample time for questions and comments.

Phases of the Group Life Cycle

Forming Phase

The initial phase of group development is the forming phase. When the group has just formed, members experience much anxiety (Jacobson, 1989). The basic need of members is acceptance. Time and effort must be given to developing commitment and trust before the actual work of the group takes place. Getting to know each other and finding common threads in personal experience seem to be important aspects of beginning group life that cannot be shortchanged without having a serious impact on the evolving effectiveness of the group (Yalom, 2005).

Developing Trust. People enter group relationships as strangers to each other. Communication is superficial, and trust is at a surface level as members get to know one another. Regardless of the importance of the identified task, the emphasis in the beginning is on getting to know other group members; their interpersonal boundaries; and their basic orientation to the sharing of responsibility, collaborative decision making, and control. Common initial questions of members include the following:

- Will I be accepted for who I am as a person in this group?
- Can I really say what I feel? What happens if I am honest with my feelings?
- Will I be expected to perform, or can I just be myself in this group?
- Am I enough like the other members to feel comfortable participating?
- Can I count on the leader to establish norms that respect my uniqueness as a person?

The leader takes an active role in helping the group members feel acceptance. The leader might initially ask the members to introduce themselves and give a little of their background or their reason for coming to the group. Either the leader or the person who looks most at ease can start the introduction. This can be followed by a general leading question, if appropriate, to the group focus: "As we begin, I would like to ask each of you, what does (stress, having a baby, a diagnosis of cancer, being in this group) mean to you?" or "I'm sure everyone here has a different mental image of what a (therapy, support, educational) group is like. I wonder if you would be willing to share your perceptions." Finding that others have the same fears and perceptions decreases anxiety. Clients need to be educated about the nature of the group process and the behaviors required to achieve group goals.

The group leader's role is to facilitate group interaction. In the first session, the group leader identifies the purpose and goals of the group and allows ample time for questions. Although members may know the purpose ahead of time, taking the time to verbalize the purpose allows group members to hear it in the same way. Sometimes members' responses and questions related to purpose or goals provide important information to individual group members as well as to the group's leader. Next, the leader clarifies how the group will be conducted and what the group can expect from the leader and other members in achieving group goals. Knowing what to expect helps to reduce anxiety.

Case Example

Nurse Leader (prenatal group): **I will be giving you information about taking the best care of yourself before the baby comes and what to expect during labor** and delivery. This is a special time, and the more you know about yourself and your baby, the more you will get out of the group experience. It is very important that you ask questions and provide your ideas as we go along.

Fostering Mutual Identification (Universality). Identification with others is an important element in the formation of bonds (Eibl-Eibesfeldt, 1975). As people talk about themselves, their hopes, and their fears, other group members hear the echo of their own experience. They both understand and feel understood when this occurs. Knowing that you are not alone and that other people have the same fears and reactions helps put difficult health issues in perspective (Brandman, 1996). The leader may start with asking clients to talk about their expectations (e.g., "It's useful at the start of a group to have an idea of what each of you would like to get out of the group. I'd like to start with Jack and ask what each of you hopes to get out of being here"). In addition to enhancing mutual identification among members, this strategy also gives the leader an opportunity to correct misperceptions about group goals. As members develop a growing group identification, content and process issues tend to carry over from one group session to another. There is a developing sense of continuity within the group as the group begins to assume active responsibility for its own functioning.

Establishing the Group Contract. The group leader develops a working agreement with group members that specifies the time and place of meetings, the nature of the group interaction, and behavioral expectations of members. The group contract becomes a shared commitment to and with the group.

The leader identifies universal or explicit behavioral norms such as confidentiality, attendance, and mutual respect (Corey & Corey, 2006); group-specific norms are negotiated as the group matures. From the beginning, nurse group leaders model an attitude of caring, objectivity, and integrity in their communication with group members. Other common explicit behavioral norms include focusing on "here and now" interactions, giving feedback to each other, sharing personal thoughts and feelings, and listening to each other (Corey & Corey, 2006).

Storming Phase

Once people feel comfortable with each other, a transitional stage in group development follows in which people strive to understand themselves and other group members at a deeper level. Referred to as the storming phase, group members cope with power and control issues. People use testing behaviors to elicit boundaries, communication styles, and personal reactions from other members and from the leader. Such behaviors might include disagreement with the group format, the topics for discussion, the best ways to achieve group goals, and certain member contributions compared with other member offerings. Although this stage is uncomfortable, it leads to the development of group norms and thus is a very important stage in group development.

The leader plays an important role in the storming phase by accepting differences in group member perceptions as normal and growth producing, and by balancing group forces when one member threatens to sabotage group efforts or becomes the target of group reaction. For example, the leader can follow a different opinion made by a member with a statement such as, "That is a good point" or, "That comment is right on target with the next issue we need to take up" or, "Thank you for clarifying your position." The group leader models effective group behaviors and directly confronts sabotage behavior with statements that deal with behavior rather than motivation.

Case Example

Leader: As I understand it, you agree with John that he should take his medication when he needs it, but you don't think he is paying enough attention to the times when his symptoms are getting out of control. Is that correct?

In this way, the participants are challenged to express differences, and the leader demonstrates an appropriate way to word statements of disagreement. Focusing on the positive comments of members and linking the constructive themes of members are effective modeling behaviors.

The group leader can also ask for group input, a particularly useful strategy when one group member is monopolizing the conversation. For example, the nurse might reflect out loud in the group, "I wonder if others in the group share Bob's reservations" or, "How would other group members respond to what Bob is saying?" Looking in the direction of positive group members as the statements are made also encourages member response. It is important for the group leader to remain nonreactive and to redirect provocative remarks back to their maker or to the group, for example, "Bill, I wonder if you might be able to tell us a little more about how you personally feel about this project without bringing anyone else into it."

If a member continues to monopolize the conversation, the leader can respectfully acknowledge the person's comment and refocus the issue within the group: "I appreciate your thoughts, but I think it would be important to hear from other people as well. What do you think about this, Jane?" or, "That sounds like a strong position on __________. I'm wondering if others agree or disagree."

Members who test boundaries through sexually provocative, overly flattering, or insulting remarks need to have limits set promptly: "That behavior isn't appropriate in the group. Our purpose as a group is to help each other, and your behavior is preventing that from happening." Resolution of this stage may be seen in the willingness of members to take stands on their personal preferences without being defensive and in accepting the comments of other members. Gradually, the group will begin to seek compromises: "I think we should consider our first proposal" or, "Maybe we should consider a number of options before we decide on this." When such comments are made, the group is ready to establish group norms, which are needed for the group to reach its goals.

Norming Phase

As the group enters the norming phase, feedback becomes more spontaneous and group members begin to share more responsibility for the leadership of the group. Out of the conflict and newfound cooperation emerge behavioral standards that will help the group achieve its task. Group members exchange more personal information about each other and begin to think more about the task at hand. Common agreement develops about the behavioral standards expected if the group is to achieve its goals. Individual goals become aligned with group goals. Once the group norms are established, the group holds members accountable and challenges individual members who fail to adhere to them. When this occurs, the leader can help the erring member see that it is because he or she is important to the functioning of the group that this matters.

Table 12-4 Leader Strategies in the Performing (Working) Phase

Strategic Action	Sample Leader Statement
Maintain focus on main themes related to group goals	"I think that maybe we're straying a little away from our discussion of the triggers that make people feel like drinking. I wonder what people are feeling right now."
Emphasize the here and now	
Between members	"I wonder if we could look at what happened between Barbara and Bill just now."
Between a group member and the group as a whole	"Would you be willing to let the members of the group give you some feedback about how they experienced your story tonight?"
Leader self-disclosure	"May I share some of my personal reactions about what I experienced when you told your story?" This can be followed by a statement such as, "I wonder how other group members experienced what you were saying."
Summarize at critical points and at the end of each session (this helps the group members to feel heard, allows correction of distortions, and provides transitions to future topics)	"I think we did a lot of good work tonight. My sense is that the group is saying that . . ." Alternatively, the group leader can ask group members if anyone would like to summarize what they think happened in the group.

Performing Phase

Most of the group's work is accomplished in the performing phase. Cohesiveness develops to a stronger degree so that the group is free to work on issues as they relate to the accomplishment of group goals. Working together on a project or participating in another person's personal growth allows members to experience one another's personal strengths and the collective caring of the group. Therefore, there is an esprit de corps and a possibility of affirmation. Affirmation is an abstract feeling that people experience as feeling validated, respected, and cared about as a person. The experience of affirmation occurs unexpectedly and emotionally rather than intellectually. Affirmation usually occurs in a way one never would have anticipated, yet it normally exceeds one's fondest expectations. Of all the possibilities that can happen in a group, feeling affirmed and respected is most highly valued by group members (Table 12-4).

Adjourning Phase

The final phase of group development is termination or adjournment, which ideally occurs when the group members have achieved desired outcomes. The leader encourages the group members to express their feelings about one another as significant group members and their perception of personal contributions to attainment of identified objectives. Each member can do this in turn, perhaps ending with the leader, who adds his or her own personal observations and feelings. Any concerns the group may have about an individual member or suggestions for future growth can be stated with a constructive purpose. By waiting until the group ends to share closing comments, the leader has an opportunity to soften or clarify previous comments, to connect cognitive and feeling elements, and to summarize the group experience. The leader needs to remind members that the norm of confidentiality does not end with the completion of the group. Exercise 12-8 considers group closure issues.

Types of Therapeutic Groups

The term *therapeutic*, as it applies to group relationships, refers to more than simply the treatment of emotional and behavioral disorders. The broad purpose of therapeutic groups is to increase knowledge of oneself and others, helping to clarify the changes that are wanted and to develop the tools needed to make changes (Corey & Corey, 2006). Support groups for mentally healthy individuals who are seeking personal growth or emotional support are considered in the broad category of therapeutic groups. Psychoeducational, parenting, and medication groups have a therapeutic purpose because they empower people to take responsibility for important aspects of their health and well-being. In today's

Exercise 12-8 Group Closure, Expressing Affection

Purpose: To experience summarizing feelings about group members.

Procedure:

1. Focus your attention on the group member next to you and think about what you like about the person, how you see him or her in the group, and what you might wish for that person as a member of the group.
2. After five minutes, your instructor will ask you to tell the person next to you to use the three themes in making a statement about the person. For example, "The thing I most like about you in the group is . . ."; "To me you represent the __________ in the group"; and so on.
3. When all of the group members have had a turn, discussion may start.

Discussion:

1. How difficult was it to capture the person's meaning in one statement?
2. How did you experience telling someone about your response to him or her in the group?
3. How did you feel being the group member receiving the message?
4. What did you learn about yourself from doing this exercise?
5. What implications does this exercise have for future interactions in group relationships?

health care arena, short-term groups are being designed for a wide range of different client populations as a first line intervention to either remediate problems or prevent them (Corey & Corey, 2006).

In a group, a client can feel a deep sense of identification with other members who are dealing with issues that are similar to the one that concerns the client (Goldstein, Alter, & Axelrod, 1996). The group becomes a valued resource (cohesiveness). The social contact and support that clients experience with other group members who are in the same predicament as they and who have the same supposedly unacceptable feelings provide a different perspective of self that simply is not available in a one-to-one interpersonal relationship (Kreidler & Carlson, 1991). Within a natural, safe setting, the person can hear and see from the experiences of others that he or she is not unique or alone, and that difficulties can be resolved. Feeling understood by peers who are struggling with similar issues (universality) helps people feel tremendous relief that the struggle is not unique or incomprehensible to others. Having a regular, safe place to talk about problems helps. A woman undergoing chemotherapy in a breast cancer support group expressed the value of the group experience in the following way:

> I'm hopeful that this treatment will work, but I'm also dealing with the fact that I might not make it. But I can't talk with my husband about it because he doesn't want to see me cry. Mom has had enough. I have to keep a stiff upper lip with my friends and children because they can't handle my talking about dying. They think I'm giving up. I'm not, but I need to talk about it with someone who understands. I have no one to turn to . . . This group is my lifeline.

Therapeutic groups offer a structured format that encourages a person to experience his or her natural healing potential (instillation of hope), and other group members reinforce individual group member's resolve. When six other people are supportive and understanding and, even more important, when they think there are solutions a client may have overlooked, it is difficult to deny the warmth and obvious caring that can foster hope. Sharing intimate feelings with one another (catharsis), coupled with the respect others have for the worth and uniqueness of the individual, strengthens personal resources (self-responsibility) and stimulates creative solutions to a problem.

Therapeutic groups provide reality testing. People under stress lose perspective. Loss of perspective compromises effective problem solving because the problem seems too big to manage. In groups, other group members usually scrutinize a member's global statements and gently suggest alternative explanations. They rarely accept universal statements at face value and can say things to the client that friends and relatives are afraid to say for fear of offending the client.

Case Example

Client: I have been worthless since I had this heart attack. I can't do anything anymore.

This global statement represents a real and pervasive feeling, but the statement reveals little else about the remaining capabilities of the individual. It probably is not true that the person has lost all value. In a group, others might challenge the validity of this client's statement.

Nurse: I can appreciate that the shock of having a heart attack can leave you feeling off balance, but I wonder how others see your situation.

Generally, other group members will give the client specific feedback that offers insights the client has not considered. Coming from peers in similar circumstances, the feedback has a special credibility. After discussion, the client might develop a more specific problem-centered statement (self-understanding) that accurately reflects his or her situation.

Client: Six weeks ago, I had a heart attack. I feel worthless because my activities are restricted.

Individuals tend to act in groups as they do in real life. The group provides a mirror with which clients can learn how others perceive them so that they can learn more adaptive responses (Brandman, 1996). When situations cannot be changed, therapeutic groups help clients accept that reality and move on with their lives. They empower clients, providing needed emotional reinforcement and comfort for clients through the supportive framework of caring words and caring actions (Dobrof, Umpierre, Rocha et al., 1990). A hidden benefit of the therapeutic group experience is the opportunity for clients to experience giving as well as receiving help from others. A satisfaction in helping others enhances self-esteem (altruism). Finding value as a resource and making a difference in someone else's life is particularly beneficial for clients who, in the throes of their own misfortune, feel they have little to offer others (Murphy, 1975).

In a number of studies, clients ranked their group therapy as one of the most valuable components of their treatment protocol (Hoge & McLoughlin, 1991). The goals of group psychotherapy directly relate to personal growth and the modification of maladaptive interpersonal behaviors. Clients are expected to verbally share personal feelings, develop insights about personal behaviors, and practice new and more productive interpersonal responses. Psychotherapy groups proliferate in outpatient mental health centers as a primary form of treatment for many clients and are used in inpatient settings for short-term stabilization of mental disorders.

Therapeutic Groups in Psychiatric Settings

Because of personnel shortages, nurses without advanced degrees often lead or co-lead unit-based group psychotherapy with clients who are experiencing major psychiatric illness (Clarke, Adamoski, & Joyce, 1998). Because they commonly spend the most time with psychotic clients, they are in an excellent position to develop effective, formal group relationships with them and to understand their painful conflicts. For the hospitalized psychotic client, life becomes incomprehensible and without meaning. Group therapy offers a safe place for exploring the client's natural healing processes (Birckhead, 1984). The client can reexperience life differently through the eyes of the nurse leader and the conversations that take place in the group, limited and halting though they may be. Therapeutic groups in the community are particularly effective for adolescents as a preventive strategy because peer group interaction is such an intrinsic part of the adolescent's life (Aronson, 2004).

Leading a group with psychotic members is anxiety-provoking. The leader needs to take an active role and a proactive approach. Before each session, the nurse may need to remind group members individually of the meeting. It may appear to the leader that psychotic clients are not willing to attend. More often, this is not the case; their seeming reluctance is part of the passivity that characterizes psychotic clients in interpersonal situations. Holding the group session in the same room at the same time is particularly important for the psychotic client, who relies on structural cues despite being seemingly oblivious to them.

A flexible leadership approach is needed. Spontaneous sharing among group members is not the rule, at least in the early stages of group development. If a topic is not forthcoming from the group, the leader can introduce a relevant, concrete, problem-centered topic and elicit discussion about how group members view the issue or have handled a similar problem. Patience, using minimal encouragers, and helping people feel comfortable by acknowledging each and every contribution help. Over time, the conversation will increase. Offering refreshments in the group session is appropriate with regressed clients because it represents another form of nurturing that enhances socialization.

A primary goal of the leader in group psychotherapy with clients suffering from a major psychiatric illness is to understand each person as a unique human being with needs disguised as symptoms. If the person chooses to use delusions, repetitive questions, or schizophrenic images in speaking, the nurse can try to "decode" the psychotic message by uncovering the underlying theme and translating it into understandable language. Sometimes other members will translate the message if called on by the nurse leader. The leader might say to the group, "I wonder if anyone in the group can help us understand better what John is trying to say." At other times, the leader decodes the message: "I wonder if your fear that the Martians are coming and will destroy you has anything to do with your parents' visit tomorrow?" Changes in physical appearance are noted. For example, one client, after being told she was attractive, appeared at the next meeting wearing makeup.

As with any chronic illness, the seriously mentally ill client suffers setbacks and remission of symptoms. Understanding that this is a dynamic of the illness and not a resistant response to group interaction is essential. It is important to recognize how difficult it is for the psychotic client to tolerate close interaction and how necessary it is to do so if the client is to succeed in the outside environment. With patience and a genuine regard for each client, the nurse can treat inevitable regressions as temporary setbacks capable of being reversed.

Because the demands of leadership are so intense with psychotic clients, co-leadership is recommended. Co-therapists can share the group process interventions, offset negative transference from group members, and provide useful feedback to each other. In addition, co-therapy provides additional opportunities for modeling cooperative behaviors in healthy relationships, behaviors that are so commonly missing in the psychotic client's interpersonal experience. If there is more than one leader, every group session should be processed immediately after its completion.

Therapeutic Groups in Long-Term Settings

Nurses often lead therapeutic groups in long-term settings. They provide a chance for the elderly to get together in a structured format designed to encourage interaction. They provide needed stimulation for people who have much more limited resources to draw from for social interaction. A balance of stimuli is needed to arouse but not overwhelm the elderly client. When making referrals or organizing such groups, the nurse should match the purpose of the group with the client's level of functional ability. For example, groups aimed at increasing insight would not be appropriate or helpful for clients who are confused. Some of the different therapeutic groups available to the elderly are discussed next.

Reality Orientation Groups. Used most often with the confused, elderly client, reality orientation groups help clients maintain contact with the environment and reduce confusion about time, place, and person. Such groups are usually held each day for approximately a half hour, and the focus of the discussion is on the immediate environment; when possible, the group is led by the same person. The nurse uses props such as a calendar, a clock, and pictures of the seasons to stimulate interest. The group should not be seen as an isolated activity; what occurs in the group needs to be reinforced throughout the 24-hour period. For example, on one unit, the nurses placed pictures of the residents in earlier times on the doors to their bedrooms.

Resocialization Groups. Because of their step-by-step structure, resocialization groups are quite useful for withdrawn, elderly clients. Resocialization groups focus on providing a simple social setting for clients to experience basic social skills again. For example, a group might settle around a table with silverware and simple foods. The nurse would provide modeling and guidance to make basic conversational requests for food. Resocialization groups are used with clients who might not be able to get involved with a remotivation group but who need companionship and involvement with others. Improvement of social skills contributes to an improved sense of self-esteem. Although the senses and cognitive abilities may diminish in the elderly, basic needs for companionship, interpersonal relationships, and a place where one is accepted and understood remain the same throughout the life span.

Remotivation Groups. Remotivation groups have a more directed focus. They are helpful in counteracting the isolation and apathy resulting from long-term institutionalization. Remotivation groups are deliberately designed to stimulate thinking about activities required for everyday life. Originally developed by Dorothy Hoskins Smith for use with chronic mental patients, remotivation groups represent an effort to reach the unwounded areas of the patient's personality (i.e., those areas and interests that have remained healthy). "Her approach to treatment was aimed at strengthening this healthy aspect of the personality and restoring a sense of self-worth and dignity" (Sullivan, Bird, Menekse et al., 2001, p. 137).

Nurses, nursing students, and nonprofessional staff with an understanding of group dynamics and interest in the elderly can lead such groups. Typically composed of 10 to 15 members, remotivation groups focus on everyday topics, such as the way plants or trees grow, or they might consist of poetry reading or art appreciation. Visual props engage the participant and stimulate more responses.

The steps the leader takes with remotivation groups, presented in Box 12-4, are easy to follow, and the project is rewarding to those nurses willing to take the time.

Reminiscence Groups. Reminiscence groups offer powerful sources of self-esteem for cognitively intact, elderly clients. Kovach (1991) described reminiscence as

Box 12-4 Steps for Conducting Remotivation Groups

1. Provide an accepting environment and greet each member by name.
2. Offer a bridge to reality by discussing topics of interest, such as news items and historical items.
3. Develop topic with group members through the use of questions, props, or visual aids.
4. Encourage members to discuss the topic in relation to themselves.
5. Express verbal appreciation to members for their contributions, and plan the following session.

a cognitive process of recalling personally significant events from the past. Sharing past achievements with others in a group helps the person remember personal life experiences that can be integrated into the individual's current self-concept. The knowledge that one has lived a meaningful life and has been loving and loved enhances self-esteem.

Nurses sometimes worry that the recalled memories will be unpleasant. Sometimes the memories are indeed bothersome or anxiety-provoking, but the reminiscence group can help the individual rework unresolved issues from the past in a positive way and integrate them into the present reality. Jonsdottir, Jonsdottir, Steingrimsdottir, and colleagues (2001) note, "Recalling the past helps people to adjust to life's changes and thus provides a sense of continuity, integrity and purpose within the person's current life context" (p. 80). Research also supports the fact that for most people reminiscences are pleasant and ego-enhancing (Hyland & Ackerman, 1988). Topics most likely to stimulate positive self-esteem include those that confirm personal meaning and those that validate personal capabilities and strengths (Kovach, 1991).

Reminiscence groups can follow a highly structured format wherein themes are decided beforehand. For example, themes can be developed using a life span approach that includes first memory, special times in childhood or adolescence, child-rearing or work experience, and handling of a crisis. The leader then guides the group in telling their stories, asking questions, and pointing out common themes to stimulate further reflections. Members create for themselves a shared reality by revealing to one another what life has meant and can be for them. In the process of remembering critical incidents, people can reconnect with sometimes forgotten parts of their life that held meaning for them.

Therapeutic Activity Groups

Activity groups are often overlooked as a legitimate form of therapeutic group, yet they account for the majority of nurse-led group modalities in psychiatric inpatient settings (Van Servellen et al., 1991). More commonly found in extended-care, mental health, or rehabilitation health care settings than in acute care or community hospitals, they offer clients a variety of self-expressive opportunities through creative activity rather than through words. The nurse may function as group leader or as a support in encouraging client participation. Activity groups include the following:

- Occupational therapy groups allow clients to work on individual projects or to participate with others in learning life skills. Examples are cooking or activities of daily living groups. Other clients go to the occupational therapy area to make items such as ceramics or leather-tooled objects. Tasks are selected for their therapeutic value as well as for client interest. Life skills groups use a problem-solving approach to interpersonal situations.
- Recreational therapy groups offer opportunities to engage in leisure activities that release energy and provide a social format for learning interpersonal skills. Some people never learned how to build needed leisure activities into their lives.
- Dance therapy groups, originally developed by Marion Chase, are a form of group therapy in which participants can experience movement in a safe environment. Dance therapy provides companionship without demands, and physical movement shared with others often prompts conversation about its meaning.
- Art therapy groups encourage clients to reveal feelings through drawing or painting. Such groups can focus on individual artwork, which is then described by each member, or on a combined group effort in the form of a mural. Psychological interpretations of artwork require advanced preparation in art therapy, but nurses can assist by modeling health behaviors that can be useful to the entire group. Often clients will be able to reveal feelings through expression of color and abstract forms that they initially cannot talk about.
- Poetry and bibliotherapy groups select readings of interest and invite clients to respond to literary works. Sluder (1990) describes an expressive therapy group for the elderly in which the nurse leader first read free verse poems and then invited the clients to compose group poems around feelings such as love or hate. Members were asked to describe the feeling in a few words, and the contributions of each member were recorded. Clients then wrote writing free verse poems and read them in the group. In the process of developing their poetry, clients got in touch with their personal creativity.
- The nurse can lead an exercise group to stimulate body movement and group interaction. Usually the nurse models the exercise behaviors, either with or

without accompanying music. This type of group works well with chronically mentally ill clients.

Community Support Groups

Support or self-help groups provide emotional and practical support to clients and their families who are experiencing chronic illness, crises, or the ill health of a family member. They can offer participants a sense of understanding, belonging, and social support in coping with difficult social and psychological issues associated with health problems or bereavement. Held in the community, these groups are led informally by group members rather than professionals, although often a health professional acts as an adviser. Self-help and support groups are commonly associated with hospitals, clinics, and national health organizations (Adamsen & Rasmussen, 2001). The meetings are free and open to anyone with a specified diagnosis or problem. Examples of familiar support groups are found in Box 12-5.

Members attend when they wish to and are not penalized for nonattendance. Support groups rarely have a formal ending, and group membership is not conditional on personality characteristics or interpersonal suitability. Nurses are encouraged to contact support group networks in their community to become informed of the countless groups available to clients and their families (Exercise 12-9). Referral to community-based support groups will become increasingly important as cost containment continues to drive health care delivery.

Nurses often lead support groups on the unit. Examples of support groups for family members are Alzheimer's

Box 12-5 Examples of Mutual Aid Support Groups in the Community

Alcoholics Anonymous
Al-Anon
Adult Children of Alcoholics
Anorexia nervosa and bulimia support groups
Chemically Dependent Anonymous
Chronic Pain Outreach
Compassionate Friends (bereaved parents of dead children)
Emotions Anonymous
Make Today Count
Men to End Spouse Abuse
Narcotics Anonymous
Neurotics Anonymous
On Our Own
Overeaters Anonymous
Parents Anonymous (parents of child abuse victims)
Parents Club of Children with Asthma
Seasons: Suicide Bereavement
Threshold: Alliance for the Mentally Ill
Tough Love (parents of teenagers)
United Ostomy Association

Exercise 12-9 **Learning About Support Groups**

Purpose: To provide direct information about support groups in the community.

Procedure:

1. Contact a support group in your community. (Ideally, students will choose different support groups so that a variety of groups are shared.)
2. Identify yourself as a nursing student and ask for information about the support group (e.g., the time and frequency of meetings, purpose and focus of the group, how a client joins the group, types of services provided, who sponsors the group, issues the group might discuss, and fee schedules).
3. Write a two-paragraph report including the information you have gathered and describe your experience in asking for the support group information.

Discussion:

1. How easy was it for you to obtain information?
2. Were you surprised by any of the informants' answers?
3. If you were a client, would the support group you chose to investigate meet your needs?
4. What did you learn from doing this exercise that might be useful in your nursing practice?

Table 12-5 Sample Format for Leaders of Support Groups

Steps	Examples
Introduce self.	"I am Christy Atkins, a staff nurse on the unit, and I am going to be your group facilitator tonight."
Explain purpose of the group.	"Our goal in having the group is to provide a place for family members to get support from each other and to provide practical information to families caring for victims of Alzheimer's disease."
Identify norms.	"We have three basic rules in this group: (1) We respect one another's feelings; (2) we don't preach or tell you how to do something; and (3) the meetings are confidential, meaning that everything of a personal nature stays in this room."
Ask members to identify themselves and have each one tell something about his or her situation.	"I'd like to go around the room and ask each of you to tell us your name and something about your situation."
Link common themes.	"It seems as if feeling powerless and out of control is a common theme tonight. What strategies have you found help you to feel more in control?"
Allow time for informal networking (optional).	Providing a 10-minute break with or without refreshments allows members to talk informally with each other.
Provide closure.	"Now I'd like to go around the group and ask each of you to identify one thing you will do in the next week for yourself to help you feel more in control."

disease support groups for family caregivers, support groups for clients with a specific diagnosis (e.g., cancer, AIDS, or learning disabilities), aftercare groups for families of former clients who are having emotional difficulties, parent groups, and bereavement groups. A suggested format for leading a support group is presented in Table 12-5.

Educational Groups

Educational groups are used in community and hospital settings to help clients develop skills in taking care of themselves (Schilling, El-Bassel, Haden et al., 1995). They also provide families of clients with serious or chronic illness with the knowledge and skills they need to care for their loved ones.

Educational groups are reality-based and focus on the present situation (Esplen, Touer, Hunter et al., 1998). They are time-limited group applications (e.g., the group might be held as four one-hour sessions over a two-week period or as an eight-week, two-hour seminar). Examples of primary prevention groups are childbirth education, parenting, stress reduction, and professional support groups for nurses working in critical care settings. Suitable adolescent groups include those that deal with values clarification, health education, and sex education as well as groups to increase coping skills (e.g., avoiding peer pressure to use drugs) (Griffith, 1986).

Medication groups are an excellent example of educational group formats used in hospitals and community clinics. Clients are taught effective ways to carry out a therapeutic medication regimen while learning about their disorder. A typical sequence would be to provide clients with information about the following: their disorder; purpose of the medication; how long before the medication will take effect; what to look for with side effects; when to call the physician; what to do when they do not take the medication as prescribed; what to avoid while on the medication (e.g., some medications cause sun sensitivity); and tests needed to monitor the medication. The nurse would present the didactic material in an informal manner, starting with what clients already know about their disorder and the medication. Giving homework and materials to be read between sessions can be helpful if the medication group is to last more than one session. The group leader allows sufficient time for questions and, by encouraging an open informal discussion of the topic, engages individual members in the group activity.

Focus Discussion Groups

Clark, Cary, Diemert et al. (2003) describe a focus group as "a group of people who have personal experience of a topic of interest and who meet to discus their perceptions and perspectives on that topic" (p. 457). Both health care providers and consumers use focus discussion groups for a variety of purposes in health care. They provide group input that is useful to caregivers in planning health care for particular populations. Through discussion of a specific topic, clients learn more about health care issues affecting them and have the opportunity to reflect on their own perceptions (Laube & Wieland, 1998). Careful preparation, formulation of relevant questions, and use of feedback ensure that personal learning

Table 12-6 Elements of Successful Discussion Groups

Element	Rationale
Careful preparation	Thoughtful agenda and assignment establish a direction for the discussion and the expected contribution of each member.
Informed participants	Each member should come prepared so that all members are communicating with relatively the same level of information, and each is able to contribute equally.
Shared leadership	Each member is responsible for contributing to the discussion.
Relevant questions	Focused questions keep the discussion moving toward the meeting objectives.
Useful feedback	Thoughtful feedback maintains the momentum of the discussion by reflecting different perspectives of topics raised and confirming or questioning others' views.

Table 12-7 Characteristics of Effective and Ineffective Listening Habits in Discussion Groups

10 Keys to Effective Listening	The Bad Listener	The Good Listener
Find areas of interest.	Tunes out dry subjects	Opportunizes; asks, "What's in it for me?"
Judge content, not delivery.	Tunes out if delivery is poor	Judges content, skips over delivery errors
Hold your fire.	Tends to enter into argument	Does not judge until comprehension is complete
Listen for ideas.	Listens for facts	Listens for central themes
Be flexible.	Takes intensive notes using only one system	Takes fewer notes; uses four or five different systems
Work at listening.	Shows no energy output; fakes attention	Works hard; exhibits active body state
Resist distractions.	Is easily distracted	Fights or avoids distractions; tolerates bad habits; knows how to concentrate
Exercise your mind.	Resists difficult expository material; seeks light, recreational material	Uses heavier material as exercise for the mind
Keep your mind open.	Reacts to emotional words	Interprets color words; does not get hung up on them
Capitalize on fact: thought is faster than speech.	Tends to daydream with slow speakers	Challenges, anticipates, and weighs the evidence; listens between the lines to tone of voice

From Sperry Corporation: Your listening profile. In Cathcart R, Samover L, editors, *Small group communication: a reader*, ed 5, Dubuque, IA, 1988, William C. Brown, p. 382. Reprinted with permission of Unisys Corporation.

needs are met. Functional elements appropriate to discussion groups are found in Table 12-6.

Group leadership is divided equally among the group members. Although the level of participation is never quite equal, discussion groups in which only a few members actively participate are disheartening to group members and limited in learning potential. Because the primary purpose of a discussion group is to promote the learning of all group members, other members are charged with the responsibility of encouraging the participation of more silent members. Allowing enough interpersonal space for dialogue to occur and asking for—but not demanding—the reluctant member's opinion encourage communication.

Sometimes, when more verbal participants keep quiet, the more reticent group member begins to speak. It is just as important to learn when to stop talking as it is to know when to present material. Cooperation, not competition, needs to be developed as a conscious group norm in all discussion groups. Characteristics of effective and ineffective listening habits in discussion groups are found in Table 12-7.

Discussion group topics use prepared data and group-generated material. New information is integrated with more established data. This new information requires the client to synthesize data into a relevant whole rather than simply parroting major themes and topics. Before the end of each meeting, the leader or a group member should summarize the major themes developed from the content material.

A discussion of group principles applied to task and work groups is found in Chapter 22.

> **Ethical Dilemma ■ *What Would You Do?***
> Mrs. Murphy is 39 years old and has had multiple admissions to the psychiatric unit for bipolar disorder. She wants to participate in group therapy but is disruptive when she is in the group. The group gets angry with her monopolization of their time, but she says it is her right as a patient to attend if she chooses. Mrs. Murphy's symptoms could be controlled with medication, but she refuses to take it when she is "high" because it makes her feel less energized. How do you balance Mrs. Murphy's rights with those of the group? Should she be required to take her medication? How would you handle this situation from an ethical perspective?

SUMMARY

This chapter looks at the ways in which a group experience enhances clients' abilities to meet therapeutic self-care demands, provides meaning, and is personally affirming. The rationale for providing a group experience for clients is described. Group dynamics include individual member commitment, functional similarity, and leadership style. Group concepts related to group dynamics consist of purpose, norms, cohesiveness, roles, and role functions. Communication variables such as clarifying, paraphrasing, linking, and summarizing build and expand on techniques used in individual relationships.

Group processes refer to the structural phases of group development as described by Tuckman (1965): forming, storming, norming, performing, and adjourning. In the forming phase of group relationships, the basic need is for acceptance. The storming phase focuses on issues of power and control in groups. Behavioral standards are formed in the norming phase that will guide the group toward goal accomplishment, and the group becomes a safe environment in which to work and express feelings. Once this occurs, most of the group's task is accomplished during the performing phase. Feelings of warmth, caring, and intimacy follow; members feel affirmed and valued. Finally, when the group task is completed to the satisfaction of the individual members, or of the group as a whole, the group enters an adjourning (termination) phase.

Different types of groups found in health care include therapeutic, support, educational, and discussion focus groups.

REFERENCES

Adamsen L, Rasmussen J: Sociological perspectives on self-help groups: reflections on conceptualization and social processes, *J Adv Nurs* 35(6):909–917, 2001.

Agapetus L: Yalom's model applied to an outpatient better breathers group, *J Psychosoc Nurs Ment Health Serv* 32(12): 11–24, 1996.

Aronson S: Where the wild things are: the power and challenge of adolescent group work, *Mt Sinai J Med* 71(3):174–180, 2004.

Benne KD, Sheats P: Functional roles of group members, *J Soc Issues* 4(2):41–49, 1948.

Bertcher H, Maple F: Elements and issues in group composition. In Sundel M, Glasser S, Vinter R, editors, *Individual change through small groups*, New York, 1985, Free Press.

Birckhead L: The nurse as leader: group psychotherapy with psychotic patients, *J Psychosoc Nurs Ment Health Serv* 22(6): 24–30, 1984.

Brandman W: Intersubjectivity, social microcosm and the here-and-now in a support group for nurses, *Arch Psychiatr Nurs* 10(6):374–378, 1996.

Brilhart J, Galanes G: *Effective group discussion*, ed 9, New York, 1997, McGraw-Hill.

Budman S, Soldz S, Demby A et al.: Cohesion, alliance and outcome in group psychotherapy, *Psychiatry* 52:339–350, 1989.

Clark M, Cary S Diemert G et al.: Involving communities in community assessment, *Public Health Nurs* 20(6):456–463, 2003.

Clarke D, Adamoski E, Joyce B: In-patient group psychotherapy: the role of the staff nurse, *J Psychosoc Nurs Ment Health Serv* 36(5):22–26, 1998.

Corey M, Corey G: *Groups: process and practice*, ed 7, Pacific Grove, CA, 2006, Brooks/Cole.

Dallam S, Manderino M: "Free to be" peer group supports patients with MPD/DD, *J Psychosoc Nurs Ment Health Serv* 35(5):22–27, 1997.

Dobrof J, Umpierre M, Rocha L et al.: Group work in a primary care medical setting *Health Soc Work* 15(1):32–37, 1990.

Eibl-Eibesfeldt I: *Ethology: the biology of behavior*, New York, 1975, Holt, Rinehart & Winston.

Esplen M, Touer B, Hunter J et al.: A group therapy approach to facilitate integration of risk information for women at risk for breast cancer, *Canadian Journal of Psychiatry* 43(4):375–380, 1998.

Gans J, Alonso A: Difficult patients: their construction in group therapy, *Int J Group Psychother* 48(3):311–326, 1998.

Goldstein J, Alter C, Axelrod R: A psychoeducational bereavement support group for families provided in an outpatient cancer center, *J Cancer Educ* 11(4):233–237, 1996.

Griffith LW: Group work with children and adolescents. In Janosik EH, Phipps LB, editors, *Life cycle group work in nursing*, Monterey, CA, 1986, Wadsworth.

Hawkins D: An invitation to join in difficulty: realizing the deeper promise of group psychotherapy, *Int J Group Psychother* 48(4):423–438, 1998.

Hoge M, McLoughlin K: Group psychotherapy in acute treatment settings: theory and technique, *Hosp Community Psychiatry* 42(2):153–157, 1991.

Hyland D, Ackerman A: Reminiscence and autobiographical memory in the study of the personal past, *J Gerontol* 43(2): 35–39, 1988.

Jacobson L: The group as an object in the cultural field, *Int J Group Psychother 39*(4):475–497, 1989.

Janis I: Groupthink, *Psychol Today* 5:43–46, 74–76, 1971.

Jonsdottir H, Jonsdottir G, Steingrimsdottir E et al.: Group reminiscence among people with end-stage chronic lung diseases, *J Adv Nurs* 35(1):79–87, 2001.

Kovach C: Reminiscence: exploring the origins, processes, and consequences, *Nurs Forum* 26(3):14–19, 1991.

Kreidler MC, Carlson RE: Breaking the incest cycle: the group as a surrogate family, *J Psychosoc Nurs Ment Health Serv* 29(4):28–32, 1991.

Laube J, Wieland V: Nourishing the body through use of process prescriptions in group therapy, *Int J Eat Disord* 24(1):1–11, 1998.

McGinley S, Baus E, Gyza K et al.: Multidisciplinary discharge planning: developing a process, *Nurs Manage* 27(10):55, 57–60, 1996.

Murphy G: Group psychotherapy in our society. In Rosenbaum M, Berger M, editors, *Group psychotherapy and group function*, New York, 1975, Basic Books.

Prehn R, Thomas P: Does it make a difference? The effect of a women's issues group on female psychiatric in-patients, *J Psychosoc Nurs Ment Health Serv* 28(11):34–38, 1990.

Rogers C: The process of the basic encounter group. In Diedrich R, Dye HA, editors, *Group procedures: purposes, processes and outcomes*, Boston, 1972, Houghton Mifflin.

Rosenblum EH: Groupthink: one peril of group cohesiveness, *J Nurs Adm* 12(4):27–31, 1982.

Schilling R, El-Bassel N, Haden B et al.: Skills training groups to reduce HIV transmission and drug use among methadone patients, *Soc Work* 40(1):91–101, 1995.

Sluder H: The write way: using poetry for self-disclosure, *J Psychosoc Nurs Ment Health Serv* 28(7):26–28, 1990.

Sullivan F, Bird E, Menekse A et al.: Remotivation therapy and Huntington's disease, *J Neurosci Nurs* 33(3):136–142, 2001.

Tannenbaum R, Wechsler I, Massarik F: Leadership: a frame of reference. In Cathcart R, Samovar L, editors, *Small group communication*, ed 5, Dubuque, IA, 1988, William C. Brown.

Tuckman B: Developmental sequence in small groups, *Psychol Bull* 63:384, 1965.

Van Servellen G, Poster E, Ryan J et al.: Nurse-led group modalities in a psychiatric in-patient setting: a program evaluation, *Arch Psychiatr Nurs* 5(3):128–136, 1991.

Yalom I, with Leszcz M: *The theory and practice of group psychotherapy*, ed 5, New York, 2005, Basic Books.

Yalom I, Yalom V: Brief interactional group psychotherapy, *Am Psychiatry* 43:440, 1990.

Zahniser J, Coursey R: The self-concept group: development and evaluation for use in psychosocial rehabilitation settings, *Psychiatr Rehabil J* 19(2):59–64, 1995.

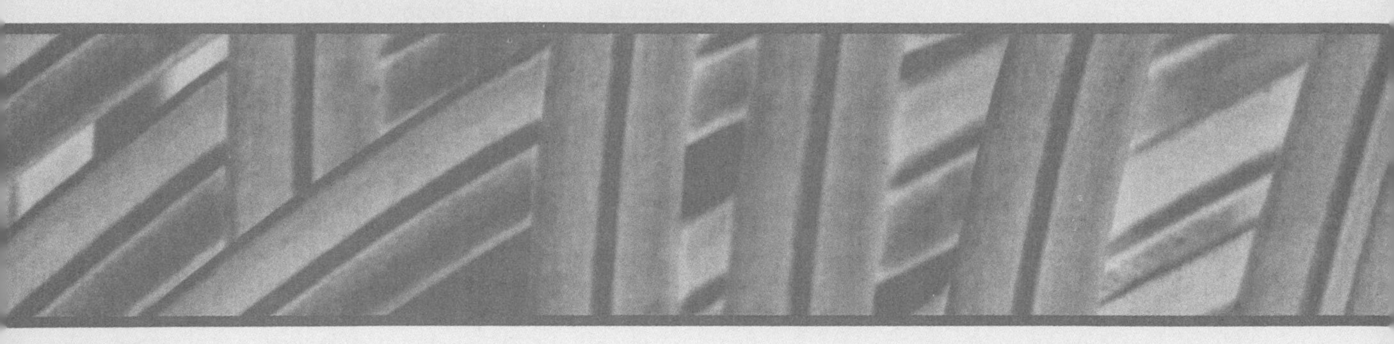

Chapter 13

Communicating with Families

Elizabeth Arnold

OUTLINE

OBJECTIVES

At the end of the chapter, the reader will be able to:

1. Define and describe family.
2. Compare and contrast theoretical frameworks used to study family communication and family dynamics.
3. Apply the nursing process in caring for the family as client.
4. Identify selected communication strategies to use in interacting with families.

I know I'm hot tempered like my father, but still I believe it's important to remember relatives' birthdays with cards the way my mother always did. My interest in world affairs comes from her, but I learned from my father how to unwind from gardening. His pride in a paycheck made me want always to have one of my own. Her pride in a tastefully furnished home gave me a yen for interior decorating.

(McBride, 1976)

Chapter 13 focuses on concepts and guidelines the nurse can use to communicate effectively with families. The chapter is based on a fundamental assumption that family communication in health situations is systemic and process-based. Nurse-family relationships require a strong understanding of the reciprocal nature and the complexity of family communication, in part because of the number and variety of communicators.

The family is described as "the principal sociocultural system in which behavior patterns are learned, adapted or altered" (Novilla, Barnes, De La Cruz et al., 2006, p. 31). Therapeutic relationships with families operate on the premise that individual clients can best be understood within the psychosocial context of their family's goals, developmental history, and current social milieu. The family has a strong influence on the development of health beliefs that shape health behaviors and on the interpretation of health information (Friedman, 1998). Although people later marry and create new family groups, family-of-origin values and patterns continue to influence their lives. Some family therapists believe that "the family of origin is the most powerful force in organizing and framing later life experiences and choices" (Framo, 1992, p. 128). The functions of family communication are presented in Box 13-1.

Nurses act as a primary human resource for families in health care. Sometimes the entire family *becomes* the client. Understanding the centrality of the family in supporting individual client family members and in making effective health care decisions is critical to formulating and implementing effective treatment plans. Learning about family communication is important for several reasons: (a) it provides an awareness of the important relationships in a client's life that can be rallied for support or that need special attention because of a negative impact on the client's situation; (b) it is helpful to know who else in the family may have had a similar illness or medical problem and how the family coped with it; and (c) the information gained can assist the health care provider in recognizing cultural and family factors that influence the client's attitudes, beliefs, and actions in his or her health care (Cole-Kelly & Seaburn, 1999).

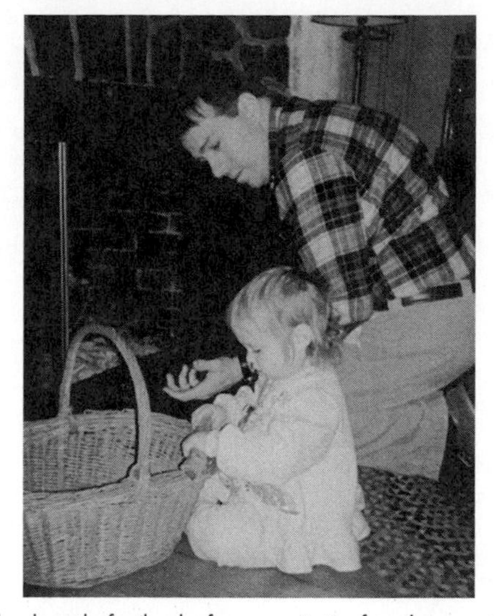

Young children learn the family rules for communication from their parents.

Box 13-1 Functions of Family Communication

- Help children learn about the environment
- Communicate rules about how family members should think and act
- Resolve family conflict
- Nurture and develop self-esteem
- Transmit cultural values and traditions
- Express emotions within the family unit

BASIC CONCEPTS

Definition of Family

Today there are so many combinations of people living together and calling themselves **family** that Wright and Leahey (2000) simply state, "a family is who they say they are" (p. 70). Family has also been defined as "those closest to the patient in knowledge, care and affection" (Kristjanson & Aoun, 2004). For health care purposes, family can be considered as those persons living with the client, or identified by the client as capable of providing family-type support. Strong emotional ties and durability of membership characterize family relationships regardless of how uniquely they are defined. How a family functions is viewed on a continuum ranging from optimal function to disintegration as a family unit. Psychologically healthy families are resilient and adaptable (Goldenberg & Goldenberg, 2002; Green & Werner, 1996).

The common belief that a family consists of one household with two parents and their biological children is outdated. Many children today are members of more than one family unit and are linked biologically and

Box 13-2 Forms of Family Units

Nuclear family: A father and mother, with one or more children, living together but apart from both of their parents.
Extended family: Nuclear family unit's combination of second- and third-generation members related by blood or marriage but not living together.
Three-generational family: Any combination of first-, second-, and third-generation members living within a household.
Dyad family: Husband and wife or other couple living alone without children.
Single-parent family: Divorced, never married, separated, or widowed male or female and at least one child; most single-parent families are headed by women.
Stepfamily: Family in which one or both spouses are divorced or widowed with one or more children from a previous marriage who may not live with the newly reconstituted family.
Blended or reconstituted family: A combination of two families with children from one or both families and sometimes children of the newly married couple.
Common law family: An unmarried couple living together with or without children.
No kin: A group of at least two people sharing a nonsexual relationship and exchanging support who have no legal, blood, or strong emotional tie to each other.
Polygamous family: One man (or woman) with several spouses.
Gay family: A homosexual couple living together with or without children.
Commune: More than one couple living together and sharing resources.
Group marriage: All individuals are "married" to one another and are considered parents of all the children.

emotionally to people who may or may not be part of their daily lives. The composition of the family can take any one of several forms, as presented in Box 13-2.

Knowledge of what constitutes the family unit is important for health care planning. For example, single-parent families must accomplish the same developmental tasks as two-parent families, but in many cases they do it without the support of the other partner or equal financial resources (Mailick & Vigilante, 1997). Children in blended families often have a different life experience than those in an unbroken family because their family structure is more complex. Their "family" may include two or more sets of grandparents, step- or half-brothers and sisters, and multiple aunts and uncles (Byng-Hall, 2000). Table 13-1 displays some of the differences between biological and blended families. Issues for blended families include discipline, money, use of time, birth of an infant, death of a stepparent, inclusion at graduation, and marriage and health care decisions.

Theoretical Models

Systems Theory

Systems theory is the foundation for most other theories of family communication, assessment, and intervention (Barker, 1998). General systems theory is based on the idea that there are universal principles of organization governing the functioning of all systems. Von Bertalanffy (1968) identifies the following principles as being applicable to all systems:

- A system is a unit in which the *whole* is greater than the sum of its parts.
- Certain *rules* govern the operation of such systems; these rules can be identified through observation of the system functioning.

Table 13-1 Comparing Differences Between Biological and Blended Families

Biological Families	Blended Families
Family is created without loss.	Family is born of loss.
There are shared family traditions.	There are two sets of family traditions.
One set of family rules evolves.	Family rules are varied and complicated.
Children arrive one at a time.	Instant parenthood of children at different ages occurs.
Biological parents live together.	Biological parents live apart.

- Each system and its environment are separated by a *boundary*, which operates much as skin does in separating the outside environment from the internal system of the body in human systems. Boundaries control what enters and leaves the family system.
- Boundaries allow exchange of information, energy, and resources into the system (*inputs*). The system actively processes the input received so that it is usable by the system (*throughput*) and transforms it into behaviors, information, energy, or matter that leave the system and reenter the environment in a new form (*output*).
- *Communication* and *feedback* mechanisms between parts of the system are important in the function of the system. Feedback provides information to the system in ways that allow it to maintain a steady state of functionality.
- *Circular causality* asserts that a change in one part of the system creates change in the whole system. Consequently, each person in the family influences every other family member and impacts the functioning of the family as a whole.
- Systems operate on the principle of *equifinality*, that is, the same endpoint can be reached from a number of starting points.
- Systems are made up of *subsystems* and are themselves parts of *suprasystems*. Subsystems describe member-unit relationships within the family, such as spousal and child-parent subsystems. Suprasystems represent outside influences and relationships in the community.
- There is a natural inclination for systems to push the unit back to its original state of equilibrium in the face of any disruption (*homeostasis*).
- Energy that promotes order within the system is termed *negentropy*. Energy that creates disorganization and chaos within the system is termed *entropy*. Functional systems are able to maintain a balance between negentropy and entropy (*morphogenesis*). When this occurs, a system steady state results. *Equilibrium* is the term used to indicate a steady state.

Bowen's Systems Theory. Murray Bowen's (1913–1990) theory of human family systems is based on general systems theory, and is perhaps the best-known theory of family functioning (Innes, 1996). Bowen (1978) conceptualized "family" as the immediate family with whom the individual lives (nuclear family), plus relatives living outside the family unit (extended family). In some cultures, Native American for example, the family can include a much larger group of non-blood-related "aunts and uncles."

Bowen viewed the family as a single emotional unit in which energy (anxiety) from its emotional process influences the behavior of every member in it. Individual family members react to each other in predictable and reciprocal ways. Until one family member is willing to challenge the dysfunction of an emotional system by refusing to play his or her reactive part, the emotional energy fueling a family's rigid dysfunctional communication pattern persists.

Differentiation of self within the system is the primary means of changing family process (Bowen, 1978). **Self-differentiation** is a term used to describe the capacity to stay involved in one's family without losing one's identity (Bohlander, 1995). Personal energy is directed toward changing the self rather than others. A self-differentiated family member equally respects the rights of self and others. By contrast, a person who is poorly self-differentiated requires the acceptance and approval of others for his or her self-identity. This person automatically reacts to what others do or say rather than take a position on important family and social issues. Lack of self-differentiation creates vulnerability.

Bowen used the term *multigenerational transmission process* to describe an emotional transmission of patterns of behaving and communicating from generation to generation. Families develop spoken and unspoken agreements of what are acceptable roles, as well as ways of communicating with each other that are handed down through one's family of origin. Unacknowledged losses and family secrets can continue to be a part of future generations, often without the contemporary family's awareness. People continue to react in the ways they learned from their families. Unspoken family rules such as "family comes first" or "appearances are the only thing that counts" can operate so strongly within a family that they dominate family functioning even when they do not fit current family circumstances.

Another key concept is the *family projection process*. This occurs when family tensions escalate and a family may unconsciously try to reduce its anxiety by "projecting" it on to one of its members. Examples of the projection process include the family hero, the dysfunctional child, and the family scapegoat.

Building on the earlier work of Toman (1992), Bowen believed that *sibling position* helped account for the take-charge qualities of oldest children and the more laid-back, spontaneous, fun-loving characteristics of the youngest child. Sibling position is simply a guideline; behavioral expectations and characteristics can be altered by illness, significant gaps between births, and other factors.

Bowen defined *emotional cutoffs* within the family as a situation in which an individual breaks off contact with family members either physically, psychologically, or both. Sometimes other family members not directly involved in the original cutoff have no idea why it exists. Making contact with cut-off parts of the family allows family members to create new relationships and roles within their family.

The concept of triangles is a critical element in Bowen's theory as a way of neutralizing family anxiety (Glasscock & Hales, 1998). Present to some degree in all families, a **triangle** represents a three-person emotional system that begins when there is tension between two members. A third person or object is brought in to stabilize the two-person relationship and reduce the anxiety. Triangles can be positive as well as negative (Tarnowski, Hanson, & May, 1999). For example, when a nurse offers information and support to a family, it can help reduce the family's anxiety about a sick or injured family member and reduce the burden of care for a family member.

Bowen's theory also can be applied to assessment and intervention with dysfunction in nonfamily systems such as work and social organizations. According to Bowen, societies go through similar periods of increased anxiety and dysfunctional communication similar to that of family dysfunction when the socioemotional process takes over principled thinking. With the level of world chaos present in today's society, one would wonder what Bowen would say! Symptoms of dysfunction in the larger social system can include increased crime and violence, escalating divorce rate, a litigious society, polarization of majority and minority cultures, increase in drug use, and improper behaviors by national leaders. Societies can practice self-differentiation similar to that of the family by taking responsibility and acting on reasoned judgment rather than automatically reacting to emotionally charged situations.

Systems-Related Terminology

Subsystems. Originally conceptualized by Minuchin (1974), subsystems help the clinician to organize the ways in which family members interact with each other. The family carries out its functions through subsystem alliances and coalitions in order to maintain the system as a whole (homeostasis). Some alliances are helpful; others are nonproductive in health care situations.

Subsystems represent family alignments formed within the family unit on the basis of generation, sex, interest, or function. Examples of subsystems include the spousal subsystem, parent/child subsystem, sibling subsystem, and male/female subsystem. Individual family members belong to more than one family subsystem at a time. For example, a person may be part of a spousal subsystem and a parent/child subsystem. Family members have different levels of power, and need to use different skills to successfully negotiate their position within each subsystem. A woman may participate in various alliances and assume different roles as mother, spouse, and daughter in her own family of origin. Being in multiple subsystems can generate conflict when the expectations of one subsystem interfere with those of another. Understanding the structure of the family and the subsystem alliances present within it is useful in providing quality health care.

Boundaries. Another important family system concept is that of **boundaries**, defined as invisible lines that protect the integrity of the family system by differentiating the family from the external environment. Boundaries also operate within the family unit by differentiating individuals and subunits within the family from one another. Their function is to define the level of participation between family members. Boundaries, then, "exist around the family as a whole, around its subsystems, and around individual family members" (Goldenberg & Goldenberg, 2002, p. 37).

Ideally, generational boundaries clearly differentiate child and parent roles. Boundaries are described as diffuse, rigid, or permeable. Diffuse boundaries are evidenced with family overinvolvement, while rigid boundaries are operative in families with little interaction between members and with family secrets. In either case, boundaries that are not clear and permeable promote family dysfunction and poor communication. Exercise 13-1 provides an opportunity to look at the structure and communication process of family life.

Family Developmental Stage Theory

Another way of looking at the family is by focusing on the life tasks the family is dealing with at the time health care is sought. Duvall (1958) viewed the family as a

Exercise 13-1 Family Structures and Processes

Purpose: To develop an awareness of the different structures and processes within families.

Procedure:
Each student will attempt to spend time with a family other than his or her own family of origin. (Family can be any two or more persons of relation.) Students should observe the communication patterns, roles, and norms of the family and write a descriptive summary of their experience. How do you think this family would cope with one of the members becoming ill? Think about how this family differs from your own regarding structure and process.

Discussion:
Each student will share experiences with the group. Identify how families are different and similar. What are some of the coping strategies that you predicted based on observations? Discuss how the nurse can interface with families and assist them with coping.

system moving through time. She proposed a family life cycle framework for understanding normal family development. Her stage theory focused on eight stages of development related to nodal events of age-related changes. Family stages are presented in Table 13-2. Developmental milestones tell the nurse about possible con-

Table 13-2 Duvall's Eight-Stage Family Life Cycle and Family Developmental Tasks

State Family Life Cycle Stage	Family Development Tasks
I. Beginning families (married couples without children)	Establishing a mutually satisfying marriage; adjusting to pregnancy and the promise of parenthood; fitting into the kin network
II. Child-bearing families (oldest child birth through 30 months)	Having, adjusting to, and encouraging the development of infants; establishing a satisfying home for both parents and infants
III. Families with preschool-age children (oldest child 2½-6 years of age)	Adapting to the critical needs and interests of preschool-age children in stimulating, growth-promoting ways; coping with energy depletion and lack of privacy as parents
IV. Families with school-age children (oldest child 6-13 years of age)	Fitting into the community of school-age families in constructive ways; encouraging children's educational achievement
V. Families with teenagers (oldest child 13-20 years of age)	Balancing freedom with responsibility as teenagers mature and emancipate themselves; establishing postparental interests and careers as growing parents
VI. Families launching young adults (first child leaving home through last child leaving home)	Releasing young adults into work, college, marriage with appropriate rituals and assistance; maintaining supportive home base
VII. Middle-age parents (empty nest to retirement)	Rebuilding the marriage relationship; maintaining kin ties with older and younger generations
VIII. Family during retirement and aging (retirement)	Adjusting to retirement; closing the family home or adapting it to aging; coping with bereavement and living alone

From Duvall EM, Miller BC: *Marriage and family development*, ed 6, Boston, 1985, Allyn and Bacon. Copyright © 1985 by Pearson Education. Adapted by permission of the publisher.

cerns and suggest ways to adapt interventions to meet the needs of families experiencing them. The better equipped a family is to meet life's developmental transition tasks, the more successful is family development.

Duvall (1958) identifies nine family characteristics indicative of successful family development. She suggests that the family must be able to establish and maintain the following:

1. An independent home
2. Satisfactory ways of earning and spending money
3. Mutually acceptable patterns in the division of labor
4. Continuity of mutually satisfying sexual relationships
5. An open system of communication
6. Workable relationships with relatives
7. Ways of interacting with the larger social community
8. Competency in child-bearing and child-rearing
9. A workable philosophy of life

McCubbin's Resiliency Model of Family Coping

The way in which a family responds to a crisis helps identify its coping pattern and level of adaptation. McCubbin's Resiliency Model of Family Stress, Adjustment, and Adaptation is considered the most extensively studied model of family coping with traumatic and chronic illness (Clark, 1999). In this model, A (the event) interacts with B (resources) and with C (family's perception of the event) to produce X (the crisis). McCubbin and colleagues (McCubbin, Cauble, & Patterson, 1982; McCubbin, McCubbin, & Thompson, 1993) expanded this model in a double A-B-C-X model that adds concepts of *pileup of demands*, *family system resources*, and *postcrisis behavior* to the original model. The most recent resiliency model incorporates these earlier understandings and emphasizes family *adaptation* to facilitate family coping (Figure 13-1). This enhancement of the original McCubbin model explores the family's "blueprint" for functioning and the ways in which each family's capabilities, strengths, resources, and methods of coping could be used or developed to successfully meet a family crisis (McCubbin, McCubbin, & Thompson, 1998). McCubbin's model attempts to explain why some family systems fall apart while others with similar circumstances are able to recover without significant psychological sequelae (Greeff & Human, 2004). Exercise 13-2 provides an opportunity to look at the differences between positive and negative family interactions.

McCubbin and colleagues (1998) stressed that "the family system and its functioning involve a very complex process of interacting individuals, personalities, and family unit characteristics, all of which influence each other to shape the family's course of changing itself" (p. 25). Knowledge of these key factors enables the nurse to understand the client's health problems in its larger context and provides a solid base for developing family-based nursing diagnoses amenable to nursing intervention. Using this model, the nurse might inquire about how the family is able to work together in dealing with the challenges of the current illness. Other questions would focus on how each family member is coping with the situation and what role he or she would like to play—how they see themselves contributing productively to the situation. Then the nurse might help the family explore the types of coping strategies, the changes needed in family functioning to cope with the illness over time, and the degree to which the family is able to meet the requirements of the crisis situation. The understanding that family coping is a process that changes over time can be communicated to the family. Exercise 13-3 examines coping strategies that families use in crisis situations.

The concept of family resilience offers a way of looking at families through the lens of family strengths and potential. Walsh (1996) identifies four characteristic beliefs held by resilient families: capacity to derive meaning from adversity, a positive outlook, the capacity to affirm strengths and consider alternative possibilities, transcendent and spiritual beliefs that allow families to connect with a larger purpose, and commitment to help others. Family resilience is more likely to occur in a healthy family atmosphere of warmth and affection.

Emotional support for individual family members and reasonable, clear-cut limits provide the foundation for positive coping strategies. The support person(s) can be a grandparent, family friend, or leader in a community agency. Other strategies to foster family resiliency include encouraging collaboration among family members, reinforcing teamwork and sharing of experiences, and referring to support groups. The concept of resilience is closely aligned with that of using personal and family strengths in responding to the stress of health disruptions and physical or mental illness.

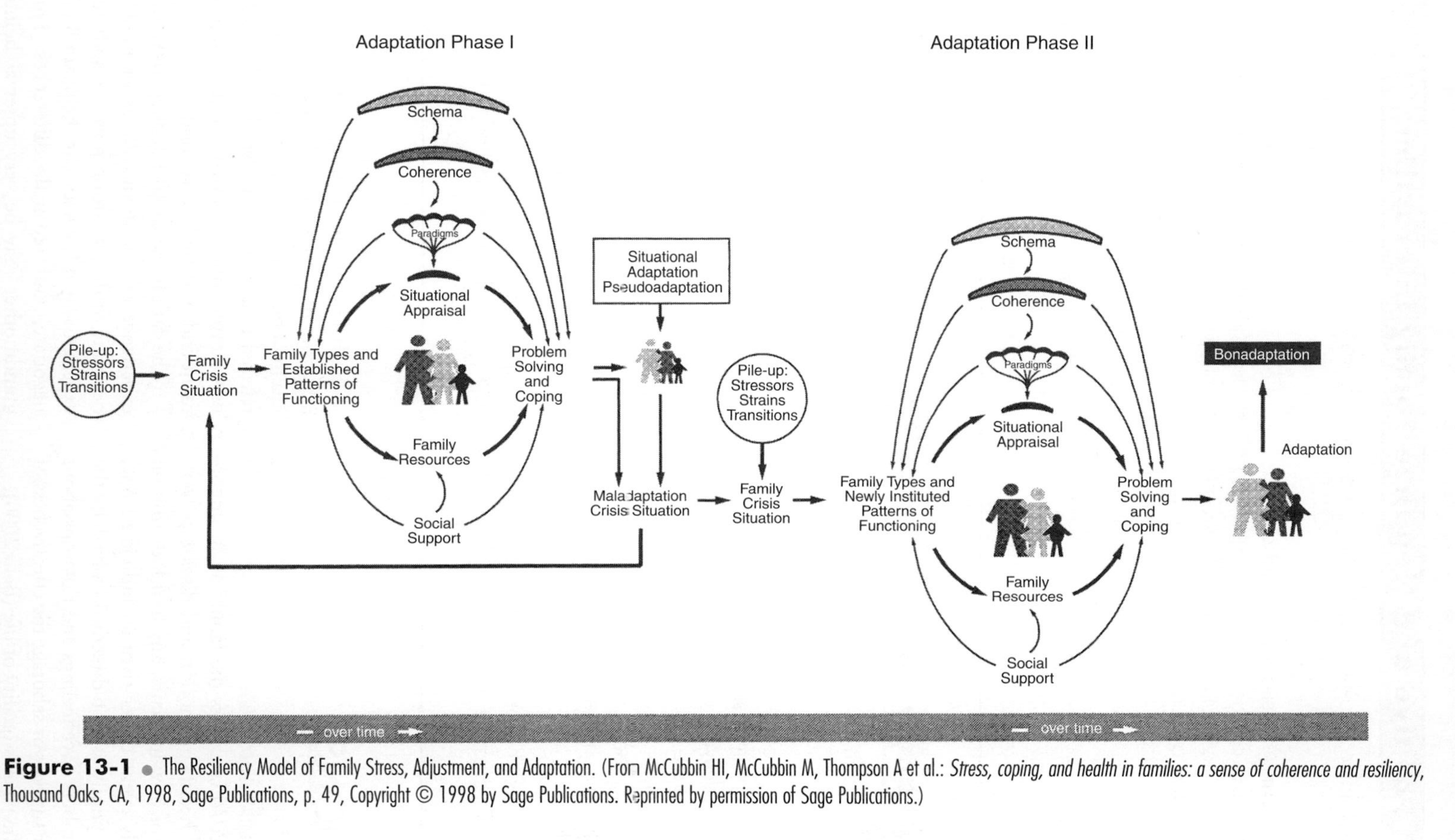

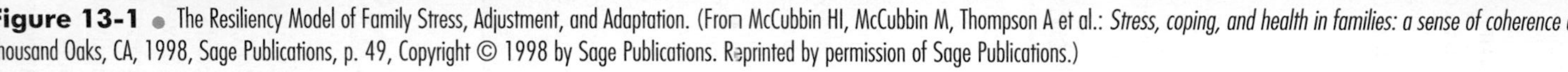

Figure 13-1 ● The Resiliency Model of Family Stress, Adjustment, and Adaptation. (From McCubbin HI, McCubbin M, Thompson A et al.: *Stress, coping, and health in families: a sense of coherence and resiliency,* Thousand Oaks, CA, 1998, Sage Publications, p. 49, Copyright © 1998 by Sage Publications. Reprinted by permission of Sage Publications.)

Exercise 13-2 Positive and Negative Family Interactions

Purpose: To examine the effects of functional versus dysfunctional communication.

Procedure:

Answer the following questions in a brief essay:

1. Do you remember a situation in dealing with a client's family that you felt was a positive experience? What characteristics of that interaction made you feel this way?
2. Do you remember a situation in dealing with a client's family that you felt was a negative experience? What characteristics of that interaction made you feel this way?

Discussion:

Compare experiences, both positive and negative. What did you see as the most striking differences? In what ways were your responses similar or dissimilar from those of your peers? What do you see as the implications of this exercise for enhancing family communication in your nursing practice?

Exercise 13-3 Family Coping Strategies

Purpose: To broaden awareness of coping strategies among families.

Procedure:

Each student is to recall a time when his or her family experienced a significant health crisis and how they coped. (Alternative strategy: Pick a health crisis you observed with a family in clinical practice.) Respond to the following questions:

1. Did the crisis cause a readjustment in roles?
2. Did it create tension and conflict, or did it catalyze members, turning to one another for support? Look at individual members' behavior.
3. What would have helped your family in this crisis? Write a descriptive summary about this experience.

Discussion:

Each student shares his or her experience. Coping strategies and helpful interventions will be compiled on the board. Discuss the differences in how families respond to crisis. Discuss the nurse's role in support to the family.

APPLICATIONS

Assessment

Indications for Family Assessment

Healthy People 2010 considers the family as an important resource in health promotion and disease prevention. Regardless of how it occurs, any health disruption becomes a family event rather than an individual one. Even when the family is not directly involved in the client's care, members have feelings and reactions about it that can either support or sabotage the effectiveness of treatment and the client's quality of life (Bell, 2000).

Each family unit is unique. Health care issues will affect not only an individual's health but also the family's health, a bidirectional interaction among family members referred to as reciprocity (Novilla et al., 2006). Box 13-3 lists sample indicators that could warrant family assessment and nursing intervention.

The family needs to tell their own story and their experience of the client's illness or injury, which may be quite different from how an individual client is experiencing it. Nurses can help families understand, negotiate, and reconcile differences. For example, a grandmother may be very upset at being placed in a

Developing an Evidence-Based Practice

Smith C, Pace K, Kochinda C et al.: Caregiving effectiveness model evolution to a midrange theory of home care: a process for critique and replication, *Adv Nurs Sci* 25(1):50-64, 2003.

This article describes the processes used to develop, validate, revise and test a caregiving nursing model that could be used to explain and predict outcomes of home care given by family members to technology-dependent clients. These data could help nurses better address the needs of clients to ensure positive clinical outcomes. Caregiving effectiveness was defined as "the provision of technical, physical and emotional care by family members that results in outcomes of optimal patient condition, yet maintains caregivers' well-being" (pp. 52-53). The study used a descriptive correlational design and incorporated both quantitative and qualitative methodologies to describe the relationship among treatment outcomes, as well as model concepts conceptualized as family adaptation, family economic stability, caregiver health status, and reactions to caregiving. Data was collected over an 18-month period. Caregiving effectiveness related to caregiver quality of life, client quality of life, client's physical condition, and side effects of the technological treatments.

Results: Study findings supported a statistically significant relationship between caregiving effectiveness outcomes and independent variables identified in the model. The higher the level of the clinical nurses' overall adaptation ratings, the greater were the fundamental caregiver and client quality of life responses.

Application to Your Clinical Practice: Informal caregivers are an important segment of health care providers today. Understanding the factors that contribute to caregiving effectiveness for both the client and caregiver can help nurses with carefully targeted interventions.

nursing home after fracturing her hip. However, the family may feel that the placement is necessary because they can't take care of her. To be helpful, the nurse will need to balance the family's position and concerns with the client's needs in helping them talk with each other and in developing the most realistic solutions.

Assessing Family Instrumental and Expressive Function. Wright and Leahey (2000) describe two ways of examining family functioning: instrumental and expressive. Instrumental functioning refers to task activities of daily living (e.g., eating, sleeping, or caring for a sick member). The second aspect, expressive functioning, looks at the communication, problem-solving skills, roles, beliefs, spheres of influence, and power that govern how individual members interact with one another. In assessing for family function, you will need to assess the functional status of each family member, as well as looking at the family unit as a whole.

Disruptive challenges to the functioning of the family system can include normative crises such as divorce, retirement, marriage, remarriage, or placement of an elderly parent in a nursing home. Existing or unexpected challenges can include sudden job loss, trauma, or the untimely death of an important or conflictual family member (Walsh, 1996). The nurse will want to assess current family functioning in comparison with past patterns for a fuller picture of family dynamics.

Box 13-3 Indicators for Family Assessment

- Initial diagnosis of a serious physical or psychiatric illness/injury in a family member
- Family involvement and understanding needed to support recovery of client
- Deterioration in a family member's condition
- Illness in a child, adolescent, or cognitively impaired adult
- A child, adolescent, or adult child having an adverse response to a parent's illness
- Discharge from a health care facility to the home or an extended-care facility
- Death of a family member
- Health problem defined by family as a family issue
- Indication of threat to relationship (abuse), neglect, or anticipated loss of family member

Assessing Family Relationships Within the Larger Social System

Assessment of family relationships within the larger social system is important, as many families will need to use community agencies and support groups to successfully manage the illness of their family member. Interactions between the family and the larger social system are tracked by means of the *ecomap*, which examines the intensity and frequency of contact between the family and its social environment. Extended family assessment data consist of information about the family of origin and its relationship with the current (nuclear) family unit. In some families, the extended family is a significant support; in other families, it can be an irritant or obstacle to independent family function. In assessing for external structure, the nurse studies the social context of the family system with regard to community supports in the larger social environment that can enhance or limit family functioning, for example, church, school, social services, and community agencies.

Assessment Tools

Commonly used family assessment tools include the genogram, ecomap, and family time line.

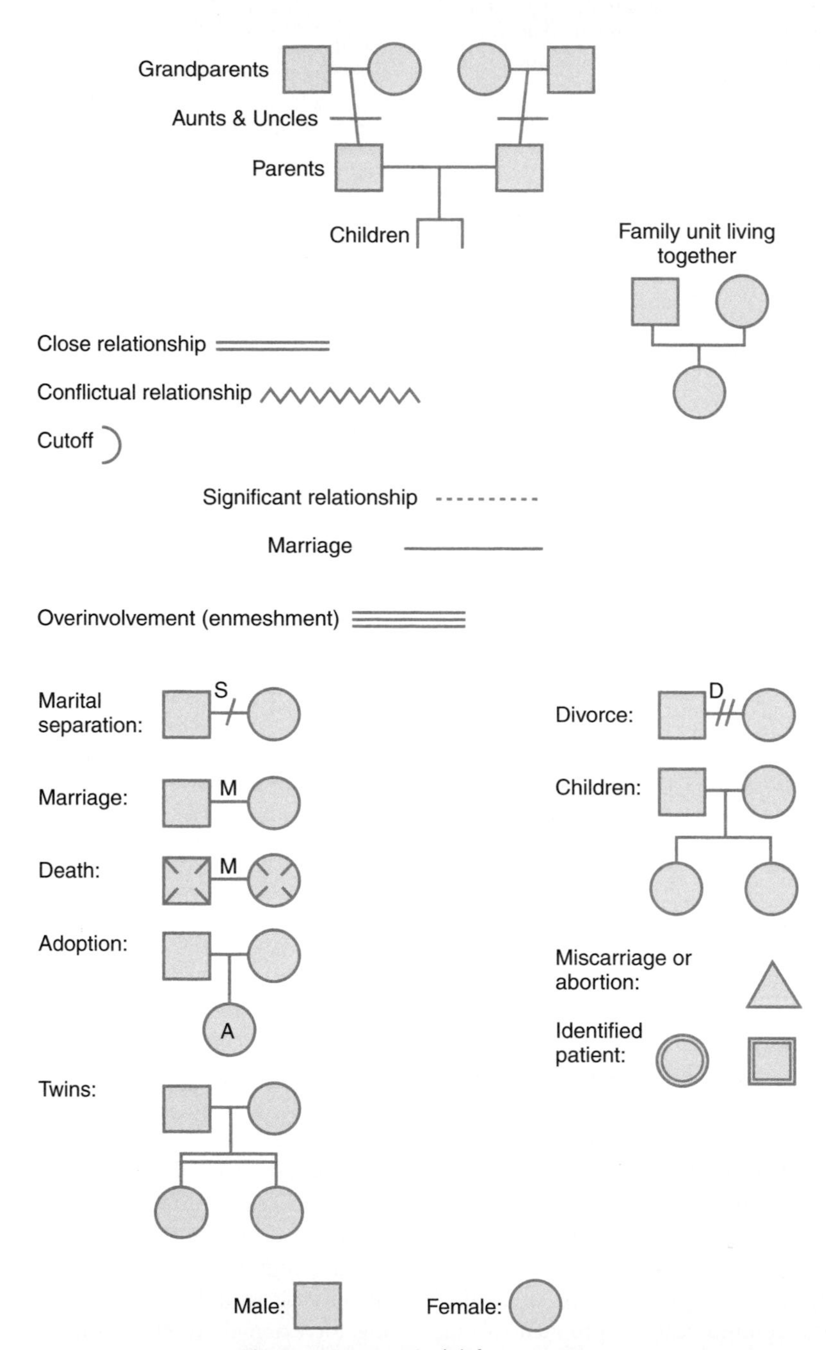

Figure 13-2 ● Symbols for a genogram.

Genograms. A **genogram** is a family diagram that records information about family members and their relationships over three generations. Most family members enjoy constructing a genogram and learn a lot about themselves in the process (Cole-Kelly & Seaburn, 1999). There are three parts to genogram construction: mapping the family structure, recording family information, and describing the nature of family relationships. A diagram of family members placed in each generation is drawn using horizontal and vertical lines. Symbols are used to map the family structure, with different symbols representing pregnancies, miscarriages, marriages, deaths, and other nodal family events (Figure 13-2). Males are placed on the left of the horizontal line as a small square and females on the right as small circles. Placing the oldest sibling on the far left and progressing toward the right represents descending birth order. In the case of multiple marriages, the earliest is placed on the left and the most recent on the right.

The genogram should include informational data about ages, birth and death dates for all family members, relevant illnesses, immigration, geographical location of current members, occupations and employment status, educational levels, patterns of family members entering or leaving the family unit, religious affiliation or change, and military service (McGoldrick, Gerson, & Shellenberger, 1999). These are written near the symbols for each involved person. Critical family events and transitions such as moves, marriages, divorces, losses, and successes are recorded. Family members' physical, emotional, and social problems or illnesses—particularly a history of drug use, abuse, incest, or mental disorder, because of their impact on family communication—are identified. Relationship patterns can be recorded as

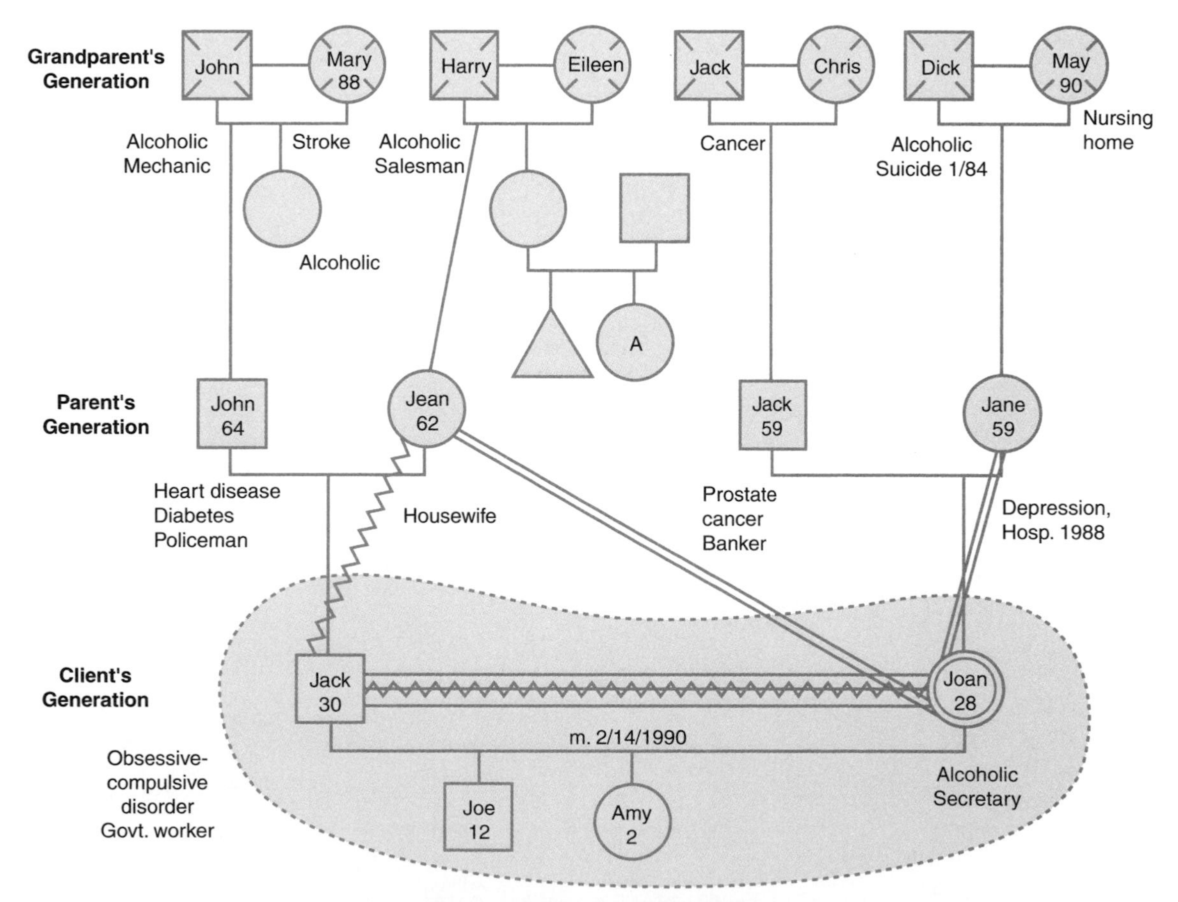

Figure 13-3 ● Basic family genogram.

overly close, close, distant, cut off, or conflictual, with the intensity of the pattern emphasized by adding or decreasing the number of lines between family members.

In helping the nurse construct the genogram, family members are reminding themselves of important members of their family, their strengths and weaknesses, and how these may relevant for the current situation. The picture of the family that is presented on the genogram helps the nurse think about the family systematically and over time. An example of a family genogram is presented in Figure 13-3.

Exercise 13-4 Family Genogram

Purpose: To learn to create a family genogram.

Procedure:
Students will break into pairs and interview one another to gain information to develop a family genogram. The genogram should include demographic information, occurrence of illness or death, and relationship patterns for three generations. Use the symbols for diagramming in Figure 13-2 to create a visual picture of the family information. Ask the author for validation of accuracy as you develop the genogram.

Discussion:
Each person will display their genogram and discuss the process of obtaining information. Discuss strategies for obtaining information expediently yet sensitively and tactfully. Discuss how genograms can be used in a helpful way with families.

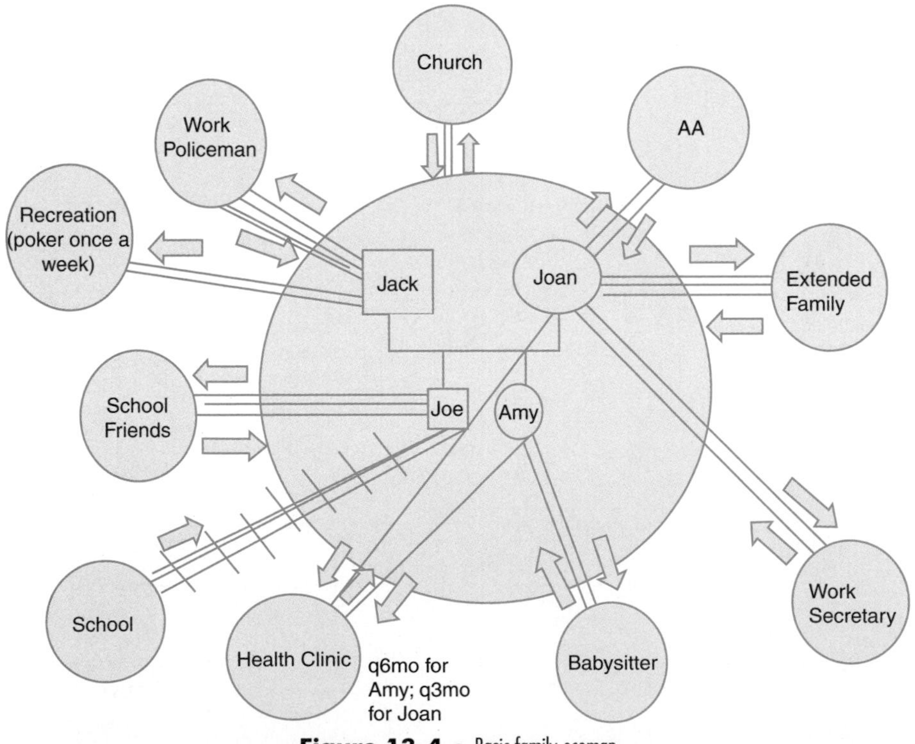

Figure 13-4 • Basic family ecomap.

Exercise 13-4 provides practice with developing a family genogram.

Ecomaps. The ecomap enhances the family information learned from the genogram and is used in assessment, planning, and intervention. An **ecomap** illustrates the relationships between family members and community-based systems such as school, work, health care system, neighborhood, and church affiliations. Information about the extent of time spent in relationships outside the family is valuable in helping to identify actual and potential family resources available through friends and community systems. Figure 13-4 shows an example of an ecomap. Exercise 13-5 provides an opportunity to explore the advantages of using an ecomap.

To develop an ecomap, start with an inner circle labeled with the family's name in the middle of the page. This represents the family unit. Smaller circles outside the family circle represent other significant people, agencies, and social institutions with whom the family interacts either as a whole or individually. Examples include school, work, church, neighborhood friends, recreation activities, health care facilities or home care, extended family, and exercise gym. Lines are drawn from the inner family circle to outer circles indicating the strength of the contact and relationship. Straight lines indicate relation, with additional lines used to indicate the strength of the relationship. Dotted lines suggest fragile relationships. Stressful relationships are represented with slashes placed through the relationship line. Directional arrows indicate the flow of the relational energy.

Family Time Lines. Time lines are another way of diagramming family life events and patterns. Family patterns that develop through multigenerational transmission and evolving community culture are represented as vertical lines. Horizontal lines indicate events occurring over the current life span. They include such milestones as marriages, illnesses, or births. Family time lines may show patterns of early death, marriage at an early age, or high educational level (Figure 13-5). This diagram is useful in looking at how the family history and concurrent life events might interact with the current health concern.

Less common assessment tools include a spirituality genogram (Frame, 2000) and a spiritual ecomap (Hodge, 2000). These more specialized tools can be useful in helping families understand the origin and development of spiritual beliefs within their family. This type of assessment is particularly useful with families and clients who are interested in exploring spirituality as a support in difficult health care situations.

Case Example

Gretchen was 49 years old when she was diagnosed with pancreatic cancer. She had been raised as a Methodist, but over the years had lost all connection with the church and no longer considered it a resource. She raised this as an issue in the past. The hospice nurse explored her feelings about this and helped her to see that she could be angry with God but still have a relationship with a higher being who could be of comfort to her. As Gretchen talked about her early years, she brought out a small prayer book she had when she was 9 years old.

Exercise 13-5 Family Ecomap

Purpose: To learn to create a family ecomap.

Procedure:

Using the interview process, students will break into pairs and interview one another to gain information to develop a family ecomap. The ecomap should include information about resources and stressors in the larger community system, such as school, church, health agencies, and interaction with extended family and friends for each student's family.

Discussion:

Each person will display his or her ecomap and discuss the process of obtaining information. Discuss strategies for obtaining information expediently yet sensitively and tactfully. Discuss how ecomaps broaden the structural information about a family and can be used in a helpful way with families.

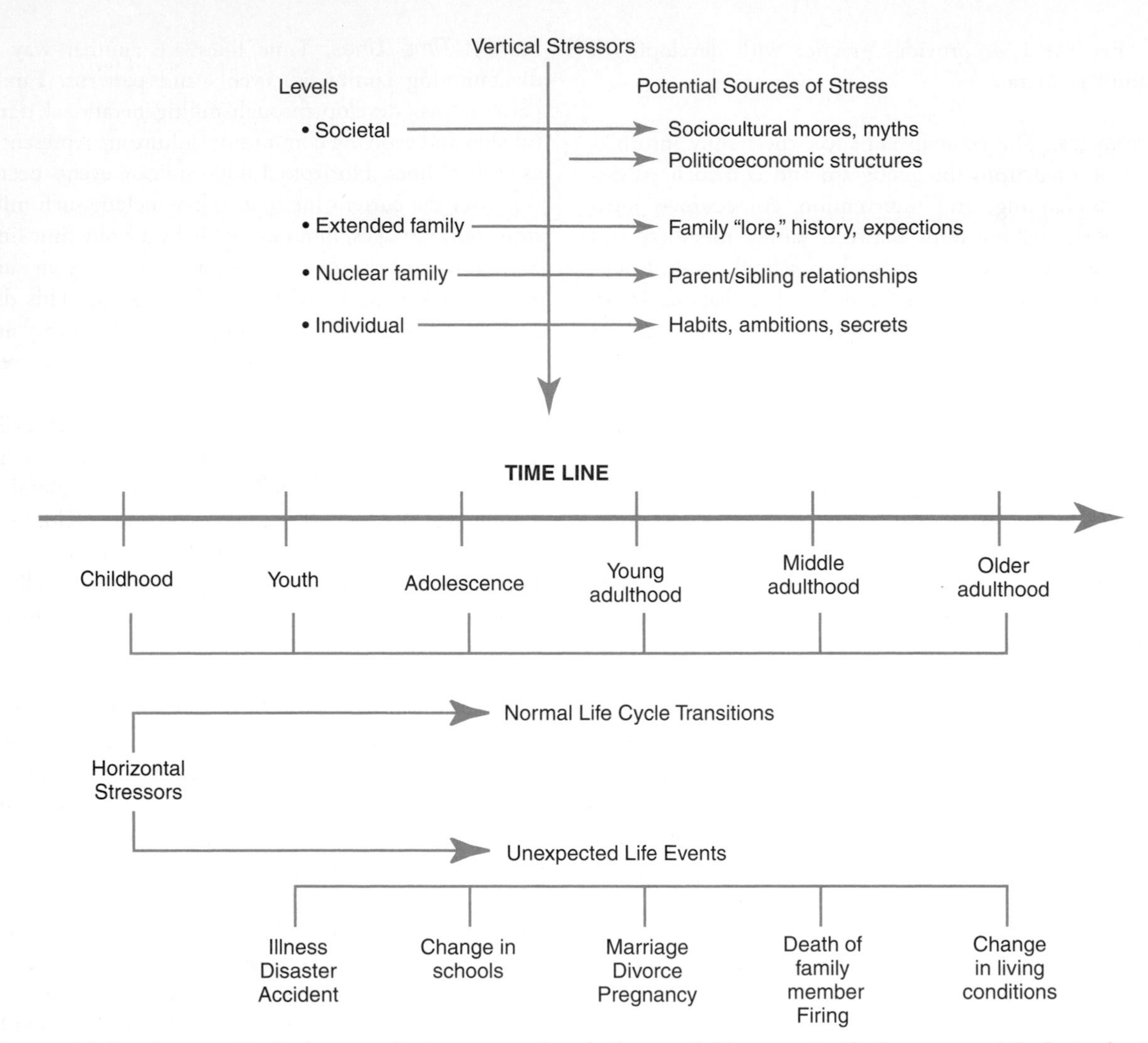

Figure 13-5 • Learning activity: Develop a comprehensive assessment of your family composed of three-generational family genograms and identification of vertical and horizontal stressors.

Together, the nurse and client looked at the little book. Over the next few weeks, Gretchen began to find comfort in a relationship she thought no longer existed. One afternoon she confided to the nurse that she had been napping and feeling frightened about the unknown quality of her dying. Suddenly she felt a sense of warmth and comfort that she equated with God. When the nurse asked what this was like, she said, "I don't know, but I'm not afraid anymore."

Another specialized tool is the gendergram (White & Tyson-Rawson, 1995), which traces the implications of **gender roles** in family dynamics. Exercise 13-6 demonstrates the use of the gendergram in assessing how gender roles can develop within a family.

Gathering Assessment Data

Family participation in data assessment enhances the therapeutic relationship (Mailick & Vigilante, 1997). Assessment of relevant family experiences provides a way of understanding the client within a socioenvironmental context that surrounds and supports his or her recovery. Meaningful involvement in the client's care not only differs from family to family, but it also differs among individual family members (Sydnor-Greenberg, Dokken, &

Exercise 13-6 Constructing a Gendergram

Purpose: To assist students in developing an understanding of family contributions to gender role development.

Procedure:
Each student should ask older family members of the same sex (e.g., mother, aunt, grandmother or father, uncle, grandfather) to talk about their experience growing up as a girl or a boy. Dialogue about what they see as different about gender roles today and how their gender has influenced who they are today. Compare their impressions with your own gender role development in a short essay.

Discussion:
Each student will share his or her findings with the larger group. Discussion can focus on how gender role expectations are different and similar to those held in the past. Discuss differences and similarities in the gender role development of men and women. Discuss implications of this exercise for health care delivery.

Ahmann, 2000). The nurse needs information about each family's usual responses to stress and coping strategies. Data about their communication styles in decision making, their perceptions of family strengths and weaknesses, value beliefs, roles, activities, environmental characteristics, and knowledge of community resources provides a comprehensive look at family dynamics.

Box 13-4 provides a comprehensive family database tool that the nurse can use to quickly gather information about these issues in non–acute care settings. In acute care situations, the nurse can ask the following key questions:

- How does the family view the current health crisis?
- How did it develop?
- Has anyone else in the family experienced a similar problem?
- What do family members believe would be most helpful to the client at this time?
- What part of the current situation worries each family member most?
- Are there any other recent changes or sources of stress in the family that make the crisis worse?
- How has the family handled the problem to date?
- What would the family like to achieve with the nurse's help in resolving the problem?

Recognizing Families at Risk. Not all families act in the best interests of their members. Marital discord, parental mental illness, overcrowded housing conditions, and limited parenting skills place children at risk for faulty development (Hawley & DeHaan, 1996). Abuse of family members, violence, substance abuse, neglect, and dysfunction are on the increase as families become more and more stressed while trying to cope with the demands of today's world. The nurse must also be able to recognize families who are providing unsafe environments for their members. Referring families to professionals able to deal with these complex problems and notifying protective service authorities when necessary are other roles of nurses who work with families. Nurses are considered reporting agents in most states and therefore are *required* by law to report suspicion of child physical or sexual abuse to child protection agencies.

Planning

Once a family assessment has been completed, the nurse analyzes the data and summarizes the family's needs. According to Wright and Leahey (2000), nurses can only *offer* interventions; it is up to the family to accept them. Selekman (1997) identifies the following four elements to consider when selecting and designing therapeutic tasks for families:

- The family's definition of the problem
- Key family characteristics (e.g., language, beliefs, and strengths)
- Unique cooperative response patterns of family members
- Family treatment goals

The family's definition of the problem as a whole may be different than that of individual family members. For

Box 13-4 Family Assessment for Client Entering Cardiac Rehabilitation

Coping/Stress

Who lives with you? ______________________________

How do you handle stress? ______________________________

Have you had any recent changes in your life (e.g., job change, move, change in marital status, loss)? ______________________________

On whom do you rely for emotional support? ______________________________

Who relies on you for emotional support? ______________________________

How does your illness affect your family members/significant other? ______________________________

Are there any health concerns of other family members? ______________________________

If so, how does this affect you? ______________________________

Communication/Decision Making

How would you describe the communication pattern in your family? ______________________________

How does your family address issues/concerns? ______________________________

Can you identify strengths/weaknesses within the family? ______________________________

Are family members supportive of each other? ______________________________

How are decisions that affect the entire family made? ______________________________

How are decisions implemented? ______________________________

Role

What is your role in the family? ______________________________

Can you describe the roles of other family members? ______________________________

Value Beliefs

What is your ethnic/cultural background? ______________________________

What is your religious background? ______________________________

Are there any particular cultural/religious healing practices in which you participate? ______________________________

Leisure Activities

Do you participate in any organized social activities? ______________________________

In what leisure activities do you participate? ______________________________

Do you anticipate any difficulty with continuing these activities? ______________________________

If so, how will you make the appropriate adjustments? ______________________________

Do you have a regular exercise regimen? ______________________________

Box 13-4 Family Assessment for Client Entering Cardiac Rehabilitation—*cont'd.*

Environmental Characteristics

Do you live in a rural, suburban, or urban area? ______________________________

What type of dwelling do you live in? ______________________________

Are there stairs in your home? ______________________________

Where is the bathroom? ______________________________

Are the facilities adequate to meet your needs? ______________________________

If not, what adjustments will be needed? ______________________________

How do you plan to make those adjustments? ______________________________

Are there any community services provided to you at home? (explain) ______________________________

Are there community resources available in your area? ______________________________

Do you have any other concerns at this time? ______________________________

Is there anything that we have omitted? ______________________________

Signature ______________________________ (must be completed by RN) Date/Time

Developed by Conrad J, Williamson J, Mignardi D: University of Maryland School of Nursing, 1993.

this reason, it is important to get each member's perspective and then help the family develop a coherent understanding. Each family treatment plan should be tailored to acknowledge important family goals, values, and priorities. Setting realistic and achievable goals that the family helps to construct makes it easier for the family to accomplish them with a sense of mastery and self-efficacy about the process. Taking little steps that are achievable is preferred to giant steps that misjudge what the family can realistically do. When treatment goals are unrealistic, goals do not get achieved, and the family is left with feelings of defeat or inadequacy. Incorporating identifiable cultural and religious beliefs in care plans increases familiarity and reassures clients of the nurse's understanding of each family's unique set of circumstances (see Chapter 11). Exercise 13-7 provides practice with developing family nursing care plans.

It is important to be sensitive to the viewpoints of each family member (even when they conflict with one another), and to facilitate the family in making informed choices. Commend individual family members and the family as a whole on specific positive actions taken to date or ones that could be used to support the client (Wright & Leahey, 2000). Whenever possible, nurses should respect the family's values and priorities, remembering that the primary goal is to help families become empowered to take as much responsibility as possible for a quality health care outcome.

Change occurs more readily when at least one member of the system, often a person who is the most free from constraints and has some power in the family, changes his or her way of functioning within the family. In this way of thinking, interventions for families are not always directed at the member who is ill, injured, or at risk but at family members who are most able to engineer necessary change. Family change—working through family strengths rather than focusing on its deficits—is useful. Helping a family to become aware of information from the environment and to use what is available from outside itself often promotes family health. By showing interest in the coping strategies that have and have not worked, the nurse can help the family see how it has reorganized itself around the stressful situation.

Incorporating Family Strengths

Otto (1963) first described the value of family strengths as a healing strategy. He labels them as personal potential and actual resources families can use to make their life more satisfying and fulfilling to its members. Nursing theorists also have identified family strengths as

Exercise 13-7 Nursing Process Applied to Family Interactions

Purpose: To practice skills needed with difficult family patterns.

Procedure:
Read the case study and think of how you could interact appropriately with this family.

Mr. Monroe, age 43 years, was chairing a board meeting of his large, successful manufacturing corporation when he developed shortness of breath; dizziness; and a crushing, viselike pain in his chest. An ambulance was called, and he was taken to the medical center. Subsequently, he was admitted to the coronary unit with a diagnosis of an impending myocardial infarction (MI).

Mr. Monroe is married, with three children: Steve, age 14; Sean, age 12; and Lisa, age 8. He is the president and majority stockholder of his company. He has no history of cardiovascular problems, although his father died at the age of 38 of a massive coronary occlusion. His oldest brother died at the age of 42 from the same condition, and his other brother, still living, became a semi-invalid after suffering two heart attacks, one at the age of 44, and the other at 47.

Mr. Monroe is tall, slim, suntanned, and very athletic. He swims daily; jogs every morning for 30 minutes; plays golf regularly; and is an avid sailor, having participated in every yacht regatta and usually winning. He is very health-conscious and has had annual physical checkups. He watches his diet and quit smoking to avoid possible damage to his heart. He has been determined to avoid dying young or becoming an invalid like his brother.

When he was admitted to the coronary care unit, he was conscious. Although in a great deal of pain, he seemed determined to control his own fate. While in the unit, he was an exceedingly difficult patient, a trial to the nursing staff and his physician. He constantly watched and listened to everything going on around him and demanded complete explanations about any procedure, equipment, or medication he received. He would sleep in brief naps and only when he was totally exhausted. Despite his obvious tension and anxiety, his condition stabilized. The damage to his heart was considered minimal, and his prognosis was good. As the pain diminished, he began asking when he could go home and when he could go back to work. He was impatient to be moved to a private room so that he could conduct some of his business by telephone.

When Mrs. Monroe visited, she approached the nursing staff with questions regarding Mr. Monroe's condition, usually asking the same question several times in different ways. She also asked why she was not being "told everything."

Interactions between Mr. Monroe and Mrs. Monroe were noted by the staff as Mr. Monroe telling Mrs. Monroe all of the things she needed to do. Very little intimate contact was noted.

Mr. Monroe denied having any anxiety or concerns about his condition, although his behavior contradicted his denial. Mrs. Monroe would agree with her husband's assessment when questioned in his company.

Discussion:
1. What questions would you ask the client and family to obtain data regarding their adaptation to crisis?
2. What family nursing diagnosis would apply with this case study?
3. What nursing interventions are appropriate to interact with this client and his family?
4. How would you plan to transmit the information to the family?

Developed by Conrad J: University of Maryland School of Nursing, 1993.

an important resource in planning intervention (Allen, 1999; Tapp & Moules, 1997). Viewing the family as having strengths to cope with a problem rather than *being* a problem is a particularly helpful strategy because it gives a family hope that the problem is not the end point but rather only a circumstance in need of a solution. Feeley and Gottlieb (2000) identify four different types of strengths nurses can help the family use to achieve important health outcomes:

- Traits that reside within an individual or a family (e.g., optimism, resilience)
- Assets that reside within an individual or a family (e.g., finances)
- Capabilities, skills, or competencies that an individual or a family has developed (e.g., problem-solving skills)
- A quality that is more transient in nature than a trait or asset (e.g., motivation)

The nurse should look for physical, emotional, and spiritual strengths present in the family that can help them experience the current health alteration as potentially growth-producing for the entire family. Often a family has unique strengths that are temporarily overshadowed by the health need, so these strengths lie outside of the family's awareness. Reinforcement and amplification of family strengths in times of crisis can both enhance and maintain behavioral changes needed in recovery.

Questions you can use to elicit family strengths include the following (Tapp & Moules, 1997):

- What has the family been doing so far that has been helpful?
- What is going well for this family?
- How have they (family) been able to do as well as they have done?
- What beliefs or previous experiences or relationships are sustaining them and preventing the problem from being worse?
- What advice would they give to other people in the same situation?

The responses to these questions can help nurses and families develop strategies specifically inclusive of identified client family strengths. Incorporating family strengths in problem solving and commitment to family goals facilitates goal achievement (Mailick & Vigilante, 1997).

Exercise 13-8 Using Intervention Skills with Families

Purpose: To provide practice with using intervention skills with families.

Procedure:

Each student will work with a family related to a specific problem. This can be a current or previous situation for the family. Talk with the family about the problem, and learn how they have dealt with the problem, their perception of the problem, and its impact on their family. Use some of the approaches identified in the text to help them explore the problem in more depth and begin to develop viable options.

Write a descriptive summary of your experiences, including a self-evaluation. Evaluate the experience with the family as well, specifically for feedback regarding your approach. Did they feel you were too intrusive or not assertive enough? Did you validate all members' perceptions and perspectives? Did you clarify information and feelings? Did you remain nonjudgmental and objective? Did you respect the family's values and beliefs without imposing your own? Did you assist the family in clarifying and understanding the problem in a way that could lead to resolution?

Discussion:

Students share their experience and the feedback they received from the family. Discuss the obstacles encountered when communicating with families. Discuss strategies to facilitate goal-directed communication and resolution of problems. How can nurses best provide support to families? How could families learn to use leveling most of the time? How does one influence this in one's own family?

Interventions

The nurse enters the family system as a teacher, counselor, and advocate to help the family adjust itself to often-dramatic change in life circumstances. Nurses use communication principles to help families solve problems and find external resources to support their functioning during times of stress. Nursing interventions can include facilitating and role modeling healthy family communication, helping the family solve problems, linking the family with other parts of the health care system, providing information, and supporting and strengthening family coping. More experienced nurses with specialized graduate training may counsel families experiencing serious problems in family dynamics. Exercise 13-8 provides an opportunity to examine nursing interactions with families.

Wright and Leahey (2000) suggest the following examples of nursing action areas that can be used to promote positive change in family functioning:

- Commending family and individual strengths
- Offering information and opinions
- Validating or normalizing emotional responses
- Encouraging the telling of illness narratives
- Drawing forth family support
- Encouraging family members as caregivers
- Encouraging respite
- Devising rituals

Change occurs more easily when at least one member of the system, often the person who is the most free from constraints and has some power in the family, changes his or her way of functioning within the family. In this way of thinking, interventions for families are not always directed at the member who is ill, injured, or at risk but at family members who are most able to engineer necessary change. Family change—working through family strengths rather than focusing on deficits—is useful. Helping a family to become aware of information from the environment and to use what is available from outside often promotes family health. By showing interest in the coping strategies that have and have not worked, the nurse can help the family see how they have reorganized themselves around the stressful situation.

Educating and Problem Solving During Developmental Crises

Families traditionally care for their members during times of life transitions such as pregnancies, births, marriages, and deaths. Whereas most families come to the situation with an expectation of what they will be doing, they often need support or education when they are experiencing new developmental challenges (Curtis, Patrick, Shannon et al., 2001). See Chapter 21 for strategies to use with families in crisis. Everyone knows that an infant will demand that the family make some adjustments; however, it is not until the infant actually arrives that the family may realize it needs information or ideas about how to rearrange the activities of daily living. When more than one crisis occurs simultaneously (e.g., the birth of a child with a congenital problem), the family who appeared to be prepared may need additional resources to cope with the pileup of demands.

A nurse who is aware of developmental family theory will attempt to locate the family within a stage in the life cycle and to assess the family's knowledge of the current developmental demands, the strategies it is using to meet these demands, and its success in meeting them. Some families need information about the "usual" course that can be expected. Others benefit from interventions that help them find balance between the developmental demands and situational stressors such as illness or job loss. Sometimes in families with an ill member, the needs of a healthy child become lost in the shuffle. The goal is to enable the family to accomplish its function for all its members, not just the ones who are ill or otherwise in the forefront. Strategies to help the family in stressful situations or crisis are described in Chapters 20 and 21.

Caregiving and the Family

Family caregivers most often are the primary caregivers for older people who can no longer take care of themselves or who require additional support to maintain their independence (McKenry & Price, 2005). Caregiving responsibilities for family members with dementia can become all-consuming and last for many years. Other family members are often the identified caregivers for any family member who becomes ill. The family member may be homebound, and family members may need to offer all the care or to coordinate it with health professionals. In other situations, the ill member is more able to care for himself or herself, but may need to enlist family support when changes are required (e.g., in diet and activity).

Healthy family members have concurrent demands on their time from their own nuclear families, work, church, and community responsibilities. This is particularly true when spouses have to become caregivers in younger families (Gordon & Perrone, 2004). A significant change in health status can give rise to previous unresolved relationship issues, which may need advanced intervention in addition to the specific health care issues. This can be particularly true in times of developmental family transitions, for example, departure of a spouse, entrance of a new spouse, departure of the last adult child, or an untimely death of a family member. Nurses need to consider the broader family responsibilities people have as an important part of the context of health care in providing holistic care to a particular family.

Families often act as the client's advocate during hospitalization, either informally or as the formal surrogate decision maker identified by law to make health care decisions on behalf of the client. The nurse is a primary health care provider agent in working with families facing these issues. Nurses need to help the family as a whole and its individual members to recognize its limitations and hidden strengths and to maintain a balance of health for all members. Curtis and Dixon (2005) recommended distinguishing between situational, transitional, and chronic health problems, as this will affect the type of planning and interventions most likely to be successful. For example, helping a family determine whether a grandmother should be placed in a nursing facility raises significant emotional issues, whereas a cancer diagnosis in a young child may require a number of interventions at different levels—care of the child with cancer, responding to the needs of healthy members simultaneously, and processing difficult emotional information. Aldridge (2005) identifies parental needs in the pediatric intensive care unit in Box 13-5.

Box 13-5 Summary of Parental Needs in the Pediatric ICU

Information/Illness Progression

- Knowing the prognosis
- Knowing why things were being done
- Having questions answered honestly
- Being called at home when the child's condition changes
- Knowing about equipment and tubes being used for the child
- Feeling that there is hope

Being a Parent to the Child

- Knowing the child is comfortable
- Participating in the child's care in any way possible
- Feeling that the child is getting the best care
- Feeling that the staff care about the child

Access to the Child

- Being able to be with the child at all times
- Being able to see the child frequently without limitations on visiting hours
- Being able to stay with the child during procedures

Physical Needs

- Having food and drink nearby
- Having a place to rest that is near the intensive care unit

Adapted from Aldridge M: Decreasing parental stress in the pediatric intensive care unit, *Crit Care Nurse*, 25(6):41, 2005.

Supporting Family Coping

The importance of supporting the family caregivers is reinforced in a study by Cannuscio, Jones, Kawachi et al. (2002) in which findings demonstrated that individuals caring for their disabled spouse were six times more likely to experience clinical depression or anxiety.

Starting with the family's information about itself, the nurse often is able to help members reframe a situation so that there is a healthier balance between self-needs and those created by the current stressors (Modricin & Robison, 1991). Each family has a different style of coping that may or may not be helpful in time of stress. If the coping style is adequate to meet the needs of the current situation, the nurse can encourage the family's methods even if others are available. Helping the family understand the implications of the pileup of demands that leads to a sense of crisis encourages members to acknowledge role strain and think about their situation in more realistic terms. For families with chronically ill members (multiple sclerosis, cardiovascular disorders, diabetes) the demands can vary with the element of uncertainty and progression of disease not far from the forefront of caregiving considerations.

Sometimes the family's style of coping is not useful. Suppose that the way one family copes is to look to the mother for all their support, even when the mother is the one who is ill. When the nurse and the family determine that the present style of coping is not working, then alternative solutions can be sought. Focus initially on issues that are manageable within the context of home caregiving. This provides a sense of mastery and satisfaction. The nurse can encourage the family to develop new ways of coping or can list alternatives and allow the family to choose coping styles that might be useful to them. Providing emotional support is crucial to helping families cope. Remaining aware of one's own values and staying calm and thoughtful can be very helpful to a family in crisis. Remember that your words can either strengthen or weaken a family's confidence in their ability to care for an ill family member. Focus on what goes well, and ask the family to share with you their ideas about how to best care for the client. There is no one "correct" way to provide care. By enhancing a family's coping style in ways that are familiar and culturally congruent with their beliefs and expectations to whatever extent is possible, the nurse stands a better chance of family involvement in taking care of their loved one.

Family members, particularly the primary caregivers, need to have an opportunity to learn the requisite skills for managing the care of their family member at home, in addition to the emotional support nurses can provide. Discharge instructions may not be enough. Nurses should open a dialogue with clients about what to expect at home and should ask for enough feedback to ensure that the family both understands and is comfortable with health care instructions. Giving the family a contact number to call if there is a problem or if they don't fully understand something after they get home is very helpful. Families also may need to be connected with supportive community resources such as disease, trauma, or chronic illness support groups. Byng-Hall (1995) also suggests the use of family life review as a way of stimulating family member reminiscence of successful past experiences and reconnection with past positive coping strategies that could be helpful in the present health care situation.

Offering Commendations

Limacher and Wright (2003) define *commendation* as "the practice of noticing, drawing forth, and highlighting previously unobserved, forgotten, or unspoken family strengths, competencies or resources" (p. 132). Commendations can be embedded indirectly within questions and listening responses. Its use is context-specific, and it is a particularly powerful tool to use when the family seems dispirited and confused about a tragic illness or accident. Ryan and Steinmiller (2004) recommend naming family strengths in front of the family, and Wright and Leahey (2000) suggest using commendations to mirror observations of behavior patterns reflective of family strengths back to the family unit. More than a simple compliment, commendations should reflect *patterns* of behavior existing in the family

Exercise 13-9 Offering Commendations

Purpose: To provide practice with using commendation skills with families.

Procedure:

Students will work in groups of three students. Each student will develop a commendation about the two other students in the group. The commendation should reflect a personal strength that the reflecting student has observed over a period time. Examples might include kindness, integrity, commitment, persistence, goal-directedness, tolerance, or patience. Write a simple paragraph about the trait or behavior you observe in this person. If you can, give some examples of why you have associated this particular characteristic with the person. Each student in turn should read his or her reflections about the other two participants, starting the conversation with good eye contact, the name of the receiving student, and a simple orienting statement (e.g., "Kelly, this is what I have observed in knowing you . . .").

Discussion:

Class discussion should focus on the thought process of the students in developing particular commendations, the values they focused on, and any consideration they gave to the impact of the commendation on the other students. The students can also discuss the effect of hearing the commendations about themselves and what it stimulated in them. Other areas of focus might be how commendations can be used with families and how they can be employed to counteract family resistance to working together.

unit over time. For example, the nurse might comment on the strength of the family unit in coping with multiple problems, the capacity to stay involved even when it is difficult to do so, or the ability of the family to thoroughly research a health problem. It is important to choose strengths the family will recognize as valid and strengths that could potentially aid in the current care of the client (McElheran & Harper-Jaques, 1994). Exercise 13-9 provides practice with giving commendations.

Interventive Questioning

Wright and Leahey (2000) identify questioning as a type of nursing intervention nurses can use with their client families to identify family strengths; help family members sort out their personal fears, concerns, and challenges in health care situations; and provide a vehicle for exploring alternative options. Interventive questioning can be either linear or circular. The use of linear (sequential) questions is discussed in Chapter 10. **Circular questions** focus on the impact of an illness or injury on the functioning of the family system (Figure 13-6). Sample interventive circular questions—categorized as difference, behavior effect, hypothetical, or future-oriented questions—and follow-up questions are found in Box 13-6. The nurse uses the information the family provides as the basis for additional questions, as expressed in the following case example when the nurse asks a family coping with a terminally ill parent, "What has been your biggest challenge in caring for your mother at home?"

Case Example

Daughter: My biggest challenge has been finding a balance between caring for my mother and also caring for my children and husband. I have also had to learn a lot about the professional and support resources that are available in the community.

Son-in-law: For me, the biggest challenge has been convincing my wife that I can take over for a while, in order for her to get some rest. I worry that she will become exhausted.

Mother: I have appreciated all the help that they give me. My biggest challenge is to continue to do as much as possible for myself so that I do not become too much of a burden on them. Sometimes I wonder about moving to a palliative care setting or a hospice. (Leahey & Harper-Jaques, 1996, p. 135)

From the responses above, the nurse gains multidimensional information about the family that might not emerge with linear questions (e.g., the clear investment of this family in the mother's care, the challenge of the daughter in finding balance between caring for her mother and her family, and her husband's fear that she is becoming too tired). Finally, the mother's response to the circular question is twofold, worrying that she is becoming too much of a burden and exploring different options for care as her condition deteriorates. The open discussion occurring around the context of the illness provides a powerful way for family members to hear the

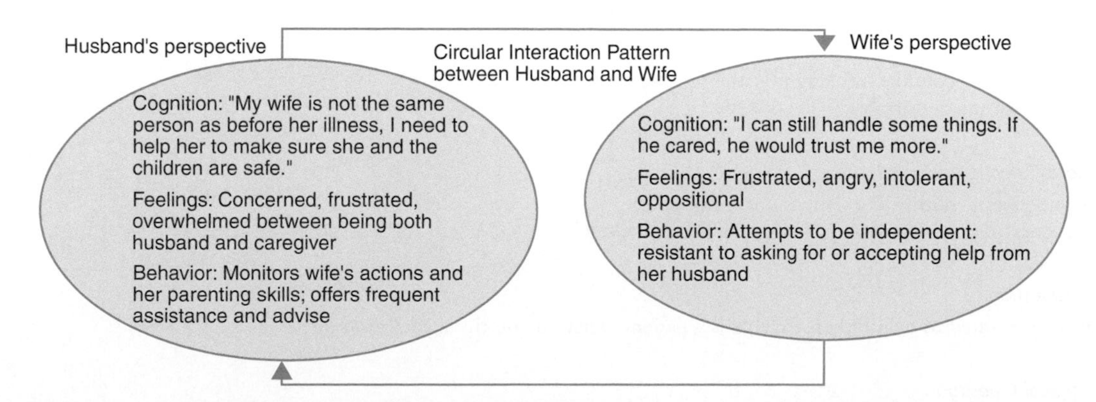

Figure 13-6 • Circular questioning applied to a family illness. (Adapted from Bell JM: Encouraging nurses and families to think interactionally: revisiting the usefulness of the circular pattern diagram, *J Fam Nurs* 6[3]:206, 2000.)

Box 13-6 Sample Interventive Circular Questions for Family of the Critically Ill

Need for Relief of Anxiety

Difference Questions

- Who will be most relieved when father wakes up/gets better?
- Who is most anxious/fearful about the illness?
- What is the worst thing that could happen because of father's illness?
- What is most helpful to mother to relieve her anxiety?
- Is mother more anxious now or when she heard about son's accident?

Behavioral Effect Questions

- How does your mother show she is anxious?
- What do you do when your mother cries?

Triadic Question

- What does your brother do to help mother relieve her anxiety?

Hypothetical Questions

- If the children stayed with you, would you be more or less anxious?
- If you went home, would you be more or less anxious?

Need for Information

Difference Questions

- Who finds the information most helpful?
- Who best understands what the doctors have explained to you?
- When a new member of the family needs to be told about the patient, who explains best?
- How do you understand what the doctors have told you?
- How is your understanding different from your mother's?

Hypothetical Questions

- If you chose to ask for more information, whom could you ask?
- If you asked for more information, who would be most helpful?

Need to Be with and Be Helpful to the Patient

Difference Questions

- Who finds most comfort in being near the patient?
- Who is most uncomfortable at the bedside?

Behavioral Effect Questions

- How does your mother show she is uncomfortable?
- What does your brother do to avoid going to the bedside?

Triadic Question

- If mother wanted to help father while he is a patient, what do you think she could do?

Hypothetical Question

- If you could do one thing to help, what would it be?

Box 13-6 Sample Interventive Circular Questions for Family of the Critically Ill—*Cont'd.*

Need to Alter and Adjust to New Roles

Difference Questions

- Now that mother is ill, who is best at disciplining the children?
- Who is best taking care of the house?
- Who is closest to mother?

Behavioral Effect Questions

- How do they show they are close?
- How does father/brother/sister help now that mother is in the hospital?

Hypothetical Question

- If son/daughter were more helpful, what would they do?

From Loos F, Bell J: Circular questions: a family interviewing strategy, *Dimens Crit Care Nurs* 9(1):49, 1990. Copyright Springhouse Corporation.

concerns of others and to reflect on the meaning of their own concern. This becomes the foundation for developing strategies mutually acceptable to all family members.

Helping Families Develop Support

Most families need some help coordinating resources. Sometimes family resources are limited or nonexistent. Other families may have plenty of financial and instrumental resources but need help finding their way through the maze of the health care system.

Providing information and linking families to available resources is a common role of the nurse. You should develop a working knowledge of community resources available to families and the best ways to access them.

Encouraging families to use natural helping systems increases the network of emotional and economic support available to the family in time of crisis. Examples include contact with other relatives, neighbors, friends, and churches. Social and emotional support among family members contribute to resilience within the family. Greeff and Human (2004) also found that spiritual beliefs and support from extended family and friends enhance family resilience in times of trauma and loss. All family members deserve communication from the health care system that recognizes their importance and worth as individuals. How the nurse interacts with each member may be as important as what he or she chooses to say.

Encouraging Self-Awareness

Helping each family member become more aware of self and of his or her impact on others in the family is a primary objective. Techniques for doing this include role-playing various positions or situations with some accompanying discussion of what that position feels like and about its continued use in the family. Circular questions are also helpful.

Reframing

Feeley and Gottlieb (2000) define cognitive reframing as "statements or questions aimed at helping the client develop a different conceptual or emotional view of a situation, person, or behavior, and it often involves sharing a perspective with the client that differs from their own" (p. 13). The reframing process helps clients and families become aware of others' points of view, often turning a negative perception into a more positive one and thereby promoting self-esteem. It detours the blaming process and often shakes up the situation just enough for the family to begin trying something different. For example, a mother who criticizes her daughter's grades may be encouraged to reframe her statements to indicate her concern about how grades can affect her daughter's future.

Giving Corrective Feedback

The nurse who takes the position of an informed observer uses corrective feedback in a neutral way. Role modeling appropriate communication is the first priority in corrective feedback, because even if you are not directly telling the family what you want, family members will be able to infer it from your behavior. Talking to all family members, not responding to someone who speaks for another member but instead addressing that person directly, modeling clear and direct communication, demonstrating techniques for getting feedback, and taking risks to deal openly with negative feelings are all examples of ways the nurse can provide this feedback. Sometimes actual comments such, as challenging generalizations ("always" and "never") or assumptions ("You assumed that he knew what you meant?") can be provided in ways that are nonthreatening and eventually perceived by the family as helpful information.

Evaluation

Terminating with Families

All things come to an end, and so will the nurse's interaction with the family. Whether the interaction has been very brief or the nurse has seen the family for a long time, the nurse will want to work toward everyone leaving the encounter with a clear sense of what has happened, and with hope that the family's progress will continue into the future. Evaluation may include examining the effectiveness of the nursing care, the quality of the nurse-family interactions, changes in the family's state that may require modification or termination of the care plan, and the family's response to the interventions. A summary note should be placed in the client's chart.

For both nurse and family, there are specific issues to consider. If nurses are committed to the value of improving communication skills, they will hope to leave the family with a better sense of how family members communicate and perhaps with more communication skills than they had before. The nurse might ask, "Did the family members become more aware of their communication styles during our interactions? Did they learn new, more effective ways of relating to each other?"

Leaving the family with a sense of what was accomplished is important and may help family members see progress that was obscure to them: "Did we summarize the progress toward goals in such a way that all family members left the encounter with a sense of knowing what happened and what was gained?"

Family needs may not have been met completely during the nursing encounter. Referrals, continuing the contact with another health professional, or family education about when to contact the health system may be needed (Wright & Leahey, 2004). The referral should include a summary of the information gained to date and should be communicated by the health team member most knowledgeable about the client's condition. The nurse should discuss with the client what will be shared with the referral resource.

Exercise 13-10 Evaluating Nurse-Family Communication

Purpose: To help students evaluate and improve their communication with families.

Procedure:

Set up an interview with a family that has volunteered to help you with this assignment. Ask the family to discuss with you a real-life problem in the family. Be prepared for the session by writing down a goal and some questions to ask the family. Ask the family's cooperation in helping you improve your communication. After the session has been conducted, ask the family members to answer the following questions:

1. Did the interviewer clarify the purpose and time limits of the meeting at the beginning?
2. Did you understand the purpose and what you were supposed to do in the meeting?
3. How did the meeting begin? What was each person doing as the meeting started?
4. Did you feel involved in the discussion? Was anyone left out?
5. Did the interviewer make you feel that what you were saying was important and that he or she valued your opinion?
6. Can you identify any feelings or emotional reactions that occurred during the discussion? How did the interviewer respond to them?
7. Did the interviewer ever ask you to validate or clarify his or her ideas of what was happening?
8. Do you have any suggestions to help this person improve communication with a family group?

Finally, the nurse needs to assess the personal behaviors that influenced the relationship.

Appraising self and using that information to adjust one's communication and interpersonal style can be growth-producing for future contacts. Exercise 13-10 provides experience with evaluating nurse-family interactions.

SUMMARY

This chapter provides an overview of family communication. Family is defined as "a self-identified group of two or more individuals whose association is characterized by special terms, who may or may not be related by bloodlines or law but who function in such a way that they consider themselves to be a family." Families have a structure, defined as the way in which members are organized. Family function refers to the roles people take in their families, and family process describes the communication that takes place within the family. Family frameworks identified in the chapter include Bowen's family systems theory and Duvall's developmental model; McCubbin's model of family coping is discussed.

The genogram is a primary assessment tool used to help families describe multigenerational transmission of family patterns. Other assessment tools include a time line and ecomap. Nursing interventions are aimed at strengthening family functioning and may include guiding family change, educating and problem solving during developmental crises, supporting family coping, enlisting the aid of family members in caring for family members, and helping family members coordinate resources. Interventive questioning and commendations are two communication strategies nurses can use to help clients cope more effectively.

Evaluation may include an estimation of the effectiveness of the nursing care, the quality of the nurse-family interactions, changes in the family's state that may require modification or termination of the care plan, and the family's response to the interventions.

Ethical Dilemma ■ *What Would You Do?*

Terry Connors is a 90-year-old woman living alone in a two-story house. Her daughter Maggie lives in another state. So far, Terry has been able to live by herself, but within the past 2 weeks, she fell down a few stairs in her house and she has trouble hearing the telephone. Terry walks with a cane and relies on her neighbors for assistance when she can't do things for herself. Maggie worries about her and would like to see her in a nursing home close to Maggie's home. Terry will not consider this option. As the nurse working with this family, how would you address your ethical responsibilities to Terry and Maggie?

REFERENCES

Aldridge M: Decreasing parental stress in the pediatric intensive care unit, *Crit Care Nurse* 25(6):40–51, 2005.

Allen EM: Comparative theories of the expanded role in nursing and implications for nursing practice, *Can J Nurs Res* 30:83–90, 1999.

Barker P: Different approaches to family therapy, *Nurs Times* 94(14):60–62, 1998.

Baumann S: Family nursing: theory–anemic, nursing theory deprived, *Nurs Sci Q* 13(4):285–290, 2000.

Bell JM: Encouraging nurses and families to think interactionally: revisiting the usefulness of the circular pattern diagram, *J Fam Nurs* 6(3):203–209, 2000.

Bohlander J: Differentiation of self: an examination of the concept, *Issues Ment Health Nurs* 16(2):165–184, 1995.

Bowen M: *Family therapy in clinical practice*, Northvale, NJ, 1978, Jason Aronson.

Byng-Hall J: *Rewriting family scripts: improvisation and system change*, New York, 1995, Guilford.

Byng-Hall J: Therapist reflections: diverse developmental pathways for the family, *J Fam Ther* 22:264–272, 2000.

Cannuscio C, Jones C, Kawachi I et al.: Reverberations of family illness: a longitudinal assessment of informal caregiving and mental health status in the Nurses' Health Study, *Am J Public Health* 92:1305–1311, 2002.

Clark S: The double ABCX model of family crisis as a representation of family functioning after rehabilitation from a stroke, *Health Med* 4(2):203–220, 1999.

Cole-Kelly K, Seaburn D: Five areas of questioning to promote a family oriented approach in primary care, *Families, Systems & Health* 17(3):341–348, 1999.

Curtis E, Dixon M: Family therapy and systemic practice with older people: Where are we now? *J Fam Ther* 27:43–46, 2005.

Curtis J, Patrick D, Shannon S et al.: The family conference as a focus to improve communication about end-of-life care in the intensive care unit: opportunities for improvement, *Crit Care Med* 29(supp 2):N26–N33, 2001.

Duvall E: *Marriage and family development*, Philadelphia, 1958, JB Lippincott.

Feeley N, Gottlieb L: Nursing approaches for working with family strengths and resources, *J Fam Nurs* 6(1):9–24, 2000.

Frame M: The spiritual genogram in family therapy, *J Marital Fam Ther* 26:211–216, 2000.

Framo JL: *Family of origin therapy: an intergenerational approach*, New York, 1992, Bruner/Mazel.

Friedman MM: *Family nursing: research, theory and practice*, ed 4, Stamford, CT, 1998, Appleton & Lange.

Glasscock F, Hales A: Bowen's family systems theory: a useful approach for a nurse administrator's practice, *J Nurs Adm* 28(6):37–42, 1998.

Goldenberg H, Goldenberg I: The family as a social unit: systems theory and beyond. In Goldenberg H, Goldenberg I, *Counseling today's families*, ed 4, Pacific Grove, CA, 2002, Wadsworth.

Gordon P, Perrone K: When spouses become caregivers: counseling implications for younger couples, *J Rehabil* 70(2):27–32, 2004.

Greeff A, Human B: Resilience in families in which a parent has died, *Am J Fam Ther* 32:27–42, 2004.

Green R, Werner P: Intrusiveness and closeness in caregiving: rethinking the concept of family enmeshment, *Fam Process* 35(2):115–131, 1996.

Hawley D, DeHaan L: Toward a definition of family resilience: integrating life span and family perspectives, *Fam Process* 35:283–298, 1996.

Hodge D: Spiritual ecomaps: a new diagrammatic tool for assessing marital and family spirituality, *J Marital Fam Ther* 26:217–228, 2000.

Innes M: Connecting Bowen theory with its human origins, *Fam Process* 35(4):487–500, 1996.

Kristjanson L, Aoun S: Palliative care for families: remembering the hidden patients, *Can J Psychiatry* 49(6):359–365, 2004.

Leahey M, Harper-Jaques S: Family-nurse relationships: core assumptions and clinical implications, *J Fam Nurs* 2(2):133–152, 1996.

Limacher L, Wright L: Commendations: listening to the silent side of a family intervention, *J Fam Nurs* 9(2):130–150, 2003.

Mailick M, Vigilante F: The family assessment wheel: a social constructionist perspective, *Families in Society* 78(4):361–369, 1997.

McBride A: *A married feminist*, New York, 1976, Harper & Row.

McCubbin H, Cauble AE, Patterson J: *Family stress, coping, and social support*, Springfield, IL, 1982, Charles C Thomas.

McCubbin HI, McCubbin MA, Thompson A: Resiliency in families: the role of family schema and appraisal in family adaptation to crisis. In Brubaker TH, editor, *Family relations: challenges for the future*, Newbury Park, CA, 1993, Sage.

McCubbin HI, McCubbin MA, Thompson AI et al.: Resiliency in ethnic families: a conceptual model for predicting family adjustment and adaptation. In McCubbin HI, McCubbin MA, Thompson AI et al., editors, *Resiliency in Native American and immigrant families*, Thousand Oaks, CA, 1998, Sage Publications.

McElheran N, Harper-Jaques S: Commendations: a resource intervention for clinical practice, *Clin Nurse Spec* 8:7–10, 15, 1994.

McGoldrick M, Gerson R, Shellenberger S: *Genograms: assessment and intervention*, ed 2, New York, 1999, Norton.

McKenry P, Price S: Families and change: *Coping with stressful events and transitions*, Thousand Oaks, CA, 2005, Sage.

Minuchin S: *Families and family therapy*, Boston, 1974, Harvard University Press.

Modricin MJ, Robison J: Parents of children with emotional disorders: issues for consideration and practice, *Community Ment Health J* 27(4):281–292, 1991.

Novilla M, Barnes N, De La Cruz et al.: Public health perspectives on the family, *Fam Community Health* 29(1): 28–42, 2006.

Otto H: Criteria for assessing family strength, *Fam Process* 2:329–338, 1963.

Rivera-Andino J, Lopez L: When culture complicates, *RN* 63(7):47–49, 2000.

Ryan E, Steinmiller E: Modeling family-centered pediatric nursing care: strategies for shift report, *Journal for Specialists Pediatric Nursing* 9(4):123–129, 2004.

Selekman M: *Solution focused therapy with children: harnessing family strengths for systemic change*, New York, 1997, Guilford Press.

Sydnor-Greenberg N, Dokken D, Ahmann E: Coping and caring in different ways: understanding and meaningful involvement, *Pediatr Nurs* 26(2):185–190, 2000.

Tapp D, Moules N: Family skills labs: facilitating the development of family nursing skills in the undergraduate, *J Fam Nurs* 3(3):247–267, 1997.

Tarnowski GT, Hanson H, May S: Nurse-family interactions in adult critical care: a Bowen family systems perspective, *J Fam Nurs* 5(1):72–92, 1999.

Toman W: *Family therapy and sibling position*, New York, 1992, Jason Aronson Publishers.

Von Bertalanffy L: *General systems theory*, New York, 1968, George Braziller.

Walsh F: The concept of family resilience: crisis and challenge, *Fam Process* 35(3):261–279, 1996.
White MB, Tyson-Rawson KJ: Assessing the dynamics of gender in couples and familes: the gendergram, *Fam Relat* 44:253–260, 1995.
Wright LM, Leahey M: *Nurses and families: a guide to family assessment and intervention*, ed 3, Philadelphia, 2000, FA Davis.
Wright L, Leahey M: How to conclude or terminate with families, *J Fam Nurs* 10(3):379–401, 2004.

Chapter 14

Resolving Conflict Between Nurse and Client

Kathleen Underman Boggs

OUTLINE

OBJECTIVES

At the end of the chapter, the reader will be able to:

1. Define conflict and contrast the functional with the dysfunctional role of conflict in a therapeutic relationship.
2. Recognize and describe personal style of response to conflict situations.
3. Discriminate among passive, assertive, and aggressive responses to conflict situations.
4. Specify the characteristics of assertive communication.
5. Identify four components of an assertive response and formulate sample assertive responses.
6. Identify appropriate assertive responses and specific nursing strategies to promote conflict resolution in relationships.
7. Discuss how findings from one research study can be applied to clinical practice.

> *Creative confrontation is a struggle between persons who are engaged in a dispute or controversy and who remain together, face to face, until acceptance, respect for differences, and love emerge; even though the persons may be at odds with the issue, they are no longer at odds with each other.*
>
> (Moustakis, 1974)

Conflict is a natural part of human relationships. We all have times when we experience negative feelings about a situation or person. When this occurs in a nurse-client relationship, clear, direct communication is needed. This chapter emphasizes awareness of the dynamics associated with conflicts and the skills needed for successful resolution.

Knowing how to respond in emotional situations allows a nurse to use feelings as a positive force rather than a negative one. Nurses often find themselves in dramatic situations in which a calm, collected response is required. To listen and to respond creatively to intense emotion when your first impulse is to withdraw or to retaliate demands a high level of skill. It requires self-knowledge, self-control, and empathy for what the client may be experiencing. It is difficult to remain cool under attack, and yet your willingness to stay with the angry client may mean more than any other response.

Assertive skills, described in this chapter, can help you deal constructively with conflict.

The literature describes workplace conflicts, which deal with conflicts between the nurse and other professionals (e.g., managers, peers, and physicians). In Chapter 22 we will discuss the nurse's role in communicating during conflicts with other professionals. The focus of this chapter will be on conflicts between nurse and client.

BASIC CONCEPTS

Conflict has been defined as tension arising from incompatible needs, in which the actions of one frustrate the ability of the other to achieve a goal (Valentine, 1995). Conflicts in any relationship are inevitable: they serve as warning that something in the relationship needs closer attention. All conflict produces stress. But we can use conflict to improve lives.

Nature of Conflict

All conflicts have certain things in common: (a) a concrete *content problem issue*; and (b) relationship or *process issues*, which involve our emotional response to the situation. It is immaterial whether the issue or associated feelings make realistic sense to the nurse. They feel real to the client and need to be addressed, or they will interfere with success in meeting goals. Most people experience conflict as uncomfortable, disquieting feelings about a person or situation. Previous experiences with conflict situations, the importance of the issue, and possible consequences for the client all play a role in the intensity of our reaction. For example, a client may have great difficulty asking appropriate questions of the physician regarding treatment or prognosis, but experience no problem asking similar questions of the nurse or family. The reasons for the discrepancy in comfort level may relate to previous experiences. Alternatively, it may have little to do with the actual persons involved. Rather, the client may be responding to anticipated fears about the type of information the physician might give.

Causes of Conflict

Psychological causes of conflict include misunderstanding, poor communication, differences in values or goals, personality clashes, and stress. Clashes occur between nurse and client or even between two clients.

Case Example

Two women who gave birth this morning are moved to a semiprivate room on the postpartum floor. Ms. Patton is 19 years old, likes loud music, and is feeling fine. Her roommate, Mrs. Busky, is 36 years old, has four children at home, and wants to rest as much as possible (*latent*). The music and visitors to Ms. Patton repeatedly wake up Mrs. Busky (*perceived*), who yells at them (*overt*). The nurse arranges to transfer Mrs. Busky to an unoccupied room (*resolution*).

Understanding Personal Responses to Conflict

Conflicts between nurse and client are not uncommon. Once a conflict is identified, it becomes your responsibility to work to resolve the conflict. If the conflict continues, the relationship process will become blocked.

Energy is transferred to conflict issues instead of being used to build the relationship. To accomplish conflict resolution, you first need to have a clear understanding of your own personal response patterns to conflict. No one is equally effective in all situations. Completing Exercise 14-1 may help you identify your personal responses.

Most interpersonal conflicts involve some threat to the nurse or client's sense of control or self-esteem. Situations producing conflict between client and nurse include the following:

- Having your statements discounted
- Being asked to give more information than you feel comfortable sharing
- Being pressured to give more time than you are able
- Encountering sexual harassment
- Being the target of a personal attack
- Wanting to do things the old way instead of trying something new

Ways you may behave that create anger or conflict with your client could include the following:

- Speaking to the client in an accusing or blaming tone
- Offering false sympathy or unrealistic reassurances
- Conveying your lack of understanding of the client's viewpoint
- Exerting too much pressure on the client to change unhealthy behavior
- Using an authoritarian tone of voice, implying you think of yourself as an infallible expert

Exercise 14-1 Personal Responses to Conflict

Purpose: To increase awareness of how students respond in conflict situations and the elements in situations (e.g., people, status, age, previous experience, lack of experience, or place) that contribute to their sense of discomfort.

Procedure:

Break up into small groups of two. You may do this as homework or create an Internet discussion room. Think of a conflict situation that could be handled in different ways.

The following feelings are common correlates of interpersonal conflict situations that many people say they experienced in conflict situations that they have not handled well:

Anger	**Competitiveness**	**Humiliation**
Annoyance	**Defensiveness**	**Inferiority**
Antagonism	**Devaluation**	**Intimidation**
Anxiousness	**Embarrassment**	**Manipulation**
Bitterness	**Frustration**	**Resentment**

Although these feelings generally are not ones we are especially proud of, they are a part of the human experience. By acknowledging their existence within ourselves, we usually have more choice about how we will handle them.

Using words from the list, describe the following as concretely as possible:

1. The details of the situation: How did it develop? What were the content issues? Was the conflict expressed verbally or nonverbally? Who were the persons involved, and where did the interaction take place?
2. What feelings were experienced before, during, and after the conflict?
3. Why was the situation particularly uncomfortable?

Discussion:

Suggest different ways to respond. Might these lead to differences in outcome?

No one likes to be criticized. Negative reactions might include anger, rationalization, or blaming others (Davidhizar, 1991).

Four Styles of Personal Conflict Management

Studies have repeatedly identified several distinct styles of response to conflict. Although not specifically addressing nurse-client conflict, the literature shows that, in the past, corporate managers felt that any conflict was destructive and needed to be suppressed. Current thinking holds that conflict can be healthy and can lead to growth. These concepts can be applied to nursing.

Avoidance is a common response to conflict. Sometimes an experience makes you so uncomfortable that you want to avoid the situation or person at all costs, so you withdraw. Studies have shown that nurses, especially female nurses, most often demonstrate this style of reaction to conflict (Valentine, 2001). This style is appropriate when the other individual is more powerful or the cost of addressing the conflict is higher than the benefit of resolution. Sometimes you just have to "pick your battles," focusing your energy on the most important issues. However, use of avoidance can just postpone the conflict, turning it into a *lose-lose situation* (McElhaney, 1996).

Accommodation is another common response; it is characterized by a desire to smooth over the conflict. The response is cooperative but nonassertive. Sometimes this involves a quick compromise or giving false reassurance. By giving in to or obliging others, the person maintains peace but does not actually deal with the issue, so it will likely resurface in the future. It is appropriate when the issue is more important to the other person. This is a *lose-win situation*. Harmony results and credits may be accumulated that can be used at some future time (McElhaney, 1996).

Competition is the response style characterized by domination. This is a contradictory style in which one party exercises power to gain his or her own personal goals regardless of the needs of the other. It is characterized by aggression and lack of compromise. Authority may be used to suppress the conflict in a dictatorial manner. This response style was commonly used in the past by corporate managers and leads to increased stress among subordinates (Dallinger & Hample, 1995). It is an effective style when there is a need for a quick decision, but it leads to problems in the long term, making it a *lose-lose situation*.

Collaboration is a solution-oriented response. It is a cooperative style of problem solving. To manage the conflict, both parties commit to finding a mutually satisfying solution. This involves directly confronting the issue, acknowledging the feelings, and using an integrative method to solve the problem. Jones, Bushardt, and Cadenhead (1990) suggested four steps for productive confrontation: identify concerns of each party; clarify assumptions; identify the real issue; and work collaboratively to find a solution that satisfies both parties. This is considered to be the most effective style for genuine resolution. This is a *win-win situation*.

Factors That Influence Responses to Conflict

Gender. Ample research demonstrates gender differences in managing conflict. Expression of emotion differs between genders (Brooks, Thomas, & Droppleman, 1996). Women have been socialized to react in ways that will assuage the other person's anger. The female response to conflict has been labeled as "tend and befriend" (Johnson & Arneson, 1991; Mayo Health Clinic, 2001). Studies have shown that women tend to use more accommodative conflict management styles such as compromise and avoidance, whereas men tend to use collaboration more often and to prefer "competitive, unyielding and aggressive strategies" (Valentine, 1995, p. 144). However, the literature is inconclusive regarding the effects of gender and style on the outcome of conflict resolution.

Culture. Many of a nurse's responses are determined by cultural socialization, which prescribes proper modes for behaviors. Personal style and past experiences influence the typical responses to conflict situations. Individuals from societies that emphasize group commitment and cooperation tend to use more avoidance and less confrontation in their conflict resolution styles. People from cultures that value individualism more tend to more often use competing/dominating styles (Trubisky, Ting-Toomey, & Lin, 1991). Of course, nurses are individuals and have different attitudes toward the existence of conflict, and therefore respond to conflict differently, although the underlying feelings generated by conflict situations may be quite similar. Common emotional responses to conflict (see Exercise 14-1) include anger, embarrassment, and anxiety. Awareness of how we cope with conflict is the first step in learning assertiveness strategies. Fortunately, assertiveness and other skills essential to conflict resolution are learned behaviors that any nurse can master.

Professional Ethics and Role Socialization. Studies have shown that up to 75% of the ethical dilemmas reported in nurse surveys involve their perceptions about inadequate client care (Redman & Fry, 1996). Nurses traditionally were socialized to follow orders. Women in general were socialized to "not make waves." Other sources suggest that intrapersonal conflict arises when nurses are faced with two different choices, each supported by a different ethical principle.

Types of Conflict: Intrapersonal Versus Interpersonal

A conflict can be internal (intrapersonal), that is, it can represent opposing feelings within an individual. Alternatively, the conflict may occur between two or more people (interpersonal).

Functional Uses of Conflict

Traditionally, conflict was viewed as a destructive force to be eliminated (Booth, 1985). Current thinking holds that conflict can serve either a functional or a dysfunctional role in relationships. In fact, conflict is thought to be an inevitable part of today's changing health care environment (Jones et al., 1990; Porter, 1996). The critical factor is the willingness to explore and resolve it mutually. Appropriately handled, conflict can provide an important opportunity for growth. Box 14-1 gives helpful guidelines regarding your responsibilities when involved in a conflict.

Box 14-1 Personal Rights and Responsibilities in Conflict Situations

- I have the right to respect from other people as a unique human being.
- I have the responsibility to respect the human rights of others.
- I have the right to make my own decisions.
- I have the responsibility to allow others to make their own decisions.
- I have the right to have feelings.
- I have the responsibility to express those feelings in ways that do not violate the rights of others.
- I have the right to make mistakes.
- I have the responsibility to accept full accountability for my mistakes.
- I have the right to decide how I will act.
- I have the responsibility to act in ways that will not be harmful to myself or to others.
- I have the right to my own opinions.
- I have the responsibility to respect the rights of others to hold opinions different from mine.

Nature of Assertive Behavior

Assertive behavior is defined as setting goals, acting on those goals in a clear and consistent manner, and taking responsibility for the consequences of those actions. The assertive nurse is able to stand up for the rights of others as well as for his or her own rights. Box 14-2 lists characteristics of assertive behaviors. Four components of assertion include the following four abilities: (1) to say no, (2) to ask for what you want, (3) to appropriately express both positive and negative thoughts and feelings, and (4) to initiate, continue, and terminate the interaction. This honest expression of yourself does not violate the needs of others, but does demonstrate self-respect rather than deference to the demands of others.

Two goals of assertiveness are to stand up for your personal rights without infringing on the rights of others and to reduce anxiety, which often prevents us from behaving assertively (Angel & Petronko, 1987).

Assertive behaviors range from making a simple, direct, and honest statement about one's beliefs to taking a very strong, confrontational stand about what will and will not be tolerated in the relationship. Assertive responses contain "I" statements that take responsibility. This behavior is in contrast to **aggressive behavior**,

Box 14-2 Characteristics Associated with the Development of Assertive Behavior

- Express your own position, using "I" statements.
- Make clear statements.
- Speak in a firm tone, using moderate pitch.
- Assume responsibility for personal feelings and wants.
- Make sure verbal and nonverbal messages are congruent.
- Address only issues related to the present conflict.
- Structure responses so as to be tactful and show awareness of the client's frame of reference.
- Understand that undesired behaviors, not feelings, attitudes, and motivations, are the focus for change.

which has a goal of dominating while suppressing the other person's rights. Aggressive responses often consist of "you" statements that fix blame and undue responsibility on the other person.

Assertiveness is a learned behavior. Many nurses, especially women, have been socialized to act passively. Passive behavior is defined as a response that denies our own rights in order to avoid conflict. An example is remaining silent and not responding to a client's demands for narcotics every 4 hours when he displays no signs of pain out of fear that he might report you to his physician. Passivity can be evidenced by the acceptance of a negative, unfair comment without any further discussion of the impact the comment had on you.

Assertiveness needs to be practiced to be learned (Exercises 14-2, 14-3, and 14-4). Effective nursing encompasses the mastery of assertive behavior (see Box 14-2). Studies show that nonassertive behavior in a professional nurse is related to lower levels of autonomy (Schutzenhofer, 1992). Continued patterns of nonassertive responses have adverse psychological effects on the nurse and a negative influence on the standard of care the nurse

Exercise 14-2 Responding Assertively

Purpose: To help students define their position in a conflict situation in an assertive manner.

Procedure:

Think of an interpersonal situation in which you wished you had acted more assertively. What behaviors would you alter? Specify how you would relate in an assertive manner. (Example: Your employer schedules you to work overtime, or your teacher incorrectly gives you a lower grade than you believe you earned. Sample response: "I would tell my boss that I had exams at school and I wasn't going to be able to continue to work every weekend.")

If you are like most people, you find it difficult to express yourself clearly about your position in conflict situations. Sometimes you may not recognize that you are involved in a conflict situation until the situation is well under way.

Discussion:

1. What were some of the variables that made it difficult for you to express yourself assertively?
2. As you listen to other students' responses, what common themes emerge?
3. How could you use this information in your professional responses to conflict?

Exercise 14-3 Pitching the Assertive Message

Purpose: To increase awareness of how the meaning of a verbal message can be significantly altered by changing one's tone of voice.

Procedure:

Place individual slips of paper in a hat so that every student in class can draw one. On each slip of paper should be written one of the five vocal pitches commonly used in conversation: whisper, soft tone with hesitant delivery, moderate tone and firm delivery, loud tone with agitated delivery, and screaming. Divide into groups, and have each student take a turn drawing and demonstrating the tone while the others in the group try to identify correctly which person is giving the assertive message.

Discussion:

How does tone affect perceptions of a message's content?

Courtesy Saretha Boggs.

Exercise 14-4 Assertiveness Self-Assessment Quiz

Purpose: To help students gain insight into their own responses.

Procedure:
Read and answer "yes" (2 points); "sometimes" (1 point); or "no" (0 points). A score of more than 10 points suggests the need to practice assertiveness.
Do you

1. Feel self-conscious if someone watches you work with a client?
2. Not feel confident in your nursing judgment?
3. Hesitate to express your feelings?
4. Avoid questioning people in authority?
5. Feel uncomfortable speaking up in class?
6. Ever say, "I hate to bother you…"?
7. Feel people take advantage of you at work?
8. Ever feel reluctant to turn down a classmate who asks you to do his or her work?
9. Avoid protesting an unfair grade or evaluation?
10. Have trouble starting a conversation?

Exercise 14-5 Assertive Responses

Purpose: To increase awareness of assertiveness.

Procedure:
Have three students volunteer to read each answer to the following scenario:

You are working full time, raising a family, and taking 12 credits of nursing classes. The teacher asks you to be a student representative on a faculty committee. You say the following:

1. "I don't think I'm the best one. Why don't you ask Karen? If she can't, I guess I can."
2. "Gee, I'd like to, but I don't know. I probably could if it doesn't take too much time."
3. "I do want students to have some input to this committee, but I am not sure I have enough time. Let me think about it and let you know in class tomorrow."

Discussion:
Ask students to choose the most assertive answer and comment about how other options could be altered.

delivers (McCanton & Hargie, 1990). Evaluate your own assertiveness with Exercise 14-5.

Dysfunctional Conflict

Several identifiable elements may occur in **dysfunctional conflict**. The dysfunction occurs when emotions distort the content issue (e.g., when some information is withheld so one of the participants must guess at what is truly going on in the mind of the other participant in the interaction). Sometimes the conflict is obscured by a double message or when feelings are denied or projected onto others. Nonproductive conflicts are characterized by feelings that are misperceived or stated too intensely.

In other dysfunctional conflicts, the feelings are stated accurately, but they are expressed so strongly that the listener feels attacked. The listener then tends to respond in a defensive manner. Consequently, the relationship is damaged. In dysfunctional communication, the outcomes provide little sense of satisfaction or accomplishment. Conflicts are not resolved, so issues build up.

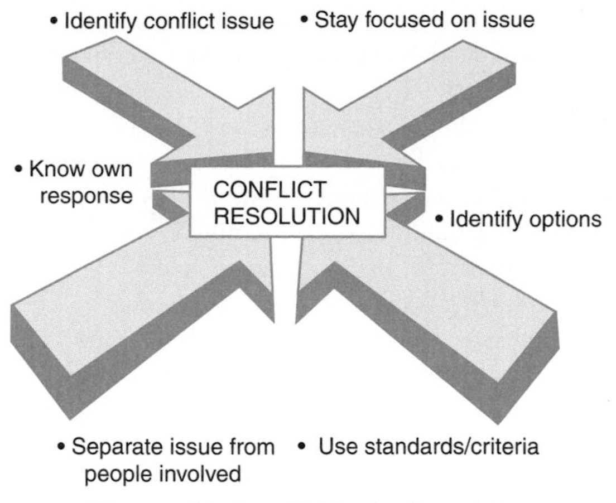

Figure 14-1 ● Principles of conflict resolution.

Principles of Conflict Resolution

Figure 14-1 describes the principles of conflict resolution.

1. *Identify conflict issues.* This has already been discussed.
2. *Know your own response to conflict.* The styles of conflict management have already been described. Recognize your own "trigger" or "hot buttons." What words or client actions evoke an immediate emotional response from you? Reflect on what triggers can provoke you. These could include having a finger pointed at you, having someone throw something at you, or having someone yelling at you or speaking to you in an angry tone of voice. Once you recognize the triggers, you can better control your own response.
3. *Separate the problem from the people involved.* Focus on the substantive issue: the problem. Put aside issues associated with the relationship. Above all, don't bring up past history. Listing prior problems that occurred in your relationship will raise emotions and prevent both of you from clearly identifying and problem solving the issue in conflict.
4. *Stay focused on the issue and on the underlying motivations behind the position the other person took.* Try to understand the reason each of you took your position. It is essential to stay focused on the current issue and not bring in old gripes.
5. *Identify available options.* Rather than immediately trying to solve the problem, look at the range of possible options. Create a list of these options and work with the other party to evaluate the feasibility of each option. By working together, the expectation shifts from adversarial conflict to an expectation of a win-win outcome. After discussing possible solutions, the best one is used to resolve the conflict (Feeney & Davidson, 1996).
6. *Try to identify established standards to guide the decision-making process.* Rather than one party exerting his or her will in a win-lose process, try to determine the outcome based on fair, objective criteria.

APPLICATIONS

Assessing the Presence of Conflict in the Nurse-Client Relationship

To foster resolution, you need to acknowledge the presence of conflict. Often the awareness of our own feelings of discomfort is an initial clue. Evidence of the presence of conflict may be *overt,* that is, observable in the client's behavior and expressed verbally. The conflict issues may be identified, expressed, and allowed to reach resolution so that constructive changes may take place. The relationship progresses and deepens.

Developing an Evidence-Based Practice

Isikhan V, Comez T, Danis MZ: Job stress and coping strategies in health care professionals working with cancer patients, *Eur J Oncol Nurs* 8(3):234-244, 2004.

In this study conducted in Turkey, 109 health professionals identified stressors and coping strategies employed in working with oncology patients.

Results: The 52 physicians and 57 nurses reported nearly the same levels of stress on two self-report questionnaires (the Job Stress Inventory and the Ways of Coping Inventory). Among the sources of stress reported were problems interacting with the relatives of cancer patients as well as with patients. Physician and nurse participants were found to use similar strategies to cope with stress.

Application to Your Clinical Practice: The authors cite the need for agency-sponsored training programs for all health care professionals working with cancer patients and with their family members. Do you think all agencies should have some support for staff nurses to help them manage job-related stress?

More often, conflict is *covert* and not so clear-cut. The conflict issues are hidden or buried among distracting feelings or tangential issues. The client talks about one issue, but talking does not seem to help, and the issue does not seem to get resolved. The client continues to be angry or anxious. Often the first clue to the existence of a conflict situation occurs when one of you becomes aware of a generalized sense of personal uneasiness. Often, the reasons for this feeling are not clear. In a covert conflict situation, the conflict acts as a hindrance to the progress of the relationship and the ultimate treatment goals. The conflict usually cannot be resolved until the issues can be revealed and explored.

Subtle behavioral manifestations of covert conflict might include the following: a reduced effort by the client to engage in the process of self-care; frequent misinterpretation of the nurse's words; behaviors that are out of character for the client; and excessive anger or undue praise. For example, when the client seems unusually demanding, has a seemingly insatiable need for your attention, or is unable to tolerate reasonable delays in having needs met, the problem may be anxiety stemming from conflictive feelings. It is important to realize that clients may intellectually want to change, but emotionally might find it difficult to let go of the old behavior.

Exercise 14-6 Defining Conflict Issues

Purpose: To help students begin to organize information and define the problem in interpersonal conflict situations.

Procedure:
In every conflict situation, it is important to look for specific behaviors (including words, tone, posture, and facial expression); feeling impressions (including words, tone, intensity, and facial expression); and need (expressed verbally or through actions).

Identify the behaviors, your impressions of the behaviors, and needs that the client is expressing in the following situations. Then suggest an appropriate nursing action. Situation 1 is completed as a guide.

Situation 1
Mrs. Patel, an Indian client, does not speak much English. Her baby was just delivered by cesarean section, and it is expected that Mrs. Patel will remain in the hospital for at least four days. Her husband tells the nurse that Mrs. Patel wants to breast-feed, but she has decided to wait until she goes home to begin because she will be more comfortable there and she wants privacy. The nurse knows that breast-feeding will be more successful if it is initiated soon after birth.

Behaviors: The client's husband states that his wife wants to breast-feed but does not wish to start before going home. Mrs. Patel is not initiating breast-feeding in the hospital.

Your impression of behaviors: Indirectly the client is expressing physical discomfort, possible insecurity, and awkwardness about breast-feeding. She may also be acting in accordance with cultural norms of her country or family.

Underlying needs: Safety and security. Mrs. Patel probably will not be motivated to attempt breast-feeding until she feels safe and secure in her home environment.

Suggested nursing action: Provide family support and guarantee total privacy for feeding.

Situation 2
Mrs. Moore is returned to the unit from surgery after a radical mastectomy. The doctor's orders call for her to ambulate, cough, and deep breathe and to use her arm as much as possible in self-care activities. Mrs. Moore asks the nurse in a very annoyed tone, "Why do I have to do this? You can see that it is difficult for me. Why can't you help me?"

As nurses, we affect the behavior of our clients through our actions, which can lead to positive or negative outcomes. See Exercise 14-6 for practice in defining conflict issues.

Sometimes the feelings themselves become the major issue, so that valid parts of the original conflict issue are obscured. There is complete focus only on the feelings. The context issue is discounted or denied. These feelings can become a major obstacle and conflict can escalate. At best, confusing feelings with the issue clouds communication and makes it more difficult to respond appropriately. Usually conflictive feelings have to be put into words and related to the issue at hand before the client can understand the meaning of the conflict. Consider yourself as the nurse in the following situation.

Case Example

Mr. Cody is scheduled for surgery at 8 a.m. tomorrow. As the student nurse assigned to care for him, you have been told that he was admitted to the hospital 3 hours ago and that he has been examined by the house resident. The anesthesia department has been notified of the client's arrival. His blood work and urine have been sent to the laboratory. As you enter his room and introduce yourself, you notice that Mr. Cody is sitting on the edge of his bed and appears tense and angry.

Client: **I wish people would just leave me alone. Nobody has come in and told me about my surgery tomorrow. I don't know what I'm supposed to do—just lay around here and rot, I guess.**

At this point, you probably can sense the presence of conflictive feelings, but it is unclear whether the emotions being expressed relate to anxiety over the surgery or to anger over some real or imagined invasion of privacy because of the necessary lab tests and physical exam. The client might also be annoyed by you or by a lack of information from his surgeon. He may feel the need to know that hospital personnel see him as a person and care about his feelings. Before you can respond empathetically to the client's feelings, his feelings will have to be decoded.

Nurse (in a concerned tone of voice): **You seem really upset. It's rough being in the hospital, isn't it?**

Notice that the nurse's reply is nonevaluative and tentative. The nurse does not suggest specific feelings beyond those the client has shared. There is an implicit request for the client to validate the nurse's perception of his feelings and to link the feelings with concrete issues. Verbal as well as nonverbal cues are included in the nurse's reply. Concern is expressed through the nurse's tone of voice and words. The content focus relates to the client's predominant feeling tone, because this is the part of the conflict the client has chosen to share with the nurse. It is important for the nurse to maintain a nonanxious presence. Recognizing client resistance can be a way to maintain personal stability, even though it may appear counterproductive to the relationship.

Nursing Strategies to Enhance Conflict Resolution

Strategies that have been found to be useful in conflict resolution are described here. Successful use of these strategies varies with the skill level of the participants and the nature of the situation. Mastery takes practice. While this seems like a lot of information, Susanne Gaddis, the "Communications Doctor," refers to the primary strategies as using a "4-second rule" to improve communications (n.d.).

Prepare for the Encounter

Careful preparation often makes the difference between being successful and failing to assert yourself when necessary. Clearly identify the issue in conflict. In dis-

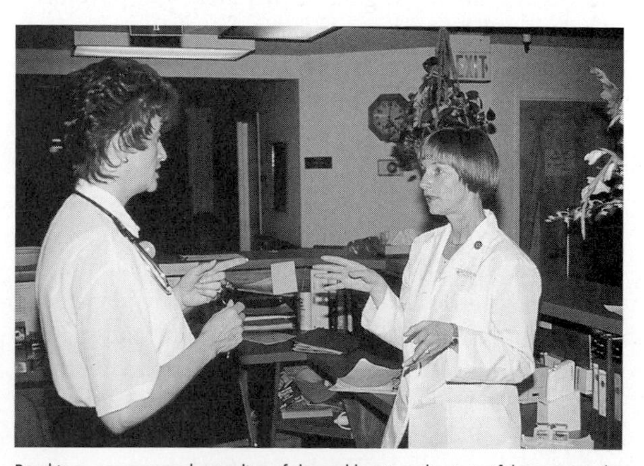

Reaching a common understanding of the problem in a direct, tactful manner is the first step in conflict resolution. (From Potter PA, Perry AG: *Fundamentals of nursing*, ed 5, St Louis, 2001, Mosby.)

cussing assertive communication, Flanagan (1990) notes that for communication to be effective it must be carefully thought out in terms of certain basic questions:

- *Purpose.* What is the purpose or objective of this information? What is the central idea, the one most important statement to be made?
- *Organization.* What are the major points to be shared, and in what order?
- *Content.* Is the information to be shared complete? Does it convey who, what, where, when, why, and how?
- *Word choice.* Has careful consideration been given to the choice of words?

If you wish to be successful, you must consider not only what is important to you in the discussion but also what is important to the other person. Bear in mind the other person's frame of reference when acting assertively. The following clinical example illustrates this idea.

Case Example

Mr. Pyle is an 80-year-old bachelor who lives alone. He has always been considered a proud and stately gentleman. He has a sister, 84 years old, who lives in Florida. His only other living relatives, a nephew and his wife, also live in another state. He recently changed his will so that it excludes his relatives, and he refuses to eat. When his neighbor brings in food he eats it, but he won't fix anything for himself. He tells his neighbor that he wants to die and that he read in the paper about a man who was able to die in 60 days by not eating. As the visiting nurse assigned to his area, you have been asked to make a home visit and assess the situation.

The issue in this case example is not one of food intake alone. The nurse's attempts to talk about why it is important for the client to eat or to express a point of view in this conflict immediately on arriving is not likely to be successful. The client's behavior suggests that he feels there is little to be gained by living any longer. His actions suggest further that he feels lonely and may be angry with his relatives. Once you correctly ascertain his needs and identify the specific issues, you may be able to help Mr. Pyle resolve his intrapersonal conflict. His wish to die may not be absolute or final, because he eats when food is prepared by his neighbor and he has not yet taken a deliberate, aggressive move to end his life. Each of these factors needs to be assessed and validated with the client before an accurate nursing diagnosis can be made.

Organize Information

Organizing your information and validating the appropriateness of your intervention with another knowledgeable person who is not directly involved in the process is useful. Sometimes it is wise to rehearse out loud what you are going to say. Remember to adhere to the principle of focusing on the conflict issue. Avoid bringing up past history.

Manage Own Anxiety or Anger

If you experience stage fright before engaging in a conflict situation that calls for an assertive response, know that you are in good company. Most people experience some variation of a physical response when taking interpersonal risks. A useful strategy for managing your own anger is to vent to a friend using "I" statements, as long as this does not become a complaining, whining session. Another strategy to manage your own anger is to "take a break." A cooling-off period, doing something else for a few minutes or hours until your anger subsides, is okay. Take care that you reengage, however, so that this doesn't become just an avoidance response style. Communicate with the correct person; don't take out your frustration on someone else. Focus on the one issue with the client involved. Try saying, "I would like to talk something over with you before the end of shift/before I go." Before you actually enter the client's room, do the following:

- Cool off. Wait until you can speak in a calm, friendly tone.
- Take a few deep breaths. Inhale deeply and count "1-2-3" to yourself. Hold your breath for a count of 2 and exhale, counting again to 4 slowly.
- Fortify yourself with positive statements (e.g., "I have a right to respect"). Anticipation is usually far worse than the reality.
- Defuse your own anger before confronting the patient.
- Focus on one issue.

Time the Encounter

Timing is a determinant of success. Know specifically the behavior you wish to have the client change. Make sure that the client is capable physically and emotionally of changing the behavior. Select a time when you both can discuss the matter privately and use neutral ground, if possible. Conflictive situations lead to varying degrees of energy depletion. Once fatigue sets in, the value of any assertive behavior on your part may be diminished. Select a time when the client is most likely to be receptive. Nonverbal support of verbal statements adds strength to the meaning of the communication.

Timing is also important if an individual is very angry. The key to assertive behavior is choice. Sometimes it is better to allow the client to let off some "emotional steam" before engaging in conversation. In this case, the assertive thing to do is to choose silence accompanied by a calm, relaxed body posture and eye contact. These nonverbal actions convey acceptance of feeling and a desire to understand. Validating the anger and reframing the emotion as adaptive is useful. Comments such as, "I'm sorry you are feeling so upset" recognize the significance of the emotion being expressed without enlarging the frame of reference beyond what is being expressed.

Put Situation into Perspective

Don't play the blame game. Put the issue into perspective. Will the issue be significant in a year? In 10 years? Will there be a significant situational change with resolution? This is another way of saying pick your battles. Not every situation is worth using up your time and energy.

Use Therapeutic Communication Skills

Refer to the discussion on therapeutic communication in Chapter 10. Particularly useful is *active listening*. Really trying to understand what the client is upset about requires more skill than just listening to his or her words. Repeat to assure the client you have heard what was said (Brixey, 2004).

Use Clear, Congruent Communication

Choose direct, declarative sentences. Use objective words, directly state your wants, and honestly convey your emotions. Listening closely to what the client is saying may help you understand his or her point of view. This understanding may decrease the stress.

Make sure verbal and nonverbal communication is congruent. Maintain an open stance and omit any gestures that might be interpreted as criticism, such as rolling your eyes or sighing heavily. Avoid mixed messages. One example of inappropriate communication might be found in the case of Larry, a staff nurse who works the 11-7 shift. Larry needs to get home to make sure his children get on the bus to school. A geriatric client routinely asks for a breathing treatment while Larry is reporting off. Instead of setting limits, Larry uses a soft voice and smiles as he tells her he can be late to begin the report. Another example is Mr. Carl, the 29-year-old client in Room 122 who constantly makes sexual comments to a young student nurse. She laughs as she tells him to cut it out.

Take One Issue at a Time

Fritchie (1995) and others suggest that you may need to first focus on acknowledging the feelings associated with the conflict, because it is these that generally escalate conflict. It is always best to start with one issue at a time.

- Choose words that may lead to a positive outcome.
- Focus only on the present issue. The past cannot be changed.

Limiting your discussion to one topic issue at a time enhances the chance of success. It usually is impossible to resolve a conflict that is multidimensional in nature with one solution. By breaking the problem down into simple steps, enough time is allowed for a clear understanding. In the case example just given, the nurse might paraphrase the client's words, reflecting the meaning back to the client to validate accuracy. Once the issues have been delineated clearly, the steps needed for resolution may appear quite simple.

Mutually Generate Some Options for Resolution

Focus on ways to resolve the problem by listing possible options. You are familiar with the "fight or flight" response to stress: many people can only respond to conflict by either fighting or avoiding the problem. But brainstorming possible options and discussing pros and cons can turn the "fight" response into a more mutual "seeking a solution" mode of operations.

Make a Request for a Behavior Change

Avoid blaming. This would only make your client feel defensive or angry. Clearly ask him or her for the needed behavior change. This is handled best when the request takes into consideration the person's developmental stage, cultural and value orientation, and other life factors likely to be affected by the change. The person's level of readiness to explore alternative options also needs to be considered. Additionally, for an ill client, level of self-care as well as outside support systems are factors. To approach the task without this information is risky and haphazard.

Rather than just stating your position, try to use some objective criteria to examine the situation. Saying, "I understand your need to________, but the hospital has a policy intended to protect all our clients" might help you talk about the situation without escalating into anger.

There obviously will be situations in which such a thorough assessment is not possible, but each of these variables affects the success of the confrontation. For example, a client with dementia who makes a pass at a nurse may simply be expressing a need for affection in much the same way that a small child does; this behavior needs a caring response rather than a reprimand. A 30-year-old client with all his cognitive faculties who makes a similar pass needs a more confrontational response.

Client readiness is vital. The behavior may need to be confronted, but the manner in which the confrontation is approached and the amount of preparation or groundwork that has been done beforehand may affect the outcome.

Understand Cultural Implications

Often what appears to be an inappropriate response in our culture is a highly acceptable way of interacting in a different culture. For example, some clients experience conflict related to taking pain medication. In the cultures of these clients, pain is supposed to be endured with a stoicism that is incompatible with reality. It is often necessary to help such clients express their discomfort when it occurs and to give them guidelines as well as explicit permission to develop a different behavior. It is easier for these clients to take such medication when they can assure their families that the nurse said it was necessary to take it. By focusing on the behavior required to meet the client's physical needs, the nurse bypasses placing a value on the rightness or wrongness of the behavior. Refer to other chapters for a more detailed discussion of cultural differences that can create conflict.

Evaluate the Conflict Resolution

Evaluation of the degree to which an interpersonal conflict has been resolved depends somewhat on the nature of the conflict. Sometimes a conflict cannot be resolved in a short time, but the willingness to persevere is a good indicator of a potentially successful outcome. Accepting small goals is useful when large goal attainment is not possible. The ideal interactive process is one in which a climate of openness and trust leads to an increase in communication in the form of feedback and increased problem solving (Jones et al., 1990).

For a client, perhaps the strongest indicator of conflict resolution is the degree to which he or she is actively engaged in activities aimed at accomplishing tasks associated with treatment goals. As the nurse, there are two questions you might want to address if modifications are necessary:

- What is the best way to establish an environment that is conducive to conflict resolution? What else needs to be considered?
- What self-care behaviors can be expected of the client if these changes are made? These need to be stated in ways that are measurable.

Both the nurse and the client benefit from conflict resolution. Successful resolution permits movement toward treatment goals and increases confidence and self-esteem.

Identify Client Intrapersonal Conflict Situations

The initial interpersonal strategy used to help clients reduce strong emotion to a workable level is to provide a neutral, accepting, interpersonal environment. Within this context, the nurse can acknowledge the client's emotion as a necessary component of adaptation to life. The nurse conveys acceptance of the individual's legitimate right to have feelings. Telling a client, "I'm not surprised that you are angry about . . ." or simply stating, "I'm sorry you are hurting so much" acknowledges the presence of an uncomfortable emotion in the client, conveys an attitude of acceptance, and encourages the client to express the feeling and the circumstances generating the emotion. Once a feeling can be put into words, it becomes manageable because it has concrete boundaries.

Talk About It

The second step in defusing the strength of an emotion is to talk the emotion through with someone. For the client, this someone is often the nurse. For the nurse, this might be a nursing supervisor or a trusted colleague. Unlike complaining, the purpose of talking the emotion through is to help the person connect with all of his or her personal feelings surrounding the incident. If one client seems to produce certain negative emotional reactions on a nursing unit, the emotional responses may need the direct attention of all staff on the unit.

Use Tension-Reducing Actions

The third phase is to take action. The specific needs expressed by the emotion suggest actions that might help the client come to terms with the consequences of the emotion. This responsibility might take the form of obtaining more information or of taking some concrete risks to change behaviors that sabotage the goals of the relationship. Convey mutual respect and avoid any "put-down" type of comment about yourself or the client.

Sometimes the most effective action is simply to listen. Active listening in a conflict situation involves concentrating on what the other person is upset about. Listening can be so powerful that it alone may reduce the client's feelings of anxiety and frustration (Shearer & Davidson, 1997).

Physical activity can reduce tension. Taking a walk, going to the gym to use the punching bag, taking a warm bath, and writing are all neutralizing interventions the nurse in psychiatric settings can suggest to control a client's initial anxiety behaviors. Stepping in before the client's behaviors escalate to the point at which they are no longer under the client's conscious control can defuse an emotionally tense situation. If the client is so consumed by emotion that he or she constitutes a danger to himself or others and talking is futile, the nurse should allow a significant amount of physical space and face the client but avoid backing the client into a corner. The nurse should speak in a low, calm tone to the client and move slowly to the nurses' station. Many hospitals and psychiatric units have a "code blue" that is used to summon trained help.

Humor is frequently used by nurses to engage a client or to initiate an interaction (Nursing Standard, 2004). Humor can also be used as a means of reducing tension. To paraphrase a famous advice columnist, two of the most important words in a relationship are "I apologize." And she recommended making amends immediately when you've made a mistake, since it is easier to eat crow while it is still warm. Is this advice easier to take (we won't say swallow) since it comes with a chuckle? Humor serves as an immediate tension reliever.

Defuse Intrapersonal Conflict

Intrapersonal conflicts develop when you hold opposing feelings within yourself. The client with a myocardial infarction who insists on conducting business from the bedside probably feels conflicted about the restraints placed on his or her activities, as does the diabetic client who sneaks off to the food vending machine for a candy bar.

There are times when the conflictive feelings begin intrapersonally within the nurse (e.g., in working with parents of an abused child or treating a foul-mouthed alcoholic client in the emergency room). Such situations often stir up strong feelings of anger or resentment in us. In this case, we may need to defuse destructive emotions before proceeding further. The following are interventions you can use to defuse intrapersonal conflicts:

- Identify the presence of an emotionally tense situation.
- Talk the situation through with someone.
- Provide a neutral, accepting environment.
- Take appropriate action to reduce tension.
- Evaluate the effectiveness of the strategies.
- Generalize behavioral approaches to other situations.

For the nurse, the first step in coping with difficult emotional responses is to recognize their presence and to assess the appropriateness of expressing emotion in the situation. If expressing the emotion does not fit the circumstances, one must deliberately remain unruffled when every natural instinct argues against it. Ambivalence, described as two opposing ideas or feelings related to any life situation or relationship coexisting within the same individual, is a relatively common phenomenon.

It is not the responsibility of the nurse to help a client resolve all intrapersonal conflict. Deal only with those that occur within the context of the immediate clinical situation and threaten to sabotage the goals of the therapeutic relationship. Long-standing conflicts require more expertise to resolve. In such cases, the nurse identifies the presence of possible conflict, refers the client to the appropriate resource, communicates with the personnel chosen, and supports the client's participation.

Evaluate

The final step in the process is to evaluate the effectiveness of responses to emotions and to generalize the experience of confronting difficult emotions to other situations. Each step in the process may need to be taken more than once and refined or revised as circumstances dictate.

Interpersonal Conflict Interventions

Developing Assertive Skills

Demonstrate Respect. Responsible, assertive statements are made in ways that do not violate the rights of others or diminish their standing. They are conveyed by a relaxed, attentive posture and a calm, friendly tone of voice. Statements should be accompanied by the use of appropriate eye contact.

Use "I" Statements. Statements that begin with "You" sound accusatory and always represent an assumption because it is impossible to know exactly, without validation, why someone acts in a certain way. Because such statements usually point a finger and imply a judgment, most people respond defensively to them.

"We" statements should be used only when you actually mean to look at an issue collaboratively. Thus, the statement, "Perhaps we both need to look at this issue a little closer" may be appropriate in certain situations. However, the statement, "Perhaps we shouldn't get so angry when things don't work out the way we think they should" is a condescending statement thinly disguised as a collaborative statement. What is actually being expressed is the expectation that both parties should handle the conflict in one way—the nurse's way.

Use of "I" statements are one of the most effective conflict management strategies you can use. Assertive statements that begin with "I" suggest that the person making the statement accepts full personal responsibility for his or her own feelings and position in relation to the presence of conflict. It is not necessary to justify your position unless the added message clarifies or adds essential information. "I" statements seem a little clumsy at first and take some practice. The traditional format is this:

"I feel _____ (use a name to claim the emotion you feel) when ______ (describe the behavior nonjudgmentally) because _____ (describe the tangible effects of the behavior)."

Example:

"I feel uncomfortable when a client's personal problems are discussed in the cafeteria because someone might overhear confidential information."

Make Clear Statements. Statements, rather than questions, set the stage for assertive responses to conflict. When questions are used, "how" questions are best because they are neutral in nature, they seek more information, and they imply a collaborative effort. "Why" questions ask for an explanation or an evaluation of behavior and often put the other person on the defensive. It is always important to state the situation clearly; describe events or expectations objectively; and use a strong, firm, yet tactful manner. The following example shows how a nurse can use the three levels of assertive behaviors to meet the client's needs in a hospital situation without compromising the nurse's own needs for respect and dignity.

Case Example

Mr. Gow is a 35-year-old executive who has been hospitalized with a myocardial infarction. He has been acting seductively toward some of the young nurses, but he seems to be giving Miss O'Hara an especially hard time.

Client: Come on in, honey, I've been waiting for you.

Nurse (using appropriate facial expression and eye contact and replying in a firm, clear voice): Mr. Gow, I would rather you called me Miss O'Hara.

Client: Aw, come on now, honey. I don't get to have much fun around here. What's the difference what I call you?

Nurse: I feel that it does make a difference, and I would like you to call me Miss O'Hara.

Client: Oh, you're no fun at all. Why do you have to be so serious?

Nurse: Mr. Gow, you're right. I am serious about some things, and being called by my name and title is one of them. I would prefer that you call me Miss O'Hara. I would like to work with you, however, and it might be important to explore the ways in which this hospitalization is hampering your natural desire to have fun.

In this interaction, the nurse's position is defined several times using successively stronger statements before the shift can be made to refocus on underlying client needs. Notice that even in the final encounter, however, the nurse labels the behavior, not the client, as unacceptable. Persistence is an essential feature when first attempts at assertiveness appear too limited. After careful analysis, if you find that a client's behavior is infringing on your rights, it is essential that the issues be addressed directly in a tactful manner. If they are not, it is quite likely that the undesirable behavior will continue until you are no longer willing to tolerate it.

Use Proper Pitch and Tone. The amount of force used in delivery of an assertive statement depends on the nature of the conflict situation as well as on the amount of confrontation needed to resolve the conflict successfully. Starting with the least amount of assertiveness required to meet the demands of the situation conserves energy and does not place the nurse into the bind of overkill. It is not necessary to use all of one's resources at one time or to express ideas strongly when this type of response is not needed. You can sometimes lose your effectiveness by becoming long-winded in your explanation when only a simple statement of rights or intent is needed. Long explanations detract from the true impact of the spoken message. Getting to the main point quickly and saying what is necessary in the simplest, most concrete way cuts down on the possibility of misinterpretation. This approach increases the probability that the communication will be constructively received.

Pitch and tone of voice contribute to another person's interpretation of the meaning of your assertive message. A soft, hesitant, passive presentation can undermine an assertive message as much as vocalizing the message in a harsh, hostile, and aggressive tone. A firm but moderate presentation often is as effective as content in conveying the message (see Exercise 14-3).

Analyze Personal Feelings. As mentioned before, part of an initial assessment of an interpersonal conflict situation includes recognition of the nurse's intrapersonal contribution to the conflict as well as that of the client. It is not wrong to have ambivalent feelings about taking care of clients with different lifestyles and values; however, this needs to be acknowledged to yourself.

Focus on the Present. The focus of assertive responses should always be on the present. Because it is impossible to do anything about the past except learn from it, and because the future is never completely predictable, the present is the only reality in which we have much decision-making power as to how we act.

To be classified as assertive, behavior must reflect deliberate choice. It is not always necessary to use words to be assertive. Sometimes it is better to listen quietly to what someone has to say, to think carefully about the message, and to plan to come back later when the person is in a more receptive frame of mind. Assertive communication is open, direct, honest, and appropriate to the interpersonal demands of the situation.

To be assertive in the face of an emotionally charged situation demands thought, energy, and commitment. Assertiveness also requires the use of common sense, self-awareness, knowledge, tact, humor, respect, and a sense of perspective. Although there is no guarantee that the use of assertive behaviors will produce desired interpersonal goals, the chances of a successful outcome are increased because the information flow is optimally honest, direct, and firm. Often the use of assertiveness brings about changes in ways that could not have been anticipated. Changes occur because the nurse offers a new resource in the form of objective feedback with no strings attached.

Structure Your Response. In mastering assertive responses, it may be helpful initially to use the four steps of an assertive response first presented by Angel and Petronko (1987), who also provided the following example:

1. Express empathy: "I understand that __________"; "I hear you saying ______."
2. Describe your feelings or the situation: "I feel that __________"; "This situation seems to me to be __________."
3. State expectations: "I want __________"; "What is required by the situation is __________."
4. List consequences: "If you do this, then ___________ will happen" (state positive outcome); "If you don't do this, then ___________ will happen" (state negative outcome).

For example, the nurse might do the following:

1. Express empathy: "I understand that things are difficult at home."
2. Describe your feelings or the situation: "But your 8-year-old daughter has expressed a lot of anxiety, saying, 'I can't learn to give my own insulin shots.'"
3. State expectations: "It is necessary for you to be here tomorrow when the diabetic teaching nurse comes so you can learn how to give injections and your daughter can, too, with your support."
4. List consequences: "If you get here on time, we can be finished and get her discharged in time for her birthday on Friday."

Clinical Encounters with Demanding, Difficult Clients

Every nurse encounters clients who seem overly demanding of your limited time and resources. While this may reflect a personality characteristic, most often it is sign of their anxiety. Box 14-3 describes behaviors that increase anger in others. People are difficult to deal with because our normal way of dealing with them has failed. We cannot change other's personalities, but we can change the way we react to them (Salazar, 2004). Refer to Box 14-4 for intervention tips.

Box 14-3 Top 10 Behaviors That Create Anger in Others

- Providing unsolicited advice
- Conveying ideas that try to create guilt
- Offering reassurances that are not realistic
- Communicating using "gloss it over" positive comments
- Offering fake sympathy
- Exerting pressure to make a person change their behavior
- Placing blame
- Portraying self as infallible
- Using excessive, histrionic language
- Using "hot button" words that have heavy emotional connotations

From Bacal R: Conflict prevention in the workplace: Using Cooperative Communication, 2000; available online: http://work911.com.

Box 14-4 Potential Approaches for Dealing with Anxious or Difficult Clients

- Use active listening skills to identify issues of concern to the client.
- Respond in a calm tone and avoid conveying irritation.
- Provide education; explain all options, with outcomes.
- Explain the limits of your role.
- Develop a nursing care plan: involve patient in care and set goals; review and reevaluate whether nurse and client have same goals; focus on mutual goals and progress.
- Work with staff so all use the same uniform approach to the client's demands.
- Preempt demands by stopping by to offer assistance.
- Use incentives and withdrawal of privileges to modify unacceptable behavior.
- Use medical and nonmedical interventions to decrease anxiety (e.g., medicine, touch, relaxation, and guided imagery).
- Set limits, give family permission (e.g., to rest or to leave).
- Promote trust by providing immediate feedback.

Clinical Encounters with Angry Clients

Newspaper, television, and radio news stories abound with what is seen by many as an epidemic level of destructive anger leading to violence. Because health care is an aspect of the larger society, you can expect to encounter clients who refuse to comply with the treatment plan, who exhibit hostile behaviors toward staff, and who act out their anger or perhaps withdraw from any positive interaction with you as their nurse. When dealing with a difficult client, ask yourself what the client is gaining from such behavior. Some people have not learned successful communication, so they revert to behavior which has gained them something in the past. For example, as children they may have only gotten needed attention when they acted out in a negative way or when they pouted or sulked. Ask yourself if the client behaving in a difficult way is getting rewarded by focusing a lot of staff attention on himself or herself, for example. Does the client just need to learn a more effective way of communicating?

As Maynard (2006) says, there are numerous nonverbal clues to anger, including clenched jaws or fists, turning away, "forgetting" or being late for appointments, and refusing to maintain eye contact. Verbal cues by a client may, of course, include use of an angry tone of voice, but they may also be disguised as witty sarcasm or as condescending or insulting remarks. To become comfortable in dealing with client anger, the nurse must first become aware of his or her own reactions to anger so that the nurse does not threaten or reject the individual expressing anger, or respond in anger. Interventions include those listed in Box 14-5.

Help the client own the angry feelings by getting the client to verbalize things that make him or her angry. Acknowledging a client's anger may prevent an expression of abusive ranting. It is essential that you use empathetic statements or active listening to acknowledge the client's anger *before* moving on to try to discuss the issue.

Box 14-5 Strategies for Dealing with an Angry Client

- Use active listening while allowing client to ventilate some of his or her anger.
- Take a deep breath and respond in a low tone of voice (avoid being defensive).
- Restate the issue.
- Help client identify his or her own anger, for example: "I notice you are clenching your fists and talking more loudly than usual. These are things people do when angry. Are you feeling angry right now?"
- Give permission within limits: "It's okay to feel angry about..., but not okay to act on it" or, "It's natural to feel angry about...".
- Offer to work with client to help him or her deal with the issue.
- Get help *immediately* if you feel in danger of physical harm.

Defuse Hostility. Avoid responding to a client's anger by getting angry yourself. Verbal attacks follow certain rules, in that the abusive person expects you to react in specific ways. Usually people will respond by becoming aggressive and attacking back or by becoming defensive and intimidated. Keep your cool using strategies discussed above. Take a deep breath! Remember: if you lose control, you lose! If you become defensive, you lose! Abusive people want to provoke confrontations as a means of controlling you. If the client persists, you need to assert limits, saying, for example, "Jim, I want to help you sort this out, but if you continue to raise your voice, I'm going to have to leave. Which do you want?" or, "Yelling at me isn't going to get this worked out. I will not argue with you. Come back when you can talk calmly and I will try to help you."

- An angry client needs to have you acknowledge both the issue and his or her feelings about that issue. Only then can the client begin to interact in a meaningful way.
- Deliberately begin to lower your voice and speak more slowly. When we get upset, we tend to speak quickly and use a higher tone of voice. If you do the opposite, the client may begin to mimic you and thus calm down.
- Realistically analyze the current situation that is disturbing the client.
- Assist the client in developing a plan to deal with the situation (e.g., the nurse could use techniques such as role-playing to help the client express anger appropriately, using "I" statements such as "I feel angry" rather than "You make me angry"). Bringing behavior up to a verbal level should help alleviate the need for other acting out of destructive behaviors.

Prevent Escalation of Conflict. Depending on the type of feedback received, an intrapersonal conflict can take on interpersonal dimensions. In the following example, the mother initially experiences an intrapersonal conflict. The wished-for perfect infant has not appeared, and her personal ambivalence related to coping with her infant's defect is expressed indirectly through her partial noncompliant behavior. If the nurse interprets the client's behavior incorrectly as poor mothering and acts in a manner that reflects this attitude, the basically intrapersonal conflict can become interpersonal.

Case Example

A mother with her first infant is informed soon after delivery that her child has a cleft palate (missing roof of mouth). The physician explains the infant's condition in detail and answers the mother's questions. The mother requests rooming in and seems genuinely interested in the infant. Each time the nurse enters the client's room, the mother complains that her child does not seem hungry and states how difficult it is to feed the baby. Although the nurse spends a great deal of time teaching the mother the special techniques necessary for feeding, and the mother seems interested at the time, she seems unable or unwilling to follow any of the nurse's suggestions when she is by herself. Later, the nurse finds out that the mother has been asking for guidance and appears to be resisting what is offered. Although she may simply need further instruction in technique, the presence of an underlying intrapersonal conflict is worth investigating. Before proceeding with teaching, the nurse needs to find out about the mother's perceptions. Does she feel competent in the mothering role? What does having a less than perfect child mean to her? What are her fears about caring for an infant with this particular type of defect? Until the underlying feelings are identified, client teaching is likely to have limited success.

This client appears to reframe the experience from her own perspective. In this situation, a client strength would be the mother's ability and willingness to express her uncomfortable feelings so that they can be addressed. Even though the mother may be unclear about the nature of her feelings, reframing the issues in this way builds on strengths instead of on personal deficits. It is hoped that the client provides more specific input about her fears and the nurse provides acceptance of the client's right to have all types of feelings, so that together they may seek a solution.

Prevent any escalation in interpersonal conflict. Hurt feelings, misunderstandings, and misperceptions about the situation being discussed can quickly escalate a conflict. If your vocal pitch is rising as you talk to an angry client, make an effort to lower your pitch. As the client's voice rises, lower yours. If eye contact seems confrontational, then break eye contact. If the client is acting out by throwing or hitting, set limits: "No hitting (spitting, or other physical behavior) is allowed here." If you set limits, be sure to follow through. Ask the client to verbalize his or her anger (e.g., "Talk about how you feel, instead of throwing things"). Studies show that talking will dramatically reduce aggressive behavior. Use other strategies described in this book for defusing conflict situations. Active listening (i.e., really listening to your client's viewpoint), using attentive body language, and summarizing the client's viewpoint can defuse some of the tension of the conflict.

Clinical Encounters with Violent Clients

Some clients have mental problems or are truly confused. It helps you to respond more positively if you perceive that their behavior is not "evil" but a result of their illness.

A few clients may be asocial. In no case is violence acceptable. Limits must be set. Failing this, you need to remove yourself from a potentially harmful situation. Starcher (1999) describes the behavior of an emotionally disturbed client admitted to a geriatric unit. Sam's behavior ranged from bullying or pushing other clients to noncompliance with his treatment. Staff tried setting clear limits and identifying specific negative outcomes, including restraints and medication, without success. Eventual successful interventions included consistent response by all staff members and using written patient contracts for each of his unacceptable behaviors. Outcomes were specifically stated for both negative behaviors (restrictions) and positive acceptable behaviors (rewards with his favorite activities).

Box 14-5 lists some useful strategies for coping with angry clients. An additional strategy for helping nurse-client problem interactions is the staff-focused consultation. Consider the following situation.

Case Example

Mr. Plotsky, age 29 years, has been employed for 6 years as a construction worker. About 4 weeks ago, while operating a forklift, he was struck by a train, leaving him paraplegic. After 2 weeks in intensive care, he was transferred to a neurological unit. When staff members attempt to provide physical care, such as changing his position or getting him up in a chair, Mr. Plotsky throws things, curses angrily, and sometimes spits at the nurses. Staff members become very upset; several nurses have requested assignment changes. Some staff members try bribing him with food to encourage good behavior; others threaten to apply restraints. The manager schedules a behavioral consultation meeting with a psychiatric nurse or clinical specialist. The immediate goal of this staff conference is to bring staff feelings out into the open and to facilitate increased awareness of the staff's behavioral responses when confronted with this client's behavior. The outcome goal is to use a problem-solving approach to develop a behavioral care plan, so that all staff members respond to Mr. Plotsky in a consistent manner.

Students are particularly prone to feeling rebuffed when they first encounter negative feedback from a client. Support from staff, instructors, and peers, coupled with efforts to understand the underlying reasons for the client's feelings, help you resist the trap of avoiding the relationship. To develop these ideas further, practice Exercise 14-6.

Defusing Potential Conflicts When Providing Home Health Care

Recognizing potential situations lending themselves to conflict is, of course, an important initial step. Caregivers have been shown to experience conflict through incompatible pressures suffered between caregiver demands and demands from their other roles, such as parenting their children or maintaining employment (Stephens, Townsend, Martire et al., 2001). In addition to this interrole conflict, caregivers suffer pressures when a nurse comes into their home to participate in the care of an ill relative. A Canadian study of home health nurses and family caregivers of elderly relatives identified four evolving stages in the nurse-caregiver relationship. The initial stage is "worker-helper," with the nurse providing care to the ill client and the family helping. Next comes "worker-worker," when the nurse begins teaching the needed care skills to family members. Third is "nurse as manager; family as worker," as the family members learn needed care skills. In the final stage, "nurse as nurse for family caregiver," occurs as the family member becomes exhausted (Butt, 2000). A source of conflict for nurses was the dual expectation of the family that the nurse would provide care not only for the identified client but also provide relief for the exhausted primary caregiver. When the nurse operated as manager and treated the caregiver as worker, the discrepancy in expectations and values resulted in increased tension in the relationship. Discussion of role expectations is essential. Because of the high cost of providing direct care to chronically ill clients, home health nurses may be expected to quickly shift to teaching the necessary skills to the family members. The nurse can clarify that this shift in responsibility results in a reduction of expensive professional time but not in the nurse's emotional commitment to the family.

SUMMARY

Conflict represents a struggle between two opposing thoughts, feelings, or needs. It can be intrapersonal in nature, deriving from within a particular individual; or interpersonal, when it represents a clash between two or more people.

All conflicts have certain things in common: a concrete content problem issue and relationship issues arising from the process of expressing the conflict. Generally, intrapersonal conflicts stimulate feelings of emotional discomfort. A neutral, supportive interpersonal environment helps reduce emotions to a workable level. Other strategies to defuse strong emotion include talking the emotion through with someone and temporarily reducing stress through the use of distraction or additional information.

Most interpersonal conflicts involve some threat, either to one's sense of power to control an interpersonal situation or to ways of thinking about the self. Giving up ineffective behavior patterns in conflict situations is difficult; such patterns are generally perceived to be safer because they are familiar. The principles of conflict management were described.

Behavioral responses to conflict situations fall into four categories. Nurses most commonly choose avoidance. However, this chapter describes other strategies (e.g., assertion) that have been more successfully used by nurses to manage client-nurse conflicts. Assertive behaviors range from making a simple statement, directly and honestly, about one's beliefs; to taking a very strong, confrontational stand about what will and will not be tolerated.

To apply conflict management principles, nurses need to identify their own conflictive feelings or reactions. For internal conflict, feelings usually have to be put into words and related to the issue at hand before the meaning of the conflict becomes understandable. In conflict between nurse and client, the nurse needs to think through the possible causes of the conflict as well as his or her own feelings about it before making a response. To resolve these kinds of conflict, you need to use "I" statements and respond assertively.

Ethical Dilemma ■ *What Would You Do?*

You are caring for Kim, born at the gestational age of 24 weeks in a rural hospital and transferred this morning to your neonatal intensive care unit. Today her father arrives on the unit. Seeing you taking a blood sample from one of the many intravenous lines attached to her body, he yells at you to "Stop poking at her! What are you trying to prove by keeping her alive? Turn off those machines." This is both a communication and an ethics problem. How do you respond to his anger?

REFERENCES

Angel G, Petronko DK: *Developing the new assertive nurse: essentials for Advancement*, ed 2, New York, 1987, Springer.

Bacal R: Eleven things that create resistance and anger in others [online article], 2000; available online: http://work911.com/articles/11things.htm.

Booth R: Conflict and conflict management. In Mason DJ, Talbot SW, editors, *Political action handbook for nurses*, Menlo Park, CA, 1985, Addison-Wesley.

Brixey L: The difficult task of delivering bad news, *Dermatol Nurs* 16(4):347–348, 356, 2004.

Brooks A, Thomas S, Droppleman P: (1996) From frustration to red fury: a description of work-related anger in male registered nurses, *Nurs Forum* 31(3):4–15, 1996.

Butt G: Nurses and family caregivers of elderly relatives engaged in 4 evolving types of relationships, *Evid Based Nurs* 3:134, 2000.

Dallinger JM, Hample D: Personalizing and managing conflict, *Int J Conflict Manag* 6(3):273–289, 1995.

Davidhizar R: Impressing the boss who criticizes you, *Adv Clin Care* 6(2):39–41, 1991.

Feeney MC, Davidson JA: Bridging the gap between the practical and the theoretical: an evaluation of a conflict resolution model, *Peace Conflict* 2(3):255–269, 1996.

Flanagan L: *Survival skills in the workplace: what every nurse should know*, Kansas City, MO, 1990, American Nurses Association.

Fritchie R: Conflict and its management, *Br J Hosp Med* 53(9):471–473, 1995.

Gaddis S: The four-second rule for improved communications [online article], accessed 8/21/06; available online: http://www.communicationsdoctor.com/articles/foursec.pdf.

Isikhan V, Comez T, Danis MZ: Job stress and coping strategies in health care professionals working with cancer patients, *Eur J Oncol Nurs* 8(3):234–244, 2004.

Johnson J, Arneson P: Women expressing anger to women in the workplace, *Wom Stud Comm* 14(2):24–41, 1991.

Jones MA, Bushardt SC, Cadenhead G: A paradigm for effective resolution of interpersonal conflict, *Nurs Manage* 21(2):64B, 64F–64K, 1990.

Maynard C: Personal communication, 2006.

Maynard C, Chitty K: Dealing with anger: guidelines for nursing intervention, *J Psychiatr Nurs Ment Health Serv* 17(6):36–41, 1979.

Mayo Health Clinic: Tips on dealing with co-worker conflict; retrieved 5/1/05 from http://www.mayohealth.org

McCanton PJ, Hargie O: Assessing assertive behavior in student nurses: a comparison of assertive measures, *J Adv Nurs* 15(12):1370–1376, 1990.

McElhaney R: Conflict management in nursing administration, *Nurs Manage* 27(3):49–50, 1996.

Moustakis C: *Finding yourself, finding others*, Englewood Cliffs, NJ, 1974, Prentice Hall.

Nursing Standard: Nurses are better at getting patients to talk, *Nurs Stand* 18(49):5, 2004.

Porter L: Conflict. *Semin Perioper Nurs* 5(3):119–126, 1996.

Potter PA, Perry AG: *Fundamentals of nursing*, ed 5, St Louis, 2001, Mosby.

Redman BK, Fry ST: Ethical conflicts reported by RN/certified diabetes educators, *Diabetes Educ* 22(3):219–224, 1996.

Salazar J: Dealing with difficult people, *Mich Nurse*; retrieved 5/05 from http://www.minurses.org

Schutzenhofer KK: Nursing education and professional autonomy, *Reflections* 18:7, 1992.

Shearer R, Davidson R: When a co-worker complains, Can Nurse 93(1):47–48, 1997.

Starcher S: Sam was an emotional terrorist, *Nursing* 99(2): 40–41, 1999.

Stephens MA, Townsend AL, Martire LM et al.: Balancing parent care with other roles: interrole conflict, *Journal of Gerontol B Psychol Sci Soc Sci* 56(1):24–34, 2001.

Trubisky P, Ting-Toomey S, Lin S: The influence of individualism-collectivism and self-monitoring on conflict styles, *Int J Intercult Relat* 15:65–84, 1991.

Valentine PE: Management of conflict: do nurses/women handle it differently? *J Adv Nurs* 22:142–149, 1995.

Valentine PE: A gender perspective on conflict management strategies, *J Nurs Scholarsh* 33(1):69–74, 2001.

Chapter 15

Health Promotion and Client Learning Needs

Elizabeth Arnold

OUTLINE

OBJECTIVES

At the end of the chapter, the reader will be able to:

1. Define health promotion.
2. Compare and contrast theory frameworks in health promotion.
3. Identify factors related to a client's readiness to learn.
4. Describe factors related to a client's ability to learn.
5. Discuss the nurse's role in population-focused health education.

The unique function of the nurse is to assist the individual, sick or well, in the performance of those activities contributing to his health or recovery (or to peaceful death) that he would perform unaided if he had the necessary strength, will, or knowledge.... [The nurse] is temporarily the consciousness of the unconscious, the love of life for the suicidal, the leg of the amputee, the eyes of the newly blind, a means of locomotion for the infant, knowledge and confidence for the young mother, the [voice] for those too weak or withdrawn to speak.

(Henderson, 1961)

Chapter 15 focuses on health promotion as the basis for health education that can be applied at all practice levels. It outlines communication strategies that the nurse can use to help individual clients, families, and targeted populations within the community promote their health and well-being. The chapter describes theoretical models related to health promotion and disease prevention, and considers factors influencing readiness to learn at the individual and community level. Health promotion is important to focus on in the nurse client relationship, as "treatment alone is unlikely to have marked effects on health inequities or health status" (Frankish, Moulton, Rootman et al., 2006, p. 271).

National health recommendations and health agendas have provided strong support for the nation's move from a predominantly medical model of health care to a public health model, and from a treatment approach offered by individual health providers to a preventive approach provided by an interdisciplinary team. In 2001, the publication of a report from the Institute of Medicine's (IOM's) Committee on Quality Health Care in America titled *Crossing the Quality Chasm: A New Health System for the 21st Century* produced recommendations for a sweeping redesign of the health care system with specific recommendations for safe, effective, patient-centered, timely, efficient, and equitable care and a preference for the development of population-based care standards (IOM, 2001).

BASIC CONCEPTS

Health Promotion

Health promotion in clinical practice is defined as "organized actions or efforts that enhance, support, or promote the well-being or health of individuals, families, groups, communities or societies" (Kulbok, Baldwin, Cox, et al., 1997, p. 17). Based on the premise that health is a basic human right intimately related to the nation's social and economic development, health promotion focuses on an individual's health and well-being and the self-management skills necessary to achieve maximum functioning and satisfaction, with a preference for primary prevention. The emphasis is on diverting health problems *before* they occur or worsen. Today, promoting a healthy lifestyle is recognized as an essential component of comprehensive health care (Fraser, 1998).

The World Health Organization (WHO) describes health promotion as a process of enabling people to increase control over and improve their health. Optimal health and well-being are considered the desired outcomes of health promotion activities. **Well-being** is a personal experience associated with personal satisfaction in six personal dimensions: intellectual, physical, emotional, social, occupational, and spiritual (Chandler, Holden, Kolander et al., 1992; Omizo, Omizo, & d'Andrea, 1992). Even for people with chronic health problems and terminal diagnosis, health promotion activities can improve well-being (Saylor, 2004).

Health promotion is concerned with factors that influence health and well-being, including "the living and working conditions that enable and support people in making healthy choices and services that promote and maintain health" (Vail, 1995, p. 59). It is a broader concept than health education because it also includes a combination of political, regulatory, and organizational supports for achieving targeted health outcomes (Huff & Kline, 1999). For example, marketing of health supports, sociopolitical measures that create supportive social and environmental change, and a set of community values that enhance a healthy lifestyle are interdependent parts of health promotion activities needed at the community and system levels.

A health promotion focus proposes that health care consumers achieve optimal health and well-being through taking personal responsibility for healthy lifestyles and actively cooperating in their health maintenance. A health promotion/disease prevention focus views the client as an informed consumer and a valued partner in health care. Health promotion activities focus on individuals and their families, communities, and larger ecosystems. *Community* is defined as "any group of citizens that have either a geographic, population-based, or self-defined relationship and whose health may be improved by a health promotion approach" (Frankish et al., 2006, p. 174).

In the 21st century, health promotion should be part of everyday nursing care (Beckford-Ball, 2006). Often people with the greatest health burdens have the least access to information, communication technologies, health care, and supporting social services. To meet this challenge, effective health promotion strategies require nurses to be leaders in inspiring people to make significant lifestyle changes and to be teachers in inviting people to follow through with the changes needed for a healthy lifestyle. Health promotion activities are viewed as a community resource that can affect personal lifestyle choices, coping skills, and health behaviors such as regular medical checkups and health screening to promote health and prevent disease (Maltby & Robinson, 1998).

Disease Prevention

Health promotion activities involve proactive decision making at all levels of prevention (Edelman & Mandel, 1998). Ideally, nursing takes into account three aspects of prevention—primary, secondary, and tertiary prevention—in a seamless continuum of health promotion and health care delivery.

Primary prevention, defined as actions taken to preclude illness or to prevent the natural course of illness from occurring, focuses on teaching people how to establish and maintain lifestyles conducive to optimal health. Primary prevention goals focus on populations who are basically healthy but who could improve factors that determine, promote, or protect health. These goals include understanding health-related threats to vulnerable populations, ensuring equity in health care, and preserving and enhancing quality of life for all health care consumers. The nurse teaches clients how to avoid exposure to controllable risk factors and how to steer clear of health-related problems in their particular age, cultural, or social group. Examples include prenatal clinics, parenting classes, stress management programs, genetic screening, and healthy eating in old age.

Secondary prevention involves interventions designed to promote early diagnosis of symptoms or timely treatment after the onset of the disease. The purpose of secondary preventive teaching programs is to catch health problems early, thus minimizing their effects on a person's life. They target populations with common risk factors. Examples include screening surveys; mammograms; purified protein derivatives; and glaucoma, diabetes, respiratory, and blood pressure screenings.

Tertiary prevention describes rehabilitation strategies designed to minimize the handicapping effects of a disease. Strategies are designed to keep problems from getting worse and are targeted toward populations who already have experienced an injury or disease process. Examples include teaching a cancer victim to manage chemotherapy symptoms, helping a stroke victim with bladder retraining to avoid infection, and teaching a client to cope effectively with the necessary adjustments a serious physical, social, or emotional illness imposes.

Box 15-1 Recommendations of the U.S. Preventive Services Task Force: Strategies in Health Education and Counseling

- Frame the teaching to match the client's perceptions.
- Fully inform clients of the purposes and expected outcomes of interventions, and when to expect these new effects.
- Suggest small changes and baby steps rather than large ones.
- Be specific.
- Add new behaviors rather than eliminating established behaviors whenever possible.
- Link new behaviors to old behaviors.
- Obtain explicit commitments from the client and client family support regarding actions.
- Refer clients to appropriate community resources.
- Use a combination of strategies to achieve outcomes.
- Monitor progress through follow-up contact.

Guidelines proposed by the U.S. Preventive Services Task Force for health promoting education and counseling are presented in Box 15-1.

Health Promotion and Disease Prevention Agendas for the Nation

The Committee on Assuring the Health of the Public in the 21st Century (2003) cited three major trends influencing health care in the United States:

1. Demographic changes with the "population growing larger, older, and more racially and ethnically diverse, with a higher incidence of chronic disease"
2. Technical and scientific advances, which "create new channels for information and communication, as well as novel ways of preventing and treating disease"
3. "Globalization and health, to include the geopolitical and economic challenge of globalization, including international terrorism" (pp. 34-41)

Healthy People 2010 (U.S. Department of Health and Human Services, 2000) represents the health promotion and disease prevention agenda for the nation. The third document of its kind, it puts forth 28 focus areas with corresponding national health objectives designed to identify and reduce the most significant preventable threats to health. Federal agencies intimately involved with health care developed the document with input from more than 350 national membership organizations and 250 state health, mental health, substance abuse, and environmental agencies. Thus the document represents the most relevant scientific expertise on health care. It contains a set of health objectives to provide direction for and outcome benchmarks related to preventive health care over the next decade. The overarching goals of *Healthy People 2010* relate to increasing the years and quality of life for people and reducing the health disparities that exist in this country. Leading health indicators proposed by *Healthy People 2010* include the following:

- Physical activity
- Overweight and obesity
- Tobacco use
- Substance abuse
- Responsible sexual behavior
- Mental health
- Injury and violence
- Environmental quality
- Immunization
- Access to health care

Centers for Disease Control and Prevention

Surveillance of health events is an important component of population-focused health promotion and disease prevention because it alerts health care providers to potential and actual health problems and provides morbidity and mortality rates for evaluation purposes. The *Centers for Disease Control and Prevention (CDC)* is "the nation's premiere health promotion, prevention and preparedness agency and a global leader in public health" (CDC, 2006). It is the operational part of the Department of Health and Human Services (DHHS), which is directly responsible for protecting the health and safety of the nation's citizens and committed to achieving improvement in people's health. As such, it is an important resource for health promotion activities.

The CDC collects data such as the incidence and prevalence of diseases and chronic illnesses, and ranks illnesses that kill Americans. It tracks the development of new disorders appearing in the United States and is recognized globally for its dedication to promoting people's health and well-being. This agency provides funding to states to implement health programs for Americans, and funding to developing countries related to prevention and treatment of AIDS. The CDC applies research findings to improve people's daily lives. State and municipal health departments receive support from the CDC to detect and reduce health threats from bioterrorism. The CDC has four health promotion impact goals:

- Healthy People in Every Stage of Life: All people, and especially those at greater risk of health disparities, will achieve their optimal life span with the best quality of life in every stage of life.
- Healthy People in Healthy Places: The places where people live, work, learn, and play will protect and promote their health and safety, especially those at greater risk of health disparities.
- People Prepared for Emerging Health Threats: People in all communities will be protected from infectious, occupational, environmental, and terrorist threats.
- Healthy People in a Healthy World: People around the world will live safer, healthier, and longer lives through health promotion, health security, and health diplomacy. (CDC, n.d.)

Nurses and other health care providers interested in population-focused health care and health promotion can find complete data online at http://www.cdc.gov.

At the community level, nurses help locate populations at risk for health problems. They design and provide health education, social marketing, and screening services to targeted populations with unrecognized health risk factors. They instruct targeted populations about the nature of the concern, what supports are available, and how services can be obtained. Examples include drug prevention and teenage pregnancy prevention programs. At the individual level, nurses use case finding strategies to identify specific individuals and families with identified risk factors and connect them with needed supports, resources, and services.

Theory Frameworks for Health Promotion

Pender's Health Promotion Model

Pender's (1996) health promotion model expands on an earlier health belief model developed by Rosenstock and his associates in the 1950s. Pender views health promotion as "increasing the level of well-being and self-actualization of a given individual or group" (Pender,

Murdaugh, & Parsons, 2002, p. 34) (see Figure 15-1). The health belief model proposes that a person's willingness to engage in health promotion behaviors is best understood through examining a person's beliefs about the seriousness of a health condition and his or her ability to influence the disease progression or outcome of treatment. For example, a client's belief about a diabetic condition and the condition's resolution with or without diet and exercise treatment protocols or insulin medication is a significant factor in predicting adherence.

Pender's health promotion model emphasizes movement toward a positive valuing of health and well-being. Cognitive perceptual factors, which include a person's definition of health, perceptions of health status, benefits, and barriers to health-promoting behaviors, strengthen or weaken interest in engaging in health-promoting behaviors. Pender calls them "the primary motivational mechanisms for acquisition and maintenance of health-promoting behaviors" (p. 60). Modifying factors are internal or external inputs that serve as "cues to action" in a person's decision to seek health care or to engage in health-promoting activities. Examples of modifying factors are schools that require immunizations, family experiences with a disorder or preventive measures, and interpersonal reminders, such as a family member's experience with the health care system, the mass media, demographic characteristics, and ethnic approval.

Case Example

Mary Nolan knows that walking will help diminish her potential for developing osteoporosis, but the threat of having this disorder in her 60s is not sufficient to motivate her to take action in her 40s. Mary does not feel any signs or symptoms of the disorder, and it is easier to maintain a sedentary life. The nurse will have to understand the client's internal value system and other factors that influence readiness to learn to create the most appropriate learning conditions and types of teaching strategies Mary will need to effect positive change in health habits. The nurse might show Mary a video of the changes osteoporosis creates in spinal structure or ask an older adult with this disease to share her experience.

Exercise 15-1 provides practice with applying Pender's health promotion model to common health problems.

Transtheoretical Model of Change

Prochaska, DiClemente, and Norcross (1992) describe motivation to change as a state of readiness that

Exercise 15-1 Pender's Health Promotion Model

Purpose: To help students understand the value of the health promotion model in assessing and promoting healthy lifestyles.

Procedure:

1. Using the health promotion model as a guide, interview a person in the community about his or her perception of a common health problem (e.g., heart disease, high cholesterol, osteoporosis, breast or prostate cancer, obesity, or diabetes).
2. Record the person's answers in written diagram form following Pender's model of health promotion. Identify individualized modifying factors and the appropriate cues to action that would best fit the person's situation.
3. Share your findings with your classmates, either in a small group of four to six students with a scribe to share common themes with the larger class, or in the general class.

Discussion:

1. Were you surprised by anything the client said, his or her perception of the problem, or interpretation of its meaning?
2. As you compare your findings with other classmates, do common themes emerge?
3. How could you use the information you obtained from this exercise in future health care situations?

fluctuates and can be influenced by external encouragement. The transtheoretical model describes intentional behavioral change and identifies five stages through which people make a decision to make a change and implement it. Motivational strategies that match the stages of change proposed by these authors increase the likelihood that the client will follow the recommended course of action toward change. The transtheoretical model is particularly effective for use with clients who are resistant to standard teaching strategies because it recognizes how hard it is for people to modify long-established health patterns. Many people will cycle through one or more of the stages several times before a permanent change is in place. Table 15-1 presents Prochaska's Model of Change with suggested approaches for each stage and corresponding sample statements.

Case Example

Nurse: I know that you think you can manage yourself at home. But most people really need some rehabilitation after a stroke to help them regain their strength. If you go home now without the rehabilitation, you may be shortchanging yourself by not taking the time to develop the skills you need to be independent at home. Is that something important to you? (*Precontemplation approach to raise awareness of the problem*)

Table 15-1 Prochaska's Stages of Change with Suggested Approaches and Sample Statements Applied to Alcoholism

Client Stage	Characteristic Behaviors	Suggested Approach	Sample Statement
Precontemplation	Client does not think there is a problem; not considering the possibility of change.	Raise doubt; give informational feedback to raise awareness of a problem and health risks.	"Your lab tests show liver damage. These tests can be predictive of serious health problems and premature death."
Contemplation	Client thinks there may be a problem; thinking about change; goes back and forth between concern and unconcern.	Tip the balance; allow open discussion of pros and cons of changing behavior; build motivation for change; help client justify a positive commitment.	"It sounds as though you think you may have a drinking problem, but are not sure you are an alcoholic. What would your life be like without alcohol?"
Determination	Client decides there is a problem and is willing to make a change: "I guess I do need to stop drinking."	Help the client choose the best course of action to take in resolving the problem.	"What kinds of changes will you need to make to stop drinking? Most people find Alcoholics Anonymous (AA) helpful as a support. Have you heard of them?"
Action	Client engages in concrete actions to effect needed change.	Help the client take active steps to resolve health problem; review progress; give feedback.	"I am impressed that you went to two AA meetings this week and have not had a drink either. What has this been like for you?"
Maintenance	Client perseveres with positive behavioral change.	Help client identify and use strategies to sustain progress; point out positive changes; accept temporary setbacks and use steps in determination phase, if needed.	"It's hard to let go of old habits, but you have been abstinent for three months now, and your liver tests are significantly improved."

Exercise 15-2 Assessing Readiness Using Prochaska's Model

Purpose: To identify elements in teaching that can promote readiness using Prochaska's Model.

Procedure:
Identify as many specific answers as possible to the following questions:

1. Patrick drinks four to six beers every evening. Last year he lost his job. He has a troubled marriage and few friends. Patrick does not consider himself an alcoholic and blames his chaotic marriage for his need to drink. There is a strong family history of alcoholism.
   What kinds of information might help Patrick want to learn more about his condition?
2. Lily has just learned she has breast cancer. Although there is a good chance that surgery and chemotherapy will help her, she is scared to commit to the process and has even talked about taking her life.
   What kinds of health teaching strategies and information might help Lily become ready to learn about her condition?
3. Shawn has just been diagnosed as having epilepsy. He is ashamed to tell his friends and teachers about his condition. Shawn is considering breaking up with his girlfriend because of his newly diagnosed illness.
   How would you use health teaching to help Shawn cope more effectively with his illness?

Exercise 15-2 provides an opportunity to work with the transtheoretical model in understanding learning readiness.

Social Learning Theory

Motivation is a fundamental component of learner readiness. Before implementing teaching strategies related to content, the nurse must help the client see a need to learn the required information (Vitousek, Watson, & Wilson, 1998). Social learning theory provides another way of understanding the types of motivators a nurse can use with clients to improve learning readiness.

Bandura (1987, 1997) considers learning to be a social process. Bandura identifies three sets of motivating factors that promote the learning necessary to achieve a predetermined goal: physical motivators, social incentives, and cognitive motivators.

Case Example

Francis Edison agrees wholeheartedly with his nurse that smoking is bad and is likely to cause an earlier death from emphysema. However, in his mind, it is impossible for him even to contemplate giving up smoking. His mind-set precludes learning until he can see the connection between giving up cigarettes and avoiding painful symptoms. A severe bronchitis creating air hunger and a hacking cough finally convinces Francis to give up cigarettes.

Physical motivators can be internal, such as memory of previous discomfort or a symptom that the client cannot ignore. Social incentives such as praise and encouragement increase self-esteem and give the client reason to continue learning. Below, the nurse combines the concept of a physical motivator with a social incentive related to something the client values (his grandson). The intervention is designed to help Francis recognize how changes in his health behavior can not only improve his health and well-being but also give him a social outlet that could be important to him.

Case Example

Nurse: I'm a little worried that you are continuing to smoke, because it does affect your breathing. There is nothing you can do about the damage to your lungs that is already there, but if you stop smoking it can help preserve the healthy tissue you still have (*physical motivator*) and you won't have as much trouble breathing. I bet your grandson would appreciate it if you could breathe better and be able to play with him (*social incentive*).

Bandura refers to a third set of motivators as cognitive motivators, describing them as internal thought processes associated with change. For example, as Francis notices that he is coughing less when he gives up smoking, this perception can act as an internal cognitive incentive to remain abstinent.

Bandura (1997) believes that *self-efficacy*, described as a personal belief in one's ability to execute the actions required to achieve a goal, also is a powerful mediator of behavior and behavioral change. Self-efficacy and motivation are reciprocal processes; increased self-efficacy strengthens motivation, which in turn strengthens the client's capacity to complete the learning task. This is a critical concept because clients and family caregivers both may have reservations about their competence to carry out treatments in the home or make changes in lifestyle without the guidance and support of the nurse.

Community-Based Models of Health Promotion: PRECEDE-PROCEED Model

Although health promotion at the individual level is associated with improved health and well-being, health promotion must occur at the community level as well. So many social and environmental factors affect health, including income, education, insurance, cultural health practices, social support, accessibility of health services, just to name a few. Frankish et al. (2006) make the point that it is difficult to change attitudes and lifestyles to promote health when a client's environment does not support these changes. Unless the community as a whole can collectively challenge and eradicate inequities in health care access and treatment provision, health promotion activities will fall short of their targeted goals (Messias, De Jong, & McLoughlin, 2005). To be successful, community-based health promotion activities must begin with the engagement and buy-in of the community in which the activity is to take place. Box 15-2 presents principles nurses can use to engage the community in health promotion activities.

The PRECEDE-PROCEED community-based health model developed by Green and Kreuter (2005) has a health promotion/disease prevention emphasis in developing appealing health education programs designed to produce targeted population-focused behavioral, environmental, and social changes that reduce risk of disease. The model is based on two fundamental assumptions: health and health risks are multidetermined, and health teaching must likewise be multidimensional and participatory (Green & Kreuter, 2005).

Box 15-2 Principles of Community Engagement

Before Starting a Community Engagement Effort

- Be clear about the purposes or goals of the engagement effort and the populations and/or communities you want to engage.
- Become knowledgeable about the community in terms of its economic conditions, political structures, norms and values, demographic trends, history, and experience with engagement efforts. Learn about the community's perceptions of those initiating the engagement activities.

For Engagement to Occur, It Is Necessary To

- Go into the community, establish relationships, build trust, work with the formal and informal leadership, and seek commitment from community organizations and leaders to create processes for mobilizing the community.
- Remember and accept that community self-determination is the responsibility and right of all people who make up a community. No external entity should assume it can bestow to a community the power to act in its own self-interest.

For Engagement to Succeed

- Partnering with the community is necessary to create change and improve health.
- All aspects of community engagement must recognize and respect community diversity. Awareness of the various cultures of a community and other factors of diversity must be paramount in designing and implementing community engagement approaches.
- Community engagement can only be sustained by identifying and mobilizing community assets, and by developing capacities and resources for community health decisions and action.
- An engaging organization or individual change agent must be prepared to release control of actions or interventions to the community, and be flexible enough to meet the changing needs of the community.
- Community collaboration requires long-term commitment by the engaging organization and its partners.

From CDC/ATSDR Committee on Community Engagement: Principles of community engagement, Atlanta, 1997, Centers for Disease Control and Prevention Program Office; available online: http://www.cdc.gov/phppo/pce/part3.htm.

Table 15-2 Examples of PRECEDE Diagnostic Behavioral Factors

Factors	Examples
Predisposing factors	Previous experience, knowledge, beliefs, and values that can affect the teaching process (e.g., culture and prior learning)
Enabling factors	Environmental factors that facilitate or present obstacles to change (e.g., transportation, scheduling, and availability of follow-up)
Reinforcing factors	Perceived positive or negative effects of adopting the new learned behaviors, including social support (e.g., family support, risk of recurrence, and avoidance of a health risk)

The PRECEDE (Predisposing, Reinforcing, Enabling Causes in Educational Diagnosis and Evaluation) component of the model focuses on assessment of the predisposing, reinforcing, and enabling factors associated with the targeted problem area (Table 15-2). It is an outcome-based model emphasizing a population rather than an individual focused educational approach to health promotion and disease prevention. The PRECEDE component is a health education model used to plan programs for a target population and/or problem. The assessment of multiple factors to determine the type of program and content most likely to engage the interest of very diverse learners in community-based settings takes place as a part of the planning process *before* the educational program is offered. Nurses also determine population needs and establish evaluation methods prior to implementation.

Table 15-3 PRECEDE/PROCEED Model Definitions

Phase	Definition
PRECEDE Components	
1. Social Diagnosis	People's perceptions of their own health needs, quality of life
2. Epidemiological Diagnosis	Determination of the extent, distribution, causes of health problem in target population
3. Behavioral and Environmental Diagnosis	Determination of specific health-related actions likely to affect problem (behavioral); systematic assessment of factors in the environment likely to influence health and quality-of-life outcomes (environmental)
4. Educational and Organizational Diagnosis	Assessment of all factors that must be changed to initiate or sustain desired behavioral changes and outcomes
5. Administrative and Policy Diagnosis	Analysis of organizational policies, resources, circumstances relevant to the development of the health program
PROCEED Components	
6. Implementation	Converting program objectives into actions taken at the organizational level
7. Process Evaluation	Assessment of materials, personnel performance, quality of practice or services offered, and activity experiences
8. Impact Evaluation	Assessment of program effects of intermediate objectives inclusive of all changes as a result of the training
9. Outcome Evaluation	Assessment of the teaching program on the ultimate objectives related to changes in health, well-being, and quality of life

Adapted from Green L, Kreuter M: *Health program planning: an educational and ecological approach,* ed 4, New York, 2005, McGraw Hill.

Achievement of program objectives is evaluated throughout the educational experiences.

The PROCEED component (Policy, Regulatory, Organizational Constructs in Educational and Environmental Development) was added to the model by Green in the late 1980s to augment the educational model with essential political, managerial, and administrative elements needed for full implementation of a community-based approach to health promotion and disease prevention. The utility of this model is that, in addition to population characteristics, it considers critical environmental and cost variables such as budget, personnel, and critical organizational relationships as part of the planning process. Having the resources in place and assessing their sustainability is important in health promotion planning, though it is not always thought through in the planning phase. Bernard (2006) notes that since health promotion and disease prevention activities do not generate the same level of revenue, they may not be as sustainable when resources become tight. The full PRECEDE-PROCEED model is presented in Table 15-3.

Exercise 15-3 provides an opportunity to think about community health problems that could be addressed with the PRECEDE/PROCEED model in planning appropriate health promotion interventions.

APPLICATIONS

To help clients achieve the goal of optimal well-being, the nurse uses one-to-one counseling and community-based group education formats to meet educational health care objectives related to health promotion and maintenance of health, prevention of illness, restoration of health, coping with impaired functioning, and rehabilitation.

Learning Readiness

The teachable moment takes place when the learner feels that there is a need to know the information and has the capacity to learn it. Learners differ in their abilities, intellectual curiosity, motivation for learning, learning styles, and rate of learning. Learner variables important in the teaching-learning process generally fall into

Exercise 15-3 Analysis of Significant Health Problems for Health Promotion Interventions

Purpose: To develop an appreciation for the multidimensional elements of a community health problem.

Procedure:

In small groups of four to six students, brainstorm about health problems you believe exist in your community and develop a consensus about one public health problem that the group would prioritize as being most important.

Use the following questions to direct your thinking about developing health promotion activities for a health-related problem in your community.

What are the most pressing health problems in your community?
What are the underlying causes or contributing factors to this problem?
In what ways does the selected problem impact the health and well-being of the larger community?
What is the population of interest you would need to target for intervention?
What types of additional information would you need to have in order to propose a solution?
Who are the stakeholders, and how should they be involved?
What step would you recommend as an initial response to this health problem?
What is one step the nurse could take to increase awareness of this problem as a health promotion issue?

Discussion:

How hard was it for your group to arrive at a consensus about the most pressing problem? Were you surprised with any of the discussion that took place about this health problem? How could you use what you learned in doing this exercise in your nursing practice?

Developing an Evidence-Based Practice

Markle-Reid M, Weir R, Browne G et al: Health promotion for frail older home care clients, *J Adv Nurs* 54(3):381-395, 2006.

This experimental study was designed to evaluate the comparative effects and costs of a proactive health promotion intervention provided to frail, elderly, home care clients. The sample, with an 84% completion rate, were randomly assigned to a control group (N = 120) or the experimental group (N = 120), who received health promotion nursing care in addition to their normal home care. This health promotion strategy consisted of a health assessment combined with their regular home visits or telephone contacts, education about the management of their illness, coordination of community services, and the use of empowerment strategies to enhance their independence.

Results: The frail elderly home care clients receiving the health promotion strategy in addition to their usual health care demonstrated significantly better mental health functioning, a reduction in depression, and enhanced perceptions of social support. Offering home-based health promotion activities can enhance the quality of life without increasing overall cost of services to homebound clients.

Application to Your Clinical Practice: As a profession, nurses are providing more and more community services reflective of a public health model. The frail elderly are a population that is growing exponentially. Finding creative, cost-effective ways to promote health and independence for this population needs to be a goal of professional nursing. What are some ways you can think of to promote health and quality of life for homebound clients with chronic illnesses?

two categories: readiness to learn and ability to learn. DiClemente, Schlundt, and Gemmell (2004) define *readiness* as "a willingness or openness to engage in a particular process or to adopt a particular behavior that represents a more pragmatic and focused view of motivation as preparedness" (p. 104). Teaching cannot begin until the client is ready.

Factors Affecting Readiness to Learn

Typically, health teaching is done with clients who are trying to adjust to recent and problematic life events, often accompanied by personal rejection, compromised body function, loss of a job, or end of an intimate relationship. The emotional fallout from these situations has a significant bearing on the learning process. Nurses need to identify any potential barriers that could interfere with motivation to learn.

Case Example

Nurse: I notice that we don't seem to be making much headway in applying what you are learning about dietary changes required by your high cholesterol. I wonder if there are some issues that we have not addressed that may be getting in the way.

Nurses need to remember that learning is never smooth or linear in its development. Rather than challenge the client's learning pattern, the nurse needs to understand it and incorporate it into new opportunities for learning (Blackie, Gregg, & Freeth, 1998). This is the art of health teaching. Psychosocial and physical factors that can affect the learner's ability to learn include previous knowledge and experience about the illness as well as its personal and cultural meaning.

Level of Anxiety. High levels of anxiety can be seriously detrimental to the teaching/learning process by interfering with the client's ability to focus attention and comprehend the material. Failure to fully comprehend recommended treatment options can compromise the full disclosure required for informed consent. Accurately assessing and managing a client's level of anxiety prior to health teaching is essential. Stephenson (2006) developed a pathway decision tree for exploring and managing high levels of anxiety in clients with a cancer diagnosis prior to providing health education (Figure 15-1). Developing a relationship with the client helps, and in some instances, medication may be required to mitigate debilitating anxiety symptoms before the nurse provides a teaching session.

Level of Social Support. Changes in social support or the health status of significant others can affect the client's willingness or ability to learn. Many elderly clients have depended on others for direction and for overseeing treatment. When these supports are no longer available through death or incapacity, the client may lack not only motivation but also the skills to cope with complex health problems.

Case Example

Edward Flanigan, an 82-year-old man who was recently widowed, has moderately severe diabetes. There is no evidence of memory problems, but there are some significant emotional components to his current health

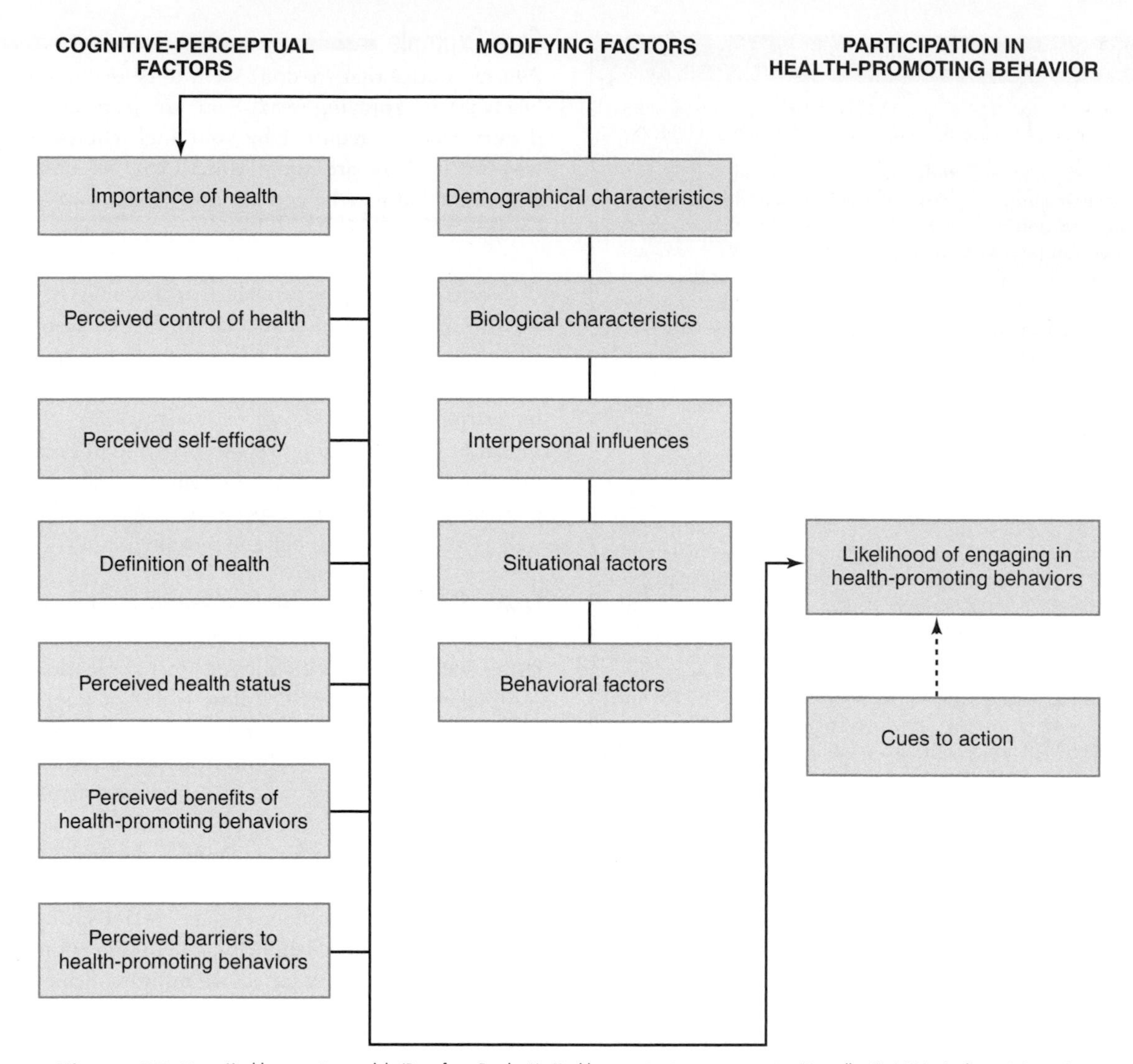

Figure 15-1 • Health promotion model. (Data from Pender N: *Health promotion in nursing practice*, Norwalk, CT, 1996, Appleton & Lange.)

care needs. All his life, his wife pampered him and did everything for him, from meal preparation to monitoring his diabetes. Now that his wife is dead, Edward takes no interest in controlling his diabetes. The home care nurse who visits him on a regular basis is discouraged because, despite careful instruction and seeming comprehension, Edward appears unwilling to follow the prescribed diabetic diet and is not consistent in taking his medication. Predictably, he goes into diabetic crisis. His family worries about him, but he is unwilling to consider leaving his home of 42 years.

Emotional issues of loss and change complicate the learning needs of this client. Edward could function and maintain his health as long as he could rely on his wife for support. To enhance Edward's learning readiness, the nurse might initially have to assess for depression, and then help him find alternative ways to meet his dependency needs, for example, by expanding his social support system.

Information to empower clients in learning about healthy lifestyles, treatment, potential side effects, and so on is now readily available through the Internet (Coward, 2006). For many disorders, clients and families can find specific information, regardless of the stage of their illness. Online support groups, chat rooms, and sharing of patient and family stories provide additional social support and practical learning tips for people who live in areas that are not geographically convenient to person-to-person contact. In the community, there are support groups available for a wide variety of diagnoses that can provide an important resource for clients and/or their families.

Active involvement of the learner enhances learning. Most people learn best when they engage more than one sense in the learning process and have an opportunity to practice essential skills. A highly participatory learning format, with the opportunity to try out new behaviors, is far more effective than giving simple instructions to a client or family or doing it for them because it is easier and faster to do so. Willison, Mitmaker, and Andrews (2005) advise that an integrative health care approach "encourages the use of varied streams of thought (i.e., different ways of thinking), to enable varied means of problem solving" (p. 4).

Your first priority in working with a client or family is to find out what the client already knows. The best way to find out the client's perceptions and attitudes is simply to ask the client and family what they already know about the topic or what they associate with it. The more obvious the links between previous experiences and new knowledge, the deeper the learning (Glover & Bruning, 1990). Strategies should demonstrate a sensitive appraisal and choice of specific strategies, unique in every case and matched to the relevant needs of the individual, family, or group. When time is short, you will need to focus on the health teaching that addresses the most pressing of health needs. Exercise 15-4 provides an opportunity to use Maslow's theory in structuring health promotion activities.

Case Example

Soon Mrs. Hixon began learning how to dress herself. At first she took an hour to complete this task. But with guidance and practice, she eventually dressed herself in 25 minutes. Even so, I practically had to sit on my hands as I watched her struggle. I could have done it so much faster for her, but she had to learn, and I had to let her. (Collier, 1992, p. 63)

Factors Affecting Ability to Learn

Many factors affect a client's capacity to learn new information and ways of behaving. Some clients are ready to learn but are unable to do so with traditional learning formats (Hemmings, 1998). Assessing the client's ability to learn and adapting the learning format to the learner's unique characteristics makes a difference. If the client cannot understand what is being taught, learning does not take place. Ochieng (2006) also contends that socioeconomic factors, level of education, age, and social networks are important contributors to understanding client preferences and working with clients to enable them to make the changes needed for a healthy lifestyle.

Exercise 15-4 Applying Maslow's Theory to Learning Readiness

Purpose: To develop skill in facilitating learning readiness.

Procedure:

Students will break into four groups and receive a case scenario that depicts a client learning need. Using Maslow's hierarchy of needs, determine where the client is and plan your teaching approach based on the client's current level. Include in your plan the supportive measures that would be necessary to foster readiness to learn.

Discussion:

Each group will present their case and plan. Discuss how the use of Maslow's hierarchy can be effective in addressing learning needs and determining nursing approach. Discuss factors that contribute to resistance to learning and noncompliance. Discuss the supportive measures that nurses must include as part of the learning process with clients.

Physical Barriers. Sometimes the client's physical condition or emotional state temporarily precludes teaching. A client in pain can focus on little else. A client emerging from the shock of a difficult diagnosis may require teaching in small segments or postponement of serious teaching sessions until the physical problems are under greater control and time to absorb the diagnosis has elapsed. Certain physical and mental conditions limit attention or compromise cognitive processing abilities. The client with significant thought disorders may need very concrete instructions and frequent prompts to perform adequately. Nausea, weakness, or speech or motor impairments may make it difficult for the client to maintain motivation. Medications or the period of disorientation after a diagnostic test or surgical procedure can influence the level of the client's ability to participate in learning. Careful assessment will usually reveal when the client's physical or emotional condition is a barrier to learning.

Comorbid health problems that could interfere with the goals or process of teaching are important pieces of data that influence what can and should be taught. For example, an exercise program might be useful for an overweight person, but if the client also has a cardiac condition or other problem that would limit activity, this information has a direct impact on the goals and strategies of the intervention.

Sometimes physical or emotional issues favor learning. Mezirow (1990) noted that crisis and life transitions provide a format for the most significant adult learning because the anxiety associated with the crisis situation (if it is not extreme) can create the need to learn, and attention is likely to be more intense. Crisis learning is particularly effective with many homeless and Medicaid clients, who frequently do not voluntarily seek health care at any other time. Health teaching for these clients should be immediate, practical, designed to resolve the crisis situation, and carefully organized to maximize client attention.

Health Literacy. Parker, Ratzan, and Lurie (2003) define **health literacy** as "the degree to which people have the capacity to obtain, process, and understand basic health information and services needed to make appropriate health decisions" (p. 147). Approximately 21% of U.S. adults would be classified as functionally illiterate, which means they read at or below a ninth grade level and would have trouble comprehending written instructions on medication bottles, negotiating the health care system, and fully understanding consent forms (Davis, Michielutte, Askov et al., 1998). Low health literacy is associated with medication nonadherence, greater presence of side effects, and poor understanding of the impact of a medication on health outcomes (Ownby, 2006).

Low health literacy is not the same as having below average intelligence, although people frequently confuse the two and they sometimes do coexist. People with English as a second language can exhibit a much lower level of functional health literacy that is directly attributable to language limitations. A persistent stigma about low literacy and learning disabilities exists even though it is unfounded. For this reason, many people try to hide the fact that they cannot read or do not know the meaning of complex words. They feel ashamed, so they fake their inability to understand by appearing to agree with the nurse educator, by saying they will read the instructions later, or by not asking questions.

There is an assumption that educationally disadvantaged or functionally illiterate people are less-responsible learners. However, just because a person is educated does not mean he or she will be more ready to assume responsibility for changing difficult behaviors than a less-educated individual. Nor does it mean that an illiterate person cannot learn. Nor does it mean that the low-literacy client does not have an interest in learning. It does mean that the nurse will need to adapt the teaching situation to compensate for the literacy deficiency. Some of the problems clients with low literacy skills have in accessing health information include the following (Doak, Doak, & Root, 1996):

- Taking instructions literally
- Having a limited ability to generalize information to new situations
- Decoding one word at a time rather than reading a passage as a whole
- Skipping over uncommon or hard words
- Thinking in individual rather than categorical terms

These problems limit the client's ability to effectively analyze or synthesize educational materials. Using symbols and images with which the client is familiar helps overcome the barriers of low literacy. Simple, concrete words convey the same message as more sophisticated language. Taking the time to understand the client's use of words and phrases provides the nurse with words and ideas that can be used as building blocks in helping the client understand difficult health-related concepts. Otherwise, the client may misunderstand what the nurse is saying.

Case Example

The discharge nurse said to a new mother, "Now you know to watch the baby's stools to be sure they're normal. You do know what normal stools look like, don't you?" The mother replied, "Oh, yeah, sure...I've got four of them in my kitchen" (Doak, Doak, & Root, 1985).

The nurse should keep instructions as simple as possible, presenting ideas in an uncomplicated, step-by-step format. Advance organizers help low-literacy clients remember important concepts (see Chapter 16). Familiar words supplemented by common pictures provide an extrasensory input for the client and improve retention. Drawings, diagrams, and photographs provide additional cues, allowing the client to understand meanings he or she would be unable to grasp through words alone.

Use commonly understood language rather than abstract or medical terminology and examples, for example, "Call the doctor on Monday if you still have pain or swelling in your knee." These same instructions, written exactly as they were spoken, act as a reminder once the person leaves the actual teaching situation. In addition to using simple words and literal interpretations, the nurse should use the same words to describe the same thing. For example, if you use "insulin" in one instance and "medicine" or "drug" later to describe the same medication, the client may become confused.

Logical sequencing of content is particularly important in teaching the low-literacy client. Doak et al. (1985) suggest thinking about the order of a teaching session from the client's perspective and advocate using the following series of questions as a framework for instruction about medication:

- What do I take?
- How much do I take?
- When do I take it?
- What will it do for me?
- What do I do if I get a side effect?

By selecting small, related pieces of data and structuring them into informational chunks, the client can remember the information better through association even if one fact is forgotten. Whenever possible, link new tasks and information with what the client already knows. This strategy, important with all clients, is particularly advantageous with the low-literacy client. It takes advantage of previous learning and helps reinforce self-esteem by reminding the client of competencies learned in the process of instruction.

When technical words are necessary for clients to communicate about their condition with other health professionals, clients need direct instruction about appropriate words to use. As with culturally diverse clients, keeping sentences short and precise and using active verbs help clients understand what is being taught. Box 15-3 provides guidelines for the nurse in teaching low-literacy clients.

Box 15-3 Guidelines for Teaching Low-Literacy Clients

- Teach the smallest amount necessary to do the job for each session.
- Sequence key behavior information first.
- Make your point as vividly as you can (e.g., use visual aids and examples for emphasis).
- Incorporate as many senses as possible in the learning process.
- Include interaction; have the client restate and demonstrate the information.
- Review repeatedly.

Adapted from Doak CC, Doak LG, Root JH: Tips on teaching patients. In Doak CC, Doak LG, Root JH, editors, *Teaching patients with low literacy skills*, ed 2, Philadelphia, 1996, JB Lippincott.

Developmental Level. Developmental level affects both teaching strategies and subject content, and the nurse will find that clients are at all levels of the learning spectrum with regard to their social, emotional, and cognitive development. Developmental learning capacity is not always age-related and is easily influenced by culture and stress. Parents can provide useful information about their child's immediate life experiences and commonly used words to incorporate into the teaching.

Teaching strategies should reflect an individual's developmental level. For example, focusing teaching on the development of competency, whether physical, psychological, or cognitive, takes advantage of the child's natural stage of development in Erikson's stage development for the school-aged child. Children of this age are eager to learn about better ways of taking care of themselves.

Andragogy refers to the "art and science of helping adults learn" (Knowles, 1980). According to Knowles, adult learners favor a problem-focused approach to learning. They are interested in learning skills and knowledge that will help them master life problems. Self-directedness is a key component of the adult teaching/learning process. Adults like to be in control of their learning processes.

Individual responsibility through taking action and reflecting on the consequences ensures ownership and stimulates learning in the adult client. The adult's orientation to learning is "life-centered." Adult learners need to be able to see the practicality of what they are learning. Experience is a rich resource that can be used wisely in planning nursing interventions. The adult client

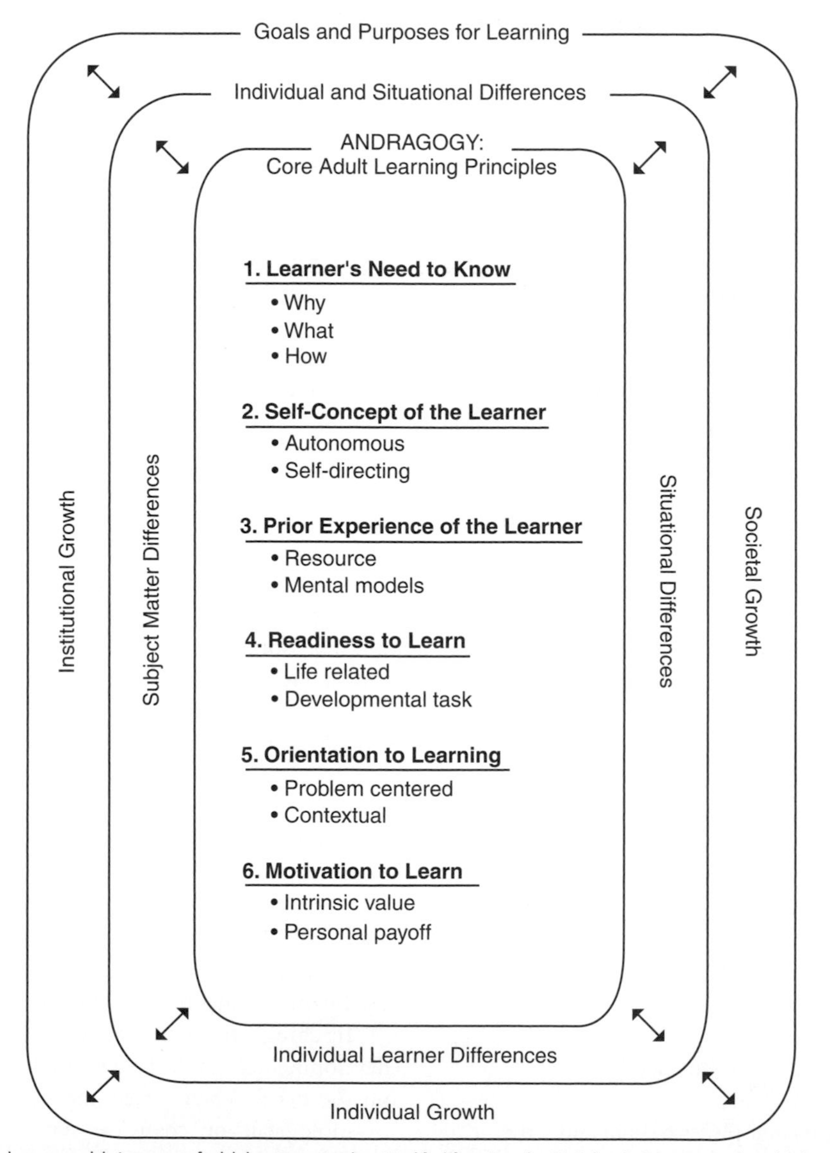

Figure 15-2 ● Andragogy model: A core set of adult learning principles. (Modified from Knowles M, Holton E, Swanson R: *The adult learner: the definitive classic on adult education and training,* Terre Haute, IL, 1998, Butterworth-Heinemann.)

expects the nurse to inquire about previous life experience and to incorporate this knowledge into the teaching plan. Figure 15-2 describes the natural learning process elements required for adult learners.

Healthy elderly clients are similar to other adult learners, except that they may need more time to think about how they want to handle a situation. The elderly client responds best in a learning milieu in which the nurse faces the client when talking, speaking clearly and slowly in a low-pitched voice. Frequent, shorter learning sessions are better than long formats. The elderly client may have difficulty with some psychomotor tasks (e.g., removing bottle caps or filling syringes) because of dexterity loss. The nurse needs to be sensitive to this possibility, as pride may prevent the client from revealing this deficit.

Assuming that elderly clients lack the capacity to understand instructions is a common error. Health care providers often direct instruction to the elderly client's younger companion, even when the client has no cognitive impairment. This action disconfirms the elderly client and diminishes self-worth. The sensitive nurse observes the client before implementing teaching and gears teaching strategies to meet the individual learning needs of each elderly client. Table 5-4 presents teaching strategies for use with clients at different developmental levels.

Culture. Culture adds to the complexity of the teaching/learning process in health care. It can and does present "major barriers to effective health care intervention" (Huff & Kline, 1999, p. 6). Culturally transmitted values regarding health and health care services affect health issues at both individual and population levels. Including the client's cultural beliefs about health into teaching promotes better acceptance. Such beliefs include assumptions about health and illness, the causes of and treatments for different types of illnesses, and traditionally accepted health actions or practices to prevent or treat illness.

Language barriers can make learning significantly more difficult for a client. Pictures, the use of dictionaries, and the help of translators may be necessary to support the learning process. It is important to design educational materials that are culturally relevant to the target group and to use well-trained bilingual health workers in health teaching.

In many cultures, the family assumes a primary role in the care of the client even when the client is physically

Table 15-4 Recommended Teaching Strategies at Different Development Levels

Developmental Level	Recommended Teaching Strategies
Preschool	Allow child to touch and play with safe equipment. Relate teaching to child's immediate experience. Use child's vocabulary whenever possible. Involve parents in teaching.
School-age	Give factual information in simple, concrete terms. Focus teaching on developing competency. Use simple drawings and models to emphasize points. Answer questions honestly and factually.
Adolescent	Use metaphors and analogies in teaching. Give choices and multiple perspectives. Incorporate the client's norm group values and personal identity issues in teaching strategies.
Adult	Involve client as an active partner in learning process. Encourage self-directed learning. Keep content and strategies relevant and practical. Incorporate previous life experience into teaching.
Elderly	Incorporate previous life experience into teaching. Accommodate for sensory and dexterity deficits. Use short, frequent learning sessions. Use praise liberally.

and emotionally capable of self-care. All parties needing information, especially those expected to support the learning process of the client, should be included from the outset in developing a realistic teaching plan as well as implementing and evaluating the plan. Otherwise, the teaching plan may be sabotaged when the client goes home. (See Chapter 16 for more information about role of culture in health teaching.)

Chen (1999) recommends that "empowering ethnocultural communities through informal care may be the most culturally appropriate approach for improving the health status of ethnocultural populations" (Chiu, Balneaves, Barroetavena et al., 2006, p. 3). Client motivation and participation increase with the use of indigenous teachers and cultural recognition of learning needs. The culturally sensitive nurse develops knowledge of the preferred communication style of different cultural groups and uses this knowledge in choosing teaching strategies. For example, Native Americans like stories. Their tradition of telling stories orally is a primary means of teaching that the nurse can use as a teaching methodology.

Self-Awareness. The nurse has an ethical and legal responsibility in health teaching to maintain the appropriate expertise and interpersonal sensitivity to client needs required for effective learning. It is easy enough to remain engaged and to provide interesting teaching formats for the self-directed, highly motivated learner. It takes much more energy and imagination to impart hope to clients and to stimulate their emotions and interest when they see little reason to participate in learning about self-care management. Although the nurse is responsible for the quality of health teaching, only the client can assure the outcome. At all times, the nurse respects the client's autonomy. Some clients want symptom relief, whereas others want more in-depth teaching. Nurses have an ethical responsibility to provide appropriate health teaching and the right to hope that if the information is not used now, perhaps later it will be.

SUMMARY

Chapter 15 focuses on health promotion as the basis for health education that can be applied at all practice levels. The World Health Organization describes health promotion as a process of enabling people to increase control over and improve their health. Optimal health and well-being are considered the desired outcomes of health promotion activities. A health promotion/disease prevention focus views the client as an informed consumer and a valued partner in health care.

Health promotion activities are viewed as a community resource that can affect personal lifestyle choices, coping skills, and health behaviors. *Healthy People 2010* represents the health promotion and disease prevention agenda for the nation. Health promotion activities involve proactive decision making at all levels of prevention (primary, secondary, and tertiary). Surveillance of health events is an important component of population-focused health promotion and disease prevention because it alerts health care providers to potential and actual health problems, and provides morbidity and mortality rates for evaluation purposes.

Theory models relevant to health promotion include Pender's health promotion model, Prochaska's transtheoretical model, and Bandura's social learning theory. Learner variables important to the success of health promotion activities can be categorized as readiness to learn and ability to learn. Physical factors, level of anxiety, level of social support, active involvement of the learner and inclusion of family members are identified as elements of readiness to learn. Lack of appropriate supports, physical barriers, health literacy, culture, and developmental status are factors that may influence the client's ability to learn. Nurses participate routinely in community health promotion and disease prevention activities. They have an ethical and legal responsibility in health teaching to maintain the appropriate expertise and interpersonal sensitivity to client needs required for effective learning. Although the nurse is responsible for the quality of health teaching, only the client can assure the outcome.

Ethical Dilemma ■ *What Would You Do?*

Jack Marks is a 16-year-old male who comes to the clinic complaining of symptoms of a sexually transmitted disease (STD). He receives antibiotics, and you give him information about safe sex and preventing STDs. Two months later, he returns to the clinic with similar symptoms. It is clear that he has not followed instructions and has no intention of doing so. He tells you he's a regular jock and just can't get used to the idea of condoms. He really can't tell you the names of his partners—there are just too many of them.

REFERENCES

Bandura A: Human agency in social cognitive theory, *Am Psychol* 44:1175–1184, 1987.

Bandura A: *Self-efficacy: the exercise of control*, New York, 1997, WH Freeman.

Beckford-Ball J: The essence of care benchmark for patient health promotion, *Nurs Times* 102(14):23–24, 2006.

Bernard M: Health promotion/disease prevention: tempering the giant geriatric tsunami, *Geriatrics* 61(2):5–7, 2006.

Blackie C, Gregg R, Freeth D: Promoting health in young people, *Nurs Stand* 12(36):39–46, 1998.

Centers for Disease Control: CDC: our story, n.d.; available online: http://www.cdc.gov/about/ourstory.htm.

Chandler C, Holden J, Kolander C: Counseling for spiritual wellness: theory and practice, *J Counsel Dev* 71:168–175, 1992.

Chen MS: Informal care and the empowerment of minority communities: comparisons between the USA and the UK, *Ethn Health* 4(3):139–151, 1999.

Chiu L, Balneaves L, Barroetavena M et al.: Use of complementary and alternative medicine by Chinese individuals living with cancer in British Columbia, *J Compl Integr Med* 3(1):1–21, 2006.

Collier S: Mrs. Hixon was more than “the C.V.A. in 251,” *Nursing* 22(5):62–64, 1992.

Committee on Assuring the Health of the Public in the 21st Century (Institute of Medicine): *The future of the public's health in the 21st century*, Washington, DC, 2003, National Academies Press.

Coward D: Supporting health promotion in adults with cancer, *Fam Community Health* 29(supp 1):52S–60S, 2006.

Davis T, Michielutte R, Askov E et al.: Practical assessment of adult literacy in health care, *Health Educ Behav* 22(5):613–624, 1998.

DiClemente C, Schlundt B, Gemmell B: Readiness and stages of change in addiction treatment, *Am J Addict* 13(2): 103–119, 2004.

Doak CC, Doak LG, Root JH: *Teaching patients with low literacy skills*, Philadelphia, 1985, JB Lippincott.

Doak CC, Doak LG, Root JH: *Teaching patients with low literacy skills*, ed 2, Philadelphia, 1996, JB Lippincott.

Edelman C, Mandel C: *Health promotion throughout the lifespan*, ed 4, St Louis, 1998, Mosby Year Book.

Frankish CJ, Moulton G, Rootman I et al.: Setting a foundation: underlying values and structures of health promotion in primary health care settings, *Prim Health Care Res Dev* 7:172–182, 2006.

Fraser A: Health promotion for everyone, *Nurs Stand* 12(25):19, 1998.

Glover J, Bruning R: *Educational psychology: principles and applications*, ed 3, Glenview, IL, 1990, Scott, Foresman.

Green L, Kreuter M: *Health program planning: an educational and ecological approach*, ed 4, New York, 2005, McGraw Hill.

Henderson V: *Basic principles of nursing care*, London, 1961, International Council of Nurses.

Hemmings D: Health promotion for people with learning disabilities in the community, *Nurs Times* 94(24):58–59, 1998.

Huff R, Kline M: *Promoting health in multicultural populations: a handbook for practitioners*, Thousand Oaks, CA, 1999, Sage Publications.

Institute of Medicine: *Crossing the quality chasm: a new health system for the 21st century*, Washington, DC, 2001, Author.

Knowles M: *The adult learner: a neglected species*, ed 2, Palo Alto, CA, 1980, Mayfield.

Kulbok P, Baldwin J, Cox C et al.: Advancing discourse on health promotion: beyond mainstream thinking, *Adv Nurs Sci* 20(1):12–20, 1997.

Levine M: The child with learning disabilities. In Scheiner A, Abroms I, editors, *The practical management of the developmentally disabled child*, St Louis, 1980, Mosby.

Maltby H, Robinson S: The role of baccalaureate nursing students in the matrix of health promotion, *J Community Health Nurs* 15(3):135–142, 1998.

Markle-Reid M, Weir R, Browne G et al.: Health promotion for frail older home care clients, *J Adv Nurs* 54(3):381–395, 2006.

Messias D, De Jong M, McLoughlin K: Being involved and making a difference: empowerment and well-being among women living in poverty, *J Holist Nurs* 23(1):70–88, 2005.

Mezirow J: *Fostering critical reflection in adulthood: a guide to transformative and emancipatory learning*, San Francisco, 1990, Jossey-Bass.

Ochieng B: Factors affecting choice of a healthy lifestyle: implications for nurses, *Br J Community Nurs* 11(2):78–81, 2006.

Omizo M, Omizo S, d'Andrea M: Promoting wellness among elementary school children, *J Counsel Dev* 71(3):194–198, 1992.

Ownby L: Medication adherence and cognition: medical, personal and economic factors influence level of adherence in older adults, *Geriatrics* 61(2):30–35, 2006.

Parker R, Ratzan S, Lurie N: Health illiteracy: a policy challenge for advancing high-quality health care, *Health Aff* 22(4):147–153, 2003.

Pender N: *Health promotion in nursing practice*, ed 3, Norwalk, CT, 1996, Appleton & Lange.

Pender N, Murdaugh C, Parsons M: *Health promotion in nursing practice*, ed 4, Upper Saddle River, NJ, 2002, Prentice Hall.

Prochaska J, DiClemente C, Norcross J: In search of how people change: applications to addictive behaviors, *Am Psychol* 47(9):1102–1114, 1992.

Saylor C: The circle of health: a health definition model, *J Holist Nurs* 22(2):98–115, 2004.

Stephenson P: Before the teaching begins: Managing patient anxiety prior to providing education, *Clin J Oncol Nurs* 10(2):241–245, April 2006.

U.S. Department of Health and Human Services: *Healthy people 2010,* Washington, DC, 2000, U.S. Government Printing Office.

Vail S: Issues and trends: clarifying population health, *Can Nurse* 91(7):59–60, 1995.

Vitousek K, Watson S, Wilson G: Enhancing motivation for change in treatment-resistant eating disorders, *Clin Psychol Rev* 18(4):391–420, 1998.

Willison K, Mitmaker L, Andrews G: Integrating complementary and alternative medicine with primary health care through public health to improve chronic disease management, *J Compl Integr Med* 2(1):1–24, 2005.

Chapter 16

Health Teaching in the Nurse-Client Relationship

Elizabeth Arnold

OUTLINE

OBJECTIVES

At the end of the chapter, the reader will be able to:

1. Define health teaching and describe the role of the nurse.
2. Contrast selected theoretical frameworks used in health teaching.
3. Identify different types of formats found in health teaching.
4. Use the nursing process to develop, implement, and evaluate a teaching care plan.
5. Specify teaching strategies relevant to health teaching.
6. Describe applications in different care settings.

When adults teach and learn in one another's company, they find themselves engaging in a challenging, passionate, and creative activity. The acts of teaching and learning allow for the creation and alteration of our beliefs, values, actions, relationships, and social forms. Through this interactive process we realize our humanity.

(Brookfield, 1986)

Chapter 16 describes health teaching principles that nurses can use in the nurse-client relationship to enhance the health and well-being of clients, families, and communities. Health teaching is a vital nursing function (Mason, 2001). It has always been an integral part of the nurse-client relationship, but is even more so in a managed-care health care delivery system with mandated limitations on time and resources (Greiner & Valiga, 1998). Nurses today carry much larger caseloads and generally have much less time to spend with their clients. They must help their clients achieve favorable health outcomes with fewer visits. Effective teaching strategies are an *essential* means to achieve this goal.

The radical shift in health care delivery from a medical model, hospital-based approach to a community-based, public health emphasis creates new learning conditions. Today's health care requirements mandate a broader base of health teaching content that includes primary prevention and quality-of-life issues (Ragland, 1997).

Technology has exponentially expanded the depth and breadth of health information available to the health consumer. The health information available on the Internet provides an avenue for individuals and families to become very well informed about their health problems and the latest treatment. The Internet provides instant health information and a wide range of learning resources that accommodate different levels of knowledge and learning styles. Information contained on the Internet is searchable, up to date, inexpensive to obtain, and accessible at any time of day from a variety of places. This powerful teaching tool can be used wisely to increase knowledge, but it has its limitations. Increasingly nurses will be called on to act as client advocates, not only to help clients access the health information they need but also to interpret its meaning and to help them sort out relevant information that fits their particular health issues.

BASIC CONCEPTS

Taylor, Lillis and Lemone (2005) define teaching as "a planned method or series of methods used to help someone learn" (p. 477). **Health teaching** is a specialized form of teaching, defined as a focused, creative, interpersonal nursing intervention whereby the nurse provides information, emotional support, and health-related skill training to clients for the purpose of helping them cope effectively with health problems and achieve maximum well-being. Health teaching is an important methodology in all aspects of health care, ranging from health promotion activities in the community to acute care and working with families and clients at end of life. Health teaching takes place in the community, schools, parish nursing, the home, the hospital, and clinics.

Although health teaching is a term with many definitions, most do not address the complexity of the teaching process in health care (Wellard, Turner, & Bethune, 1998). For example, the "learner" in a health care setting can be a client, the client's family, a caregiver, or a community.

The context of health teaching is also different. Whereas most teaching situations engage learners having a similar level of education and knowledge, health teaching must be designed to meet the diverse learning needs of individuals from markedly different socioeconomic, educational, and experiential backgrounds. In health care, a highly educated client, a noncompliant client, and a low-literacy client may have the same medical condition with similar needs for health teaching. The teaching may take place under less-than-ideal circumstances, and the individualized learning needs of everyone involved in the care of the client may be quite different. Specific teaching strategies, type of involvement of others, and level of content will need to reflect these unique learning needs.

Professional, Legal, and Ethical Mandates of Health Teaching

The importance of health teaching as a *fundamental* nursing function is indisputable. The Joint Commission on Accreditation of Healthcare Organizations (JCAHO) has established educational standards requiring health care agencies to provide systematic health education in the following areas:

- *Standard PF 1* specifies that the client and family must be provided with appropriate education to increase their knowledge of their diagnosis, illness, treatment needs, and the skills and behaviors needed to promote their recovery and rehabilitation.
- *Standard PF 2* specifies that the client and family receive education in line with their assessed learning needs, abilities, and readiness to learn as well as appropriate to their length of stay. Implicit in this standard is the need to use individualized teaching strategies.

- *Standard PF 3* specifies that discharge instructions given to the client and family are also provided to the care provider who will be responsible for the client's continuing care.
- *Standard PF 4* specifies that the health care agency must have an identifiable education plan demonstrating coordinated learning activities and resources based on client and family needs. Implicit in this standard is ongoing health care team involvement in the educational process (Miller & Capp, 1997).

Professional nursing standards, developed by the American Nurses Association (ANA), reinforce the importance of health teaching as an essential nursing intervention (ANA, 2004). Most state Nurse Practice Acts mandate health teaching as an independent professional nursing function; third-party reimbursement for Medicare defines health teaching as a skilled nursing intervention. Mason (2001) identifies health teaching as a vital nursing function.

Educating clients about their health conditions and treatment options also is a legal and ethical responsibility of the nurse related to **informed consent**. Health teaching requirements specifically related to informed consent include the following: (a) explanation of the procedure, test, and treatment; (b) description of possible risks and adverse effects; (c) description of potential benefits; and (d) disclosure of possible alternative procedures or treatments (Usher & Arthur, 1998). Individuals and families must be given the opportunity to ask questions and to receive knowledgeable answers specifically related to their unique health care situation.

The primary purpose of health teaching is to assist clients and families to develop the knowledge, attitudes, and skills they need to promote and/or restore their health and well-being, and to enhance their quality of life. For example, a person with recent myocardial infarction will (a) need to learn about the disease process; the medications, diet and exercise regimes required to improve cardiac function; and the periodic checkups required of a client who experienced a heart attack; (b) develop lifestyle attitudes that embrace regular exercise and a healthy diet; and (c) learn the skills needed to incorporate a scheduled plan of activity, stress reduction strategies, and medication management required for health.

The process of health teaching involves assessing client/learner needs, selecting appropriate content, planning and implementing the health teaching, and evaluating whether the desired behavioral or attitudinal change has occurred. Written documentation of all phases of the teaching/learning process is necessary. Always included in the documentation is the client's response to the health teaching.

Health Teaching Domains

Health teaching involves connecting with three interrelated human domains: *cognitive* (understanding content); *affective* (changing attitudes and promoting acceptance); and *psychomotor* (hands-on skill development). For example, when people practice a skill, they also develop "cognitive knowledge" about the factors that contribute to success.

Cognitive learning is essential when the client has a knowledge deficit related to his or her illness or treatment. For example, objectives in the cognitive domain for a client with a nursing diagnosis of knowledge deficit related to a recent diagnosis of diabetes would include understanding the disease; the role of diet, exercise, and insulin in diabetic control; and trouble signs that would require immediate attention. Learning outcomes would consist of having a basic understanding of the disease process and treatment protocols and being able to apply new information to meet personal health needs. A teaching outcome in the cognitive domain might read, "The client will be able to translate instructions on a medicine bottle into action" (Redman, 1997, p. 39). The information clients and families need related to informed consent falls into the cognitive domain.

Affective learning refers to the emotional component of learning. It focuses on the attitudes needed for successful treatment outcomes, with desired outcomes of acceptance, compliance, and taking personal responsibility for health care. This type of learning is necessary to change health and lifestyle viewpoints to ones that encourage development of the behaviors required for optimal health and well-being. Behavioral change in the affective domain usually takes longer than learning in the cognitive domain (Leahy & Kizilay, 1998).

Case Example

Jack cognitively understands that adhering to his diabetic diet is essential to control of his diabetes. He can tell you everything there is to know about the relationship of diet to diabetic control. Although he follows his diet at home because his wife does the cooking, he eats

snack foods at work and insists on extra helpings at dinner. This is because he resents having a lifelong health condition that he has to think about all the time. His problem with compliance lies in the affective domain, and it is in this domain that the nurse must concentrate teaching efforts. Desired outcomes for Jack's learning in the affective domain include his accepting responsibility for treatment compliance despite his reservations. During the course of teaching Jack about his diet, the nurse will need to allow him time to vent his frustration and help him figure out ways to cope with a chronic illness in less self-destructive ways. If you were Jack's nurse, what health teaching strategies could you use to help him become more comfortable with the changes he needs to make to promote his health and well-being?

The psychomotor domain refers to learning a skill through *hands-on practice*. **Psychomotor learning** is a critical prerequisite for skills related to self-care management of health. People retain information best when they are actively involved with hands-on learning and problem solving. The problem solving of obstacles encountered in practicing a skill can be invaluable when the client replicates the skill in his personal context. Supervised practice of a skill is one of the best ways for the nurse to evaluate the client's mastery of an essential skill. The nurse can demonstrate the skill, followed by a return demonstration by the client with coaching from the nurse (e.g., teaching a diabetic client to titrate the dosage, fill the syringe, and self-inject). Outcomes of learning in the psychomotor domain relate to being able to perform the motor skill; developing personal confidence and proficiency in performing health care skills; and being able to adjust the performance of the skill when challenged with new situations.

Theoretical Frameworks

Client-Centered Health Teaching

Rogers (1983) emphasizes the primacy of the teacher-student relationship as the medium through which learning occurs. He describes client-centered teaching as an interactive process integrating the teacher's knowledge of the content area, self-awareness, and a good understanding of teaching and learning principles with knowledge of the client's learning needs and provision of emotional support. A client-centered teaching approach involves engaging clients as active partners in the learning process and helping them take responsibility for their own learning. Rogers insists that the teacher must start where the learner is, structuring the learning process to support the learner's natural desire to learn and mindful of learner characteristics that enable or impede the process.

There is no single correct way to teach. Teaching methodologies vary from situation to situation as the nurse strives to make new content comprehensible and interesting to the client. The nurse acts as a guide, information provider, and resource support. As a *guide*, the nurse coaches clients on actions they can take to improve their health and offers suggestions on the modifications needed as their condition changes. As *information provider*, the nurse helps clients become more aware of why, what, and how they can learn to take better care of themselves. As a *resource support*, the nurse engages the client as a partner in learning in order to understand barriers to treatment and to promote those behaviors that maintain or enhance optimal well-being.

The same conditions of empathy, authenticity, and respect required for a successful therapeutic relationship apply to health teaching. Through the nurse-client teaching relationship, clients begin to challenge old, unworkable ideas and habits; transform unproductive understandings and actions; and act on new perspectives (Hansen & Fisher, 1998). Clients enter a learning situation with a story model of their illness or disability, which helps them make sense of what is happening to them. By asking questions that demonstrate a genuine interest getting to know what is important to clients and families, nurses can tailor their teaching to each client's unique needs. The following case example illustrates the impact of a client-centered teaching encounter on a client.

Case Example

There was Nadine, who was an excellent preoperative teacher. She was the first person who clearly explained what a bladder augmentation entailed. She described different tubes I'd have and the purpose of each. When I returned from surgery, she helped me cope with my body image by teaching me how to use my bladder and by being a compassionate listener. (Manning, 1992, p. 47)

An important goal of client-centered health teaching is to empower clients and their families to function at their highest potential for maximum health and well-being. As with other aspects of nursing care, empowerment principles place the learner in charge of his or her learning and build on personal strengths to achieve learning objectives. A highly participative learning environment, in which the nurse provides the teaching while the learner assumes primary responsibility for the learning process, encourages empowerment (Post-White, 1998).

To empower clients through the learning process, nurses provide sufficient information, specific instructions, and emotional support—but no more than is required—to allow each client to take charge of his or her health care to whatever extent is possible. By providing health information in unambiguous, concrete, objective terms using the client's terminology, the nurse allows the client to integrate the health teaching in his or her unique way.

Setting mutual goals with clients and following up with periodic reviews help to motivate clients and serve as a benchmark for evaluating change. Reinforcement of successful performance encourages clients to continue learning because it offers immediate positive feedback and builds the client's confidence and self-esteem.

Behavioral Models

Many people look at behavioral models of learning with suspicion. The reality is that we all learn behaviors as the result of behavioral cues. Paychecks, performance appraisals, and disciplinary actions, for example, all reinforce desired behavior and discourage unwanted behavior. Behavioral approaches use a structured learning format in which learning occurs by linking a desired behavior with reinforcement for performing the behavior.

Behavioral approaches are based on the theoretical framework of B. F. Skinner, who believed all behavior is learned. His position was that it is possible to change specific behaviors by altering the predictable consequence or response to the behavior. **Reinforcement**, defined as anything that strengthens a desired response, is a key concept in Skinner's theory. Behaviors that are rewarded (positive reinforcement) tend to be repeated, and behaviors that are ignored tend to diminish or disappear (extinction). When behaviors are punished, by having a reward removed or by a negative consequence, they also tend to extinguish. Selecting rewards (reinforcers) that have meaning to the learner is critical because what is reinforcing to one person may not be so for another. Referred to as the **Premack principle**, the choice of reinforcer should always be something of value to the individual learner.

Reinforcement refers to the situational consequences of performing specified behaviors. Behaviorists believe that reinforcement strengthens learner responses. Reinforcement can be scheduled as continuous, at intervals, or after a certain number of positive responses. Reinforcement given immediately after successful performance is more effective. The different types of reinforcers used with behavioral approaches are found in Table 16-1. Research consistently has found that positive reinforcers are the most effective.

To be effective, reinforcers should have meaning to the client. Nurses need to choose activities and rewards that the client values. Once the behavior is learned, the nurse can introduce new content and distribute rewards

Table 16-1 Types of Reinforcement

Concept	Purpose	Example
Positive reinforcer	Increases probability of behavior through reward	Stars on a board, smiling, verbal praise, candy, tokens to "purchase" items
Negative reinforcer	Increases probability of behavior by removing aversive consequence	Restoring privileges when client performs desired behavior
Punishment	Decreases behavior by presenting a negative consequence or removing a positive one	Time outs, denial of privileges
Ignoring	Decreases behavior by not reinforcing it	Not paying attention to whining, provocative behaviors

less frequently. Progressive learning challenges with appropriate support stimulate the client's interest and desire to continue learning.

Modeling. **Modeling** is a behavioral strategy that refers to learning by observing another person performing a behavior. Nurses model behaviors both unconsciously and consciously in their normal conduct of nursing activities, as well as in actual teaching situations. Bathing an infant, feeding an older person, and talking to a scared child in front of significant caregivers all provide opportunities for informal teaching through modeling desired behaviors.

Shaping. **Shaping** is the term used to describe specific behavioral steps that result in the desired behavior. Steps build one upon the other, moving the learner from the familiar to the unfamiliar as he or she moves toward the treatment goals.

Shaping as a behavioral strategy to increase learning is a common occurrence in our lives. The grades students receive in this course, the approval or disapproval of an instructor, and written comments on care plans and papers all help "shape" student behaviors by providing positive or negative reinforcement of their learning. In health care, providing constructive feedback and verbally encouraging client efforts reinforce learning and shape future attempts.

Implementing a Behavioral Approach. The nurse starts with a careful description of a concrete behavior requiring change. Each behavior is described as a single behavior unit (e.g., failing to take a medication, cheating on a diet, or not participating in unit activities). It is important to start small so the client will experience success. Counting the number of times the client engages in a behavior as a baseline before implementing the behavioral approach allows the nurse and the client to monitor progress and to chart setbacks once it is in place.

The next step in the process is to define the problem in behavioral terms and to validate the problem statement with the client (e.g., "The client does not take his medication as prescribed" or "The client does not attend any unit activities"). A behavioral approach requires the cooperation of the client and a mutual understanding of the problem on the part of the nurse and the client. Active listening skills will alert the nurse to any concerns or barriers to implementation.

Next the nurse and client reframe the problem as a solution statement (e.g., "The client will attend all scheduled unit activities"). If the problem and solution are complex, the nurse breaks them down into simpler definitions, beginning with the simplest and most likely behavior to stimulate client interest. The nurse identifies the tasks in sequential order; defines specific consequences, positive and negative, for behavioral responses; and solicits the client's cooperation.

Once these steps are complete, the nurse establishes a learning contract with the client that serves as a formal commitment to the learning process. This contract includes the following:

- Behavioral changes that are to occur
- Conditions under which they are to occur
- Reinforcement schedule
- Time frame

Contracts spell out the responsibilities of each party and the consequences if positive behaviors are completed or, in the case of undesired behaviors, negative consequences if behaviors persist. The nurse rewards the client for each instance of expected behavior. If the client is noncompliant or needs to pay more attention to a particular aspect of behavior, the nurse can say, "This (*name the behavior or skill*) needs a little more work." One advantage of a behavioral approach is that it never considers the client as bad or unworthy.

Case Example

Peggy Braddock, a student nurse, was working with a seriously mentally ill client with diabetes. All types of strategies were used to help the client take responsibility for collecting and testing her urine. Regardless of whether she was punished or pushed into performing these activities, the client remained resistant. To avoid taking her insulin injections, the client would take urine from the toilets or would simply refuse to produce a urine sample. Peggy decided to use a behavioral approach with her. She observed that the client liked sweets. Consequently, the reward she chose was artificially sweetened Jell-O cubes. To earn a Jell-O cube, the client had to bring her urine to Peggy. After some initial testing of Peggy's resolve to give the cubes only for appropriate behavior, the client began bringing her urine on a regular basis. Once this behavior was firmly established, Peggy began to teach the client how to give her own insulin. The reward remained the same,

except that now the client received praise for what she had accomplished to date. Peggy also used the time she spent with the client to build trust and acceptance. She wrote her plan in the Kardex, and other nurses used the same systematic approach with the client. Over time, this client took full responsibility for testing her urine and for administering her own insulin. The intervention also increased her sense of independence and self-esteem.

Exercise 16-1 provides practice with a behavioral learning approach.

APPLICATIONS

Constructing a Teaching Plan

Assessment

For health teaching to be effective, the nurse and client must have a clear understanding of actual and potential health problems, specifically the following:

- What specific *information* does the client need to enhance self-management and/or compliance with treatment?
- What *attitudes* does the client hold that potentially could enable or hinder the learning process?
- What specific *skills* does this client need for self-management?

Checking out how much the client already knows aids the nurse in knowing the appropriate level and amount of knowledge the client needs to achieve treatment goals. This assessment also serves the purpose of giving the client permission to ask questions. By introducing the idea that most people do have questions, the client feels freer to question data or ask for more explanation.

Probing the learner's beliefs about his or her illness and proposed treatment is an essential aspect of the assessment process. Beliefs and values influence learning. For example, the client who believes that *any* drugs taken into the body are harmful will have a hard time learning about the insulin injection he needs to take every day.

Broad, open-ended questions help the nurse understand the learning needs of individual clients and families in a practical way. Preliminary questions in a teaching assessment could include the following:

- "Tell me what this illness has been like for you so far."

Exercise 16-1 Using a Behavioral Approach

Purpose: To help students gain an appreciation of the behavioral approach in the learning process.

Procedure:

Think about a relationship you have with one or more people that you would like to improve. The person you choose may be a friend, teacher, supervisor, peer worker, parent, or sibling.

1. Set a goal for improving that relationship.
2. Develop a problem statement as the basis for establishing your goal.
3. Identify the behaviors that will indicate you have achieved your goal.
4. Identify the specific behaviors you will have to perform to accomplish your goal.
5. Identify the personal strengths you will use to accomplish your goal.
6. Identify potential barriers to achieving your goal.
7. In groups of four or five students, present your goal-setting agenda and solicit feedback.

Discussion:

1. Do any of your peers have ideas or information that might help you reach your goals?
2. Are there any common themes, strengths, or behaviors related to goal setting that are found across student groups?
3. What did you learn about yourself that might be useful in helping clients develop goals using a behavioral approach?

Developing an Evidence-Based Practice

Ruffolo M, Kuhn M, Evans M: Support, empowerment and education: a study of multiple family group psychoeducation, *J Emot Behav Disord* 13(4):200-212, 2005.

This quasiexperimental study was designed to evaluate a multiple family group psychoeducation intervention (MFGPI) for parents and primary caregivers of children with serious emotional disturbance who were enrolled in a community-based case management program. Parents and primary caregivers (N = 94) were randomly assigned to one of two treatment conditions (intensive case management plus adjunctive MFGPI or the usual treatment of intensive case management). Parent problem solving skills, parental coping skills, perceived social support resources, and child behavior were measured initially, at 9 months, and at 18 months.

Results: At the 9-month measurement point, parents and primary caregivers in the treatment group reported significantly more people in their lives to turn to for help, and significantly more coping resources. There were no significant differences between the two groups at the 18-month marker. The children in both groups demonstrated behavioral improvements, leading the authors to draw the conclusion that the parental involvement in both the case management and teaching sessions and the social support received was the most important element in behavioral change.

Application to Your Clinical Practice: As a profession, nurses need to develop effective strategies for involving parents and caregivers in the care of their children. How could you incorporate support and education as a way of empowering the clients that you see in your clinical practice?

Box 16-1 Questions to Assess Learning Needs

- What does the client already know about his or her condition and treatment?
- In what ways is the client affected by it?
- In what ways are those persons intimately involved with the client affected by the client's condition or treatment?
- To what extent is the client willing to take personal responsibility for seeking solutions?
- What goals would the client like to achieve?
- What will the client need to do to achieve those goals?
- What resources are available to the client and family that might affect the learning process?
- What barriers to learning exist?

- "Tell me what your doctor has told you about your treatment."

Types of follow-up questions the nurse can use to assess client learning needs are found in Box 16-1. Based on the circumstances the client presents and the client's responses to key questions, teaching plans can begin. The nurse will want to explore potential *environmental factors*, such as limited health insurance, transportation difficulties, lack of follow-up facilities, and cultural dietary considerations that present obstacles to the client's implementation of the teaching plan. This knowledge ensures that both nurse and client have a realistic understanding of treatment goals based on the specific learning needs of the client.

If other family members will be involved in the care of the client, the nurse needs to assess the family's general patterns of health care behaviors, their expectations for the client, and their knowledge of the client's condition. Many well-planned teaching interventions do not produce the desired outcomes because the family fails to understand or fully support the client's efforts to implement new behaviors (*reinforcing factors*). At the conclusion of the assessment interview, the nurse needs to summarize important points. This strategy helps to identify any misinformation and reinforce the health teaching.

Planning

Each learning situation has a past as well as a present reality. Past experience and beliefs about illness, medications, certain treatments, cultural values, and the reactions of others produce assumptions that will influence the acceptance of health teaching. The nurse needs to know not only what information the client has received but also whom the client looks to and respects for health teaching purposes. Focusing on accurate information without destroying the credibility of well-meaning and influential informal health teachers in the client's life is part of the art of health teaching. Nothing is gained by injuring the reputation of the person who gave the client the information. Instead, the nurse might say, "There have been some new findings that I think you might be interested in. The most current thinking suggests that (*give example*) works well in situations like this." With this statement, the nurse can introduce a different way of thinking without challenging the person identified in the client's mind as expert.

Health teaching often includes family members either in a supportive role or as the primary recipients of the teaching process. For example, the family or caregiver would be involved as a primary learner with children and with clients who have sensory or cognitive deficits. Content presentations to these family members would be the same as those given to the client if the client were able to assume full responsibility for self-care.

When family members take supportive roles in cases involving teenagers, clients in crisis, elderly or critically ill clients with intact cognitive abilities, and adolescents, for example, the health teaching would focus on what they need to know to support the primary learner. Information and anticipatory guidance about what to expect when the client goes home and early warning signs of complications or potential problems are given to family members as well as clients.

Assessment and inclusion of previous learning continue throughout the teaching process. This allows the nurse to make the teaching meaningful to the client and relevant to changes in the client's condition. Health teaching is not a static process. As the client's condition worsens, becomes stable, or improves, you may need to modify the teaching content and strategies. Successful health teaching is interactive, using the real-life experiences of the client as the basis for determining content and strategies.

Health teaching addresses specific health care needs. Sample nursing diagnoses that respond to teaching interventions are found in Box 16-2. The nursing diagnosis clarifies the specific nature of the learning need. For example, a knowledge deficit related to signs and symptoms of hyper- and hypoglycemia requires different content and strategies from a nursing diagnosis of "deficient knowledge related to how to prefill syringes and administer insulin."

Box 16-2 Sample Nursing Diagnoses Amenable to Health Teaching

- Risk for injury or violence
- Ineffective coping
- Alternations in parenting or family process
- Self-care deficits
- Anxiety
- Noncompliance
- Impaired home maintenance
- Deficient knowledge

Although too much information puts the learner into informational overload so that critical content is not learned, not enough direction can also prove harmful. For example, a nurse on the evening shift instructed an 85-year-old man to keep his arm in an upright position after a treatment procedure. The nurse neglected to tell him that he could release his arm once the needle was securely in place. The man called his wife at 5 AM the next day to tell her he did not think he could hold his arm in that position any longer. The man had been awake all night, his arm felt numb, and he was at his wits' end because of incomplete health teaching. Had the nurse told him to keep his arm elevated for a specific period of time, e.g., 30 minutes to an hour, the outcome and level of client satisfaction could have been different. In addition to giving complete information, the nurse can ask, "Do you have any questions for me?" and suggest that if things come up that the client has questions about later, the client should ask for further clarification.

Developing Learning Goals. Learning goals are the outcomes one hopes to achieve. Setting clear learning goals that the client is interested in meeting and has the necessary resources to achieve is essential to success. It is important to set goals *with* your client rather than *for* your client. Client-centered goals tailored to the learner's needs, abilities, and interests increase the chances that the information will be understood and applied (London, 2001). After setting appropriate learning goals, the next step is to break the broad goals down into specific objectives or accomplishments the client is expected to achieve.

Motivation enhances learning. In developing relevant goals, you should focus on what the client and family *want* to know about a topic as well as what they *need* to know. Health teaching goals should be comprehensive enough to provide needed information and yet narrow enough to be achievable. Included in the development of outcome goals is a broad statement about what the client needs to achieve maximum health potential (e.g., "Following health teaching, the client will maintain dietary control of her diabetes"). An interim goal might be, "Following health teaching, the client will develop an appropriate diet plan for 1 week." Setting realistic goals prevents disappointment on the part of both nurse and client. Achieving small goals stimulates success and encourages the client to take charge. Box 16-3 summarizes guidelines to use in the development of effective health teaching goals and objectives. Exercise 16-2 provides experience with developing relevant behavioral goals.

Establishing Priorities. In today's health care environment, time is an issue. Teaching goals need to be modest and achievable in the time frame allotted. To structure the learning session, the nurse needs to reflect on the minimum information the client needs to know and what kinds of activities are absolutely essential for the client and family to have knowledge of in meeting the client's health care needs.

Health teaching can never be eliminated because the nurse lacks time, but it can be streamlined. Even in the most limited situation, scheduling a defined block of time for teaching to occur is essential, because otherwise teaching may not become a priority.

Matching teaching strategies with the client's developmental level and unique client needs is important. Those experiencing a procedure for the first time need to have more detailed information than clients who require only follow-up information. Clients with English as a second language may require additional learning time. Simple modifications that can overcome age-related barriers to learning when teaching the older adult (Mauk, 2006) are summarized in Box 16-4. There is increasing evidence that keeping the mind active, stimulating the elder client's mental process, and learning new ways to maintain a healthy lifestyle can positively affect the older person's level of health and well-being.

Box 16-3 Guidelines for Developing Effective Goals and Objectives

- Link goals to the nursing diagnosis.
- Make goals action-oriented.
- Make goals specific and measurable.
- Define objectives as behavioral outcomes.
- Design objectives with a specific time frame for achievement.
- Show a logical progression with established priorities.
- Review periodically and modify goals as needed.

Developing Measurable Objectives. Health teaching objectives describe the steps needed to accomplish identified goals. They should be achievable, measurable, and

Exercise 16-2 Developing Behavioral Goals

Purpose: To provide practical experience with developing teaching goals.

Procedure:
Establish a nursing diagnosis related to health teaching and a teaching goal that supports the diagnosis in each of the following situations:

1. Jimmy is a 15-year-old adolescent who has been admitted to a mental health unit with disorders associated with impulse control and conduct. He wants to lie on his bed and read Stephen King novels. He refuses to attend unit therapy activities.
2. Maria, a 19-year-old single woman, is in the clinic for the first time because of cramping. She is seven months pregnant and has had no prenatal care.
3. Jennifer is overweight and desperately wants to lose weight. However, she cannot walk past the refrigerator without stopping, and she finds it difficult to resist the snack machines at work. She wants a plan to help her lose weight and resist her impulses to eat.

Discussion:

1. What factors did you have to consider in developing the most appropriate diagnosis and teaching goals for each client?
2. In considering the diagnosis and teaching goals for each situation, what common themes did you find?
3. What differences in each situation contributed to variations in diagnosis and teaching goals? What contributed to these differences?
4. In what ways can you use the information in this exercise in your future nursing practice?

Box 16-4 Overcoming Age-Related Barriers to Learning

- Explain why the information will be important to the client.
- Use familiar sources to provide information.
- Draw on the client's experiences and interests in planning your teaching.
- Find out through questioning what is important and relevant to the client.
- Make teaching sessions less than an hour to avoid tiring the client.
- If the client wears glasses, make sure they are clear and in use.
- Take into account vision changes, allowing more light and different placement of materials.
- Speak slowly, naturally, and clearly.
- If the client wears a hearing aid, make sure it is in place.
- Face the client so the client can see your lips and expressions as you speak.

related to specific health outcomes. To determine whether an objective is achievable, consider the client's level of experience, educational level, resources, and motivation. Then define the specific learning objectives needed to achieve the health goal. The objectives, like the health outcome, should relate to the nursing diagnosis. For example, the nursing diagnosis for a newly diagnosed diabetic might read, "Deficient knowledge related to diabetic diet." Each learning objective should describe a single learning task related to the expected outcome of dietary control of the client's diabetes. Including the time frame in which each objective should be achieved reinforces commitment.

Examples of appropriate and progressive learning objectives related to diabetic control might include the following:

- The client will identify the purpose of a diabetic diet and appropriate foods by the end of the first teaching session.
- The client will identify appropriate foods and serving sizes allowed on a diabetic diet by the end of the second teaching session.
- The client will demonstrate actions for urine testing for sugar at home by the third teaching session.
- The client will identify foods to avoid on the diabetic diet and the rationale for compliance by the fourth teaching session.
- The client will describe symptoms and actions to take for hyperglycemia and hypoglycemia by the end of the fifth teaching session.
- The client will develop a food plan for 1 week before discharge in 2 weeks.

Structuring the Environment. Teaching sessions conducted in a quiet, well-lighted area stress the importance of the learning endeavor. If health teaching is done in the home, all of those involved in the health care of the client should be included. Small children need to be cared for elsewhere, and the telephone should not become a distraction. Stating these conditions before the home teaching session begins prevents misunderstandings and unnecessary disturbances. In hospital situations, the client often is in bed or sitting in a chair. The learning environment is relatively informal, but having enough space for equipment and demonstration is critical.

Timing. Timing is essential, because learning takes place only when the learner is ready. The nurse needs to consider how much time is needed to learn a particular skill or body of knowledge and build this into the learning situation. Complicated and essential skills need blocks of time and repeated practice with feedback. Some information can be provided as written backup material. Scheduling shorter sessions with time in between to process information helps prevent sensory overload.

Pick times for teaching when energy levels are high, the client is not distracted by other things, it is not visiting time, and the client is not in pain. Careful observation of the client will help determine the most appropriate times for learning.

People also have saturation points as to how much they can learn in one time period, no matter how interesting the topic is to them. Keep the teaching session short and to the point. Another simple strategy that helps break up learning segments is to change the pace by inserting an activity, visual aid, or discussion point.

Not all health teaching is formal. Simple, spontaneous health teaching takes minutes, yet in some instances, it can be highly effective. The following case example, taken from *Heartsounds* (Lear, 1980), illustrates this point.

Case Example

A nurse came in while he was eating dinner. "Dr. Lear," she said, "after angiography the patients always seem to have the same complaints, and I thought you might

want to know about them. It might help." (This was a good nurse. I didn't know it then, because I didn't know how scared he was. But later I understood that this was a darned good nurse.) "Thanks, it would help," he said.

"It's mostly two things. The first is, they say that during the test, they feel a tremendous flush. It's very sudden and it can be scary."

He responds to the nurse, "Okay, the flush. And what's the other thing?"

"It's … well, they say that at a certain point, they feel as though they are about to die. But that feeling passes quickly." He thanked her again. He was very grateful.

(Later, during the actual procedure, Dr. Lear remembered the nurse's words and found comfort.) "Easy. Easy. You're supposed to feel this way. This is precisely what the nurse described. The moment you feel you are dying." (pp. 120-121)

This teaching intervention probably took less than 2 minutes, yet its effect was long-lasting and healing. There are countless opportunities for this type of health teaching in clinical practice if the nurse consciously looks for them.

Timing and length of sessions are particularly important issues for learners handicapped by memory deficits, lack of insight, poor judgment, and limited problem-solving abilities. These learners respond best to a learning environment in which the content is presented in a consistent, concrete, and patient manner, with clear and frequent cues to action. Box 16-5 covers important aspects of timing in health teaching.

Box 16-5 Factors Involved in Timing

- Client readiness
- Time needed to learn skill or body of knowledge
- Possible need for attitude change by client
- Time constraints of nurse
- Client priorities about information or skill
- Client's energy level
- Atmosphere of trust

Selecting Appropriate Content. Essential content in most teaching plans includes information about the health care problem, risk factors, treatment, and self-care skills the client will need to manage at home (Lee, Wasson, Anderson et al., 1998). Attitudes that will affect the client's adjustment and compliance with treatment also require attention.

The nurse should consider the client's perception of the acceptability of the content. Is the content complicated or likely to make the client uncomfortable? If so, the nurse must be able to organize it in such a way that the client can relate to it. Clients learn more effectively when they understand the goals of the learning session and when the content helps them connect new knowledge to what they already know.

To make content comprehensible to the client is an art. Content that builds on the person's experiences, abilities, interests, motivation, and skills is more likely to engage the learner's attention. Attention to the reading level of clients helps ensure that a pamphlet can be read. Large-print pamphlets and audiotapes are helpful learning aids for those with sight problems.

Selecting Appropriate Teaching Methods. No one teaching strategy can meet the needs of all clients (Rycroft-Malone, Latter, Yerrell et al., 2000). Unlike other forms of teaching, client teaching must be individualized. Recognizing distinctive differences in client learning needs is critical in choosing the most appropriate teaching strategies.

Additionally, in health care the nurse needs to adjust teaching strategies as the client's medical condition changes. Preoperation teaching strategies should differ from those used immediately after the operation. The amount of information given, the pace of the teaching, and the level of learner involvement necessarily reflect the client's physical condition and learning needs in each time frame.

Planning to use a variety of teaching strategies is most effective. For example, mothers respond positively to posters showing normal infant features and development because they can see as well as hear that head molding and skin rashes are typical findings in newborns. The nurse might provide one-to-one instruction for the client related to diabetic teaching, with additional sessions scheduled to include the family caregiver in open discussion of dietary modifications, particularly if this person prepares the meals. Another factor to consider is how people learn best. Box 16-6 displays characteristics of different learning styles.

Box 16-6 Characteristics of Different Learning Styles

Visual
- Learns best by seeing
- Likes to watch demonstrations
- Organizes thoughts by writing them down
- Needs detail
- Looks around; examines situation

Auditory
- Learns best with verbal instructions
- Likes to talk things through
- Detail is not as important
- Talks about situation and pros, cons

Kinetic
- Learns best by doing
- Hands-on involvement
- Needs action and likes to touch, feel
- Loses interest with detailed instructions
- Tries things out

Implementation

A key element in successful health teaching is an enthusiastic presentation that demonstrates a thorough knowledge of the subject matter, a keen understanding of the client's learning needs, and a genuine interest in the client. The client must be actively involved in the process. Effective teaching involves not only a healthy exchange of information, but also plenty of opportunities to ask questions and to receive feedback.

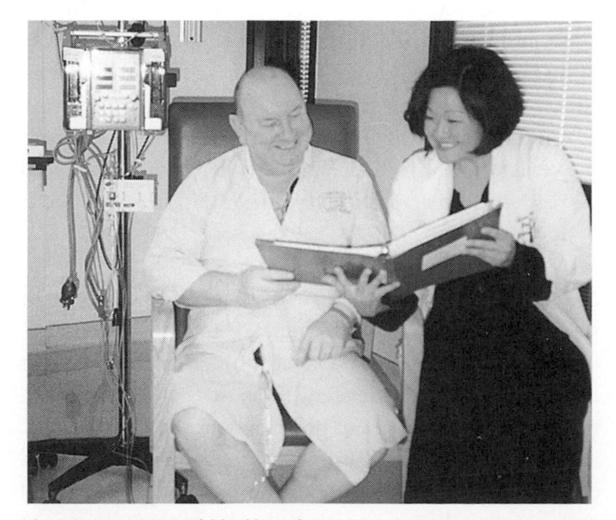

A key element in successful health teaching is an enthusiastic presentation. (From Lewis SM, Heitkemper MM, Dirksen SR: *Medical-surgical nursing: assessment and management of clinical problems*, ed 5, St Louis, 2000, Mosby.)

Sequencing the Learning Experience. People learn best when there is a logical flow and building of information from simple to complex. Information that builds on previous knowledge and experience is even better. The nurse sets the stage for the learning process by presenting a simple overview of what will be taught and why the information will be important to the learner. Deliver key points and allow an opportunity for client feedback and questions. If the material is complex, it can be broken down into smaller learning segments. For example, diabetic teaching could include the following segments:

- Introduction, including what the client does know
- Basic pathophysiology of diabetes
- Diet and exercise
- Demonstration of insulin injection with return demonstration
- Recognizing signs and symptoms of hyper- and hypoglycemia
- Care of skin and feet
- How to talk to the doctor

A strong closing, summarizing major points, reinforces the learning process. Exercise 16-3 provides practice with developing a mini teaching plan.

Using Clear Language. Using clear and precise language is critical to understanding, because many words in English have several different meanings. For example, the word "cold" can refer to temperature, an illness, an emotional tone, or a missed opportunity. Providing information with abstract and vague language leaves the learner wondering what the nurse actually meant. For example, "Call the doctor if you have any problems" can mean many different things. "Problems" can refer to side effects of the medication, a return of symptoms, problems with family acceptance, changed relationships, and even alterations in self-concept. The best way to provide information and instructions is to use clear behavioral descriptions that include the following:

- Who needs to be involved
- Identification of specific behaviors
- What needs to happen
- Under what specific circumstances

Exercise 16-3 Developing Teaching Plans

Purpose: To provide practice with developing teaching plans.

Procedure:

1. Develop a mini teaching plan for one of the following client situations.
   a. Jim Dolan feels stressed and is requesting health teaching on stress management and relaxation techniques.
   b. Adrienne Parker is a newly diagnosed diabetic. Her grandfather had diabetes.
   c. Vera Carter is scheduled to have an appendectomy in the morning.
   d. Marion Hill just gave birth to her first child. She wants to breast-feed her infant, but she does not think she has enough milk.
   e. Barbara Scott wants to lose weight.
2. Use guidelines presented in Chapters 15 and 16 in the development of your teaching plan. Include the following data: a brief statement of client learning needs and a list of related nursing diagnoses in order of priority.
3. For one nursing diagnosis, develop a long-term goal, short-term learning objectives, a teaching time frame, content to be covered, teaching strategies, and methods of evaluation.

An example of a clear statement the nurse might use is, "If you should develop a headache or feel dizzy in the next 24 hours, call the emergency room doctor right away." Avoid vague statements such as, "Take the pill three times a day" or, "Call the doctor if you feel bad." When teaching a client with English as a second language, remember that concepts from one language can not always be directly translated into another. In fact, in some cultures, word descriptors for certain concepts either do not exist or the phrases used for expressing and describing them are quite different.

Using Visual Aids. Visual aids are useful tools to supplement the words of the nurse because they help reinforce a message and provide concrete visual images. Simple images and few words work better than complex visual aids (Huntsman & Binger, 1981). Visual aids are particularly relevant in explaining complex anatomy or displaying external symptoms such as a rash or mole changes. For example, the nurse might show a client a skeleton model to explain a collapsed disc. A chart or model showing the heart might help another client understand the anatomy and physiology of a heart disorder.

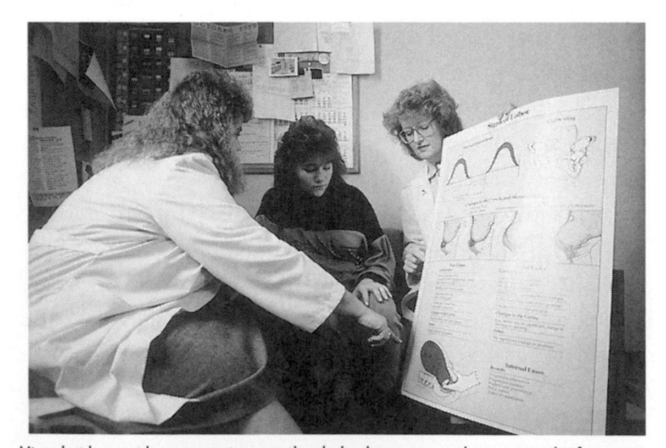

Visual aids provide concrete images that help clients remember essential information. (Courtesy University of Maryland School of Nursing.)

Low literacy (see Chapter 15) requires additional accommodations (Perdue, Degazon, & Lunny, 1999). Films and videotapes are especially useful in teaching clients with limited reading skills, and they have the advantage of allowing clients to watch at their convenience. A later discussion with the nurse helps to correct misinterpretations and emphasize pertinent points.

Storytelling. The nurse can use stories of how other people manage similar problems. Stories can help reinforce content or put a concept into a familiar context that the client can understand. The story should relate to realistic life experiences of potential interest to the client. The story should be a short vignette showing cause and effect. Finally, the story should deal with the "here and now" of the client's situation. In describing the use of stories to transmit health messages to American Indians, Hodge, Pasqua, Marquez et al. (2002) suggest using a wellness message at the end of the story "that assists participants/listeners to reflect on the story and that applies general concepts to the listener's individual experience" (p. 8). Use concrete, common words to express or strengthen the client's comprehension of the material.

Using Advance Organizers. Advance organizers, consisting of cue words related to more complex data, help clients anticipate and respond to more complex information in their own minds. A *mnemonic*, defined as a key letter, word, or phrase, helps clients organize important ideas. For example, the nurse might use the word "diabetes" to help a client remember key concepts about diabetes:

D = diet
I = infections
A = administering medications
B = basic pathophysiology
E = eating schedules
T = treatment for hyperglycemia or hypoglycemia
E = exercise
S = symptom recognition

Each letter stands for one of the concepts needed for comprehensive diabetic education. Taken together, the client has a useful tool for remembering *all* of the important concepts. A mnemonic can be letters of the alphabet, places, or words—in fact, any associations that have personal or group meanings for the persons developing them. Nursing students can use mnemonics to help them remember key points. The word association fosters identification in much the same way that linking new information to previously learned information does. For example, the four Fs (fat, forty, female, family history) can help students remember risk factors for gallbladder disorder. Developing mnemonics can be fun and creative.

Providing Transitional Cues. Sometimes people do not understand an instruction because the nurse fails to make the necessary transitions that link one idea to another. Johnson notes that "being complete and specific seems so obvious, but often people do not communicate the frame of reference they are using, the assumptions they are making, the intentions they have in communicating, or the leaps in thinking they are making" (cited in Flanagan, 1991, p. 24). Directions may seem simple and obvious to the nurse, but clients may have difficulty with elementary material simply because the information is new to them. Transition statements can help the client see how the ideas fit together.

Case Example

Statement A

Nurse: The doctor wants you to take a half a pill for the first week and increase the dose to a full pill after the first week. You should call him if you experience any side effects such as nausea or headaches.

Statement B

Nurse: This medication works well for most people, but some people tolerate it better than others. The doctor would like you to take a half a pill for the first week so that your system has a chance to adapt to it, and the doctor can see how you are responding before you take the full dose. If you have no side effects, he would like you to increase the dose to a full pill after the first week. The most common side effects are nausea or headaches. They don't occur with most people, but each person's response to medication is a little different. He would like you to call him if you notice these side effects.

Although the second statement takes a little longer, it includes clear transitions between ideas that will make it easier for the client to remember the instructions.

Repeating Key Concepts. Most learners need more than one exposure to new content or skill development. Review new information frequently. If possible, have more than one session for each learning segment. Although it may feel redundant, repeating yourself and restating key elements helps the client process material by going over it mentally. Having the opportunity to practice self-care skills that the client can apply immediately enhances the teaching process (Bohny, 1997). Allowing extra time for the client to talk about and do return demonstrations of tasks reinforces learning.

Asking for a Commitment. Asking for a commitment from the client enhances the learning process because it requires the learner to seriously consider how he or she will implement the learned material. For example, you might ask a client with a heart condition to describe a specific physical activity he will do the following week, including the time and how often he will do this during the time frame. This simple strategy encourages the client to think specifically about how a particular activity will be integrated into his or her daily routine. The more detailed the commitment, the more likely the treatment regime will be followed. If you have any doubts about the client's commitment, you might state, "Many people with newly diagnosed heart problems have trouble really following through with a regular exercise program. Do you think you might have any problems with this?"

Giving and Seeking Feedback. In a research study of factors considered necessary to a successful patient teaching program on medications, clients identified feedback as an essential element (Mullen & Green, 1985). To appreciate its significance, consider your performance if you did not receive feedback from your instructor. Feedback about how the client is accomplishing teaching goals should be descriptive, not evaluative, and should include both positive and negative elements. One way of doing this is to describe all of the behaviors that contributed to an outcome rather than selectively choosing only those in need of alteration.

Effective feedback is honest and based on concrete data. It is important to differentiate between observational data and personal interpretations or conclusions, and to focus on "what" needs to change, not the "why" of behaviors. Determining motivation is a guessing game, because most of the time noncompliance is multifactorial.

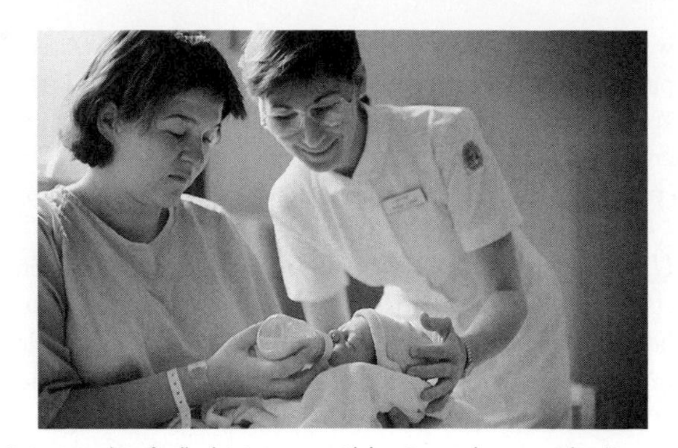

Giving immediate feedback is important with learning psychomotor tasks. (Courtesy University of Maryland School of Nursing.)

Feedback given as soon as possible after observation is more likely to be accurately reported and hence more readily accepted by the client. Behavioral statements on a continuum (e.g., "You need a little more practice" or, "You are able to draw up the medication okay, but you need a little more work with selecting sites") are more effective than absolute statements (e.g., "You still are not doing this correctly"). Exercise 16-4 provides practice with giving feedback in health teaching.

Exercise 16-4 Giving Teaching Feedback

Purpose: To give students perspective and experience in giving usable feedback.

Procedure:

1. Divide the class into working groups of three or four students.
2. Present a 3-minute sketch of some aspect of your current learning situation that you find difficult (e.g., writing a paper, speaking in class, coordinating study schedules, or studying certain material).
3. Each person in turn offers one piece of usable informative feedback to the presenter. In making suggestions, use the guidelines on feedback given in this chapter.
4. Place feedback suggestions on a flip chart or chalkboard.

Discussion:

1. What were your thoughts and feelings about the feedback you heard in relation to resolving the problem you presented to the group?
2. What were your thoughts and feelings in giving feedback to each presenter?
3. Was it harder to give feedback in some cases than in others? In what ways?
4. What common themes emerged in your group?
5. In what ways can you use the self-exploration about feedback in this exercise in teaching conversations with clients?

Indirect feedback—given through nodding, smiling, and sharing information about the process and experiences of others—reinforces learning. Acknowledging the contributions of participants in group learning provides encouragement for active participation, and repeating questions or answers emphasizes key concepts.

Another strategy is to ask the client to repeat the instructions in his or her own words and to describe for the nurse the actions that need to be taken if the instructions cannot be followed exactly or if they fail to produce the desired effect. Asking the client to repeat as you go along reinforces each piece of information and eliminates the problem of delivering a comprehensive teaching plan only to discover that the client lost your train of thought after the first few sentences.

Coaching the Client. *Webster's Ninth New Collegiate Dictionary* (1985) defines *coaching* as instructing or training, for example, of a player, in fundamental rules and strategies of a game. Clients may need coaching through unfamiliar and often painful procedures, and it is a particularly effective strategy to use when the client needs to gain control (Lewis & Zahlis, 1997). In most cases, the nurse will teach self-management problem-solving skills in primary prevention through coaching the client.

Coaching involves a number of skills presented in this and other chapters; these are displayed in Figure 16-1. It is a teaching strategy that fully respects the client's autonomy in developing appropriate solutions, because the client is always in charge of the pace and direction of the learning. In addition to giving appropriate information, coaching involves taking the client step by step through the procedure or activities in a mutual dialogue in which the client makes suggestions about care.

To coach a client successfully, the nurse must know and appreciate the client as an individual. This helps the

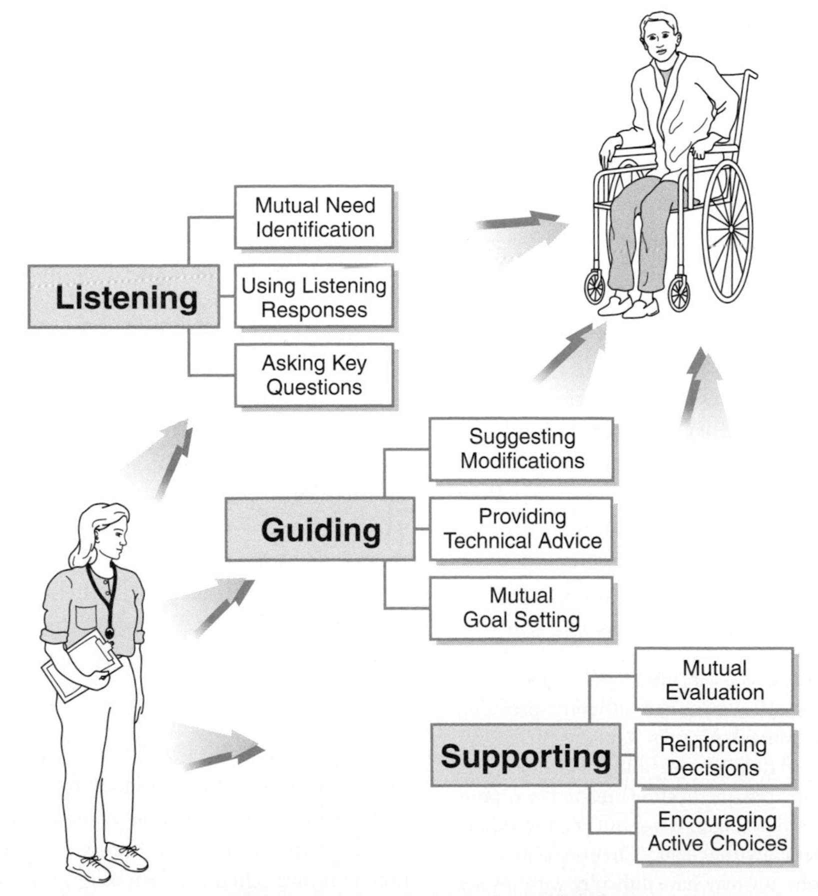

Figure 16-1 • The nurse's role in coaching clients.

Exercise 16-5 Coaching

Purpose: To help students understand the process of coaching.

Procedure:
Identify the steps you would use to coach clients in each of the following situations. Use Figure 16-1 as a guide to develop your plan.

1. A client returning from surgery, with pain medication ordered "as needed"
2. A client newly admitted to a cardiac care unit
3. A client with a newly inserted intravenous catheter for antibiotic medications
4. A child and his parents coming for a preoperative visit to the hospital before surgery

Share your suggestions with your classmates.

Discussion:

1. What were some of the different coaching strategies you used with each of these clients?
2. In what ways were your coaching strategies similar to or unlike those of your classmates?
3. How could you use the information you gained from this exercise to improve the quality of your helping?

nurse to know what information the client needs and how best to guide a particular client in taking charge of a situation. Sometimes the coaching a client needs relates to negotiating a complex health care system or developing better ways to have personal needs met.

The secret of successful coaching is to provide enough information to help the client take the next step without taking over. Exercise 16-5 provides practice with coaching as a teaching strategy.

Evaluation

The Joint Commission on Accreditation of Healthcare Organizations (JCAHO) requires documentation of client teaching. Notes about the initial assessment should be detailed, comprehensive, and objective. Included in the documentation are the teaching actions and the client response, both directly linked to nursing diagnosis. For example, the nursing documentation for ongoing home health teaching about diabetic control would start with client assessment data and might be written as follows:

> 4/8/07 Blood glucose check normal. Vital signs stable. Client on insulin for 10 years; has difficulty prefilling syringes. Lives with son who works. Nursing diagnosis: knowledge deficit related to prefilling syringes and ineffective coping in self-medication related to poor eyesight. Nurse prefilled syringes, wrote out med schedule, and discussed in detail with client. Client receptive to medication instruction, but may have difficulty with insulin prefill secondary to poor vision. Instructed client on medications, signs and symptoms to report to MD, diet and safety measures. Client able to repeat instructions. Spoke with son regarding medication supervision.
>
> M. Haggerty, RN

Accurate documentation serves another critical purpose in health teaching: it helps ensure continuity and prevents duplication of teaching efforts. The client's record becomes a secondary vehicle of communication, informing other health care workers of what has been taught and what areas need to be addressed in future teaching sessions. This is important for two reasons. First, the client can lose interest or become confused when the same information is repeated or is given in such a different way that the client is unsure which is "the correct information." Second, because many insurance carriers will not pay for parallel teaching, nurses need to share their teaching with other members of the interdisciplinary health team. This helps to avoid additional costs for the client and prevents complicating the client's life with insurance company questions about claim information.

Teaching Applications in Different Settings

Health teaching takes place in a variety of settings (e.g., informal one-to-one relationships, formal structured group sessions, and family conferences). The nurse may conduct scheduled teaching groups related to health care issues (e.g., in medication and rehabilitation discharge groups). Family conferences incorporate formal and informal teaching strategies for providing families with information they will need to help the client recover and for answering the many questions families have about their loved ones in the clinical setting. The media provide mass health teaching, particularly in primary prevention (e.g., safe sex and drug abuse prevention commercials). Written instructions, videotapes, and informational pamphlets provide supplemental health teaching. Health teaching in the home helps clients and their families in a variety of traditional and non-traditional ways. Most recently, telehealth has emerged as a technical means of providing information to clients in their homes by telecasting health information through video or interactive teaching formats using telephone and television. This type of health teaching is important in rural areas, where distance precludes ongoing nursing support.

Box 16-7 Medication Teaching Tips

- Provide clients with written drug information, particularly for metered-dose inhalants and high alert medications such as insulin.
- Include family or caregivers in the teaching sessions for clients who need extra support or reminders.
- Do not wait until discharge to begin education about complex drug regimens.
- Clearly explain directions for using each medication.
- Always require repeat demonstrations or explanations about medications to be taken at home, particularly for those requiring special drug administration techniques.
- Use the time you already spend with clients during assessments and daily care to evaluate their level of understanding about their medications.
- Keep medication administration schedule as simple and easy to follow as possible.

Adapted from Institute for Safe Medication Practices: *Patient medication teaching tips.* Huntingdon Valley, PA, 2006, Author.

Health Teaching About Medications. In today's health care arena, where much of the responsibility for health care must be assumed by clients and their families, it is essential that they be told what they can do to help with their own recovery. This means that both client and family should be advised of what to expect from treatment and medications as well as risks, benefits, prognosis, and options for treatment. This information allows clients to make better decisions about whether to take a particular drug and to be more compliant with treatment because they understand why it is important, what they can expect from following a treatment protocol, and how it can help them. There are fewer surprises and a higher level of confidence. Health care providers also need to have a clear understanding of client preferences. As preferences change—and for many clients and their families, they will—clients should be encouraged to make them known to their health care provider. Clients and families need to know the danger signals to watch for that would require a prompt call for assistance. They should be encouraged to ask questions of their health care provider and should be coached on the types of circumstances requiring a call to their health care provider.

Nurses need to assess the client's current level of knowledge and the types of information and recommendations that might be most helpful given an individual's culture, developmental level, health literacy, and motivation. You will need to clearly identify the purpose of the medication as well as side effects of the medications clients are receiving, what happens if they miss a dose or decide to stop the medication, and any pain or discomfort they may experience from either the medication or blood tests, if required, to determine efficacy or toxicity of the prescribed drug. Family members need to be given enough information to support client adherence to the treatment protocol. Box 16-7 provides medication teaching tips developed by the Institute for Safe Medication Practices that you can use in clinical practice.

Group Presentations. Group presentations offer the advantage of being able to teach a number of people at one time, and the format allows people to learn from each other as well as from the teacher. Health teaching topics that lend themselves to a group format include care of the newborn, diabetes, oncology, and pre- and postnatal care (Redman, 2001).

Formal group teaching should be structured in a space large enough to accommodate all participants. Temperature is important. A hot, stuffy room causes people to become drowsy; if a room is cold, learners tend to focus on this rather than what the instructor is saying. The learner should be able to hear and see the instructor, all of the equipment, and visual aids without strain. Space to practice and equipment to take notes give people a sense of purpose.

The nurse needs to make sure that the room is available and should plan to arrive a little early for setup. If the teaching plan calls for use of equipment or flip charts for visual aids, these need to be available and in working order. Consistency and planning help provide a structured environmental framework for the teaching process and decrease instructor anxiety. Should the equipment not work, it is better to eliminate the planned teaching aid completely than to spend a portion of the teaching session trying to fix it.

Preparation and practice can ensure that your presentation is clear, concise, and well spoken. Practice giving the information in a natural manner, particularly if the information is emotionally laden for you, the client, or both. If your teaching includes visual aids or equipment, developing an ease with incorporating them into your teaching process will make it easier, and you will appear more confident. In a group presentation, you also will need to establish rapport with your audience. This means being receptive to the learners' styles, making courteous observations, and initiating discussion appropriately. Use simple gestures such as smiling, nodding, and responding.

A quote at the beginning that captures the meaning of the presentation or a humorous opening grabs the audience's attention. Make eye contact immediately, and continue to do so throughout the teaching session. Extension of eye contact to all participants communicates acceptance and inclusion. Strengthen content statements with careful use of specific examples. Citing a specific problem and the ways another person dealt with it gives general statements credibility. Repeating key points and summarizing them again at the conclusion of the session helps reinforce learning.

If you plan to use overhead transparencies, use a font that is large enough to see from a distance (32-point is recommended) and include no more than four or five items per transparency. Gauge the number of overheads that you will need, and remember that the anticipated time for teaching may be made longer by questions from the audience.

To be a good teacher, one must also be a good listener. Asking questions confidently and thoughtfully as they relate to your understanding of participant circumstances conveys interest in the client's learning needs. Giving answers that are direct and clear reinforces the presentation. It is important for the nurse to anticipate questions and be on the alert for blank looks.

No matter how good a teacher you are, you will from time to time experience the blank look. When this occurs, it is appropriate to ask, "Does anyone have any questions about what I just said?" or, "This content is difficult to grasp; I wonder if you have any questions or concerns about what I have said so far?"

If you do not know the answer to a question, do not bluff it. It is appropriate to say, "That is a good question. I don't have an answer at this moment, but I will get back to you with it." Sometimes in a group presentation, another person will have the required information and will share it, with encouragement. Group members provide a rich learning resource that often is overlooked.

Handouts and other materials provide additional reinforcement. Make sure that the information is accurate, complete, easy to understand, and logical. Some-

Exercise 16-6 Group Health Teaching

Purpose: To provide practice with presenting a health topic in a group setting.

Procedure:

1. Plan a 15- to 20-minute health presentation on a health topic of interest to you, including teaching aids and methods for evaluation.
   Suggested topics:

   Nutrition
   Drinking and driving
   High blood pressure
   Dental care
   Weight control
   Mammograms
   Safe sex

2. Present your topic to your class group.

Box 16-8 Assessing Learning Needs at Discharge

- What potential problems are likely to prevent a safe discharge?
- What potential problems are likely to cause complications or readmission?
- What prior knowledge or experience does the patient and family have with this problem?
- What skills and equipment are needed to manage the problem at home?
- Who (what agency) will assume responsibility for continuing care?

times it is useful to have a nonprofessional who is unfamiliar with the topic review written instructions for clarity and logic before using them with clients. Asking clients for feedback also helps. Exercise 16-6 provides an opportunity to practice health teaching in a group setting.

Discharge Teaching. Discharge health teaching becomes extremely important when the client is in a health care facility for a restricted period of time, or when the number of home visits to clients in the community is limited. When the client is ready for discharge, the nurse asks a set of questions focused on the discharge process and what is likely to happen when the client returns home. Appropriate questions are found in Box 16-8.

Family conferences are used as teaching sessions during discharge planning. Topics commonly covered in discharge planning include information about the nature of the illness or injury, a summary of individual progress in meeting treatment goals, and information about care of the client once the client leaves the hospital. Reinforcement of teaching about medications and referrals to community health and support groups are part of the teaching session. For example, there may have to be some modifications in medication schedules to fit individual and family lifestyles. The family should have ample opportunity to ask questions and to have them answered completely and honestly. Written instructions and a post-discharge telephone number both support learning and provide necessary transitional support for client and family (Cagan & Meier, 1983).

Health Teaching in the Home. As health care moves to community-based care, with a case mix of unstable, acutely ill home care clients and constrained funding for

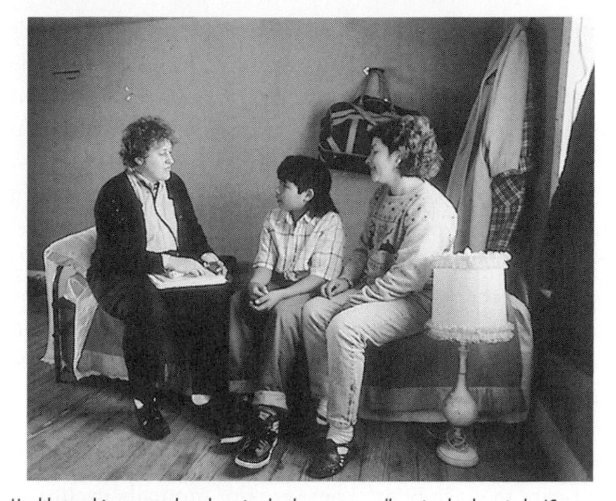

Health teaching can take place in the home as well as in the hospital. (Courtesy University of Maryland School of Nursing.)

community home-based care, skilled health teaching becomes an increasingly important component of health care delivery. In home care, the nurse is a guest in the client's home. Part of the teaching assessment includes appraisal of the home environment, family supports, and resources as well as client needs.

Although the principles of health teaching remain the same regardless of setting, the nurse implements them differently in home care settings because there is more time available and the teaching can be adapted to the client's individual situation. Teaching aids and structured teaching strategies available in the hospital setting may not be available; however, in many ways the home offers a teaching laboratory unparalleled in the hospital. The nurse can actually "see" the improvisations in equipment and technique that are possible in the home environment. Family members may have ideas that the nurse would not have thought of and that can make care easier. It is more natural for the client to reproduce teaching outcomes in the home environment when that is where he or she initially learned the procedure.

The nurse should call before going to the client's home. This is common courtesy, and it protects the nurse's time if the client is going to be out. The tools of the trade are housed in a bag the nurse carries into the home. Before setting the bag down on a table, the nurse should spread a clean paper to protect both the client's table and the bag. It is important for the nurse to talk the client through procedures and dressing changes in much the same way as was done in the hospital. The nurse models appropriate behaviors (e.g., washing hands in the bathroom sink before touching the client). Simple strategies, such as not washing one's hands in the kitchen sink where food is prepared, encourage the client to do likewise.

Caregivers often do not recognize that they have a teaching need or know what they need to ask to feel comfortable as a caregiver. Conley and Burman (1997) suggested that caregivers need information related to the client's disease "including its progression, symptoms and side effects, treatment options, and what to expect in the future" (p. 812).

Teaching outcomes for clients in their homes relate to increased knowledge, optimal functioning, and better self-care management. These are not mutually exclusive. In addition to content knowledge about the client's condition and treatment interventions, the nurse must have a working knowledge of community resources. Helping clients access supportive services, particularly when working with clients who are not by nature assertive, can be extremely helpful to families who would not otherwise do so even with the appropriate written information. The nurse must be able to select from a number of existing resources and create new ones through novel uses of family and community support systems. An understanding of Medicare, Medicaid, and other insurance matters (e.g., regulations, required documentation, and reimbursement schedules) is factored into the management of health care teaching in home health care.

The community health home care nurse works alone; consequently, there is a need for creativity as well as competence in providing health teaching. Teaching in home care settings is rewarding. Often, the nurse is the client's only visitor. Other family members often display a curiosity and willingness to be a part of the learning group, particularly if the nurse actively uses knowledge of the home environment to make suggestions about needed modifications.

Teaching in home care settings has to be short-term and comprehensive, because most insurance companies will provide third-party reimbursement only for intermittent, episodic care. Nurses need to plan teaching sessions realistically so that they can be delivered in the shortest time possible. Content must reflect specific information the client and family need to provide immediate effective care for the client, *nothing more and nothing less*. Sometimes it is tempting to include more than what is essential to know. Because there are so many regulations regarding the length and scope of skilled nursing interventions imposed by third-party reimbursement guidelines, the nurse needs to pay careful attention to health teaching content and formats.

SUMMARY

This chapter describes the nurse's role in health teaching. Theoretical frameworks, client-centered teaching, critical thinking, and behavioral approaches guide the nurse in implementing health teaching. Teaching is designed to access one or more of the three domains of learning: cognitive, affective, and psychomotor. Assessment for purposes of constructing a teaching plan centers on three areas: What does the client already know? What is important for the client to know? What is the client ready to know?

Essential content in all teaching plans includes information about the health care problem, risk factors, and self-care skills needed to manage at home. No one teaching strategy can meet the needs of all individual clients. The learning needs of the client will help define relevant teaching strategies. Several teaching strategies, such as coaching, use of mnemonics, and visual aids, are described. Repetition of key concepts and frequent feedback make the difference between simple instruction and teaching that informs. Documentation of the learning process is essential. The client's record becomes a vehicle of communication, informing other health care workers what has been taught and what areas need to be addressed in future teaching sessions.

Ethical Dilemma ▪ *What Would You Do?*

Jack is a 3-year-old boy recently admitted to your unit with a high fever, headache, and stiff neck. The physician wants to do a spinal tap on him to rule out meningitis. The family is opposed to this procedure, fearing it will further traumatize their child. What are the ethical considerations related to health teaching regarding this procedure?

REFERENCES

American Nurses Association: *Scope and standards of practice*, Washington, DC, 2004, Author.

Bohny B: A time for self-care: role of the home healthcare nurse, *Home Healthc Nurse* 15(4):281-286, 1997.

Brookfield S: *Understanding and facilitating adult learning*, San Francisco, 1986, Jossey-Bass.

Cagan J, Meier P: Evaluation of a discharge planning tool for use with families of high risk infants, *J Obstetr Gynecol Neonatal Nurs* 12:275-281, 1983.

Conley V, Burman M: Informational needs of caregivers of terminal patients in a rural state, *Home Healthc Nurse* 15(11): 808-817, 1997.

Flanagan L: *Survival skills in the workplace: what every nurse should know*, Kansas City, MO, 1991, American Nurses Association.

Greiner P, Valiga T: Creative educational strategies for health promotion, *Holist Nurs Pract* 12(2):73-83, 1998.

Hansen M, Fisher JC: Patient teaching: patient-centered teaching from theory to practice, *Am J Nurs* 98(1):56-60, 1998.

Hodge F, Pasqua A, Marquez C et al.: Utilizing traditional storytelling to promote wellness in American Indian communities, *J Transcult Nurs* 13(1):6-11, 2002.

Huntsman A, Binger J: *Communicating effectively*, Wakefield, MA, 1981, Nursing Resources.

Leahy J, Kizilay P: *Fundamentals of nursing practice: a nursing process approach*, Philadelphia, 1998, WB Saunders.

Lear MW: *Heartsounds*, New York, 1980, Pocket Books, Simon & Schuster.

Lee N, Wasson D, Anderson M et al.: A survey of patient education post discharge, *J Nurs Care Qual* 13(1):63-70, 1998.

Lewis F, Zahlis E: The nurse as coach: a conceptual framework for clinical practice, *Oncol Nurs Forum* 24(10):1695-1702, 1997.

London F: Take the frustration out of patient education, *Home Healthc Nurse* 19(3):158-160, 2001.

Manning S: The nurses I'll never forget, *Nursing* 22(8):47, 1992.

Mason D: Promoting health literacy: patient teaching as a vital nursing function, *Am J Nurs* 101(2):7, 2001.

Mauk KL: Healthier aging: Reaching and teaching older adults, *Holistic Nurs Pract* 20(3):158, 2006.

Miller B, Capp SE: Meeting JCAHO patient education standards, *Nurs Manage* (5):55-58, 1997.

Mullen P, Green L: Meta-analysis points the way toward more effective teaching, *Promot Health* 6:68, 1985.

Perdue B, Degazon C, Lunny M: Diagnoses and interventions with low literacy, *Nurs Diagn* 10(1):36-39, 1999.

Post-White J: Wind behind the sails: empowering our patients and ourselves, *Oncol Nurs Forum* 25(6):1011-1017, 1998.

Ragland G: *Instant teaching treasures for patient education*, St Louis, 1997, Mosby

Redman BK: *The practice of patient education*, ed 8, St Louis, 1997, Mosby.

Redman BK: *The practice of patient education*, ed 9, St Louis, 2001, Mosby.

Rogers C: *Freedom to learn for the '80s*, Columbus, OH, 1983, Merrill.

Rycroft-Malone J, Latter S, Yerrell P et al.: Nursing and medication education, *Nurs Stand* 14(50):35-39, 2000.

Skinner BF: *Beyond freedom and dignity*, New York, 1971, Knopf.

Taylor C, Lillis C, Lemone P: *Fundamentals of nursing: the art and science of nursing care*, ed 5, Philadelphia, 2005, Lippincott Williams & Wilkins.

Usher K, Arthur D: Process consent: a model for enhancing informed consent in mental health nursing, *J Adv Nurs* 27:692-697, 1998.

Webster's ninth new collegiate dictionary: Springfield, MA, 1985, Merriam Webster.

Wellard S, Turner D, Bethune E: Nurses as patient-teachers: exploring current expressions of the role, *Contemp Nurse* 7(1):12-14, 1998.

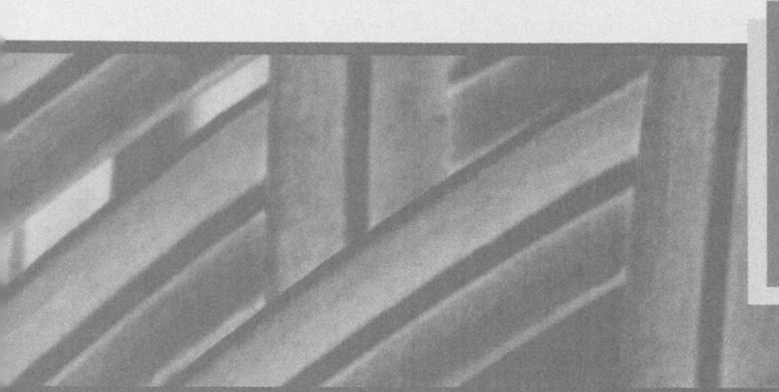

Part IV
Responding to Special Needs

Chapter 17
Communicating with Clients Experiencing Communication Deficits

Kathleen Underman Boggs

OUTLINE

OBJECTIVES

At the end of the chapter, the reader will be able to:

1. Identify common communication deficits.
2. Describe nursing strategies for communicating with clients experiencing communication deficits.
3. Discuss application of one research study's results to your clinical practice.

As Hubert Humphrey was fond of saying, the moral test of a society is how well it treats people in the dawn of life (children), people in the twilight of life (the elderly), and people in the shadows of life (the poor, the sick, the handicapped).

(Thompson, 1984)

When clients perceive that others value them, they feel more personal control and are more likely to feel emotionally comfortable.

(Williams & Irurita, 2004)

Chapter 17 presents an overview of common communication deficits. Communication deficits may involve lost function of one or more of the five senses. Examples include hearing loss, blindness, aphasia, or mental illness. Alternatively, communication deficits can arise from illiteracy, inability to speak English, or from sensory deprivation (Rutledge, 2004). When working with some clients who have sensory deficits, you may need to modify the general therapeutic communication strategies presented earlier in this book. It is important for us to remember that two individuals can be equally impaired but not equally disabled, since people compensate for their impairments in different ways. The primary nursing goal is to maximize the client's independence and ability to successfully interact with the health care system. This chapter focuses on suggested strategies for communication.

BASIC CONCEPTS

Clients with sensory or cognitive deficits are known to encounter barriers to adequate health care. Problems in communication are one of the main problems cited (O'Day, Killeen, & Iezzoni, 2004). Some clients become so frustrated that they omit needed care.

Types of Deficits

Hearing Loss

Nearly 16 million Americans have some hearing problems. Loss can be conductive, sensorineural, or functional. Nurses have both a legal and ethical obligation to provide appropriate care. Title III of the Americans with Disabilities Act (ADA) applies to communication between deaf clients and medical services (Herring & Hock, 2000).

In Children. Nearly three out of every one thousand newborns are deaf or have hearing loss. Fortunately, many of these deficits are diagnosed at birth. Newborn hearing is tested in the nursery via auditory brain stem response tests (National Institute on Deafness and Other Communication Disorders, see online references). People's sense of hearing alerts them to changes in the environment so they can respond effectively. The listener hears sounds and words and also a speaker's vocal pitch, loudness, and intricate inflections accompanying the verbalization. Subtle variations can completely change the sense of the communication. Combined with the sound and intensity, the organization of the verbal symbols allows the client to perceive and interpret the meaning of the sender's message.

In Older Adults. As we age we have an increased likelihood for experiencing sensory deficits related to the aging process. *Presbycusis* is a sensorineural dysfunction that commonly occurs as we age. British studies found that older adults, as a group, have significant decreases in hearing, poorer consonant discrimination, and changes in their conversational styles, especially in those over age 75 years (Abel, Sass-Kortsak, & Naugler, 2000; Mackenzie, 2000). Chapter 19 will discuss this.

When communication is compromised through birth defect, injury, illness, or the aging process, the client is at an enormous disadvantage in relationships with others. The extent of the loss is not always appreciated because the person looks normal, and the effects of partial hearing loss are not always readily apparent. Deprived of a primary means of receiving signals from the environment, the client with hearing loss may try to hide his or her deficit and may even withdraw from relationships.

Vision Loss

According to O'Day and colleagues, there are nearly 10 million residents of the United States who are blind or who have low vision (2004). Clients use vision to decode the meaning of messages. They watch the sender's facial expression and gestures for clues about interpreting the meaning of the message. All of the nonverbal cues that accompany speech communication (e.g., facial expression, nodding, and leaning toward the client) are lost to blind clients. Because clients cannot see our faces or observe our nonverbal signals, we need to use words to express what the client cannot see in the message.

In Older Adults. As your clients age they are more likely to have vision problems that may interfere with the communication process. As we age, the lens of our eyes becomes less flexible, making it difficult to accommodate shifts from far to near vision; this is a condition known as *presbyopia*. A British study found substantial decreases in visual acuity in older adults. These decreases ranged from 3% at age 65 years to over 35% in those over age 85 years (van der Pols, Bates, McGraw et al., 2000). Macular degeneration has become a major cause of vision loss in older adults. Chapter 19 discusses communication concerns with older adults.

Speech and Language Deficits

Clients who have speech and language deficits resulting from neurological trauma present a different type of communication problem. Normal communication allows people to perceive and interact with the world in an organized and systematic manner. People use language to express self-needs and to control environmental events. Language is the system people rely on to represent what they know about the world. When the ability to process and express language is disrupted, many areas of functioning are assaulted simultaneously.

Aphasia is defined as a neurological linguistic deficit, such as occurs following a stroke. It produces a sudden alteration of communication that invariably has an impact on the sense of self. Your client may have feelings of loss and social isolation imposed by the communication impairment. While there may be no cognitive impairment, the client may need more "think time" for cognitive processing during a conversation. Aphasia can present as primarily an expressive or receptive disorder. The client with *expressive aphasia* can understand what is being said but cannot express thoughts or feelings in words. *Receptive aphasia* creates difficulties in receiving and processing written and oral messages. With *global aphasia*, the client has difficulty with both expressive language and reception of messages.

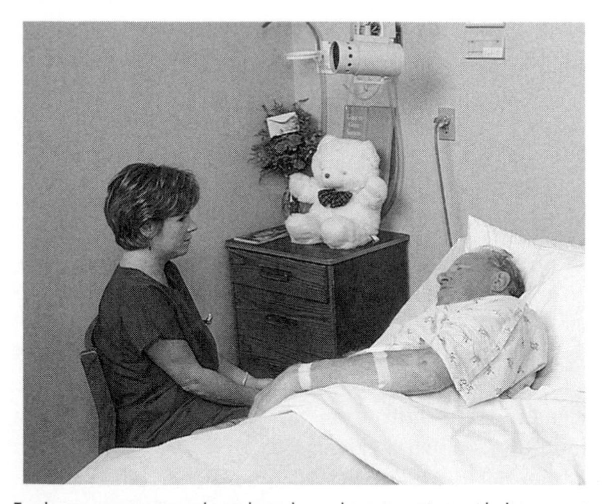

Touch, eye movements, and sounds can be used to communicate with clients experiencing aphasia. (From deWit SE: *Fundamental concepts and skills for nursing*, Philadelphia, 2001, WB Saunders.)

Impaired Cognition or Learning Delay

As your clients age, they are more likely to have cognitive losses that may interfere with the communication process. The responsibility for organizing care and overcoming communication and understanding problems rests with both social services and health care workers. Powrie's study found that effective communication between caretakers and nurses enhances (primary) health care provision (2003). While most older adults retain their mental acuity, a study by Naylor, Stephens, Bowles, and colleagues (2005) found cognitive deficits in 35% of 145 adults older than age 70 years who were hospitalized for routine medical or surgical events.

Serious Mental Illness

Clients with serious mental disorders have a different type of communication deficit resulting from a malfunctioning of the neurotransmitters that normally transmit and make sense out of messages in the brain. Social isolation, impaired coping, and low self-esteem accompany the client's inability to receive or express language signals. The emotional impact of these disabilities reflects the degree of severity of the deficits and the coping skills of the client.

The communication deficits found in clients with serious mental dysfunctions are related to their psychiatric disorders. Psychotic clients have intact sensory channels, but they cannot process and respond appropriately to what they hear, see, smell, or touch. The most serious communication difficulties are found in clients with *autism* (a childhood disorder charaterized by a profound inability to communicate) and *schizophrenia*. In these conditions, alterations in the biochemical neurotransmitters in the brain, which normally conduct messages between nerve cells and help orchestrate the person's response to the external environment, tangle messages and distort meanings. It is beyond the scope of this text to discuss in detail the psychotic client's communication deficits or the most appropriate strategies to use in communicating with these clients. This information is found in the many excellent psychiatric nursing texts available to the student. It is appropriate here, however, to appreciate the profound thought disintegration and communication problems psychotic clients face and to suggest basic guidelines for interacting with them.

The psychotic client usually presents with a poverty of speech and limited content. Speech appears blocked, reflecting disturbed patterns of perception, thought, emotions, and motivation. The client demonstrates a lack of vocal inflection and an unchanging facial expression, both of which make it difficult to truly understand the underlying message. Many clients display illogical thinking processes in the form of illusions, hallucinations, and delusions. Common words assume new meanings known only to the person experiencing them. The client thinks concretely and is unable to make abstract connections between ideas. Words and ideas are loosely connected and difficult to follow. Spontaneous movement is decreased, and the schizophrenic client exhibits inappropriate affect or appears nonresponsive to conversation (Tremeau, Malaspina, Duval et al., 2005). What the client hears may be overshadowed by the client's mental disorder, resulting in pervasive, distorted perceptions.

Environmental Deprivation as Related to Illness

Communication is particularly important in nursing situations characterized by sensory deprivation, physical immobility, and limited environmental stimuli. In the emergency room as well as the intensive care unit (ICU), perceptions and dialogue are limited by the nature of the unit and by the unstable nature of the conditions precipitating admission.

For the most part, the client is kept physically immobile, so the relationship with the critical care nurse often becomes most important. Nurses need to show concern for the client in a bewildering situation. When you empathize with your client, it helps him or her to develop meaning from the current situation. Clients are surrounded by high-tech equipment, have minimal privacy, and may not even have a window from which to orient themselves to day and night (Figure 17-1). Medical emergencies are the rule rather than the exception, and the client's usual support system is excluded except for brief visits. As Cooper (1993) points out, these units lack familiar landmarks and limit a person's ability to use environmental cues to direct behavior. Moreover, clients usually are frightened, in pain, and unable to communicate easily with others. Barriers to communication can also include intubation or sedation.

Research indicates that the absence of interpersonal stimulation and the subsequent gradual decline of cognitive abilities are related. Clients with normal intellectual capacity can appear dull, uninterested, and lacking in problem-solving abilities if they do not have frequent interpersonal stimulation.

Communication Difficulties Due to Foreign Language

Most health providers will increasingly encounter clients who do not speak the same language as the provider. Governments and health care agencies are becoming more sensitive to the need to provide quality health care to such clients. For example, the U.S. Health and Human Services Office for Civil Rights has published

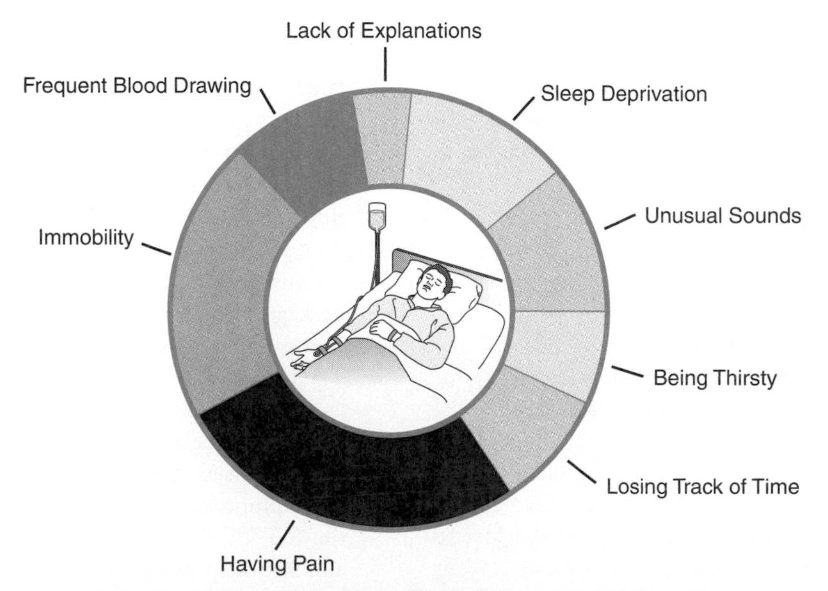

Figure 17-1 • Situational factors affecting client responses to critical care units.

Developing an Evidence-Based Practice

Naylor MD, Stephens C, Bowles KH et al.: Cognitively impaired older adults: from hospital to home, *Am J Nurs* 105(2):52-61, 2005.

This exploratory study conducted in Scotland identified the rate of cognitive impairment among 145 older adults (over age 70) undergoing acute hospitalization and described their needs.

Results: Fifty-one (35%) were found to be cognitively impaired. Five of these clients and their caregivers were interviewed in depth. Both hospital staff and family members often miss symptoms indicating the older adult is cognitively impaired. These cognitive deficits can negatively affect the client's ability to understand your teaching. Multiple needs were identified. These cognitively impaired clients averaged more than seven medications each (one client was on 21 medications). On average, they had approximately eight diagnosed health problems. It is no wonder that their greatest concerns were managing these conditions and negotiating care with multiple care providers. Memory loss interfered with the client's ability to correctly take prescribed medicines.

Application to Your Clinical Practice: While this reflects a very limited number of clients, results emphasize the need for you to assess your older clients for cognitive impairment and to individualize care both during hospitalization and during the initial 2- to 6-week postdischarge period. Family caregivers need your assistance to develop a postdischarge plan to identify and communicate worsening symptoms and to correctly manage multiple medications while recognizing their side effects.

policy guidelines that list the nurse's responsibilities under federal law when providing services to clients with limited English skills (see Online Resources). English as a second language is discussed in Chapter 11.

APPLICATIONS

Communication Strategies

Clients with Hearing Loss

The American Academy of Pediatrics (AAP) Joint Committee on Infant Hearing has endorsed universal newborn hearing screening (Finitzo & AAP Joint Committee on Infant Hearing, 2000). In older clients, assessment of auditory sensory loss can provide an opportunity for referral for nurses, who may be the first to note a client's decreased hearing (Stock, 2002). Your assessment should include the age of onset and the severity of the deficit. Hearing loss that occurs after the development of speech means that the client has access to word symbols and language skills. Deafness in children can cause developmental delays, which may need to be taken into account in planning the most appropriate communication strategies. Hearing deficits have also been shown to be associated with depression (Kalayam, Meyers, Kakuma et al., 1995). Choice of method of communication depends upon the severity of the deafness (Li, Bain, & Steinberg, 2003).

Clues to hearing loss occur when clients appear unresponsive to sound or respond only when the speaker is directly facing them. The nurse should ask clients whether they use a hearing aid and whether it is working properly. Auditory amplifiers such as assisted listening devices, hearing aids, and telephone attachments counterbalance certain types of hearing loss. Often, clients have hearing aids but fail to use them because they do not fit well or are hard to insert. Other people complain that the hearing aid amplifies all sounds indiscriminately, not just the voices of people in conversation, and they find this distracting. Exercises 17-1 and 17-2 will help you understand what it is like to have a sensory deficit.

Refer to Boxes 17-1 and 17-2 to adapt communication techniques. American Sign Language has been a standard communication tool for many years; however, few care providers use it. Communication assistance devices include the following:

- For hearing-impaired clients, there are speech amplifiers such as the pocket talker.
- Wireless text communication has become an important, basic necessity for the deaf (Power & Power, 2004). As a nurse you can use text messaging (short message service) on cell phones to communicate with deaf clients. Deaf clients use handheld electronics to exchange e-mail and receive instant alphanumeric messaging, paging, and so on. For example, various wireless service providers offer a data-only package for those who cannot use voice communication (Berke, 2005; Online Resources).
- The **Optacon** is a reading device that converts printed letters into a vibration that can be felt by the client who is both deaf and blind.
- Pictographs are laminated cards that show drawings of common foods and activities. Products such as the "AT&T Picture Guide" are commercially available and help you get your point across. These may be useful also with clients whose language you do

Exercise 17-1 Loss of Sensory Function in Geriatric Clients

Purpose: To assist students in getting in touch with the feelings often experienced by older adults as they lose sensory function. If the younger individual is able to "walk in the older person's shoes," he or she will be more sensitive to the losses and needs created by those losses in the older person.

Procedure:

1. Students separate into three groups.
2. Group A: Place cotton balls in your ears. Group B: Cover your eyes with a plastic bag. Group C: Place cotton balls in your ears and cover your eyes with a plastic bag.
3. A student from Group B should be approached by a student from Group A. The student from Group B is to talk to the student from Group A using a whispered voice. The Group A student is to verify the message heard with the student who spoke. The student from Group B is then to identify the student from Group A.
4. The students in Group C are expected to identify at least one person in the group and describe to that person what he or she is wearing. Each student who does not do the description is to make a statement to the other person and have that individual reveal what he or she was told.
5. Having identified and conversed with each other, hold hands or remain next to each other and remove the plastic bags and cotton balls (to facilitate verification of what was heard and described).

Discussion:

1. How did the loss you experienced make you feel?
2. Were you comfortable performing the function expected of you with your limitation?
3. What do you think could have been done to make you feel less handicapped?
4. How did you feel when your "normal" level of functioning was restored?
5. How would you feel if you knew the loss you just simulated was to be permanent?
6. What impact do you think this experience might have on your future interactions with older individuals with such sensory losses?

Courtesy B. J. Glenn, former member, North Carolina State Health Coordinating Council Acute Care Committee, 1998.

not speak, as well as those clients with aphasia or altered hearing.

- Pagers, which vibrate to alert the deaf person to an incoming message, convert voice mail into e-mail that can be read.
- Real-time captioning devices allow spoken words to be typed simultaneously onto a screen.
- Interactive videodiscs have signing avatars, which are onscreen figures that sign words preprogrammed into bar codes that you select (Lipton, Goldstein, Fahnbulleh et al., 1996) or that you speak into a microphone (Walker, 2001).

The recent technological explosion continues to produce other devices through which the hearing-impaired client can communicate with health providers, including the popular laptop computer, fax machine, and PDA (personal digital assistant—an electronic computer small enough to be held in one hand). Devices such as hearing-amplified stethoscopes also allow hearing-impaired nurses to care for clients!

Case Example

Two student nurses were assigned to care for 9-year-old Timmy, who is deaf and mute. When they went into his room for assessment, he was alone and appeared anxious. No information was available as to his ability to read lips, the nurses were not sure what reading skills he had, and they did not know sign language. So, instead of using a pad and paper for communication, they decided to role-play taking vital signs by using some funny facial expressions and demonstrating on a doll.

Exercise 17-2 Sensory Loss: Hearing or Vision

Purpose: To help raise consciousness regarding loss of a sensory function.

Procedure:

- Pair up with another student. One student should be blindfolded. The other student should guide the "blind" student on a walk around the campus.
- During a 5- to 10-minute walk, the student guide should converse with the "blind" student about the route they are taking.

or

- Watch the first two minutes of a television show with the sound turned off. All students should watch the same show (e.g., the news report or a rerun of a situation comedy).
- In class, students share observations and answer the questions below.

Discussion:

1. Were perceptual differences noted? What implications do you think these differences have in working with blind or deaf clients?
2. How frustrating was it for you to be sensory-deprived? How did it make you feel?
3. What did you learn about yourself from this exercise that you can apply to your nursing clinical practice?

Box 17-1 Suggestions for Helping the Client with Sensory Loss

- Always maximize use of sensory aides, such as hearing aid, pictures, sign language, regular or laser cane (which vibrates a warning if an obstacle is within 5 feet).
- Pick the means of available communication best suited to your client.
- Keep the client informed; explain procedures in advance.
- Develop and use your own special sign to identify yourself to the client who is both blind and deaf.

For Hearing-Impaired Clients

- Always have a writing pad available.
- Always face the client when communicating, so the client can see your lips move.
- Tap on the floor or table to get client's attention via the vibration.
- Arrange for TTY (amplified telephone handset) for client with partial hearing loss.
- If unable to hear, rely primarily on visual materials.
- Arrange for closed-captioned television.
- Use text messaging on client's cell phone or e-mail at his or her computer.
- Encourage the client with hearing loss to verbalize speech, even if the person uses only a few words or the words are difficult to understand at first.

For Vision-Impaired Clients

- Let the person know when you approach by a simple touch, and always indicate when you are leaving.
- Adapt teaching for low vision by using large print, audiotaped information, or Braille.
- Do not lead or hold the client's arm when walking; instead, allow the person to take your arm.
- Use touch and close physical proximity while you are with the client; give the person something substantial to touch in your absence.
- Develop and use signals to indicate changes in pace or direction while walking.

Box 17-2 Specific Strategies to Maximize the Quality of the Communication Process

- Stand or sit so that you face the client and the client can see your facial expression and mouthing of words. Communicate in a well-lighted room.
- Use facial expressions and gestures that reinforce verbal content.
- Use gestures and speak distinctly without exaggerating words. Partially deaf clients respond best to well-articulated words spoken in a moderate, even tone.
- Write important ideas and allow the client the same option to increase the chances of communication.
- Help elderly clients adjust hearing aids. Lacking fine motor dexterity, the elderly client may not be able to insert aids to amplify hearing.
- Allow more time to communicate information.
- Become familiar with the client's communication pattern, likes, and dislikes.
- For patients with memory loss or just fatigue, present small amounts of information at a time. For print materials, use short, bulleted lists.
- Use an intermediary, such as a family member who knows sign language, to facilitate communication with deaf clients who sign.

Clients with Vision Loss

The blind person experiences the world as full of shadows and lacking in detail. Use of vocal cues (e.g., speaking as you approach) helps prevent startling the blind client. It also is helpful to mention your name as you enter the client's room. Even people who are partially blind appreciate hearing the name of the person to whom they are speaking. If computer screens are involved, a screen reader with voice synthesizer can be used, as can Braille keypads (Mates, 2000). For partially sighted clients, screen enlargers or magnifying machines are available to magnify prescription or treatment instructions.

You can use words to supply additional information to counterbalance the missing visual cues. For example, a blind, elderly client commented to the student nurse that she felt the student was uncomfortable talking with her and perhaps did not like her. Not being able to see the student, the client interpreted the hesitant uneasiness in the student's voice as evidence that the student did not wish to be with her. The student agreed with the client that she was quite uncomfortable but did not explain further. Had the client been able to see the apprehensive body posture of the student, she would have realized that the student was quite shy and might have been ill at ease with *any* interpersonal relationship. To avoid this serious error in communication, the student might have clarified the reasons for her discomfort, and the relationship could have moved forward. Clients with decreased vision, such as those with macular degeneration, can be reading-enabled via use of electronic magnifier machines. However, it may be better to rely on auditory teaching materials, such as on an audiocassette. When caring for clients with macular degeneration, remember to stand to their side, an exception to the "face them directly" rule applied with hearing loss clients. Macular degeneration clients often still have some peripheral vision.

Use of Touch. The social isolation experienced by blind clients can be profound, and the need for human contact is important. Touching the client lightly as you speak alerts the client to your presence. Voice tones and pauses that reinforce the verbal content are helpful. The client needs to be informed when the nurse is leaving the room. Compensatory interventions for the blind include a plentiful assortment of auditory stimuli, such as books on tape and music, as well as tactile stimuli.

Orientation to Environmental Hazards. When a blind client is being introduced to a new environmental setting, the nurse should orient the client by describing the size of the room and the position of the furniture and equipment. If other people are present, the nurse should name each person. A good communication strategy is to ask the other people in the room to introduce themselves to the client. In this way, the client gains an appreciation for their voice configurations. The nurse should avoid any tendency to speak with a blind client in a louder voice than usual or to enunciate words in an exaggerated manner. This may be perceived by some clients as condescending or insensitive to the nature of the handicap. Voice tones should be kept natural.

The blind client needs guidance in moving around in unfamiliar surroundings. One way of preserving the client's autonomy is to offer your arm to the client instead of taking the client's arm. Mention steps and changes in movement as they are about to occur to help the client navigate new places and differences in terrain. The client will be less socially isolated if you help him or her maintain contact with as much of the environment as the client's capabilities will allow.

Use of Braille. More sophisticated tactile methods of communication (e.g., Braille) can be used with clients who have the skills to understand. The Braille Alphabet Card has letters in both print and Braille, so nurse or client can spell out words to communicate. The **Tellatouch** is a portable machine into which the nurse types a message that emerges in Braille. It can be used by the nurse to convert a message into a punched-out paper in Braille format.

Clients with Speech and Language Deficits

Assessment of the type of aphasia a client is experiencing aids in selecting the most appropriate intervention. Expressive language problems are evidenced in an inability to find words or to associate ideas with accurate word symbols. In some instances, clients can find the correct word if given enough time and support. Other clients have difficulty organizing their words into meaningful sentences or describing a sequence of events. Clients with receptive communication deficits have trouble following directions, reading information, and writing. They hear the words but have difficulty classifying data or relating data to previous knowledge. Common properties of familiar items are not connected. This inability limits short-term memory and is sometimes misinterpreted as a short-term memory deficit associated with dementia. These clients appreciate the nurse who helps them supply the missing connections. Clients who lose both expressive and receptive communication abilities have global aphasia. Even though they appear not to understand, the nurse should explain in very simple terms what is happening. Using touch, gestures, eye movements, and squeezing of the hand can improve communication and should be attempted.

Clients with speech and language deficits become frustrated when they are not understood and may refuse to repeat themselves. The level of concentration required by the nurse to capture every word and its meaning is tiring. Clients fatigue easily and need short, positive sessions to reinforce their efforts. Otherwise, they may become nonverbal as a way of regaining energy and composure. Changes in self-image occasioned by physical changes, the uncertain recovery course and outcome of strokes, shifts in family roles, and the disruption of free-flowing verbal interaction among family members all make the loss of functional communication particularly agonizing for clients. The inability to talk about these profound changes increases the client's feelings of social isolation and fear. Even more important than verbal interaction with the aphasic client is the attitude you bring to the interaction. When you are sensitive to these concerns and able to express them, clients feel supported and reassured.

When the capacity to communicate through words is lost through illness or injury, the client must learn different ways to compensate for normal speech production skills. Any language skills that are preserved should be exploited. Other means of communication (e.g., pointing, gesturing, using pictures, and repeating phrases) can be used. Sounds and eye movements can develop into unique communication systems between nurse and client.

Case Example

Your client Mr. Lopez is totally paralyzed immediately following a rupture of a blood vessel in his brain, except he can still blink his eyes. You tell him, "Blink once for yes and twice for no."

Flexibility and accurate assessment of learning needs are key to developing the most effective teaching strategies with aphasic clients. It does not matter if the sentence does not make complete grammatical sense or is expressed in a halting way; the important thing is that the client is communicating and the communication is understandable. Anything you can do to encourage and support verbal expressive abilities is useful (Box 17-3).

Box 17-3 Strategies to Assist the Client with Speech and Language Difficulties

- Avoid prolonged, continuous conversations; instead, use frequent, short talks.
- When clients falter in written or oral expression, supply needed compensatory support.
- Praise efforts to communicate, and make learning new ways to communicate a creative game.
- Provide regular mental stimulation in a nontaxing way.
- Help clients focus on the faculties still available to them for communication.
- Allow extra time for delays in cognitive processing of information.
- Encourage the client to practice what is learned in speech therapy.

If the client is in speech therapy, you can be an important source of support. Exposure to varied social environments without the pressure to talk helps the client with a communication deficit remain connected. Point out familiar objects in the immediate environment.

Clients with Impaired Cognition or Learning Delay

Depending on the degree of delay, adaptations in nursing care would include simplifying explanations and using comforting touch, familiar objects, and so on. One study found the best pain measurement scale is the Visual Analog Scale, where your client need only to point to a picture depicting his or her level of pain (Benini, Trapanotto, Gobber et al., 2004). However, another study of older adults with cognitive impairment showed no difference among the various formats of pain scale rating instruments (Closs, Barr, Broggs et al., 2004).

Clients with Serious Mental Illness

When working with psychotic or demented clients, the nurse faces a formidable challenge in trying to establish a relationship. With clients out in the community, the most important modifications needed center on taking a more proactive approach to communicating. Research by Blazer, Hays, and Salive (1996) found that 1 of every 10 older adults in a community sample displayed symptoms of paranoia. Other studies suggest about a 2% incidence of more severe undiagnosed mental illness in community elders.

Rarely will the psychotic client approach the nurse directly; it is the nurse who must reach out and try different communication strategies. Patience and respect for the client are essential. The client generally responds to questions, but the answers are likely to be brief, and the client does not elaborate without further probes. Knowing this is the most common form of response helps the nurse depersonalize the impact of a response that conveys little information. Although the client appears to rebuff any social interaction, it is important to keep trying to connect (Box 17-4). People with mental illnesses such as schizophrenia are easily overwhelmed by the external environment (see Online Resources).

Tremeau and colleagues (2005) demonstrated that schizophrenic clients have the same expressive deficits as do depressed clients. Keeping in mind that the client's unresponsiveness to words, failure to make eye contact, unchanging facial expression, and monotonic voice are patterns of the disorder and not a commentary on your communication skills helps you to continue to engage with the client.

Box 17-4 Strategies to Assist the Client with Schizophrenia

- Keep contact short; avoid longer interactions.
- Use simple, concrete sentences.
- Use props and actions, such as games, magazines, going for walks, discussing simple topics, curling a client's hair, or manicuring the client's nails.
- Avoid crowding the client's personal space.
- Maintain eye contact while speaking in a calm voice.
- Express positive feelings by saying, "I like it when you...".
- Express negative feelings by saying, "I get uncomfortable when you...".

If the client is hallucinating or using delusions as a primary form of communication, you should neither challenge their validity directly nor enter into a prolonged discussion of illogical thinking. Instead, say, "I know that your sense that God is going to destroy the world tomorrow seems very real to you, but I don't see it that way."

Often you can identify the underlying theme the client is trying to convey with the delusional statement. For example, you might say to the client making the previous statement, "It sounds as though you feel powerless and afraid at this moment." The technique of listening to the client carefully, using alert posture, nodding to demonstrate active listening, and trying to make sense out of the underlying feelings, models effective communication for the client and helps you decode nonsensical messages. If you are willing to look beyond the misleading exterior to the way the individual experiences reality and wishes to be seen by others, a different picture can emerge. A mark of the growing trust in a relationship with a psychotic client is expanded rational conversation and a willingness to remain with the nurse for increasing periods of time. Exercise 17-3 may help you gain some understanding of communication problems experienced by the client with schizophrenia.

Clients Experiencing Environmental Deprivation

It is not that the client actually is forgotten, but nurses in the high-tech ICU environment often forget that the client is still a psychosocial being. The human concerns

Exercise 17-3 Schizophrenia Communication Simulation

Purpose: To gain insight into communication deficits encountered by clients with schizophrenia.

Procedure:
1. Break class into groups of three (triads) by counting off 1, 2, 3.
2. Person #1 (the nurse) reads a paragraph of rules to the client, and then quizzes him or her afterward about the content.
3. Person #2 (the client with schizophrenia) listens to everything and tries to answer the nurse's questions correctly to get 100% on the test.
4. Person #3 (representing the mental illness) speaks loudly and continuously in the client's ear while the nurse is communicating, saying things like "You are so stupid," "You have done bad things," and "It is coming to get you" over and over.

Discussion:
Did any client have 100% recall? Ask the client to share how difficult is it to communicate to the nurse when you are "hearing voices."

Courtesy Ann Newman, PhD, University North Carolina, Charlotte.

of the client assume a secondary priority, receiving less attention than the more immediate physical needs. In the rush to stabilize the client physically, communication is of poor quality; nurses verbalize less often or are less sensitive to the client's behavioral cues (Turnock, 1991).

When a client is not fully alert, it is not uncommon for nurses to speak in the client's presence in ways they would not if they thought the client could fully understand what is being said. Such situations are unfortunate for two reasons: first, because hearing is the last sense to go, and clients have been able to repeat whole conversations spoken when they were supposedly unconscious of their surroundings; and second, because the client may hear only parts of what is said and misinterpret it. A rule of thumb is to never say anything you would not want the client to hear.

In addition to conveying a caring, compassionate attitude, the nurse may use several of the strategies for communicating listed in Box 17-5.

An example of orienting cues would be the labeling of meals as breakfast, lunch, or dinner. Linking events to routines (e.g., saying, "The x-ray technician will take your chest x-ray right after lunch") helps secure the client in time and space. When the client is unable or unwilling to engage in a dialogue, you should continue to initiate communication in a one-way mode (Turnock, 1991).

Box 17-5 Strategies for Communicating with Clients in the ICU

- Encourage the client to display pictures or a simple object from home.
- Orient the client to the environment.
- Frequently provide information about the client's condition and progress.
- Reassure the client that cognitive and psychological disturbances are common.
- Give explanations before procedures by providing information about the sounds, sights, and feelings the client is experiencing.
- Provide the client with frequent orienting cues to time and place.

Case Example

Nurse: I am going to give you your bath now. The water will feel a little warm to you. After your bath, your wife will be in to see you. She stayed in the waiting room last night because she wanted to be with you. *(No answer is necessary if the client is unable to talk, but the sound of a human voice and attention to the client's unspoken concerns can be very healing.)*

The client should be called by name. Nurses need to identify themselves and explain procedures in simple language even if the client does not appear particularly alert. Clients who are awake or even semi-alert should not be allowed to stare at a blank ceiling for extended periods. Changing the client's position frequently benefits the person physiologically and offers an opportunity for episodic dialogue with the nurse. The nurse is often in a position to create a more stimulating environment. For example, a simple animated conversation that taps into the client's world of knowledge can provide a source of ongoing emotional support because of the indirect recognition of the client's intellectual and perceptual qualities.

If the client in the ICU becomes temporarily delusional or experiences hallucinations, you can use strategies similar to those used with the psychotic client. The client is reassured if the nurse does not appear bothered by the symptoms and is able to confirm to the client that experiencing strange sensations, thoughts, and feelings is a common occurrence in the ICU.

Clients Whose Language Differs from That of Care Providers

Many of the strategies listed above (e.g., pictographs) can be used to facilitate communication. Translators introduce a third person into the interpersonal communication process, a circumstance that can lead to difficulties. Consider the ethical implications of the process.

> **Ethical Dilemma ■ *What Would You Do?***
> Working in a health department clinic, the nurse—through a Spanish-speaking translator—interviews a 46-year-old married woman about the missing results of her recent breast biopsy for suspected cancer. Because the translator is of the same culture as the client and holds the same cultural belief that suicide is shameful, he chooses to withhold from the nurse information he obtained about a recent suicide attempt. If this information remains hidden from the nurse and doctor, could this adversely affect the client? What ethical principle is being violated?

SUMMARY

This chapter discusses the specialized communication needs of clients with communication deficits. Basic issues and applications for communicating with clients experiencing sensory loss of hearing and sight are outlined. Sensory stimulation and compensatory channels of communication are needed for clients with sensory deprivation. The mentally ill client has intact senses, but information processing and language are affected by the disorder. It is important for the nurse to develop a proactive communication approach with learning-impaired or psychotic clients. The aphasic client has trouble expressing and/or receiving communication. Nurses can develop alternative methods of communicating with these clients. Clients in the ICU can experience a temporary distortion of reality. Such clients need frequent cues that orient them to time and place as well as sensory stimulation.

REFERENCES

Abel SM, Sass-Kortsak A, Naugler JJ: The role of high frequency hearing in age related speech: understanding deficits, *Scand Audiol* 29(3):131–138, 2000.

Benini F, Trapanotto BF, Gobber D et al.: Evaluating pain induced by venipuncture in pediatric patients with developmental delay, *Clin J Pain* 20(3):156–163, 2004.

Berke J: Wireless wars: text communication for the deaf [online article], n.d.; retrieved 5/24/05 from http://deafness.about.com/cs/instantandmobile/a/wireless.htm.

Blazer D, Hays J, Salive ME: Factors associated with paranoid symptoms in a community sample of older adults, *Gerontologist* 36(1):70–75, 1996.

Closs SJ, Barr B, Broggs M et al.: A comparison of five pain assessment scales for nursing home residents with varying degrees of cognitive impairment, *J Pain Symptom Manage* 27(3):196–205, 2004.

Cooper M: The intersection of technology and care in the ICU, *Adv Nurs Sci* 15(3):23–32, 1993.

Finitzo T, AAP Joint Committee on Infant Hearing: Year 2000 position statement: principles and guidelines for early hearing detection and intervention programs, *Pediatrics* 106(4):798–817, 2000.

Herring R, Hock J: Health professionals, *N J Med* 97(2):45–49, 2000.

Kalayam B, Meyers BS, Kakuma T et al.: Age at onset of geriatric depression and sensorineural hearing deficits, *Biol Psychiatry* 38(10):649–658, 1995.

Li Y, Bain L, Steinberg AG: Parental decision making and choice of communication modality for the child who is deaf, *Arch Pediatr Adolesc Med* 157(2):162–168, 2003.

Lipton DS, Goldstein MF, Fahnbulleh FW et al.: The interactive video-questionnaire: a new technology for interviewing deaf persons, *Am Ann Deaf* 14(5):370–378, 1996.

Mackenzie C: *Adult spoken discourse, Int J Lang Commun Disorders* 35(2):269–285, 2000.

Mates BT: *Adaptive technology for the Internet*, Chicago, 2000, American Library Association.

Naylor MD, Stephens C, Bowles KH et al.: Cognitively impaired older adults: from hospital to home, *Am J Nurs* 105(2):52–61, 2005.

O'Day BL, Killeen M, Iezzoni LI: Improving health care experiences of persons who are blind or have low vision: suggestions from focus groups, *Am J Med Qual* 19(5): 193–200, 2004.

Power MR, Power D: Everyone here speaks TXT: deaf people using SMS in Australia and the rest of the world, *J Deaf Stud Deaf Educ* 9(3):333–343, 2004.

Powrie E: Primary health care provision for adults with a learning disability, *J Adv Nurs* 42(4):413–423, 2003.

Rutledge D: What strategies are nurses using to overcome communication barriers? *ONS News* 19(9):1, 4, 2004.

Stock S: When silence isn't golden, *Advance for Nurses* 4(2):22–23, 40, 2002.

Tremeau F, Malaspina D, Duval F et al.: Facial expressiveness in patients with schizophrenia compared to depressed patients and nonpatient comparison subjects, *Am J Psychiatry* 162(1): 92–101, 2005.

Turnock C: Communicating with patients in ICU, *Nurs Stand* 9(5):38–40, 1991.

van der Pols JC, Bates CJ, McGraw PV et al.: Visual acuity measurements in a national sample of British elderly people, *Br J Ophthalmol* 84(2):165–170, 2000.

Walker LA: They're breaking the sound barrier, *Parade Magazine,* May 13, 2001, pp. 4–5.

Williams AM, Irurita VF: Therapeutic and non-therapeutic interpersonal interactions: the patient's perspective, *J Clin Nurs* 13(7):806–815, 2004.

Chapter 18

Communicating with Children

Kathleen Underman Boggs

OUTLINE

OBJECTIVES

At the end of the chapter, the reader will be able to:

1. Identify how developmental levels impact the child's ability to participate in interpersonal relationships with caregivers.
2. Briefly discuss one research-based application in communicating with a child.
3. Describe modifications in communication strategies to meet the specialized needs of children.
4. Describe interpersonal techniques needed to interact with concerned parents of ill children.
5. Discuss application on one research study results to clinical practice.

A revolution is occurring in the world of pediatric medicine which will have profound effects on the way we practice and on the venue in which patients are encountered...with unique opportunities to actively prevent future illness by altering life habits at an early stage.

(Bernstein & Shelov, 2000)

If a child lives with criticism, he learns to condemn.
If a child lives with ridicule, he learns to be shy.
If a child lives with acceptance, he learns to love.
If a child lives with honesty, he learns what truth is.
If a child lives with fairness, he learns justice.

(Anonymous)

Chapter 18 is designed to help you recognize and apply communication concepts related to the nurse-client relationship in pediatric clinical situations. Each nursing situation represents a unique application of communication strategies. Tools needed by caregivers to provide effective and ethical care are cognitive, interpersonal, and attitudinal. For each of these domains, the child's and family's socioeconomic status and cultural background must be considered. As the prior quotation reveals, major changes in society are having an impact on the health care of children. Some research suggests that societal changes have also increased the communication initiatives taken by children with health care providers (Meeuwesen & Kaptein, 1996).

Communicating with children at different age levels requires modifications of the skills learned in previous chapters. By understanding the child's cognitive, developmental, and functional level, you are able to select the most appropriate communication strategies. Children undergo significant age-related changes in the ability to process cognitive information and in the capacity to interact effectively with the environment. To have an effective therapeutic relationship with a child, understand the feelings and thought processes from the child's perspective. Developing rapport requires that you understand the interpersonal world as the child perceives it and convey honesty, respect, and acceptance of feelings.

BASIC CONCEPTS

Childhood is very different from adulthood. A child has fewer life experiences from which to draw and is still in the process of developing skills needed for reasoning and communicating. Every child's concept of health and illness must be considered within a developmental framework. Erikson's (1963) concepts of ego development and Piaget's (1972) description of the progressive development of the child's cognitive thought processes together form the theoretical basis for the child-centered nursing interventions described in this chapter. Both theorists say that the child's thought processes, ways of perceiving the world, judgments, and emotional responses to life situations are qualitatively different from those of the adult. Cognitive and psychosocial development unfold according to an ordered hierarchical scheme, increasing in depth and complexity as the child matures.

Table 18-1 Stages of Cognitive Development

Age	Piaget's Stage	Characteristics	Language Development
Birth–2 years	Sensorimotor	Infant learns by manipulating objects. At birth, reflexive communication, then moves through six stages to reach actual thinking.	**Presymbolic** Communication largely nonverbal. Vocabulary of more than four words by 12 months, increases to >200 words and use of short sentences before age 2 years.
2–6 years	Preoperational	Beginning use of symbolic thinking. Imaginative play. Masters reversibility.	**Symbolic** Actual use of structured grammar and language to communicate. Uses pronouns. Average vocabulary >10,000 words by age 6 years.
7–11 years	Concrete operations	Logical thinking. Masters use of numbers and other concrete ideas such as classification and conservation.	Mastery of passive tense by age 7 years and complex grammatical skills by age 10 years.
12+ years	Formal operations	Abstract thinking. Futuristic; takes a broader, more theoretical perspective.	Near adult-like skills.

Adapted from Piaget J: *The child's conception of the world,* Savage, MD, 1972, Littlefield, Adams.

The trend toward family-centered health care of children will continue with attention to family diversity and family processes in "successful" families. A growing body of research is documenting relationships between such processes and child health (Wertlieb, 2003).

The Child's Developmental Environment

Piaget's (1972) descriptions of stages of cognitive development provide a valuable contribution toward understanding the dimensions of a child's perceptions. Cognitive development and early language development are integrally related. Although current developmental theorists expand on Piaget's theoretical model by recognizing the effects of the parent-child relationship and a stimulating environment on developing communication abilities, his work forms the foundation for the understanding of childhood cognitive development. Piaget observed cognitive development occurring in sequential stages (Table 18-1). The ages are only approximated, since Piaget himself was not specific.

Piaget's Stages

In the first stage of cognitive maturation, the **sensorimotor period**, the infant explores his or her own body as a source of information, gradually modifying reflexive responses to include more purposeful interactions with the environment. As the infant gains more motor control, cognitive behaviors become more intentional, and the infant begins to differentiate between objects in the environment. At about 8 months of age, the infant clearly is able to distinguish the primary caregiver in the environment from less familiar persons. The infant may begin to vocalize some awareness that objects may be dissimilar in nature and function. By the end of this stage, the infant is developing an understanding of symbolic thinking and thus begins to use language to communicate.

The second stage of cognitive development emerges around the age of 2 years. In this stage, known as the **preoperational period**, the toddler is markedly egocentric, unable to see another's viewpoint, and for this reason unable to engage productively in interactive, cooperative play. However, there is a genuine interest in being with other children and playing alongside them in parallel play. In the preoperational stage of cognitive development, children are not able to make cognitive connections between past events and a given end result.

The preschool child is still unable to distinguish fantasy from reality, to consider another's viewpoint, and to accept the possibility of alternative options. Images are developed through concrete devices. Verbal explanations should be accompanied by opportunities for the child to use concrete, touchable objects and to play in a cooperative, turn-taking fashion with other children. As the child makes the transition to the concrete operational stage, there is a growing ability to categorize information and to internalize more structures into thinking about things. At the end of the preoperational period in the early elementary school years, the child begins to notice the cause-and-effect relationships in situations and is able to describe differences in objects having some similarities (Crain, 1992; Piaget, 1972).

The third stage of cognitive development, referred to as the **concrete operations period**, extends from approximately 7 to 11 years of age and beyond. The child now is capable of structural cooperative play with complex rules. Children can comprehend concepts presented in graphic detail and are beginning to appreciate the possibility of developing alternative solutions to problems. The child is able to distinguish between concrete, disparate groups of objects. Health teaching with children in this stage of cognitive development should be closely aligned with reality and presented with concrete images.

The final stage of cognitive development described by Piaget is the **formal operations period**. Starting at about 12 years of age in some children and continuing through adulthood, abstract reality and logical thought processes emerge. Cooperation, collaboration, and social conscience are noted. The formal operational thinker is able to consider several alternative options at the same time and to set long-term goals. Adolescents who have developed formal operational thinking abilities are capable of making health-related judgments about their care. Whenever possible, they should be given the opportunity to exercise this right.

Wide individual differences exist in the intellectual functioning of same-age children. Variations also occur across situations, so that the child under stress or in a different environment may process information at a lower level than he or she would under normal conditions. Because two children of the same chronological age may have quite different skills as information processors, the nurse needs to assess level of functioning. Language alternatives familiar to one child because of certain life experiences may not be useful in providing health care and teaching with another. Application of nursing care to children draws heavily from Erikson's model of psychosocial development. Integrating cognitive and psychosocial developmental approaches into communication with children at different ages enhances its effectiveness.

Gender Differences in Communication

In a study by Bernzweig, Takayama, Phibbs, and colleagues (1997), children ages 4 to 14 were shown to be more satisfied when their care provider (physician) was of the same gender, whereas their parents were more satisfied if the physician was a woman. Some of the factors identified in this study were that female physicians engaged in more social conversation, spent more time giving encouragement and reassurance, and more commonly spoke directly to children when gathering information. Use of good age-appropriate communication strategies probably outweighs gender as a factor in successful communication with a child, but gender cannot be excluded as a factor affecting this communication.

Developing an Evidence-Based Practice

Bouve LR, Rozmus CL Giordano P: Preparing parents for their child's transfer from PICU to the pediatric floor, *Appl Nurs Res* 12(3):114-120, 1999.

Bouve, Rozmus, and Giordano studied the use of a written information letter to prepare 50 parents for their children's transfer from a pediatric intensive care unit to a regular pediatric floor. The study measured effects on the parents' anxiety states in both a control group and a treatment group who received a letter containing information about the transfer and emphasizing the positive aspects of the transfer. The Spielberger State-Trait Anxiety Inventory questionnaire was administered 24 hours prior to transfer, and again one hour prior to transfer.

Results: When differences in anxiety level were controlled for, the group who received the explanation letter after the first measure of their anxiety had a significantly lower anxiety at one hour prior to transfer than did members of the control group who did not receive this letter.

Application to Your Clinical Practice: Parents' levels of anxiety affect the ability of a child to adjust to in-hospital transfers. Based on these study findings, nurses could effectively reduce parental anxiety by providing written explanations prior to a child's transfer between units.

Understanding the Ill Child's Needs

Difficulties arise in adult-child communications, in part because of the child's cognitive level in an early developmental stage. Children have limited social experience in interpreting subtle nuances of facial expression, inflection, and word meanings. When illness and physical or developmental disabilities occur during formative years, situational stressors are added that affect the way children perceive themselves and the environment. Illness may lead to significant alterations in role relationships with family and peers. The nurse needs to assess not only the physical care needs of the child but also the impact of the illness on the child's self-esteem and on his or her relationships with family and friends. Factors affecting the child's response may include the chronicity of illness, its impact on lifestyle, the child's cognitive understanding of the disease process, and the family's ability to cope with care demands.

If the child needs to be hospitalized, this is a *situational crisis* for the child and the entire family. Hospitalization is always stressful. Hospitalized children have to contend not only with physical changes but also with possible separation from family and friends as well as living in a strange, frightening, and probably hurtful environment. The family needs to learn new interactional patterns and coping strategies that take into consideration the meaning of an illness and disability in family life. Keeping illness a "secret" is not an effective means of coping. *Prehospitalization preparation* needs to be done to decrease the child's anxiety. Prior to elective procedures, many hospitals now offer orientation education tours to youngsters. There are many good books designed to prepare children for their hospitalization available in most public libraries.

APPLICATIONS

While children historically have not been the focus of study, research studies have contributed to our knowledge of child learning and development. According to Berman (2003), findings are limited due to overreliance on what parents have told us. Berman feels treatment of children is characterized by perceptions that all children are similar, without consideration of differences due to age, gender, race, or culture. To give one example, many of the medicines we use to treat children have been tested only on adults by pharmaceutical companies.

Numerous descriptive studies have identified major sources of stress for parents of critically ill children. These include uncertainty about current condition or prognosis and lack of knowledge about how to best help their hospitalized child or how to deal with their child's response (Melnyk, Small, & Carno, 2004). While more nursing research is being conducted on effective communication with both parents and their ill children, many of the applications we will discuss are based more on experience than on research.

Assessment

Assessing a child's reaction to illness requires knowing the child's normal patterns of communication. Interactions are observed between parent and child. The child's behavioral responses to the entire interpersonal environment (including nurse and peers) are assessed. Are the child's interactions age-appropriate? Are behaviors organized, or is the child unable to complete activities?

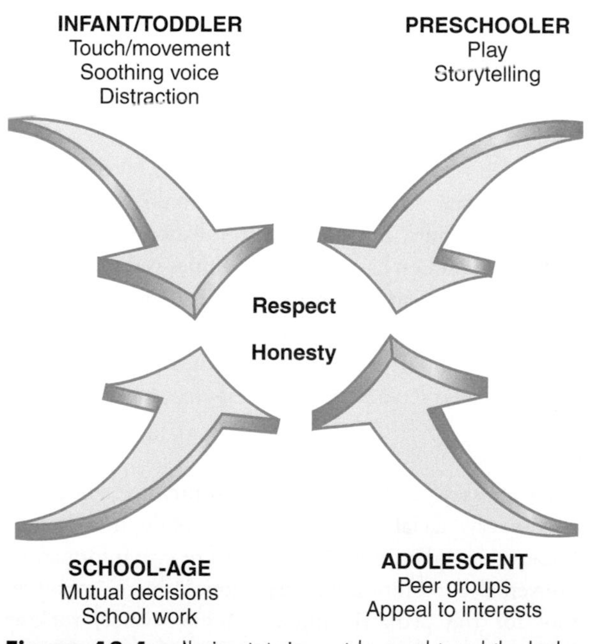

Figure 18-1 • Nursing strategies must be geared toward the developmental level of the child.

Does the child act out an entire play sequence, or is such play fragmented and disorganized? Do the child's interactions with others suggest imagination and a broad repertoire of relating behaviors, or is communication devoid of possibilities? Once baseline data have been collected, you can plan specific communication strategies to meet the specialized needs of the child client (Figure 18-1). An overview of nursing adaptations needed to communicate effectively with children is summarized in Box 18-1.

Box 18-1 Nurse-Child Communication Strategies: Adapting Communication to Meet the Ill Child's Needs

- Develop an understanding of age-related norms of development.
- Let the child know you are interested in him or her; convey respect and authenticity.
- Assess and use familiar vocabulary at the child's level of understanding.
- Assess the child's needs in relation to the immediate situation.
- Assess the child's capacity to cope successfully with change.
- Let the child know how to summon you (call bell, etc.).
- Use nonverbal communication and alternatives to verbalization (e.g., tactile [soothing strokes]; kinesthetic [rocking]; visual [eye contact]; and reassuring facial expressions).
- Work to develop trust through honesty and consistency in meeting the child's needs.
- Use "transitional objects" such as familiar pictures or toys from home.
- Interpret the child's nonverbal cues verbally to him or her.
- Use humor and active listening to foster the relationship.
- Respect the child's privacy.
- Get down to the child's height; don't tower over him or her.
- Increase coping skills by providing play opportunities; use creative, unstructured play, medical role-play, and pantomime.
- Instead of conversation, use some indirect age-appropriate communication techniques (e.g., storytelling, picture drawing, and creative writing).
- Use alternative, supplementary communication devices for children with specialized needs (e.g., sign language and computer-enhanced communication programs).

Regression as a Form of Childhood Communication

A severe illness can cause a child to show behaviors that are reminiscent of an earlier stage of development. A certain amount of regression is normal. Common behaviors include whining, teasing other children, demanding undue attention, withdrawal, or having toileting "accidents." In most cases, the underlying dynamic is the powerlessness the child feels in attempting to cope with a potentially overwhelming, frightening environment. Reassuring the parent that this is a common response to the stress of illness can be helpful.

Because children have limited life experience to draw from, they exhibit a narrower range of behaviors in coping with threat. The quiet, overly compliant child who does not complain may be more frightened than the child who screams or cries. This should alert you to the child's emotional distress. The nurse needs to obtain detailed information regarding the usual behavioral responses of the family and child. Some behaviors that look regressive may be a typical behavioral response for the child (e.g., the 2-year-old who wants a bedtime bottle). A complete baseline history offers a good counterpoint for assessing the meaning of current behaviors.

Age-Appropriate Communication

Whenever possible, you should communicate using words familiar to the child. Ask his or her parents what specific words the child uses for toileting, pain, and other conditions. Parents are also valuable resources in helping interpret behavioral data; if possible, they should be part of the nurse's interpersonal relationship with the child. An assessment of vocabulary and understanding is essential in fostering communications. You might assist a child who is having difficulty finding the right words by reframing what the child has said and repeating it in a slightly different way. Another strategy is to ask the parent what words the child uses to express specific health-related concerns.

The afflicted child's peers often have difficulty accepting individual differences created by health deviations. They lack the knowledge and sensitivity to deal with physical changes that they do not understand, as evidenced by "bald" jokes about the child receiving chemotherapy. Children with hidden disorders such as diabetes, some forms of epilepsy, or minimal brain dysfunction are particularly susceptible to interpersonal distress. For example, it may be difficult for diabetics to regulate their intake of fast foods when all of their friends are able to eat what they want. When peer pressure is at its peak in adolescence, a teenager with a newly diagnosed convulsive seizure disorder may find it difficult to tell peers he no longer can ride his bicycle or drive a car. Unless the family and nurse provide appropriate interpersonal support, such children have to cope with an indistinct assault to their self-concept all by themselves. A summary of age-appropriate strategies is provided in Box 18-2.

Communicating with Children with Psychological Behavioral Problems

One out of 10 adolescents and children in our society suffer from a mental illness These illnesses lead to some level of interactional problems, which may be encountered by nurses in schools, hospitals, or clinics treating common physical illnesses. Discussion of mental illness and appropriate interventions is beyond the scope of this book. Please refer to a multitude of hotlinks available through U.S. Health and Human Services website in the Maternal Child Health Library (see Online Resources).

Communicating with Physically Ill Children in the Hospital and Ambulatory Clinic

Overestimating a child's understanding of information about illness results in confusion, increased anxiety, anger, or sadness. Beyond physiological care, ill children of all ages need support from every member of the health team—support that they normally would receive from parents. The nurse must provide stimulation to talk, listen, and play. Children have major difficulties verbalizing their true feelings about the treatment experience. The nurse can be a primary resource in adapting interventions to meet the ill child's needs. Many agencies also have play therapists who serve as excellent resources for staff.

Infants

Cues to assessment of the preverbal infant include tone of the cry, facial appearance, and body movements. Because the infant uses the senses to receive information, nonverbal communication (e.g., touch) is an important tool for the pediatric nurse. Tone of voice, rocking motion, use of distraction, and a soothing touch can be used in addition to or in conjunction with verbal

Box 18-2 Key Points in Communicating with Children According to Age Group

Infants

Nonverbal communication is a primary mode.
Biologically "wired" to pay close attention to words. In first year are able to distinguish all conversational sounds.
Infants are bonded to primary caregivers only. Those older than 8 months may display separation anxiety when separated from parent or when approached by strangers.

Use Kinesthetic Communication

Use stroking, soft touching, holding.
Use motion (e.g., rocking) to reassure. Allow freedom of movement, and avoid restraining when possible.
Learn specifically how the primary caregiver provides care in terms of sleeping, bathing, and feeding, and attempt to mimic these approaches.

Hold Close to Adapt to Limited Vision (20/200-20/300 at Birth)

Encourage the infant's caregivers (parents) to use a lot of intimate space interaction (e.g., 8-18 inches). Mimic the same when trust is established.

Talk with Infants

Talk with infants in normal conversational tones; soothe them with crooning voice tone.

Establish Trust

Use parents to give care. Arrange for one or both parents to remain within the child's sight.

Shorten Your Stature

Sit down on chair, stool, or carpet to decrease posture superiority, so as to look less imposing.

Handle Separation Anxiety When Primary Caregiver Is Absent

Establish rapport with the caregiver (parent) and encourage them to be with child and reassure child that staff will be there if they are away. At first keep at least 2 feet between nurse and infant. Talk to and touch the infant and initially smile often. Provide for kinesthetic approaches; offer self while infant is protesting (e.g., stay with the child; pick the child up and rock or walk; talk to the child about Mommy and Daddy and how much the child cares for them).

1- to 3-Year-Olds

Child begins to talk around 1 year of age; learns nine new words a day after 18 months.
By age 2, begins to use phrases; should be able to respond to "what" and "where" type questions.
By age 3, uses and understands sentences.

Adapt to Limited Vocabulary and Verbal Skills

Make explanations brief and clear. Use the child's own vocabulary words for basic care activities (e.g., use the child's words for defecate [poop, goodies] and urinate [pee-pee, tinkle]). Learn and use self-name of the child.
Rephrase the child's message in a simple, complete sentence; avoid baby talk. Child should be able to follow two simple directions.

Continue to Use Kinesthetic Communication

Allow ambulating where possible (e.g., using toddler chairs or walkers). Pull the child in a wagon often if child cannot achieve mobility.

Facilitate Child's Struggle with Issues of Autonomy and Control

Allow the child some control (e.g., "Do you want a half a glass or a whole glass of milk?").
Reassure the child if he or she displays some regressive behavior (e.g., if child wets pants, say, "We will get a dry pair of pants and let you find something fun to do.").
Allow the child to express anger and to protest about his or her care (e.g., "It's okay to cry when you are angry or hurt.").
Allow the child to sit up or walk as often as possible and as soon as possible after intrusive or hurtful procedures (e.g., "It's all over and we can do something more fun.").

Box 18-2 Key Points in Communicating with Children According to Age Group—*Cont'd.*

Use nondirective modes, such as reflecting an aspect of appearance or temperament (e.g., "You smile so often.") or playing with a toy and slowly coming closer to and including the child in play.

Recognize Fear of Bodily Injury

Show hands (free of hurtful items) and say, "There is nothing to hurt you. I came to play/talk."

Accept Egocentrism and Possible Regression

Allow child to be self-oriented. Use distraction if another child wants the same item or toy rather than expect the child to share. Some children cope with stress of hospitalization by regressing to an earlier mode of behavior, such as wanting to suck on a bottle, etc.

Redirect Behavior to a Verbal Level

Use a nondirective approach. Sit down and join the parallel play of the child. Reflect messages sent by toddler (nonverbally) in a verbal and nonverbal manner (e.g., "Yes, that toy does lots of interesting and fun things.").

Deal with Separation Anxiety

Accept protesting when parent(s) leave. Hug, rock the child, and say, "You miss Mommy and Daddy! They miss you too." Play peek-a-boo games with child. Make a big deal about saying, "Now I am here."

Show an interest in one of the child's favorite toys. Say, "I wonder what it does" or the like. If the child responds with actions, reflect them back.

3- to 5-Year-Olds

Most children this age can make themselves understood to strangers.

They speak in sentences but are unable to comprehend abstract ideas.

Begins to understand cause-and-effect relationships; should be able to understand "If you do…, then we can…".

Can follow a series of up to four directions, unless anxious about being hurt, etc.

Use Age-Appropriate, Simple Vocabulary

Use simple vocabulary; avoid lengthy explanations. Focus on the present, not the distant future; use concrete, meaningful references. For example, say, "Mommy will be back after you eat your lunch" (instead of "at 1 o'clock").

Behave in a Culturally Sensitive Manner

In some cultures, child is unable to tolerate direct eye-to-eye contact, so use some eye contact and attending posture. Sit or stoop, and use a slow, soft tone of voice.

Attempt to Decrease Anxiety About Being Hurt

May react negatively and with increased anxiety if a long explanation is given regarding a painful procedure.

Complete the procedure as quickly as possible; give explanations about its purpose afterward. For example, say, "Jimmy, I'm going to give you a shot," then quickly administer the injection. Then say, "There. All done. It's okay to cry when you hurt. I'd complain, too. This medicine will make your tummy feel better." Some experts suggest you create a "safe zone" in the child's bed by doing all painful procedures elsewhere, perhaps in a treatment room.

Use Play Therapy

Explanations and education can be done using imagination (puppetry, drama with dress-ups), music, or drawings.

Allow the child to play with safe equipment used in treatment. Talk about the needed procedure happening to a doll or teddy bear, and state simply how it will occur and be experienced. Use sensory data (e.g., "The teddy bear will hear a buzzing sound.").

Use Distraction and a Sense of Humor

Tell corny jokes and laugh with the child.

Allow for Child's Continuing Need to Have Control

Provide for many choices (e.g., "Do you want to get dressed now or after breakfast?").

Box 18-2 Key Points in Communicating with Children According to Age Group—*Cont'd.*

5- to 10-Year-Olds

Are developing their ability to comprehend. Can understand sequencing of events if clearly explained: "First this happens…, then…".
Can use written materials to learn.

Facilitate Child to Assume Increased Responsibility for Own Health Care Practices

Include the child in concrete explanations about condition, treatment, and protocols.
Use draw-a-person to identify basic knowledge the child has, and build on it.
Use some of the same words the child uses in giving explanations.
Use sensory information in giving explanations (e.g., "You will smell alcohol in the cast room.").
Reinforce basic health self-care activities in teaching.

Respect Increased Need for Privacy

Knock on the door before entering; tell the client when and for what reasons you will need to return to his or her room.

11-Year-Olds and Older

Have an increased comprehension about possible negative threats to life or body integrity, yet some difficulty in adhering to long-term goals.
Continue to use mainly concrete rather than abstract thinking.
Are struggling to establish identity and be independent.

Verbalize Issues

Talk about treatment protocols that require giving up immediate gratifications for long-term gain. Explore alternative options (e.g., tell a diabetic adolescent who must give up after-school fries with friends that he or she could save two breads and four fats exchanges to have a milkshake). If you use abstract thinking, look for nonverbal cues (e.g., puzzled face) that may indicate lack of understanding. Then clarify in more concrete terms.

Remember That Confidentiality May Be an Issue

Reassure the adolescent about the confidentiality of your discussion, but clearly state the limits of this confidentiality. If, for example, the child should talk of killing himself, this information needs to be shared with parents and staff.

Allow Sense of Independence

Allow participation in decision making, wearing own clothes. Avoid an authoritarian approach when possible. Avoid a judgmental approach. Use a clarifying and qualifying approach. Actively listen. Accept regression.

Be Age-Appropriate

If teen uses colloquial language or street slang, you can couch your dialogue with the use of some of the client's words.

Assess Sexual Awareness and Maturation

Offer self and a willingness to listen. Provide value-free, accurate information.

Updated 2005, from material originally supplied by Joyce Ruth, MSN, University of North Carolina, Charlotte, College of Health Sciences.

explanations. Face-to-face position, bending or moving to the child's eye level, maintaining eye contact, and making a reassuring facial expression further help in interactions with infants.

Anticipate developmental behaviors such as "stranger anxiety" in infants between 9 and 18 months of age. Rather than reaching to pick a child up immediately, the nurse might smile and extend a hand toward the child or stroke the child's arm before attempting to hold the child. In this way, the nurse acknowledges the infant's inability to generalize to unfamiliar caregivers. If the child is able to talk, asking the child his or her name and pointing out a notable pleasant physical characteristic conveys the impression that the nurse sees the child client as a unique person. To a tiny child, this treatment can be synonymous with caring.

Toddlers

Almost all small children receiving invasive treatment feel some threat to their safety and security, one of Maslow's hierarchy of human needs. This need is exaggerated in toddlers and young children, who cannot articulate their needs or understand why they are ill. To help the child's comprehension, nurses use phrases rather than long sentences and repeat words for emphasis. Because the toddler has a limited vocabulary, the caretaker may need to put into words the feelings that the ill child is conveying nonverbally.

Evaluate the agency environment. Is it safe? Does it allow for some independence and autonomy? Care in the ambulatory setting is facilitated if a parent or caregiver is present. Care in the hospital is enhanced by agency policies that promote parent-child contact (e.g., unlimited visiting hours, rooming in, or use of audiocassettes of a parent's voice). Familiar objects make the environment feel safer. Use transitional objects such as a teddy bear, blanket, or favorite toy to remind the alone or frightened child that the security of the parent is still available even when he or she is not physically present. Some hospitals have a prehospital orientation in which they present small children with a familiar transitional object to bring with them when they return for the actual hospitalization.

Distraction is a successful strategy with toddlers in ambulatory settings. Use of stuffed animals, wind-up toys, or "magic" exam lights that blow out "like a birthday candle" can turn fright into delight. One advanced practice nurse recommended the use of a musical watch during otoscopic exams, telling the child that "children who sit very still can hear a song when I look into their ears" (Flarity, 1997). The author wears a small toy bear on her stethoscope and asks the child to help listen for a heart sound from the bear, so the child focuses on the toy, making it easier to listen to the child's heart.

Preschoolers

Throughout the preoperational period, young children tend to interpret language in a literal way. For example, the child who is told that he will be "put to sleep" during the operation tomorrow may think it means the same as the action recently taken for a pet dog who was too ill to live. Children do not ask for clarification, so messages can be misunderstood quite easily.

Preschool children have limited auditory recall and are unable to process auditory information quickly. They have a short attention span. Verbal communication with the preschool child should be clear, succinct, and easy to understand.

Before the age of 7 years, most children cannot make a clear distinction between fantasy and reality. Everything is "real," and anything strange is perceived as potentially harmful. Anything the nurse can do to make the child's environment stable, real, and manageable will be helpful to the preschool client.

In the hospital, young children need frequent concrete reminders to reinforce reality. Assigning the same caregiver reduces insecurity. Visiting the preschooler at the same time each day and posting family pictures are simple strategies to reduce the child's fears of abandonment. The nurse can link information to activities of daily living. For example, saying, "Your mother will come after you take your nap" rather than "at 2 o'clock" is much more understandable to the preschool client.

Assessment of the preschooler's ability to communicate involves a careful evaluation of the child's actual level of understanding. Children need to be assessed for misconceptions and troubling problems, preferably using free play and fantasy storytelling exercises. Egocentrism can be a normal developmental process that may prevent children from understanding why they cannot have a drink when they are fasting before a scheduled test. Explanations given a long time beforehand may not be remembered. If something is going to hurt, you should be forthright about it, while at the same time reassuring the child that he or she will have the appropriate support. Simple explanations reduce the child's anxiety. No child should ever be left to figure out what is happening without some type of simple explanation. Reinforce the child's communication by praising the willingness to tell you how he or she feels. Avoid judging or censuring the child who yells such things as, "I hate you" or, "You are mean for hurting me." Box 18-2 can help you focus on specific communication strategies with the hospitalized preschooler.

Play as a Communication Strategy. The preschooler lacks a suitable vocabulary to express complex thoughts and feelings. Small children cannot picture what they have never experienced. Play is an effective means by which a puzzling and sometimes painful real world can be approached. Play allows the child to create a concrete experience of something unknown and potentially frightening. By constructing a situation in play, the child is able to put together the components of the situation in ways that promote recognition and make it a concrete reality. When the child can deal with things that are small or inanimate, the child masters situations that might otherwise be overwhelming. Cartoons, pictures, or puppets can be used to demonstrate actions and terminology. Dolls with removable cloth organs help children understand scheduled operations.

Preschoolers tend to think of their disabilities or illnesses, their separation from parents, and any painful treatments as punishment. Play can be used to help children express their feelings about an illness and to role-play coping strategies. Allowing the young child to manipulate syringes, give "shots" to a doll, or put a bandage or restraint on a teddy bear's arm allows the child to act out his or her feelings. The child becomes "the aggressor." Play can be a major channel for communication in the nurse-client relationship involving a young child. Preschool children develop communication themes through their play, and work through conflict situations in their own good time; the process cannot be rushed. As the child develops trust in the interpersonal environment, themes are clarified and goals can be accomplished.

Exercise 18-1 Using a Mutual Storytelling Technique

Purpose: To give practical experience with the mutual storytelling technique.

Procedure:

1. Use the mutual storytelling process described in the text with a 5- to 8-year-old child in your neighborhood.
2. Write down the story the child told and suggest alternate endings.
3. Share your stories in turn during the next class period.

Discussion:

1. How difficult was it for you to engage the child? If you had trouble, what alternate actions would you incorporate in using the technique again?
2. Were you surprised at the story the child produced? If so, in what ways?
3. What did you learn about the child when using this technique?
4. What conclusions might you draw from hearing the other students relate their experiences about the use of this technique? In what situations was it most effective? Least effective?
5. What did you learn about yourself as a helping person in using this technique?

Sample Answer:

Nurse: Once upon a time in a land far away, there lived a...

Child: dragon

Nurse: a dragon who ate...

Child: carrots

Nurse: The dragon ate carrots and slept...

Child: in a cave

Nurse: One day he left the cave to go out and find many sweet carrots to eat, but as he walked along he ran into a...

Child: bike

Nurse: He was afraid of the bike and so he...

Child: kicked it and ran away

Nurse: After he ran away, is there any more to the story?

Child (upset): He got hit with a stick.

Nurse: What is the message to this story? What does it tell us?

Child: About running away not to be punished.

Play materials vary with the age and developmental status of the child. Simple, large toys are used with young children; more intricate playthings are used with older preschoolers. Clay, crayons, and paper become modes of expression for important feelings and thoughts about problems.

Play can be the pediatric health care professional's primary tool for assessing preschool children's perceptions about their hospital experience, their anxieties, and their fears. Play can increase their coping ability. Preschoolers love jokes, puns, and riddles; the cornier, the better. Using jokes during the physical assessment, such as, "Let me hear your lunch" or, "Golly, could that be a potato in your ear?" helps form the bonds needed for a successful relationship with the preschool client.

Storytelling as a Communication Strategy. A communication strategy often used with young children is the use of story plots. Gardner (1986) describes a mutual storytelling technique in which the caregiver asks the child whether he would like to help make up a story. If the child is a little reluctant, the nurse may begin, as described in Exercise 18-1. At the end of the story, the child is asked to indicate what lesson might be learned from the story. If the child seems a little reluctant to give a moral to the story, the nurse might suggest that all stories have something that can be learned from them. The nurse analyzes the themes presented by the child, which usually reveal important feelings. Is the story fearful? Are the characters scary or pleasing? The child should be praised for telling the story. The next step in the process is for nurses to ask themselves, "What would be a healthier resolution or a more mature adaptation than the one used by the child?" The nurse could suggest an alternative ending or plot. In the nurse's version of the story, the characters and other details remain the same initially, but the story contains a more positive solution or suggests alternative answers to problems. The object of mutual storytelling is to offer the child an opportunity to explore different alternatives in a neutral communication process with a helping person. Exercise 18-1 provides an opportunity to experiment with a mutual storytelling strategy.

School-Age Children

As children move into concrete operational thinking, they begin to internalize the reasons for illness: illness is caused by germs, or you have cavities because you ate too much candy or did not brush your teeth. In later childhood, most children become better able to work verbally with the nurse. It still is important to prepare responses carefully and to anticipate problems, but the child is capable of expressing feelings and venting frustration more directly through words. Use Exercise 18-2 to reformulate medical technology into age-appropriate expressions.

Exercise 18-2 Age-Appropriate Medical Terminology

Purpose: To help students think of terminology appropriate to use with young clients.

Procedure:
This can be fun if the instructor quickly asks students, going around the room.
Reformulate the following expressions using words a child can understand:

Anesthesia	Inflammation	NPO
Cardiac catheterization	Injection	Operating room
Disease	Intake and output	Sedation
Dressings	Isolation	Urine specimen
Enema	IV needle	Vital signs
Infection	Nausea	

Discussion:
Think of any experiences you might have had as a child client or may have observed. What were some of the troublesome words you remember from these experiences?

Assessment of the child's cognitive level of understanding continues to be essential. Search for concrete examples to which the child can relate rather than giving abstract examples. If children are to learn from a model, they must see the model performing the skill to be learned. School-age children thrive on explanations of how their bodies work and enjoy understanding the scientific rationales for their treatment. Ask questions directly to the child, consulting the parent for validation.

Using Audiovisual Aids as a Communication Strategy. Audiovisual aids and reading material geared to the child's level of understanding may supplement verbal explanations. Details about what the child will hear, see, smell, and feel are important. Diagrams can be used to help provide simple, accurate scientific information. For the younger school-age child, expressive art can be a useful method to convey feelings and to open up communication. The older school-age child or adolescent might best convey feelings by writing a poem, a short story, or a letter. This written material can assist the nurse in understanding hidden thoughts or emotions.

Mutuality in Decision Making. Children of this age need to be involved in discussions of their illness and in planning for their care. Explanations giving the rationale for care are useful. Involving the child in decision making may decrease fears about the illness, the treatment, or the effect on family life. Videos and written materials may be useful in involving the child in the management phase of care. Lewis, Pantell, and Sharp (1991) note that, although children often are included in data gathering, there is a tendency to exclude them from management and diagnostic information. In this study, when children were included in discussions of medical recommendations, the children were more satisfied with their care and recalled more information.

Adolescents

An understanding of adolescence and the intensity of the search for identity is essential for the nurse working with teenagers. Even teens enjoying good health are forced to deal with new health issues such as acne, menstrual problems, and sexual activity (Tindall, Beardsley, & Kimberlin, 1994). The adolescent vacillates between childhood and adulthood and is emotionally vulnerable. The ambivalence of the adolescent period may be expressed through withdrawal, rebellion, lost motivation, and rapid mood changes. All of these behaviors are normal in varying degrees as teenagers examine values and standards. However, identity issues become more difficult to resolve when the normal opportunities for physical independence, privacy, and social contacts are compromised by illness or handicap. Sick, well, or disabled, all adolescents have questions about their developing body and sexuality. They have the same longings and desires. Problems may be greater for ill teens because the natural outlets for their expression with peers are curtailed by the disorder or by hospitalization. Use of peer groups, adolescent lounges (separate from the small children's playroom), and a telephone in the rooms, as well as provisions for wearing one's own clothes, fixing one's hair, or attending hospital school, may help teenagers adjust to hospitalization. When the developmental identity crisis becomes too uncomfortable, adolescents may project their fury and frustration onto family or staff. Identifying rage as a normal response to a difficult situation can be very reassuring.

Assessment of the adolescent should occur in a private setting. Attention to the client's interpersonal comfort and space will have a tremendous impact on the quality of the interaction. To the teenager, the nurse represents an authority figure. The need for compassion, concern, and respect is perhaps greater during adolescence than at any other time in the life span. Often lacking the verbal skills of adults, yet wishing to appear in control, adolescents do well with direct questions. Innocuous questions are used first to allow the teenager enough space to check the validity of his or her reactions to the nurse. In caring for a teen in an ambulatory office or clinic, conduct part of the history interview without the parent present. If the parent will not leave the exam room, this can be done while walking the teen down to the laboratory. Questions about substance use, sexual activity, and so on demand confidentiality.

To assess a teen's cognitive level, find out about his or her ability to make long-term plans. An easy way to do this is the "three wishes question." Ask the teen to name three things he or she would expect to have in 5 years. Answers can be analyzed for factors such as concreteness, realism, and goal-directness.

Questions for psychosocial assessment are provided in Box 18-3. Remember that some teens lack sufficient experience to recognize that life has ups and downs and that things will eventually be better. Suicide is the

Box 18-3 Psychosocial Assessment of Adolescents

- Level of self-care responsibility
- Quality of relationships with significant others, including health practices such as safe sex for those who are sexually active
- Self-concept, body image, and personal identity
- Threats to developmental integration of body functions, such as may occur with an ostomy
- Age-appropriate interpersonal and cognitive functioning

second leading cause of death in teenagers, and many experts think that the actual rate is higher because many deaths from the number one cause, motor vehicle accidents, may actually be attributed to this cause. Be aware of danger signs such as apathy, persistent depression, or self-destructive behavior. When faced with a tragedy, teens tend to mourn in doses, with wide mood swings. Grieving teens may need periods of privacy, but also need the opportunity for relief through distracting activities. In communicating with an ill adolescent, remember to *listen*. When a teen asks a direct question, he or she is ready to hear the answer. Answer directly and honestly (*Kindermourn News*, 2001).

Using Hobbies as a Communication Strategy. Adolescents still rely primarily on feedback from adults and from friends to judge their own competency. A teen may not yet have developed proficiency and comfort in carrying on verbal conversations with adults. The teen may respond best if the nurse uses several modalities to communicate. Using empathy, conveying acceptance, and using open-ended questions are three useful strategies (Tindall et al., 1994). Sometimes more innovative communication strategies are needed. In the following case example, the teen has a difficult time talking, so the use of another modality is appropriate.

Case Example

Ashley, a first-year student nurse, becomes frustrated during the course of her conversation with her assigned client, 17-year-old Cary, admitted 5 days ago to the psychiatric unit. Despite a genuine desire to engage him in a therapeutic alliance, the client would not talk. Attempts to get to know him on a verbal level seemed to increase rather than decrease his anxiety. The nurse correctly inferred that, despite his age, this adolescent needed a more tangible approach. Knowing that the client likes cars, Ashley brought in an automotive magazine. Together they looked at the magazine; the publication soon became their special vehicle for communication, bridging the gap between the client's inner reality and his ability to express himself verbally in a meaningful way. Feelings about cars gradually generalized to verbal expressions about other situations, and Cary quickly began describing his life dreams, disappointments, and attitudes about himself. When Ashley left the unit, he asked to keep the magazine and frequently spoke of her with fondness. This simple recognition of his awkwardness in verbal communication and use of another tool to facilitate the relationship had a positive effect.

Dealing with Care Problems

Pain. The literature has identified a lack of understanding about pain in children, as well as nurses' personal beliefs that children overreport their pain, as a barrier to giving optimal nursing care (Van Hulle Vincent, 2005). For years, children's ability to feel pain has been underrated by adult caregivers. For example, newborn males were routinely circumcised for the last 50 years without pain relief. Of course, circumcisions are no longer recommended by the American Academy of Pediatrics (1999), but it may take 20 years for this to become accepted common practice (see online references). When circumcision is performed now, pain interventions are recommended, although morphine has been demonstrated ineffective for neonatal acute pain control (Carbajal, Lenclen, Jugie et al., 2005). Lack of adequate pain relief may in part be due to fears of oversedating a child, but more likely are due to the child's limited capacity to communicate the nature of his or her discomfort. Infants indicate pain with physiological changes (e.g., diaphoresis, pallor, increased heart rate, increased respirations, and decreased oxygen saturation). Migdal, Chudzynska-Pomianowska, Vause, and associates (2005) found lidocaine, a local anesthetic, effective in reducing the pain associated with venipuncture. Effective nonpharmacological interventions for pain include pacifiers, rocking, physical contact, and sometimes even swaddling (Page & Halvorson, 1991). We now use age-specific

Exercise 18-3 Pediatric Nursing Procedures

Purpose: To give practice in preparing young clients for painful procedures.

Procedure:
Timmy, age 4 years, is going to have a bone marrow aspiration. (The insertion of a large needle into the hip is a painful procedure.) Answer the following questions:
1. What essential information does Timmy need?
2. If this is a frequently repeated procedure, how can you make him feel safe before and after the procedure?
3. How soon in advance should you prepare him?

pain assessment instruments, such as smiley faces or poker chips with toddlers and preschoolers, to evaluate levels of pain with our pediatric clients. Exercise 18-3 will stimulate discussion about care for children in pain.

Anxiety. Illness is often an unanticipated event. Uncertainty and even anxiety should be expected when both treatment and outcome are unknown. Young children react to unexpected stimuli, to painful procedures, and even to the presence of strangers with fear. Older children fear separation from parents, but also may fear injury, loss of body function, or even just being perceived by friends as different because of their illness. Exercise 18-4 helps develop age-appropriate explanations that may reduce anxiety.

Acting-Out Behaviors. Behavior problems in adolescents present a special challenge to the nurse. Clear communication of expectations, treatment protocols, and hospital rules is of value. As much as possible, adolescents should be allowed to act on their own behalf in making choices and judgments about their

Exercise 18-4 Preparing Children for Treatment Procedures

Purpose: To help students apply developmental concepts to age-appropriate nursing interventions.

Procedure:
Students divide into four small groups and design an age-appropriate intervention for the following situation. As a large group, each small-group spokesperson writes the intervention on the board under the label for the age group.

Situation:
Jamie is scheduled to go to the surgical suite later today to have a central infusion catheter inserted for hyperalimentation. This is Jamie's first procedure on the first day of this first hospitalization experience.

Discussion:
Group focuses on comparing interventions across the age spans.
1. How does each intervention differ according to the age of the child? (Describe age-appropriate interventions for preschooler, school-age child, and adolescent.)
2. What concept themes are common across the age spans? (Education components; assessing initial level of knowledge; assessing ability to comprehend information, readiness to receive information; adapting information to cognitive level of child.)
3. What formats might be best used for each age group? (Role-play with tools such as dolls, pictures, comic books, educational pamphlets, peer group sessions.)

functioning. At the same time, adolescents still need limits on behavior, though it should be a collaborative experience.

Limits define the boundaries of acceptable behaviors in a relationship. Initially determined by the parents or the nurse, limits can be developed mutually as an important part of the relationship as the child matures. Determining consequences has a positive value in that it provides the child with a model for handling frustrating situations in a more adult manner.

Once the conflict is resolved and the child has accepted the consequences of his or her behavior, the child should be given an opportunity to discuss attitudes and feelings that led up to the need for limits as well as his or her reaction to the limits set.

Although communication about limits is necessary for the survival of the relationship, it needs to be balanced with time for interaction that is pleasant and positive. Sometimes with children who need limits set on a regular basis, discussion of the restrictions is the only conversation that takes place between nurse and client. When this is noted, nurses might ask themselves what feelings the child might be expressing through his or her actions. Putting into words the feelings that are being acted out helps children trust the nurse's competence and concern. Usually it is necessary for the entire staff to share this responsibility. Boxes 18-4 and 18-5 present a step-by-step proposal for setting limits within the context of the nurse-client relationship.

Box 18-5 Outline of a Limit-Setting Plan

1. Have the child describe his or her behavior.
   Key: Evaluate realistically.
2. Encourage the child to assess behavior. Is it helpful for others and himself or herself?
   Key: Evaluate realistically.
3. Encourage the child to develop an alternative plan for governing behavior.
   Key: Set reasonable goals.
4. Have the child sign a statement about his or her plan.
   Key: Commit to goals.
5. At the end of the appropriate time period, have the child assess his or her performance.
   Key: Evaluate realistically.
6. Provide positive reinforcement for those aspects of performance that were successful.*
   Key: Evaluate realistically.
7. Encourage the child to make a positive statement about his or her performance.
   Key: Teach self-praise.

From Felker D: *Building positive self-concepts*, Minneapolis, MN, 1974, Burgess Publishing.
*If the child's performance does not meet the criteria set in the plan, return to Step 3 and assist the child in modifying the plan so that success is more possible. If, on the other hand, the child's performance is successful, help him or her to develop a more ambitious plan (e.g., for a longer time period or for a larger set of behaviors).

Box 18-4 Guidelines for Developing Workable Consequences for Unacceptable Behavior

Effective consequences are
- Logical and fit the situation.
- Applied in a matter-of-fact manner without lengthy discussion.
- Situation-centered rather than person-centered.
- Applied immediately after the transgression.

Exercise 18-5 **Strategies for Conducting an Assessment on the Toddler and the Preschooler**

Purpose: To help students adapt assessment skills to younger children.

Procedure:
Each student will state one technique he or she has seen successfully used by a health care worker attempting to auscultate heart sounds in a toddler. Change this scenario to examining the child's ear with an otoscope. Change the context from hospital to ambulatory care or outpatient clinic. Then change the age to preschooler.

More Helpful Strategies for Communicating with Children

Adapting the general communications strategies studied earlier in this book to interactions with children requires some imagination and creativity. Exercise 18-5 should provoke some lighthearted activities that may strengthen pediatric care skills.

Active Listening. Knowing what a child truly needs and values is the heart of successful interpersonal relationships in health care settings. The process of active listening takes form initially from watching the behaviors of children as they play and interact with their environments. As a child's vocabulary increases and the capacity to engage with others develops, listening begins to approximate the communication process that occurs between adults, with one important difference: because the perceptual world of the child is concrete, the nurse's feedback and informational messages should coincide with the child's developmental level.

Do you agree with the message conveyed in the following poem by an anonymous writer?

> When I ask you to listen and you start giving me advice, you have not done what I asked.
>
> When I ask you to listen to me and you feel you have to do something to solve my problem, you have failed me, strange as that may seem.
>
> Listen! All that I asked was that you listen, not talk or do —just hear me.
>
> When you do something for me that I can or need to do for myself, you contribute to my fear and inadequacy.
>
> But when you accept as a simple fact I do feel what I feel, no matter how irrational, then I can quit trying to convince you and get about this business of understanding what is behind this irrational feeling.
>
> And when that's clear, the answers are obvious and I don't need advice.
>
> Irrational feelings make sense when we understand what's behind them.
>
> So, please listen and just hear me.
>
> And if you want to talk, wait a minute for your turn— and I'll listen to you.

Working with children is rewarding, hard work that sometimes must be evaluated indirectly. For instance, George was the primary care nurse who had worked very hard with a 13-year-old girl over a 6-month period while the girl was on a bone marrow transplant unit. He felt bad when, at discharge, the girl stated, "I never want to see any of you people again." However, just before leaving, the nurse found her sobbing on her bed. No words were spoken, but the child threw her arms around George and clung to him for comfort. For this nurse, the child's expression of grief was an acknowledgment of the meaning of the relationship. Children, even those who can use words, often communicate through behavior rather than verbally when under stress.

Authenticity and Veracity. Life crises are an inevitable part of life. Many parents and health professionals ignore children's feelings or else deceive them about procedures, illness, or hospitalization in the mistaken belief that they will be overwhelmed by the truth. Just the opposite is true. Children, like adults, can cope with most stressors as long as they are presented in a manner they can understand and given enough time and support from the environment to cope. In fact, very ill children often are a source of inspiration to the adults working with them because of their courage in facing the truth about themselves and dealing with it constructively. When Britto, DeVillis, Hornung, and associates (2004) surveyed adolescents with chronic illnesses, teens rated honesty, attention to pain, and respect as the three most important factors in their quality of care. Completing Exercise 18-6 may stimulate some discussion.

A nurse should never allow any individual, even a parent, to threaten a child. For example, many a parent has been heard to say, "You be good or I'll have the nurse give you a shot." It is appropriate to interrupt this parent. Children respect honest expression of emotions in adults. Being truthful and trustworthy with children is a crucial factor in the development of a therapeutic relationship.

Case Example

In a community setting, an older student nurse, with a family of her own, was monitoring a family in which the mother had terminal cancer. There were three children in the family, and the identified client of the student was a 13-year-old boy. He was abnormally quiet, and it was difficult to draw him out. Halfway through the semester, the boy's father died unexpectedly of a heart attack. When the boy and student nurse next met, the nurse asked the boy whether there was anything special that had happened between father and son that the boy would remember about his father. The boy replied that the day before his father's death he had received a letter of acceptance to the same school his

Exercise 18-6 Working with the Newly Diagnosed HIV-Positive Teenager

Purpose: To stimulate class discussion about how to deal with the adolescent with whom it is difficult to communicate.

Procedure:
Read the case situation and answer the questions that follow. Questions can be done out of class, with class time used only for discussion.

Situation:
Bill, age 17 years, seeks treatment for gonorrhea. He is hospitalized for further testing after his initial workup reveals he is seropositive for human immunodeficiency virus (HIV) type 1. For 2 days on the unit he has cried, cursed, and been uncooperative. Staff tends to avoid him when possible. A team of residents begins a bone marrow aspiration procedure in the treatment room after obtaining his absent mother's permission. (She has expressed condemnation and has not yet been to visit.) A technician walks in and out of the room to obtain supplies while the doctors concentrate on completing the procedure. A student nurse is asked to come in to help restrain Bill, who is alternately screaming, crying, and being very quiet.

1. What communication strategies could this student use while squeezing into this small room? (Clue: Verbal and nonverbal directed to the client and to the doctors)
2. What assessment might the nurse want to make? (Clue: What are Bill's feelings about his diagnosis?)
3. What can be inferred about Bill's current behavior?
4. What interventions would you suggest for initiating interaction with his single mom?
5. What additional data are needed before attempting any teaching about acquired immunodeficiency syndrome (AIDS)?

Discussion:
May be discussed in small groups.

father had attended, and he had shared this with his father. He said his father was very proud that he had been accepted. The student nurse could feel her eyes fill as the boy revealed himself to her in this special way. Her sharing of honest emotion was a significant turning point in what became a very important relationship for both participants. It was a moment of shared meaning for both of them and, from that time on, the needed common ground for communication existed.

Being authentic does not mean being overly familiar. Trying to interact with older children and adolescents as though the nurse is a buddy is confusing to the client. What the child wants is an emotionally available, calm, caring, competent resource who can protect, care about, and above all, listen to him or her.

Conveying Respect. It is easy for adults to impose their own wishes on a child. Respecting a child's right to feel and to express his or her feelings appropriately is important. Providing truthful answers is a hallmark of respect. When interacting with the older child, using the concept of mutuality will promote respect and should foster more positive and lasting health care outcomes. Confidentiality needs to be maintained unless the nurse judges that revealing information is necessary to prevent harm to the child or adolescent. In such cases, the child needs to be advised of the disclosure.

Providing Anticipatory Guidance to the Child. The nursing profession advocates client education. A physician would call similar preventive education *anticipatory guidance* (AG). As more clinics become located within schools, more emphasis is being placed on AG (Kaplan,

Calonge, Guernsey et al., 1998). The American Academy of Pediatrics has published guidelines for health care providers working with well children in the community. These suggestions focus on health promotion information to be given to caretakers at appropriate ages. Managed care has brought an increased focus on the role a child can assume in being responsible for his or her own health care. It is never too early to begin. For example, McCarthy and Hobbie (1997) provide very clear written handouts for incorporating violence prevention into well-child visits made to nurse practitioners. This shift in placing responsibility for good health practices onto the individual is in line with recommendations in *Healthy People 2010* (see Online Resources).

Interacting with Parents of Ill Children

According to some estimates, up to 20% or 30% of all children have some form of chronic illness (Sterling,

Box 18-6 Representative Nursing Problem: Dealing with a Frightened Parent

During report, the night nurse relates an incident that occurred between Mrs. Smith, the mother of an 8-year-old admitted for possible acute lymphocytic leukemia, and the night supervisor. Mrs. Smith told the supervisor that her son was receiving poor care from the nurses and that they frequently ignored her and refused to answer her questions. While you are making rounds following the report, Mrs. Smith corners you outside her son's room and begins to tell you about all the things that went wrong during the night. She goes on to say, "If you people think I'm going to stand around and allow my son to be treated this way, you are sadly mistaken."

Problem

Frustration and anger caused by a sense of powerlessness and fear related to the son's possible diagnosis

Nursing Diagnosis

Ineffective coping related to hospitalization of son and possible diagnosis of leukemia

Nursing Goals

Increase the mother's sense of control and problem-solving capabilities; help the mother develop adaptive coping behaviors.

Method of Assistance

Guiding; supporting; providing developmental environment

Interventions

1. Actively listen to the client's concerns with as much objectivity as possible; maintain eye contact with the client; use minimal verbal activity, allowing the client the opportunity to express her concerns and fears freely.
2. Use reflective questioning to determine the client's level of understanding and the extent of information obtained from health team members.
3. Listen for repetitive words or phrases that may serve to identify problem areas or provide insight into fears and concerns.
4. Reassure the mother when appropriate that her child's hospitalization is indeed frightening and it is all right to be scared; remember to demonstrate interest in the client as a person; use listening responses (e.g., "It must be hard not knowing the results of all these tests.") to create an atmosphere of concern.
5. Avoid communication blocks, such as giving false reassurance, telling the client what to do, or ignoring the concerns; such behavior effectively cuts off therapeutic communication.
6. Keep the client continually informed regarding her child's progress.
7. Involve the client in her son's care; do not overwhelm her or make her feel she has to do this; watch for cues that tell you she is ready "to do more."
8. Acknowledge the impact this illness may have on the family; involve the health team in identifying ways to reduce the client's fears and provide for continuity in the type of information presented to her and to other family members.
9. Assign a primary nurse to care for the client's son and serve as a resource to the client. Identify support systems in the community that might provide help and support to the client.

Courtesy M. Michaels, University of Maryland School of Nursing, 1987.

Peterson, & Weekes, 1997). Having an ill child is stressful for parents. Many research studies have shown that loss of the ability to act as the child's parent, to alleviate the child's pain, and to comfort the child is more stressful than factors connected with the illness, including coping with uncertainty over the outcome. Other stressors include financial and marital strains. Stress may vary across cultures. For example, Hispanic parents in the Rei and Fong study (1996) cited coping with strange sights, sounds, and equipment as being highly stressful. Other studies pointed to a lack of needed information and support from professionals as being a top stressor, exacerbating already existing family problems and resulting in feelings of fear and helplessness.

Parents often have questions about discussing their child's illness or disability with others. Telling siblings and friends the truth is important. For one thing, it provides a role model for the siblings to follow in answering the curious questions of their friends. Issues such as overprotectiveness, discipline, time out for parents to replenish commitment and energy, and the quality and quantity of interactions with the hospitalized child have a powerful impact on the child's growth and development. However, older children have a need for confidentiality and respond better if the nurse interviews and treats them away from parents' presence. Consider the ethical dilemma provided at the end of this chapter.

More frustrating to nurses are parents who are critical of the nurse's interventions, displacing the anger they feel about their own powerlessness onto the nurse (Box 18-6). The nurse may be tempted to become defensive or sarcastic or simply to dismiss the comments of the parent as irrational. However, a more helpful response would be to place oneself in the parents' shoes and to consider the possible issues. Asking the parents what information they have or might need, simply listening in a nondefensive way, and allowing the parents to vent some of their frustrations facilitate the possibility of dialogue about the underlying feelings. The listening strategies given in Chapter 10 are helpful. Sometimes a listening response that acknowledges the legitimacy of the parent's feeling is helpful: "I'm sorry that you feel so bad" or, "It must be difficult for you to see your child in such pain." These simple comments acknowledge the very real anguish parents experience in health care situations having few palatable options. If possible, parental venting of feeling should occur in a private setting out of hearing range from the child. It is very upsetting to children to experience splitting in the parent-nurse relationship.

Box 18-7 Guidelines for Communicating with Parents

- Present complex information in informational chunks.
- Repeat information and allow plenty of time for questions.
- Keep parents continually informed of progress and changes in condition.
- Involve parents in determining goals; anticipate possible reactions and difficulties.
- Discuss problems with parents directly and honestly.
- Explore all alternative options with parents.
- Share knowledge of community supports; help parents role-play responses to others.
- Acknowledge the impact of the illness on finances; on emotions; and especially on the family, including siblings.
- Use other staff for support in personally coping with the emotional drain created by working with very ill children and their parents.

You can reduce parents' stress by educating them about their child's condition. When the child has a chronic illness, the family is called on to continually adjust the family system to adapt to changing demands in the child's health. More than 10 percent of the population has a chronically ill or disabled child to care for (Clawson, 1996). Because nursing care is largely moving to care in the home, nurses will have an increasing need to help families cope with seriously chronically ill children. At times, the nurse will be called on to act as the child's advocate in giving parents helpful information, anticipatory guidance, and complex technical assistance in caring for the health and developmental needs of their child. Guidelines for communicating with parents are presented in Box 18-7.

Anticipatory Guidance in the Community

Every parent is entitled to a full explanation of his or her child's disability and treatment. Because the parents usually assume responsibility for the child's care after they leave the hospital, it is essential to encourage active involvement from the very beginning of treatment. Many parents look to the nurse for guidance and support in this process. In ambulatory well-child clinics, parents of well children need facts about normal development and milestones to expect, as well as information about prevention of illness.

Community, Family, and Nurse Partnerships

Forming a partnership with the family can be the best method a nurse has to address the complex health care needs of children with chronic illnesses. Parents' participation in the care of their child, and active involvement in decision making regarding the youngster's treatment, ensure a more stable environment for the child. Providing family support is important for those caring for chronically ill children. The study by Chernoff, Ireys, DeVet et al. (2002) demonstrates the positive effectiveness of family support groups in the community in aiding parental adjustment while raising children with chronic illnesses.

The focus of care is shifting to community partnership movements across the world. Parents are the central figures in care planning, with significant input as to which community, social, formal, and friend networks and which professionals will be mobilized to provide care to their child. Successful collaboration requires active commitment to meet client needs by all parties involved. School nurses are often crucial to the ability of the child with a chronic illness to maintain school attendance. In addition, school nurses often act as case managers by communicating about the child's needs among parent, care providers, teachers and other resource personnel. By law in the United States, children with special needs in the educational system are required to have an Individualized Education Plan. A part of this may be the health plan for children who need medical intervention/treatment during school.

Support groups in the community have been organized to assist families. Often information about the group's meeting times can be obtained from health care providers, from the national or local organization, or even from the phone book. For parents who cannot travel to meetings, a new form of support may be available via the Internet, as described in Chapter 24.

> **Ethical Dilemma ■ *What Would You Do?***
> You are caring for Mika Soon, a 15-year-old adolescent. She has confided to you that she is being treated for chlamydia. Her mother approaches you privately and demands to know if Mika has told you if she is sexually active with her boyfriend. Since Mika is a minor and Mrs. Soon is paying for this clinic visit, are you obligated to tell her the truth?

SUMMARY

Working with children requires patience, imagination, and creative applications of therapeutic communication strategies. Children's ability to understand and communicate with nurses is largely influenced by their cognitive developmental level and by their limited life experiences. Nurses need to develop an understanding of feelings and thought processes from the child's perspective, and communication strategies with children should reflect these understandings. Various strategies for communicating with children of different ages are suggested, as are strategies for communicating with their parents. A marvelous characteristic of children is how well they respond to caregivers who make an effort to understand their needs and take the time to relate to them.

REFERENCES

American Academy of Pediatrics Task Force on Circumcision: Circumcision policy statement (RE9850), *Pediatrics* 103(3): 686–693, 1999.

Berman H: Getting critical with children: empowering approaches with a disempowered group, *Adv Nurs Sci* 26(2):102–113, 2003.

Bernstein D, Shelov SP: *Pediatrics*, Baltimore, 2000, Williams & Wilkins.

Bernzweig J, Takayama JI, Phibbs C et al.: Gender differences in physician-patient communication, *Arch Pediatr Adolesc Med* 15(6):568–591, 1997.

Bouve LR, Rozmus CL, Giordano P: Preparing parents for their child's transfer from PICU to the pediatric floor, *Appl Nurs Res* 12(3):114–120, 1999.

Britto MT, DeVillis RF, Hornung RW et al.: Health care preferences and priorities of adolescents with chronic illnesses, *Pediatrics* 114(5):1272–1280, 2004.

Carbajal R, Lenclen R, Jugie M et al.: Morphine does not provide adequate analgesia for acute procedural pain among preterm neonates, *Pediatrics* 115(6):1494–1500, 2005.

Chernoff RG, Ireys HT, DeVet KA et al.: A randomized controlled trial of a community-based support program for families of children with chronic illness: pediatric outcomes, *Arch Pediatr Adolesc Med* 156(6):533–539, 2002.

Clawson JA: A child with chronic illness and the process of family adaptation, *J Pediatr Nurs* 11(1):52–61, 1996.

Crain W: *Theories of development: concepts and application*, ed 3, Englewood Cliffs, NJ, 1992, Prentice Hall.

Erikson EH: *Childhood and society*, New York, 1963: Norton.

Flarity K: Practice pointers, *Nurs Pract* 22(11):106, 1997.

Gardner R: *Therapeutic communication with children*, ed 2, New York, 1986, Science Books.

Kaplan DW, Calonge N, Guernsey BP et al.: Managed care and school-based health centers, *Arch Pediatr Adolesc Med* 152(1):25–33, 1998.

Kindermourn News: Help for adolescents, Spring, 2001.

Lewis CC, Pantell RH, Sharp L: Increasing patient knowledge, satisfaction, and involvement: randomized trial of a communication intervention, *Pediatrics* 88(2):351–358, 1991.

McCarthy V, Hobbie C: Incorporating violence prevention into anticipatory guidance for well child visits, *J Pediatr Health Care* 11(5):222–226, 1997.

Meeuwesen L, Kaptein M: Changing interactions in doctor-parent-child communication, *Psychol Health* 11(6): 787–795, 1996.

Melnyk BM, Small L, Carno M: The effectiveness of parent-focused interventions in improving coping/mental health outcomes of critically ill children and their parents: an evidence base to guide clinical practice, *Pediatr Nurs* 30(2):143–148, 2004.

Migdal M, Chudzynska-Pomianowska E, Vause E et al.: Rapid, needle-free delivery of lidocaine for reducing the pain of venipuncture among pediatric subjects, *Pediatrics* 115(4):e393–e398, 2005; available online: http://pediatrics.aappublications.org/cgi/content/full/115/4/e393.

Page GG, Halvorson M: Pediatric nurses: the assessment and control of pain in preverbal infants, *J Pediatr Nurs* 6(2):99–106, 1991.

Piaget J: *The child's conception of the world*, Savage, MD, 1972, Littlefield, Adams.

Rei RM, Fong C: The Spanish version of the parental stressor scale: pediatric intensive care unit, *J Pediatr Nurs* 11(1):3–9, 1996.

Sterling YM, Peterson J, Weekes DP: African-American families with chronically ill children, *J Pediatr Nurs* 12(5):292–300, 1997.

Tindall WN, Beardsley RS, Kimberlin CL: *Communication skills in pharmacy practice*, Philadelphia, 1994, Lea & Febiger.

Van Hulle Vincent C: Nurses' knowledge, attitudes and practices regarding children's pain, *MCN Am J Matern Child Nurs* 30(3):177–183, 2005.

Wertlieb D: Converging trends in family research and pediatrics: recent findings for the American Academy of Pediatrics Task Force on the Family, *Pediatrics* 111(6):1572–1587, 2003.

Williams BE: Reaching adolescents through portraiture photography, *Child Youth Care Q* 16(4):241–245, 1987.

Chapter 19

Communicating with Older Adults

Elizabeth Arnold and *Judith W. Ryan*

OUTLINE

OBJECTIVES

At the end of the chapter, the reader will be able to:

1. Identify age-related physical, cognitive, and psychosocial environmental changes that can affect communication.
2. Identify two theoretical frameworks used with the older adult.
3. Discuss appropriate assessment strategies and related nursing interventions.
4. Describe blocks to communication with the older adult.
5. Specify communication strategies for use in longterm care of the older adult.
6. Describe communication strategies to use with clients demonstrating cognitive impairment.

The way we treat our children in the dawn of their lives, and the way we treat the elderly in the twilight of their lives, is a measure of the quality of a nation.

Hubert Humphrey

Chapter 19 focuses on communication strategies used in the nurse-client relationship with the older adult. The term "older adult" is used in this chapter to indicate persons age 65 years and older. In 2006, the oldest old (>85) continue to be the most rapidly growing segment of our society. By the year 2030, it is anticipated that the number of people designated as older adults will double from 35 million in 2000 to 70 million and will account for 20% of the population. Four- and five-generation families will be more common as the life span for individuals increases, and family-based assistance as the primary source of long-term care for the frail elderly will continue to increase (Gavan, 2003).

The postwar baby boomer generation, which will add significantly to the number of older adults, begins to turn 65 in this decade (Curtis & Dixon, 2005). This significant age segment of the population is predicted to bring about a fundamental shift in the demographic structure such that their elder status will affect all aspects of public policy (Coughlin, 1999).

Today's older adults have had significantly different life experiences and opportunities from their parents. In the next decade the *healthy* older adult is expected to be

- More culturally diverse, and a much larger cohort than ever before.
- More active and physically fit than in past generations.
- Better educated and computer-literate.
- Healthier, with less severe functional problems and chronic disability.
- Better off financially than in previous generations (although the same racial and income health care disparities exist for elders as for other population segments).
- Likely to live much longer. (Maples & Abney, 2006)

At the same time, healthy older adults are *not* young people. Their nutrition, exercise, and other health needs are different, so health promotion and health care needs to be modified to meet the unique requirements of older adults (Nakasato & Carnes, 2006). Older adults vary greatly in capabilities, interests, and capacities for relationships. Whereas some are frail and have reduced intellectual function due to disease, many retain a high level of physical and intellectual function until relatively close to their death (e.g., consider the nursing home resident versus a Senior Olympics participant). To some extent,

> Age is a self-fulfilling prophecy. If we dread growing old, thinking of it as a time of forgetfulness and physical deterioration, then it is likely to be just that. On the other hand, if we expect it to be full of energy and anticipate that our lives will be rich with new adventures and insight; then that is the likely reality. We prescribe who we are. We prescribe what we are to become. (Bortz, 1990, p. 55)

BASIC CONCEPTS

The first goal of *Healthy People 2010* is to increase the quality and years of healthy life, which is consistent with the goals of the International Council of Nurses (2005). Communication is the primary means through which these goals can be achieved. Communication problems that many nurses experience with older adults arise from both the societal discrimination and stereotyping that occurs and a lack of understanding about the physical changes that take place in older adults. The sensory losses that occur with normal aging, especially the hearing and vision changes, contribute to alterations in developing therapeutic relationships. For example, in the nursing home population, the prevalence of hearing loss is as high as 70% (Jerger, Chmiel, Wilson et al., 1995).

Physical Changes in Normal Aging

Aging is a natural life process and is *not* reversible. The aging process affects physical strength, stamina, and flexibility, which in turn affect an individual's ability to control the physical environment. Although in many instances the impact of these physical changes can be modified with diet, exercise, and a positive attitude, they nevertheless occur with regularity in everyone (Weil, 2005). After the age of 60, people are more vulnerable to a wide category of age-related disease such as cancer, cardiac and circulatory problems, stroke, and degenerative bone loss, all of which become more frequent as people age. Older people may gradually lose control over bodily functions and movements, which interferes with their sense of dignity and self-image (Franklin, Ternestedt, & Nordenfelt, 2006). The goal of health promotion for the older adult is to help people live as long and as well as possible, with the shortest period of decline possible. Andrew Weil (2005) refers to this as "compressed morbidity" and suggests that attention to the more positive values of aging can lengthen the time of quality living and shorten the time of decline.

Age-Related Changes in Cognition

Age-related changes in cognition for *healthy* adults are minimal. Without the ravages of disease, the older adult shows no loss of intelligence but may require more time in completing verbal tasks or in retrieving information from long-term memory (Ivnik, Smith, Malec et al., 1995; Salthouse, 1993; Wilson, Bennet, & Swartzendruber, 1997). In addition, older adults are less likely to make guesses when they are presented with ambiguous testing items in mental status exams, or respond less well if they are under time pressure to perform. Therefore, communication with healthy older adults does not require special modification based on changes in their cognition. Allowing a little extra time for processing may be all that is required for successful communication.

For approximately 5% of the population over the age of 65 years, and 20% of those who reach the age of 80 years, however, there are abnormal cognitive changes. These abnormal age-related changes are profound and progressive and are referred to as Alzheimer's disease and related dementias. Dementia is characterized by memory loss, personality changes, and a deterioration in intellectual functioning that affects every aspect of the person's life. A small percentage of abnormal cognitive changes are caused by organic problems (e.g., drug toxicity, metabolic disorders, and depression) and may be reversed with treatment. The nurse can play a vital role in encouraging and directing clients and their families to seek appropriate diagnosis and treatment. Because short-term memory fades before long-term memory, family can still reach the client by talking about past events.

Psychosocial and Environmental Changes

The environment affects communication opportunities for the older adult. As they grow older, people are more likely to suffer multiple losses of people, activities, and functions that were very important to them. Occupational changes in the form of retirement can have the dual impact of significantly changing a person's lifestyle, both financially and as a source of meaning. Emotional energy that used to find expression in work, friendships, and creative activities may lose its earlier intensity as the familiar landmarks in a life tapestry are altered by age. For people who have placed a high value on their achievement in a job, there can be a perceived loss of status and self-esteem. Losses of people significant to the older adult occur with increasing regularity (e.g., through friends and family dying and adult children moving out of the area or becoming increasingly involved with their own nuclear families).

The client may express a decreased capacity for mastery in many areas of his or her life, with associated feelings of helplessness, a loss of self-esteem, and sometimes a loss of purpose. Whenever the nurse senses from the client that there is a loss of emotional energy in life and feelings of desolation about a client's situation, the nurse needs to gather more information. A life without purpose is a life without meaning, and all people need to feel that their lives have meaning. Statements of concern to the nurse that indicate a need for further exploration include the following:

"I am just useless."

"I can't do any of the things I used to do."

"I wish I were dead."

Depression is a common, often untreated, problem in older adults. Somatization of vague physical complaints may be its early presenting sign. In addition, old age is one of the strongest risk factors for suicide, especially among Caucasian males (Groh & Whall, 2001). Because age is such an important risk factor for suicide, statements reflecting helplessness and hopelessness should never be taken lightly.

Older adults face many negative situational stressors, but they also carry a lifetime of strengths that can be temporarily forgotten. Whereas deficits are real and must be acknowledged, it is the strengths of the client that form the basis for planning and interventions. Generally, people who have demonstrated resiliency in tackling life's difficult issues during earlier stages of their lives will continue to do so as they face the tasks of aging. Maples and Abney (2006) suggest attitude, creativity, positivism, and wellness are keys to empowering the older adult. Exercise 19-1 can help you understand the value of resiliency as an adaptive mechanism in promoting well-being.

Theoretical Frameworks

Erik Erikson. Erikson's (1982) model of psychosocial development can be used in the assessment of the older adult's health care needs (see Chapter 1). Erikson portrays the psychosocial maturational crisis of old age as that of ego integrity versus ego despair. Ego integrity relates to the capacity of older adults to look back on

Exercise 19-1 Psychosocial Strengths and Resiliency

Purpose: To promote an understanding of psychosocial strengths in life accomplishment.

Procedure:

1. Interview an older adult (75 years or older) who, in your opinion, has had a fulfilling life. Ask the person to describe a few of his or her most satisfying life events, and what he or she did to accomplish them. Do the same for a few of the person's most stressful events and how he or she coped with them. Ask the person to identify his or her most meaningful life accomplishments. The interview should be taped or recorded in writing immediately following the interview.
2. In a written format, reflect on this person's comments and your ideas of what strengths this person had that allowed him or her to achieve a sense of well-being and to value his or her accomplishments.

Discussion:

1. Were you surprised at any of the older adult's responses to the question about most satisfying experiences? Most stressful experiences?
2. On a blackboard or flip chart, identify the accomplishments that people have identified. Classify them as work-related or people-related.
3. What common themes emerged in the overall class responses that speak to the strengths in the life experience of older adults?
4. How can you apply what you learned from doing this exercise in your future nursing practice?

their lives with a deep sense of satisfaction and a willingness to let the next generation carry on their legacy. Threads from all of life's previous psychosocial crises—trust, autonomy, purpose, competence, identity, intimacy, and generativity—will resurface during this period.

Ego despair is defined as the failure of a person to accept one's life as appropriate and meaningful. It can be temporary, lifted by a more realistic appraisal of one's life; or permanent, leading to feelings of emotional desolation, bitterness, and hostility. Empowerment is a particularly useful concept to use as the basis for intervention. Sometimes in the throes of reverses of life, the older adult loses sight of a proven track record of coping skills. The nurse can guide clients to recognize their ability to create their own path in old age, as they have done in other situations.

Abraham Maslow. Another theoretical framework used in assessing the needs of the older adult and directing appropriate interventions is that of Maslow's hierarchy of needs (1954) (see Chapter 1).

The five levels are biological integrity (e.g., food, shelter); safety and security; belonging (e.g., friends, group affiliation); self-esteem (e.g., success, control, being needed); and self-actualization (maximization of poten-

Developing an Evidence-Based Practice

Weman K, Fagerberg I: Registered nurses working together with family members of older people, *J Clin Nurs* 15(3):281-289, 2006.

This aim of this study was to explore the perceptions of nurses working in elder care about the difficulties and problems encountered in working with families of elder clients. Positive and negative aspects of working with family members to ensure quality care of their elderly family member were examined using a latent content analysis methodology of responses to open-ended questions related to the topic.

Results: Findings stressed the need for family members and nurses to work together cooperatively as a team in their care of the elderly.

Application to Your Clinical Practice: Family members are and can be an important resource for the older adult. Keeping family members informed and having a good relationship with them is essential in building the type of cooperative working relationship needed for quality care, especially when time and/or resources are needed. As a professional nurse, what factors do you see as being most important in building an effective working relationship with family members of older adults? How would you involve the client's family in clinical decision making?

tial and future-focused). The nurse can assess where on this hierarchy of needs an older adult is positioned. To attempt to address a loneliness problem when the client does not feel safe or secure in his or her environment will meet with frustration and lack of success.

APPLICATIONS

The literature identifies three fundamental characteristics associated with successful aging (Nakasato & Carnes, 2006; Rowe & Kahn, 1998):

- Low risk of disease and disease-related disability
- High mental and physical function
- Active engagement with life

Staying engaged with life to whatever extent is possible and *stimulating the mind* are two critical strategies healthy older adults can use on a daily basis to promote health and well-being as they grow older. Older adults today can be expected to have a wider range of interests, with more time and income to devote to learning, travel, volunteering, and part-time work (Coughlin, 1999).

Nurses working with older clients need to have a great deal of patience and positive respect for the struggles of the older adult. The same person dwells within, but the capacity of that person to interact with his or her environment may become increasingly limited by physical, cognitive, and social changes over which the person has incomplete control. Exercise 19-2 provides you with an opportunity to explore your personal ideas about aging.

Assessment

The assessment of older adults should focus on their level of functioning rather than on chronological age. Functional level is a far more accurate indicator of the client's issues and relationship needs. Functional abilities in the older adult can range from vigorous, active, and independent to frail and highly dependent, with serious physical, cognitive, psychological, and sensory deficits (Bonder & Wagner, 2001).

Assessing Sensory Deficits

Sensory deficits can have a direct and significant impact on communication and cognitive processing. Anderson (2005) notes that addressing common causes of sensory impairment and providing sensory cues can help reduce the manifestation of confusion.

Hearing. Hearing deficits have been associated with perceived poor health and depression in the older adult

Exercise 19-2 What Is It Like to Be Old?

Purpose: To stimulate personal awareness and feelings about the aging process.

Procedure:

Think about and write down the answers to the following questions about your own aging process:

1. What do you think will be important to you when you are 65?
2. Prepare a list of the traits, qualities, and attributes you hope you will have when you are this age.
3. What do you think will be different for you in terms of physical, emotional, spiritual, and social perceptions and activities?
4. How would you like people to treat you when you are an older adult?

Discussion:

In groups of three to four students, share your thoughts. Have one person act as a scribe and write down common themes. Students should ask questions about anything they don't understand.

1. In what ways did doing this exercise give you some insight into what the issues of aging might be for your age group?
2. In what ways might the issues be different for people in your age group and for people currently classified as older adults?
3. How could you use this exercise to better understand the needs of older adults in the hospital and in the home?

(Wallhagen, Strawbridge, & Kaplan, 1996). Hearing loss associated with normal aging begins after age 50 years and is due to loss of hair cells (which are not replaced) in the organ of Corti in the inner ear. This change leads initially to a loss in the ability to hear high-frequency sounds (e.g., f, s, th, sh, ch) and is called presbycusis (Gallo, 2000). Later the loss includes the sounds of the explosive consonants (e.g., b, t, p, k, d), although the lower-frequency sounds of vowels are preserved longer. Older adults also have special difficulty in perceiving sounds against background noises and in understanding fast-paced speech. The most understandable speech for older adults is about 125 words per minute.

Therapeutic Strategies to Use with Hearing Changes. In addition to the strategies suggested in Chapter 17 for the hearing-impaired, several strategies can be used to improve communication with an older adult who has age-related partial hearing loss. It is important to remember that the older adult who does not hear well may very likely be cognitively intact. With a little planning in modifying communication with the hearing-impaired older adult, the relationship should not be any different from one with a client who does not have this disability. Nurses should do the following:

- Address the person by name before beginning to speak. It focuses attention.
- Determine if hearing is better in one ear, and then direct speech to that side.
- Speak distinctly but in a normal voice.
- Do not speak rapidly; about 125 words a minute is best.
- If your voice is high-pitched, lower it.
- Use gestures and facial expression to expand the meaning of the message.
- Face the older adult so he or she can see your facial expression and/or read your lips to enhance comprehension. For example, humor is often communicated by subtle facial expressions.
- If the older adult does not understand, use different words when repeating the message. If "spaghetti" does not work, say "pasta" instead.
- Help older adults adjust hearing aids. Lacking fine-motor dexterity, the older adult may not be able to insert aids to amplify hearing. Check the batteries.
- Do not talk with your hands in front of your mouth or with food or gum in your mouth.
- Keep background noises to a minimum (e.g., turn down the radio or television when talking).
- Obtain feedback periodically to monitor how much the person has heard.

Vision. Vision decreases as people grow older. Cataracts, glaucoma, and age-related macular degeneration are common diseases that can cause visual loss in this age group. Colors lose their vividness, and images can be blurred. Loss of vision can affect a person's ability to perform everyday activities (e.g., dressing, preparing meals, taking medication, driving or using other transportation, handling the checkbook, and using the telephone). It also affects functional ability to engage in many hobbies or leisure activities (e.g., reading, doing handwork, and watching television). In short, a significant decrease in visual function almost invariably affects an individual's ability to function autonomously. The nurse can play a vital role in supporting the independence of the visually impaired client by taking a few simple actions.

Therapeutic Strategies to Use with the Visually Impaired. Because visual acuity can contribute significantly to understanding the meaning of verbal as well as written communication, it will serve the client well if the nurse does the following:

- Have eyeglasses in place, if they are worn.
- Identify yourself by name when you enter the room or initiate conversation.
- Stand in front of the client and use head movements.
- Verbally explain all written information, allowing time for the client to ask questions. Do not assume that because the person appears to be reading a document that it has been read accurately. Ask questions to determine the level of comprehension.
- Provide appropriate lighting and other visual aids to enhance vision.
- Remove any hazards (e.g., obstructed pathways or glares from lighting).
- When ambulating or transporting a client, be certain to tell the client where you are going and verbally describe landmarks along the way.

Assessing Functional Ability

Medication Adherence. Medication adherence is a major problem with the elderly (Nakasato & Carnes,

2006), and effective communication is a significant determinant of compliance. As people age, they usually take multiple medications to maintain a healthy lifestyle (Gavan, 2003). Older adults are more likely to have more side effects because of age-related changes in metabolism (Cochran, 2005). If clients are not compliant with their medications, nurses should explore common risk factors for nonadherence, which can include poor eyesight or diminished cognitive ability, economic factors (including whether the client has prescription insurance coverage), level of health literacy and overall intellectual and organization skills, side effects of medications, and complexity of taking the medication or complying with the protocol.

During an assessment interview or a home visit, you should ask specifically about medication and treatment adherence. Ownby (2006) recommends using an open-ended question such as, "Tell me how you take your medications" rather than asking, "Are you taking your medication as prescribed?" (p. 33).

Use of pill boxes, reminder cues, and careful instruction as to the purpose, dosage, anticipated outcomes and side effects are helpful interventions to increase medication adherence.

Assessing and Responding to Psychosocial Needs

Beginning with the Client's Story. Assessment of the older adult always begins with the client's story. It is important to see and hear what is happening from the older person's perspective. In this way, value-laden psychosocial issues (e.g., independence, fears about being a burden, role changes, and vulnerability) can be brought to the surface.

Case Example

Nurse: You seem concerned that your stroke will have a major impact on your life.

Client: Yes, I am. I'm an old woman now, and I don't want to be a burden to my family.

Nurse: In what ways do you think you might be a burden?

Client: Well, I obviously can't move around as I did. I can't go back to doing what I used to do, but that doesn't mean I'm ready for a nursing home.

Nurse: What were some of the things you used to do?

Client: Well, I raised three children, and they're all married now with good jobs. That's hard to do in this day and age. I did a lot for the church. I held a job as a secretary for 32 years, and I got several awards for my work.

Nurse: It sounds as though you were very productive and were able to cope with a lot of things. You are right that this time in your life is different. It isn't possible to do the things you did previously, but you have a proven track record of coping with life. What you have given to your family is important, but it also is important to allow them to give some things to you. It can be very

Exercise 19-3 Hearing the Stories of Older Adults

Purpose: To promote an understanding of the older adult.

Procedure:

1. Interview an older adult in your family (minimum age 75 years). If there are no older adults in your family, interview a family friend whose lifestyle is similar to your family's.
2. Ask this person to describe what growing up was like, what is different today from the way it was when he or she was your age, what are the important values held, and if there have been any changes in them over the years. Ask this person what advice he or she would give you about how to achieve satisfaction in life. If this person could change one thing about our society today, what would it be?

Discussion:

1. Were you surprised at any of the answers the older adult gave you?
2. What are some common themes you and your classmates found related to values and the type of advice the older adult gave each of you?
3. What implications do the findings from this exercise have for your future nursing practice?

meaningful to them and to you. Let's think about some ways you can make your life more satisfying and as rewarding as it has been in the past.

Successful past achievements can be used as tools to help the client face necessary transitions and take control of his or her life. Helping the client identify sources of social support, personal resources, and coping strategies can alter the impact of physical and emotional stressors associated with age-related transitions. Exercise 19-3 provides a glimpse into the life stories of the older adult.

Using a Proactive Approach. For many reasons, the older adult needs the nurse to assume initial responsibility for directing the interview at the beginning of the relationship (Cochran, 2005). At first, new situations can cause transitory confusion for many older adults. Knowing what to expect helps decrease anxiety and build trust. Many clients are aware of the stereotypes associated with aging and are reluctant to expose themselves as inadequate in any way.

When the nurse has concern about the cognitive capability of the older adult, it is prudent to perform a mental status assessment early in the interview to avoid obtaining questionable data. The Mini-Mental State Examination (Folstein, Folstein, & McHugh, 1975) is a good example to consider. It measures several dimensions of cognition (e.g., orientation, memory, abstraction, and language). The nurse's approach in assessing cognition can contribute significantly to obtaining useful and reliable information. Suggestions for approaching mental status testing with older adults are presented in Box 19-1.

Box 19-1 Guide for Mental Status Testing with Older Adults

1. Select a standardized test such as the Mini-Mental State Examination (MMSE), which can be completed in 5 minutes.
2. Administer the test in a quiet, nondistracting environment at a time when the client is not anxious, agitated, or tired.
3. Make sure the client has eyeglasses or hearing aids, if needed, prior to testing.
4. Ask easier questions first, and provide frequent reassurance that the client is doing well with the testing.
5. Determine the client's level of formal education. If the client never learned to spell, it will be impossible to spell "world" backwards. Saying the days of the week backwards is a good alternative.
6. Document your findings clearly in the client's record, including the client's response to the testing process, so that future comparisons can be made.

The older adult appreciates having the nurse provide structure to the history-taking interview by explaining the reasons for it and the outline of what it will involve. The I-thou position stressed in earlier chapters is used to enhance connectedness. Questions that the older adult perceives as relevant and that follow a logical sequence are likely to hold the client's interest. Having an opportunity to talk about oneself can be extremely beneficial.

Of equal importance is the sensitivity of the nurse to the unexpressed fears of the older adult. Often the client has a strong concern that in accepting external or professional services, there is a loss of independence. In the client's mind, accepting help is the first step toward the nursing home. Consequently, the older adult may minimize difficulties to avoid that possibility.

The nurse may need to assess environmental supports directly and should always bear in mind the possible association in the older adult's mind between accepting any help and relinquishing independent living. For example, an older adult in cardiac rehabilitation told his nurse that he had a bedside commode and no stairs in his home. When the nurse visited the home, there was no commode, and the client's home had a significant number of stairs. He told the nurse that he was afraid she would take steps to make him move if these facts were known.

Promoting Client Autonomy and Independence. Independence is something most people take for granted as a younger adult, but it is a significant issue for elders and their caregivers. The nurse plays a critical role in helping older adults maintain their autonomy. Corey and Corey (2006) note, "We live most of our adult years with an internal locus control. As we age, we have to adjust to an increasingly external locus of control when confronted with losses over which we have little control" (p. 403).

For most older clients, being independent means that they are still in charge of their lives. It is easy for the nurse to confuse the fact that an older adult appears frail with an inability to function. As the nurse assists the client to clarify values, make choices, and take action, a stronger understanding of the unique needs and strengths of the client emerges. An open-ended approach to understanding the client as a person is helpful to both nurse and client. Often in relating their life stories and exploring options relevant to their current situation with the nurse, older adults are able to step back and look at the present in a more positive way. To whatever extent is possible, the older adult needs to take responsibility for choices and goal setting in health care.

Case Example

Nurse: Mr. Matturo, it sounds as if being in charge of your life is very important to you.

Client: Yes, it is. I grew up on a farm and was always taught that I should pull my own weight. You have to on a farm. I've lived my entire life that way. I've never asked anyone for anything.

Nurse: I can hear how important that is to you. What else has been important?

Client: Well, I was a Marine sergeant in World War II, and I led many a platoon into battle. My men depended on me, and I never let them down. My wife says I've been a good provider, and I've always taught my children to value honor and the simple way of life.

Nurse: It sounds as though you have led a very interesting and productive life. Tell me more about what you mean by honor and the simple way of life.

As the client expresses important information about values and life experiences, previous coping strategies can be identified. At the end of the dialogue, the nurse might summarize what the client has expressed and follow up with, "Do you think you might be able to use any of these life skills now?" It is easier for the client to imagine possible coping skills when they are linked to principles of coping in the past, and the care is better individualized and sensitive to the older adult's needs and values. Other simple interventions to promote independence include the following:

- Allowing elders personal choices about their bedtime, within reason
- Respecting choices in food selection
- Providing chair risers that help elders raise themselves from sitting to standing position
- Safety modifications in the home (e.g., bathtub rails, scatter rug removal, night lights)
- Including elder clients in decision making about health care and giving them the information they need to make responsible choices

While there will always be a delicate balance between the client's needs and restrictions needed for safety, usually there are at least some areas that can be negotiated.

Modern technology can support independence in the elderly. Telehealth assistive services now include virtual health visits, reminder systems, home security, social and health alarm monitors, and compensatory supports for failing functional abilities (Magnusson, Hanson, & Borg, 2004) (see Chapter 24).

Acting as the Client's Advocate. The nurse plays an important role as advocate with the older adult. When there is a breakdown in the client's ability to meet essential needs, sometimes they can be addressed with some very simple environmental modifications and referrals. It is important to engage the client in actively exploring appropriate environmental supports (e.g., homemaker services, leisure activities, home nursing support). Introducing the need for external supports, however, without first building rapport and helping the client establish a sense of his or her personal strengths, is likely to be counterproductive. Framing suggestions for external supports in terms of helping the older adult maintain independent living as long as possible often works with clients who are reluctant to use them.

Advocating for the client with the family also is important. Seen through the client's eyes, the dilemma of allowing the older adult both enough freedom and enough protection is eloquently described in the following poem:

> My children are coming today. They mean well. But they worry.
>
> They think I should have a railing in the hall. A telephone in the kitchen.
>
> They want someone to come in when I take a bath.
>
> They really don't like my living alone.
>
> Help me to be grateful for their concern. And help them to understand that I have to do what I can as long as I can.
>
> They're right when they say there are risks. I might fall. I might leave the stove on. But there is no real challenge, no possibility of triumph, no real aliveness without risk.

When they were young and climbed trees and rode bicycles and went away to camp, I was terrified, but I let them go.
Because to hold them would have hurt them.
Now our roles are reversed. Help them see.
Keep me from being grim or stubborn about it. But don't let them smother me.
Elise Maclay (1977)

Life review is another useful strategy. There is always a part of the essence of self that remains the same regardless of age-related bodily and cognitive changes. This is true even for people in the early stages of dementia. Connecting with that essential part of the self draws on the experiences we have gained through life. Nurses can assist older adults in this process with an unhurried storytelling approach to learning about the client's early life and important relationships. Helping family members connect with their loved one in this way is beneficial for all concerned.

Blocks to Communication

There are a few special considerations or cautions that are relevant when communicating with older adults. Whereas these can be problems across the life span, they seem more prevalent in interactions with older persons. It is very easy to impede communication with any of the following communication mistakes.

Offering Cliché Reassurances

An older man says, "I just got back from burying my wife; she was sick with cancer a long time." An example of a communication-blocking response might be, "Well, at least her suffering is over" or, "In time, your grief will lessen." These are not particularly helpful comments, and they certainly do not promote a response from the client. In addition, they do not contribute to an assessment of the impact of this situation on the client. A better option might be, "How are you doing?" or, "I have some time, would you like to talk?"

Giving Advice

Telling an older adult what to do in a given situation rather than exploring the options available is a common block to communication. An example of this would be, "With your bad arthritis you really do need to start a walking program or you will start to lose function." A better statement might be, "With your bad arthritis, I worry about your losing your mobility. What kinds of things do you do to stay physically active?"

Answering Your Own Questions

Sometimes older adults require more time to hear and understand the communication, so their responses are not as rapidly forthcoming as with younger persons. For example, "Which do you want: tomato, orange, or apple juice?" may be quickly followed by, "I guess you would like apple juice" if a response from the older adult did not come fast enough. Another example of not waiting for an answer is, "How would you describe your chest pain?" too quickly followed by, "Is it sharp, dull, pricking, or aching?" The older adult should be allowed the additional few seconds to determine an answer ("It's burning") before the question is made "multiple choice." Allowing the cognitively intact older adult to use his or her own words to describe a problem or concern rather than having the caregiver provide the terminology provides a much better data-gathering approach.

Giving Excessive Praise or Reprimands

Often giving effusive praise can be detrimental because it blocks most responses except "Thank you." For example, "You have done a wonderfully fantastic job in organizing your medications" does not readily allow the older adult to ask questions or raise a concern about some aspect of what has been done. A better response might be to recognize the accomplishment and ask if there are any remaining concerns about the medications. Also, reprimanding or scolding the older adult can be demeaning as well as a block to communication. For example, "Haven't you finished your lunch yet? You are the slowest one on the unit. What am I going to do with you?" could be more appropriately managed by identifying that this person eats slowly and perhaps could benefit from getting meals first.

Defending Against a Complaint

Many older adults have no difficulty in criticizing their environment or treatment by others, and it is often to the nurse that this criticism is verbalized. For example, "No one answered my call light last night, and I almost fell going to the bathroom by myself" may elicit a defensive response such as, "The unit was really busy last night. We had two admissions." A better approach is to determine what underlies the comment. Is the older adult afraid of being alone, of falling, or of something else? A better response might be, "What was happening with you last night?"

Using Parenting Approaches or Behaviors

When nurses use these approaches, older adults may be embarrassed or feel demeaned. Using terms such as "honey," "sweetie," or "doll" rather than asking them the names by which they would like to be addressed is the same as treating these adults like children. Additionally, the nurse may answer for the older adult when someone asks the person a question. For example, the chaplain asks an older woman, "How are you doing today?" and the nurse answers for her, "Oh, she is just fine." There is a simple rule to follow when communicating with older adults: the older adult is an adult and should be acknowledged as such and related to in an adult manner.

Communication Strategies in Long-Term Care Settings

Liukkonen (1993) reports that many older adults in long-term facilities suffer from loneliness and long for someone simply to listen to them. Older adults who are institutionalized in hospitals or nursing homes often appreciate short, frequent conversations. Like everyone else, the need to be acknowledged is paramount to the older adult's sense of self-esteem. Continuity of care with one primary caregiver, when possible, helps foster the development of a comfortable nurse-client relationship.

Dealing with Memories and Reminiscences

It is not uncommon for healthy older persons to share the memories from youth or earlier days with those around them. This can be a very meaningful way in which older adults review their life, establish its meaning, and confront their conflicts or negative acts. It can also provide opportunities for the older adult to reconcile these conflicts and atone (Butler, 1995). It can be frustrating for the people who have heard the older person's stories a hundred times, and so they may turn off or avoid interacting with the person. Rather than responding with, "Oh my, here he goes again with that old 'Model T' car story," it is better to respond to the story and enter it with the older adult to learn more about why it has special relevance or meaning. It is an opportunity to gain insight into the person, who he or she was, what aspirations and dreams were fulfilled or unfulfilled, what contributions are valued, and what goals are yet to be attained. Reminiscing also has been demonstrated to increase self-esteem, mood, morale, and socialization (Stater, 1995). Each time the older adult tells the story, he remembers a time when he saw himself as a valued, productive member of society.

Several suggestions have been made by Cox and Waller (1987) in connection with responding to the reminiscences of the older person, including the following:

1. *Ask exploring questions.* In the Model T car story, one might ask, "What made you buy that car?" or, "How did you get the money to buy it?"
2. *Use the memory as a bridge to other information.* "What other types of cars did you have after that? Were you usually the one in your social group who had the car? Where would you go?"
3. *Find a cue for a question within frequently heard stories.* "Cars seem very important to you. What was it like for you when you had to give up driving last year?"
4. *Practice ways to tell the person that you have heard the story before.* "Oh yes, I remember the Model T episode when you drove the car into the Madison County reservoir. What other unusual or amusing things happened to you during your life?" (This should be done only if the repetition occurs within the same conversation, or close to it—otherwise, let it go.)

Group Activities

Groups can be an important source of social support and healing for the older adult. They help restore hope and reestablish a sense of personal worth. The model of empowerment described in Chapter 5 and the variety of groups available for the older adult described in Chapter 12 offer hope to clients by helping them receive needed emotional support and keeping their minds active. The interpersonal contact in groups can be very therapeutic for lonely, isolated older adults (Henderson & Gladding, 2004). Guidelines for group communication with older adult clients are presented in Box 19-2.

Role Modeling

Role modeling is an aspect of care that indirectly affects the interpersonal relationships older adults have with their caregivers. Since ancillary personnel often constitute the largest group of primary caregivers in long-term care settings, it is particularly important for professional

Box 19-2 Working with Older Adult Groups

- Avoid keeping members busy with meaningless activities.
- Affirm the dignity, intelligence, and pride of elderly group members.
- Ask group members to introduce themselves and ask how they would like to be called.
- Make use of humor, but never at the expense of an individual group member.
- Keep the communication simple, but at an adult level.
- Call attention to the range of life experiences and personal strengths when they occur.
- Allow group members to voice their complaints, even when nothing can be done about them, and then refocus on the group task.
- Avoid probing for the release of strong emotions that neither you nor they can handle effectively in the group sessions.
- Thank each person for contributing to the group and summarize the group activity for that session.

Adapted from Corey M, Corey G: Groups for the elderly. In Corey M, Corey G, *Groups*, ed 7, Belmont, CA, 2006, Thompson/Brooks Cole, p. 406.

nurses, who commonly supervise them, to serve as positive role models. This means that the professional nurse needs to be actively involved with older adults and willing to share observations with other personnel. People learn not only what is taught but also what is "caught" in the form of attitudes toward the older adult. If professional attitudes are positive and supportive, they influence positively the care a nursing assistant gives to clients.

Health Promotion Activities

The Centers for Disease Control and Prevention maintain that health-damaging behaviors such as poor nutrition, inactivity, and alcohol and tobacco use contribute heavily to the onset of disability in the elderly. They recommend an integrated health promotion approach to address common risk factors and comorbidities in older adults (Lang, Moore, Harris et al., 2005). Through regularly scheduled health promotion activities, nurses can assist clients in learning about a healthier lifestyle. They can monitor common medical indicators such as blood pressure, blood sugar, respiratory and cardiac concerns, and medical regimens on a regular basis. Box 19-3 presents the components of health promotion activities for the older adult in the community.

Box 19-3 Examples of Health Promotion Components in Caring for the Older Adult

- Health protection: Public health approaches promoting flu vaccines
- Health prevention: Environmental or home assessments to prevent falls
- Health education: Information about healthy eating and exercise
- Health preservation: Promoting optimal levels of functioning by increasing the control older adults have over their lives and health

Adapted from Sanders K: Developing practice for healthy aging, *Nurs Older People* 18(3):18-21, 2006; Bernard M: *Promoting health in old age*, Buckingham, England, 2000, Open University Press.

Nurses can most effectively engage older adults in health promotion activities by appealing to their interests and by incorporating cultural values in the presentation. Examples of relevant activities from several resources include the following (Lang et al., 2005; Penprase, 2006):

- Preparing examples of healthy ethnic food (e.g. "soul cooking the healthy way")
- Assigning blocks of time for preventive screening specifically for older adults
- Combining multiple prevention services into one clinical visit
- Providing free flu and pneumonia immunizations at convenient times in nontraditional as well as traditional settings

Protecting Client Privacy

The Health Insurance Portability and Accountability Act (HIPAA) privacy rule introduced a significant challenge to protecting the client's privacy in long-term care settings related to relationships with family and personal representatives of the client. Lessner (2006) advises that nurses may provide information to family members involved in the resident's care or to the resident's personal representative authorized by state law to speak on behalf of the client if the client is incompetent. This is important, because when there is a change in the elder resident's health status, the family needs to be notified. Notification compliance takes precedence in this situation unless a competent resident has specifically requested that the disclosure not be made. In that case, documentation should clearly state that the client was given the opportunity to object to the disclosure.

Communication Strategies with the Cognitively Impaired Adult

Assessment of cognitive function should occur early in the communication process with older adults. If the nurse perceives the client to have diagnosable cognitive impairment, a full neurological assessment is indicated. Clients in the very early stages of dementia have enough cognition to participate in legal decisions regarding their health care and finances that they may not later be able to execute. Consultation with a lawyer regarding wills, durable and health powers of attorney, and living wills should be initiated at this time (Arnold, 2005).

Some older adults with moderately severe communication deficits retain all of their intellectual abilities. Other older adults retain enough of their sensory functions to communicate effectively, but the means of processing information, learning, and responding become dysfunctional. Most communication deficits associated with memory loss, however, are cumulative and progressive. Unfortunately, in the early stages, environmental conflicts may be heightened because of the older adult's seemingly normal, superficial verbal behaviors. Only when one tries to engage the older adult in a deeper conversation does the degree of communication deficit become apparent. For example, the client may say, "I'm feeling great; Martha and I visited the grandchildren, and we had a great time." But when asked what he actually did on the visit, he may be unable to answer with any real detail.

In a more advanced loss of cognition, the older adult is unable to express complete thoughts. He or she has difficulty finding the words to use, and sentences are unfinished. The client with dementia, unable to continue, stops in mid-sentence or continues with phrases that have little to do with the intended meaning. In such cases the nurse can help by filling in the missing words, smiling, supplying the logical meaning, and then asking the client if this is what he or she meant. Another strategy is to almost finish a sentence and have the client supply the last word. In fact, anything to help reduce the client's anxiety about groping for thoughts that do not come helps the person continue.

Another communication difficulty is **apraxia**, defined as the loss of the ability to take purposeful action even when the muscles, senses, and vocabulary seem intact. This condition causes a person to appear to register on a command, but then to act in ways that suggest he or she has little understanding of what transpired verbally. When the cognitively impaired adult fails to follow through on the agreed-upon action, the nurse may interpret the behavior as uncooperative or obstinate. Talking the client through a procedure step by step, providing

Box 19-4 Sample Clinical Situation: Nursing Process Application to Care of a Cognitively Impaired Older Adult

Problem: An 86-year-old woman exhibits disturbed attention and confusion

Nursing Diagnosis: Ineffective coping related to organic memory loss

Nursing Goals: Minimize factors that contribute to inattention

Nursing Approach: Compensatory and supportive

Method of Assistance: Guiding, supporting, and providing an understanding environment

Nursing Interventions:

1. Look directly at the client when talking.
2. Call the client by name several times.
3. Position self in the client's line of vision.
4. Rest hands on the client's hands.
5. Give clear, simple directions in a step-by-step manner.
6. Direct conversation toward concrete, familiar objects.
7. If attention lapses, let the client rest a few minutes before trying to regain his or her attention.
8. Provide simple activities that will encourage purposeful action.
9. Repeat messages slowly, calmly, and patiently until some signs of comprehension are shown.
10. Vary the words to fit the client's ability to comprehend.
11. Modify the environmental stimuli that affect attention.
12. Assist the family to understand that inattention and failure to respond is due to the inability to process information cognitively.

The evaluation of the effectiveness, appropriateness, and efficiency of the nursing actions with the dementia client does not occur through words, as it does with other nurse-client relationships. Behaviors of the client in which agitation is reduced, cooperation is obtained, and the client responds positively to the caregiver are indicators of effective nursing interventions and successful outcomes.

additional cues, and allowing additional time for processing information reduces the person's anxiety and improves performance. Box 19-4 provides a sample of how the nursing process can be applied to the care of a cognitively impaired client.

Reminiscence

Relationships with older adults with mild to moderate cognitive disability can take advantage of the simple fact that remote memory (recall of past events) is retained longer than memory for recent events. Asking older adults about their past life experiences often serves as a way to connect verbally with those who might have difficulty telling you what they had for breakfast 2 hours ago. The nurse should appreciate that when older adults share memories they are giving a gift to the nurse, sharing part of themselves when they may have little else to give. For some reason, once older adults with mild memory deficits begin to reminisce about the past, communication flows more freely and retention of messages is stronger. Mentally impaired persons become more verbal and will even assist others in remembering events when in a reminiscence group (Baker, 1985). The nurse can act as an advocate in learning about the dementia client's needs, expressed as past occurrences, and can translate them into current requirements for care.

Repetition and Instructions

The nurse should have additional means of communicating with older adults experiencing memory loss. It is very appropriate to address the older adult by his or her name several times before beginning the communication. This approach can be useful in focusing the older adult's attention on what is coming next. By selecting a simple, relevant thought from a stream of loosely connected ideas, the nurse permits the conversation to continue, often to the visible relief of the impaired dementia client. Restating ideas using the same words and sequence is a simple communication strategy that allow a conversation to continue.

By speaking in simple sentences, repeating phrases, and giving directions one at a time, the nurse enables the older adult to use his or her remaining capabilities. For example, asking the older adult to make a cup of coffee might be beyond her comprehension. But breaking the request down into smaller steps (e.g., "Open the cupboard," "Open the drawer," "Take out a spoon," "Close the drawer," "Open the jar of instant coffee") may make the activity possible and thus reinforce self-esteem.

Use of Touch

Gaining eye contact and using touch are also helpful to maintain focus. The use of appropriate touch with the cognitively impaired can be a helpful tool, but its applicability must be determined on an individual basis. For some people, being touched increases their agitation and confusion, whereas for others being touched is a calming and welcome action.

Nurses should be sensitive to their own style of touching: how it is done, to whom, when, and why. Watson (1975) reports that the older adults least likely to experience touch from nurses were men and those who have severe cognitive impairment. Thus men with cognitive impairment are likely to have limited touch experiences.

There is also a hierarchy of places on the body that are appropriate to touch (e.g., the hands, shoulders, back, and arms). Although the thigh and face are relatively personal parts of the body, they are often selected when touching older adults. These areas should not be chosen as sites for touching until rapport has been established—and even then, it is better to touch other parts of the body, which represent more equality in relationship.

Use of Multiple Modalities

Using more than one sense in communication facilitates the process. For example, touching the hand with the hairbrush in it and saying, "Now use the brush to fix your hair" provides an additional focus for the older adult. Knowing, when helping a dementia client groom and dress, that stiffening can occur due to an automatic neurological response and that this manifestation is not due to a resistive and rejecting person, enables the nurse to be more sensitive to the older adult. Sometimes, waiting 5-10 minutes and trying again can be a productive option.

Use of Distraction for Disruptive Behaviors

Because older adults with memory loss lack the cognitive ability to develop alternatives, they can have what appears to be temper tantrums in response to real or perceived frustration. These tantrums are called **catastrophic reactions** and represent a completely disorganized set of responses. They are often difficult for the nurse to comprehend or manage. Usually there is something in the immediate environment that precipitates the reaction, but fatigue, overstimulation, misinterpretations, and inability to meet expectations may also be contributing factors. The emotion may be appropriate even if its behavioral manifestation is not. In these situations, the nurse can use distraction to move the older adult away from the offending stimuli in the environment or to diffuse the troublesome feeling through postponement. For example, the nurse might say to the older adult, "We will do that later; right now, let us go out on the porch," while gently leading the person away. Direct confrontation and an appeal for more civilized behavior usually serve to escalate rather than diminish the episode.

Often there are warning signs of an impending catastrophic reaction (e.g., restlessness, refusals, or general uncooperativeness); by redirecting the dementia client, the outburst may be avoided. It is important for the nurse to model the appropriate responses to this behavior and to explain to the family members and staff what is happening and what to do to prevent or address it.

Ethical Dilemma ■ *What Would You Do?*

Mrs. Porter's mother, Eileen O'Smith, is a feisty, independent, 86-year-old. She lives alone and treasures her independence. Mrs. O'Smith is in your urgent care clinic for suturing of a lesion on her leg, which was injured in a fall. Mrs. Porter accompanies her mother and you listen to them argue; it is clear to you that Mrs. Porter wants to commit her mother to a long-term care facility. While you are alone with Mrs. O'Smith in the examination room, taking her history, she swears you to silence and confides in you that she is having increasingly frequent lapses in memory, sometimes forgetting to eat. You are aware of the need to maintain client confidentiality, but you also recognize that to ignore the ethical concept of beneficence and keep silent may well endanger Mrs. O'Smith's life. What would you do?

Courtesy Elaine Cloud, M.D., 2002.

SUMMARY

Chapter 19 emphasizes the use of therapeutic communication skills with older adults. Understanding the principles of communication as they relate to relationships with older adults requires a clear understanding of the uniqueness of older persons.

Older adults vary greatly in capabilities, interests, and capacities for relationships. Whereas some are frail, with reduction of intellectual function due to disease, others retain a high level of physical and intellectual functioning until their death. Technological advances and better nutrition have reduced mortality rates, increased the life span, and correspondingly increased the number of older adults who now require health care. Communication difficulties can occur because of changes in sensory and cognitive functioning in the older adult as well as because of significant changes in social support systems. The nurse can provide the older adult with a therapeutic environment that supports the client's independence and that helps the client compensate for failing physical, cognitive, and emotional functioning. Strategies such as reminiscing, promoting client autonomy, using a proactive approach, acting as a client advocate, and treating the older adult with dignity are proposed. Health promotion activities that take into account the unique needs and cultural values of older adults are more likely to be successful. A care plan for the cognitively impaired client is presented. As a primary provider in long-term care and in the community, the nurse is in a unique role to support and meet the communication needs of the frail older adult.

REFERENCES

Anderson D: Preventing delirium in older people, *Br Med J* 73/74:25-34, 2005.

Arnold E: Sorting out the 3 D's: delirium, dementia, depression, *Holist Nurs Pract* 19(3):99-104, 2005.

Baker N: Reminiscing in group therapy for self-worth, *J Gerontol Nurs* 11:21, 1985.

Bernard M: *Promoting health in old age*, Buckingham, England, 2000, Open University Press.

Bonder BR, Wagner MB, editors: *Functional performance in older adults*, ed 2, Philadelphia, 2001, FA Davis.

Bortz W: Use it or lose it, *Runner's World* 25:55-58, 1990.

Butler RN: Forward. In Haight BK, Webster JD, editors, *The art and science of reminiscing: theory, research, methods and applications*, Washington, DC, 1995, Taylor & Francis.

Cochran P: Acute care for elders prevents functional decline, *Nursing* 35(10):70-71, 2005.

Corey M, Cory G: Groups for the elderly. In *Groups: Process and practice*, ed 7, Belmont, CA, 2006, Thompson Brooks/Cole.

Coughlin J: Technology needs of aging boomers [online article], *Issues in Science and Technology Online* 16(1), Fall, 1999; available online: http://www.issues.org/issues/16.1/coughlin.htm.

Cox BJ, Waller L: *Communicating with the older adult*, St Louis, 1987, Catholic Health Association of the United States.

Curtis E, Dixon M: Family therapy and systemic practice with older people: where are we now? *J Fam Ther* 27:43-64, 2005.

Erikson E: *The life cycle completed*, New York, 1982, Norton.

Folstein MF, Folstein S, McHugh PR: Mini-mental state: a practical method for grading cognition state of patients for the clinician, *J Psychiatr Res* 12:189-198, 1975.

Franklin L, Ternestedt B, Nordenfelt L: Views on dignity of elderly nursing home residents, *Nurs Ethics* 13(2):130-146, 2006.

Gallo JJ: *Handbook of geriatric assessment*, ed 3, Gaithersburg, MD, 2000, Aspen.

Gavan C: Successful aging families, *Holist Nurs Pract* 17(1):11-18, 2003.

Groh CJ, Whall AL: Self-esteem disturbances. In Maas ML, Buckwalter KC, Hardy MD et al., editors, *Nursing care of older adults: diagnoses, outcomes, & interventions*, St Louis, 2001, Mosby.

Henderson DA, Gladding ST: Group counseling with older adults. In DeLucia-Waack JL, Gerrity DA, Kalodner CR et al., editors, *Handbook of group counseling and psychotherapy*, Thousand Oaks, CA, 2004, Sage.

International Council of Nurses: ICN on healthy aging: a public health and nursing challenge [*Nursing Matters* fact sheet], 2005; available online: http://www.icn.ch/matters_aging.htm.

Ivnik RJ, Smith GE, Malec JF et al.: Long-term stability and intercorrelations of cognitive abilities in older persons, *Psychol Assess* 7(2):155-161, 1995.

Jerger J, Chmiel R, Wilson N et al.: Hearing impairment in older adults: new concepts, *J Am Geriatr Soc* 43(8):928-935, 1995.

Lang J, Moore M, Harris A et al.: Healthy aging: priorities and programs of the Centers for Disease Control and Prevention, *Generations* 29(2):24-29, 2005.

Lessner J: HIPAA checkups for compliance, *Geriatr Nurs* 27(2):83-84, 2006.

Liukkonen A: The content of nurses' oral shift reports in homes for older adult people, *J Adv Nurs* 18(7):1095-1100, 1993.

Maclay E: *Green winter: celebrations of old age*, New York, 1977, McGraw-Hill.

Magnusson L, Hanson, Borg M: A literature review study of information and communication technology as a support for frail older people living at home and their family carers, *Technol Disabil* 16:223-235, 2004.

Maples MF, Abney P: Baby boomers mature and gerontological counseling comes of age, *J Counsel Dev* 84:3-9, 2006.

Maslow A: *Motivation and personality*, New York, 1954, Harper & Row.

Nakasato Y, Carnes B: Health promotion in older adults: promoting successful aging in primary care settings, *Geriatrics* 61(4):27-31, 2006.

Ownby R: Medication adherence and cognition: medical, personal and economic factors influence level of adherence in older adults, *Geriatrics* 61(2):30-35, 2006.

Penprase B: Developing comprehensive health care for an underserved population, *Geriatr Nurs* 27(1):45-50, 2006.

Rowe JW, Kahn RL: *Successful aging*, New York, 1998, Pantheon Books.

Salthouse T: Speed mediation of adult age differences in cognition, *Dev Psychol* 29:722-738, 1993.

Sanders K: Developing practice for healthy aging, *Nurs Older People* 18(3):18-21, 2006.

Stater R: *The psychology of growing old: looking forward*, Buckingham, England, 1995, Open University Press.

Wallhagen MI, Strawbridge WJ, Kaplan GA: 6-year impact of hearing impairment on psychosocial and physiologic functioning, *Nurs Pract* 21:11, 1996.

Watson W: The meaning of touch: gerontological nursing, *J Commun* 25:104-112, 1975.

Weil A: *Healthy aging: a lifelong guide to your physical and spiritual well-being*, New York, 2005, Knopf.

Weman K, Fagerberg I: Registered nurses working together with family members of older people, *J Clin Nurs* 15(3):281-289, 2006.

Wilson RS, Bennet DA, Swartzendruber A: Age-related change in cognitive function. In Nussbaum PD, editor, *Handbook of neuropsychology and aging*, New York, 1997, Plenum Press.

Chapter 20

Communicating with Clients in Stressful Situations

Elizabeth Arnold

OUTLINE

OBJECTIVES

At the end of the chapter, the reader will be able to:

1. Define stress and sources of stress.
2. Identify selected theoretical frameworks of stress and coping.
3. Identify factors influencing the impact of stress.
4. Specify the relationship between stress and disease.
5. Identify expressions of grief.
6. Identify basic concepts of coping.
7. Apply the nursing process to the care of clients in stressful situations.
8. Identify strategies for burnout prevention.

> *I knew I was being childish; still I acted terribly. I insulted nurses and doctors, repeatedly questioned their judgment . . . basically acted like a jerk. If only someone could have realized what was happening to me.*
>
> (Bluhm, 1987)

Chapter 20 provides a framework for understanding basic concepts of stress and coping in the nurse-client relationship. Stress is an inevitable, normal part of life that no human being can escape (Antai-Otong, 2001). Factors that create stress can be actual or potential, real or imagined. People feel stressed when there is (a) a threat to the person's self-integrity or well-being; (b) a loss of something important to the person's well-being and self-esteem; or (c) a challenge to be overcome. Most people struggling with health care issues are stressed. Making difficult decisions under less-than-ideal circumstances creates stress and is the rule rather than the exception in health care.

Problem-focused coping mechanisms such as negotiation, directly confronting challenging issues, and seeking out social support can alleviate some stressors, but others cannot be changed. Terminal illness, chronic pain, death of a significant person or pet, end of a relationship, or serious injury may require acceptance, a constructive outlook, and new strategies to maintain self-esteem in the face of overwhelming, often unfair, and irreversible circumstances. Helping a client explore new directions and develop a different perspective can be just as important as the more traditional problem-solving strategies used to cope with stress (Michalenko, 1998). Incorporating coping and stress management principles into the nurse-client relationship enables the nurse to communicate effectively with clients in stressful health care situations ranging from health promotion to care of the terminally ill.

BASIC CONCEPTS

Stress represents a personalized physiological, psychological, and spiritual response to the presence of a stressor. A **stressor** can be any demand, situation, internal stimulus, or circumstance that threatens a person's personal security or self-integrity. Illness, a personally significant loss (e.g., job or relationship), a move to a different city, loss of income—all can create stress. People also experience stress as a response to a positive circumstance (e.g., a promotion or the birth of a child). Stress disrupts normal functioning and contributes to people behaving in ways they ordinarily would not consider.

The intensity and duration of stress varies according to the circumstances and the emotional state of the person experiencing it. It can be brief (e.g., avoiding a car crash) or it can be episodic (e.g., the stress of studying for an exam or meeting a deadline). It can be chronic (e.g., living with an abusive relationship or caring for a relative with a debilitating illness) or it can occur as an acute experience with breakthrough flashbacks (e.g., an assault or robbery).

Stress is an individual experience. What is stressful one day for a person may not be stressful the next, and what is stressful for one person may not be for another. Cumulative stress can become chronic over time.

People experience stress as an integrated life experience, affecting both mind and body. People can experience only so much stress before it leads to permanent physiological changes. Conversely, physical illness or injury can produce emotional strain, tension, and stress. Psychological stress arouses powerful emotional reactions that can lead to depression and other mental disorders. Common sources of personal stress are identified in Box 20-1.

Stress is contagious. Parents witnessing the children of other parents die cannot help but project that experience onto their own situation and experience grieving of their own (Johnson, 1997). The nurse is a valuable resource in providing clients and their families with emotional support and health-related information that helps

Box 20-1 Personal Sources of Stress

Physical Stressors

- Aging process
- Illness
- Injury
- Pain
- Mental disorder

Psychological Stressors

- Loss of a job
- Death of a significant person
- Getting married or divorced
- Becoming a single parent
- Moving from a familiar place
- Role overload, conflict, change

Spiritual Stressors

- Loss of role
- Loss of meaning
- Questioning of values
- Change in religious affiliation

Data from McCaffery M, Beebe A: *Pain: clinical manual for nursing practice*, St Louis, 1989, Mosby.

reduce the sense of insecurity associated with not knowing what to expect or how to respond in an unfamiliar, stressful health care situation.

Personal responses to stress are as different as the people experiencing them. Men and women experience and respond to stress differently (Gadzella, Ginther, Tomcala et al., 1991). Men are more likely to respond with anger or denial, whereas women internalize stress and may experience depression. Children express stress according to their stage of development and established family patterns. Acting out behavioral changes can mask their distress.

Some people use alcohol or other drugs to dull the pain of stress. Stress can challenge spiritual beliefs. A person's language, ethnic background, religion, social support, cultural and economic level, and education will influence his or her unique behavioral response to stress (Leininger, 1991).

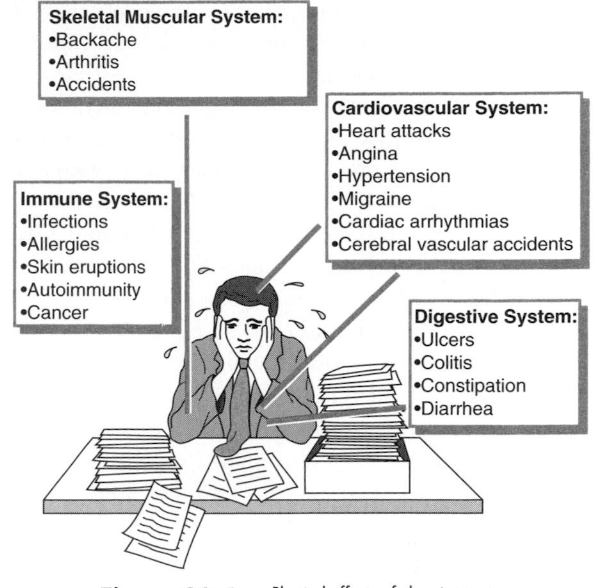

Figure 20-1 ● Physical effects of chronic stress.

Theoretical Models of Stress

Stress as a Physiologic Response

Cannon (1914) was the first to describe human stress as a threat to the body's state of physiological equilibrium. According to Cannon, when people feel physically well, emotionally centered, and personally secure, they are in a state of dynamic equilibrium or **homeostasis**. Stress upsets this homeostasis, creating an imbalance in normal physiological processes such as blood pressure, respiration, and endocrine function.

When a person is under stress, the body prepares for a "fight or flight" response by releasing adrenaline, cholesterol, and glucose into the bloodstream. Over time, stress weakens the immune system, thereby contributing to the development of stress-related illnesses such as hypertension, cardiac abnormalities, cancer, colitis, and migraine headaches (Ben-Schlomo & Chaturvedi, 1992; Gelent & Hochman, 1992; Niaura & Goldstein, 1992; Schneiderman, Antoni, Saab et al., 2001). Severe or untreated, prolonged physiological alterations caused by stress can result in death. As we develop more effective ways to study brain function and measure changes in the neuroendocrine system during acute stress, our understanding of the psychophysiological responses to stress and adaptation will become clearer (Dantzer, 1997). Figure 20-1 displays some of the currently known physical effects of stress on body systems.

General Adaptation Syndrome. Selye (1946, 1956, 1982), a physician in Canada, expanded on Cannon's work by describing the concept of stress as an internal, generalized, patterned response to environmental demands. According to Selye, not all stress is dangerous. In fact, life would be quite boring with no stress. Selye used the term **eustress** to describe a mild level of stress that acts as a positive stress response with protective and adaptive functions. The increased stress a person feels in completing a project with a deadline is an example of eustress. As a person capitalizes on the additional physiological energy created by the stress of the deadline, the stress can actually improve performance.

Distress is the word Selye used to describe negative stress. According to Selye, the same patterned response occurs regardless of whether a person experiences a physical or psychological stressor; this is referred to as the **general adaptation syndrome**. Selye developed a model that described an alarm phase, which, if unchecked, develops into a resistance phase as the body tries to restore equilibrium.

Stress as a Stimulus

A second popular model views stress as a psychological stimulus. In 1967, Holmes and Rahe developed a stress model based on the number of life change events a person experiences and subsequent development of physical illness. Theirs is a cumulative stress model centered around a list of 43 potential life events deemed capable of stimulating a stress reaction. Each life event stressor is given a numerical score. Stressors requiring a significant change in the lifestyle of the individual have a greater impact, as do cumulative stresses that occur within a short time (Steptoe, 1991).

The Holmes and Rahe scale captures the cumulative nature of stressors on an individual. The scale quantifies many different types of stressors, some of which would not be readily identified (e.g., job loss, move to a different area, or a promotion). In doing so, the contextual nature of stress becomes more visible. Although the scale has been criticized for trying to capture a major concept with a single measure, it still remains a widely used measurement of the links between mind and body under stress.

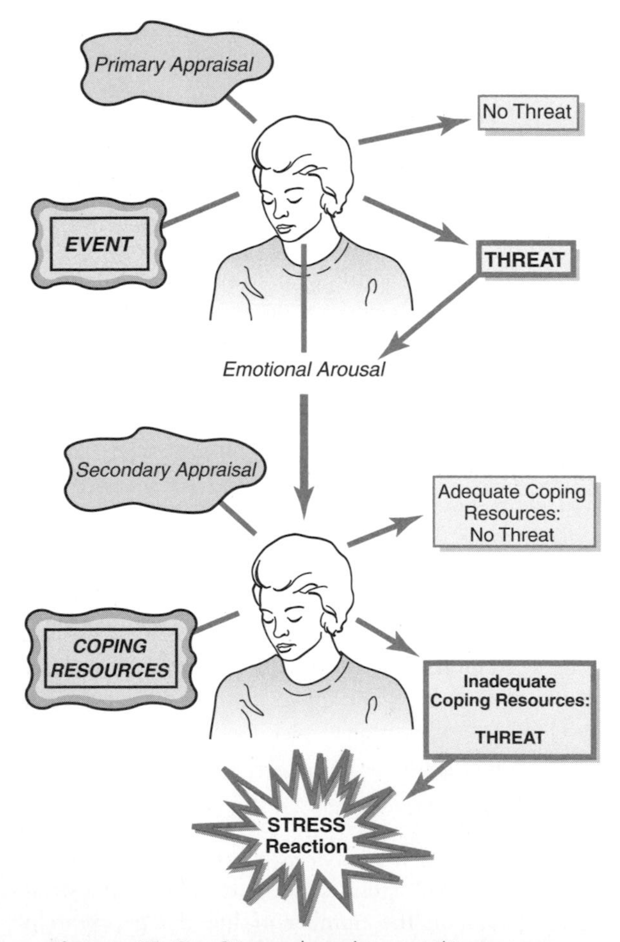

Figure 20-2 • Primary and secondary appraisal in stress reactions.

Transactional Model of Stress

Prior to the development of Lazarus and Folkman's (1984) model, stress and coping were considered primarily a biological process. Their model emphasized an interaction between person and environment that created both the impact of the stress and the person's psychological response to it as important variables. For stress to occur, there must be a dynamic relationship between a situation or circumstance in the environment (stressor) and the individual experiencing the stressor. This approach emphasizes the personal interpretation of the stressor and the subjective meaning attached to a stressful event as influencing a person's response to it (Lazarus, 1991). Each person uses primary and secondary cognitive appraisals in evaluating the magnitude of the stressor and the individual's ability to cope with it (Figure 20-2).

Primary and Secondary Appraisals. Two levels of personal appraisal (i.e., primary and secondary) influence the development of a stress response. The first level, primary appraisal, focuses on the event itself. A person determines whether an event is stressful and can draw one of three conclusions: that it is not stressful, that it is a relatively benign stressor, or that it is stressful. Stressors perceived as a major threat to self elicit a stronger stress response than those having less impact on a person's sense of self and significant relationships. Most intense are life events experienced as a personal physical threat to homeostasis (e.g., a terminal or disfiguring illness); or a psychological threat to self-concept (e.g., job loss) or to significant relationships with family or friends. Primary stress appraisals can include threat of harm or losses that are anticipated but have not yet occurred.

Primary appraisal of a stressful situation is a subjective experience influenced by a variety of factors, as shown in Box 20-2. Although some stressors are of such magnitude or number that it would be impossible not to experience them as overwhelming, most personal responses to life stress are highly individual. A set of circumstances can be overwhelmingly stressful for one person, whereas another person can cope with the same circumstances without significant distress (Lazarus & Folkman, 1984). Two college freshmen, for example, may experience their first semester away from home quite differently. For one student, the experience may be a challenging and growth-producing adventure; the other student may feel extremely confused and frightened.

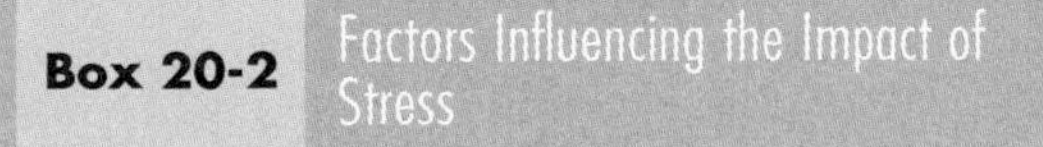

Box 20-2 Factors Influencing the Impact of Stress

- Magnitude of the stressor
- Number of stressors
- Subjective meaning of the stressor
- Developmental level of the client
- Availability of social support

How each student personally perceives the meaning of the stressor will influence its impact.

When a primary cognitive appraisal of the stressor determines it to be a threat to self, a person automatically switches to a secondary appraisal to determine how to respond. Secondary appraisals consist of a person's perception of his or her coping skills in handling the stressor. It is a dynamic concept that considers the efficacy of potential coping responses, the availability of coping resources, and the ability of the person to carry out an effective strategy to reduce the stressor. Coping resources can include health, energy, problem-solving skills, and amount and availability of social supports and other material resources to cope effectively with the stressor (Lazarus & Folkman, 1984). Primary and secondary appraisals do not occur in isolation from one another; they occur as a composite transactional response in determining the level of stress that an individual experiences.

Previous experiences, the ability to make friends, and cognitive maturity can intensify or reduce the impact of the stressor. **Social support**, defined as social environmental factors that contribute to a person's sense of well-being (Edens, Larkin, & Abel, 1992), can include family, friends, church, work, or school. These help people respond productively to stress. Social support can act as a buffer on stress by reducing its intensity (Caplan, 1981). For example, having a supportive roommate and frequent care packages from home can reduce the impact of the stressor for the student who is lonely and unsure during the first semester of college.

Behavioral Responses to Stress

Anxiety

Stress inevitably creates **anxiety**. The word anxiety derives from the Latin root *angere*, "to cause anguish or distress." Anxiety reduces a person's objectivity and makes it more difficult to envision possibilities, weigh options, make choices, and take action. Acute anxiety causes clients to become hypervigilant of their physical symptoms, particularly pain. Unlike fear, which has a direct, identifiable source of discomfort, anxiety is diffuse, and the client may not be able to relate it to an identifiable cause.

People experiencing anxiety as a response to stress have many emotions simultaneously (e.g., anger, grief, shame, embarrassment, dread, and dismay), all of which may be difficult to sort out as being anxiety. At times, anxiety is expressed directly in nervousness, pacing, inability to concentrate, or insomnia. Other psychological symptoms include inability to recall information, blocked speech, and fear of losing control (Arnold, 1997). In other circumstances, a person does not feel the anxiety directly, but experiences it as emotional numbness or as feeling images of impending doom, feelings of going crazy, or destructive fantasies. Some people describe their anxious response to a situation as deja vu, or experience it as happening to someone else and not themselves.

The consistent, calm presence of the nurse as a source of support is helpful in helping clients and their families deescalate (Hoff, 2001). People who are anxious need additional information and frequent support delivered in a calm, competent manner. Giving the family progress reports, being available to answer questions, and letting the client and family know who is available to respond to their needs and how to contact the nurse are simple interventions that keep a client and family from becoming more anxious (Hull, 1991; Rushton, 1990). Including a relevant family member in discussions and providing practical information about community resources can help reduce client and family anxiety.

Hostility

Anger and hostility are common emotions experienced in stressful situations, most commonly when the client feels helpless. Stressed people say things they do not mean and would not dream of saying in ordinary circumstances. Family members angrily blame each other for an injury, blame the physician for operating (or not operating) on a loved one, and criticize the nurse for not responding quickly enough. If the nurse can recognize the origin of the hostility and see it as a cry for help in coping with escalating stress, it is possible to defuse the stress before it becomes out of control. Verbal hostility can be deflected if the nurse is open to the expression of negative feelings and supports the hostile person without necessarily condoning the behavior. A calm attitude, with interest expressed in learning more about what is going on with a client that creates the hostility, is the best antidote for hostility.

Case Example

Client: I don't see any point in talking to you. You can't bring Jenny back, and I don't want what you have to offer me now.

Nurse (in a calm, low, slow voice): You're right, Don, I can't bring Jenny back, but what I can offer you is a chance to talk about a very tragic and frightening situation for you. My experience is that talking about it can prove to be healing, and I think this might be helpful to you.

When clients or family members are hostile, the nurse needs to regroup and consider two factors. First, hostility is a temporary emotional response displaced on you. Usually it has little to do with you, personally, other than that you are available, you are the one most involved with the care of the loved one, and you are unlikely to retaliate. Second, the experience of a serious illness is always an emotional as well as an intellectual event for families who are emotionally connected to the client (Bluhm, 1987). Although families and clients can understand intellectually why the nurse is acting in certain ways and what is happening to their loved one, their emotional understanding may be quite different in stressful situations. They can't understand why their loved one, who is now in the hospital being cared for by skilled providers, is not getting better. When there is a discrepancy between cognitive and emotional understanding, nurses will find that anger is a common response. For example, even though Mother is 95 years old and the family knows intellectually that death is imminent, the emotional remembrance of her is that of someone they do not want to lose just yet. Family members may be angry at the physician, at you, or at other family members for the decision to let her die without heroic measures. Effective nurses do not take the anger personally; rather, they help the family accept the fact that there is no way to avoid making very difficult life-and-death decisions, and they support them in their grief without judging them.

Anger projected on the nurse as primary caregiver, even when closely linked with anxiety, can threaten the nurse's energy and commitment. What a hostile person or family yearns for most—despite their behavior—is understanding, comforting, and human intimacy (Dossey, 1991). What every client and family expects from the nurse is a person who will perceive their pain and confusion and help them to decode the hostile behaviors, feelings, and thoughts that distort reality. For example, the nurse can listen calmly and suggest ways in which the client's concerns can be addressed. Acknowledging the client's right to be angry and simply listening is helpful. If client or family expectations are unrealistic or unable to be met in the current situation, alternative explanations and suggestions reduce anxiety and allow further discussion.

Case Example

Client: I'm paying a lot of money here and no one is willing to help me. The nursing care is terrible, and I just have to lie here in pain with no one to help me.

Nurse: I'm sorry you are feeling so bad. Please tell me a little more specifically what's going on with you, and maybe we can try to do something a little differently to help you.

The nurse's first statement acknowledges the feelings of the client. The second statement asks for more information and encourages the client to enter a mutual partnership in correcting the problem. The client feels heard even if the issue cannot be totally resolved as the client wishes. Exercise 20-1 helps the student address the relationship between anger and anxiety. Specific strategies to resolve conflict are presented in Chapter 14.

A major goal in implementing this nursing intervention is to help the client or family replace unrealistic expectations for self, other professionals, and the health care setting with attainable goals. It is usually useless to defend personalities or intentions. A tactful statement acknowledging the client's feeling without agreeing with it is helpful: "It sounds as though you are pretty angry with Dr. Moore, but I'd like to see if there is something we could come up with that might make this situation less frustrating for you." Such an approach takes the focus off nonproductive blaming and helps people refocus on specific, productive behaviors. It allows space to contradict false information without making the client lose face, and it doesn't put the nurse in the position of becoming defensive about the physician's actions.

Exercise 20-1

Relationship Between Anger and Anxiety

Purpose: To help students appreciate the links between anger and anxiety and understand how anger is triggered.

Procedure:

1. Think of a time when you were really angry. It need not be a significant event or one that would necessarily make anyone else angry.
2. Identify your thoughts, feelings, and behavior in separate columns of a table you construct. For example, what were the thoughts that went through your head when you were feeling this anger? What were your physical and emotional responses to this experience? Write down words or phrases to express what you were feeling at the time. How did you respond when you were angry?
3. Identify what was going on with you before experiencing the anger. Sometimes it is not the event itself, but your feelings before the incident that make the event the straw that breaks the camel's back.
4. Identify underlying threats to your self-concept in the situation (e.g., you were not treated with respect, your opinion was discounted, you lost status, you were rejected, you feared the unknown).

Discussion:

1. In what ways were your answers similar to and different from those of your classmates?
2. What role did anxiety and threat to the self-concept play in the development of the anger response? What percentage of your anger related to the actual event and to self-concept?
3. In what ways did you see anger as a multidetermined behavioral response to threats to self-concept?
4. Did this exercise change any of your ideas about how you might handle your feelings and behavior in a similar situation?
5. What are the common threads in the events that made people in group angry?
6. In what ways could experiential knowledge of the close association between anger and anxiety be helpful in your nursing practice?

This strategy is particularly helpful when the client or family blame themselves for things that are beyond their control. The nurse can help the family reframe their situation as one in which they acted with good intentions on the basis of the knowledge they had at the time. Family members sometimes feel better about circumstances they cannot erase when they can look at a situation this way.

Concepts of Coping

Coping is a conceptual term used to describe the many ways that people respond to the stressors in their lives. In their classic work, Pearlin and Schooler (1978) defined coping as "any response to external life strains that serves to prevent, avoid, or control emotional distress" (p. 2). They identify the following three purposes of coping strategies:

- To change the stressful situation
- To change the meaning of the stressor
- To help the person relax enough to take the stress in stride

Coping strategies can be either ego-enhancing or defensive. The more versatile and flexible a person's coping strategies are, the more likely it is that he or she is able to manage life's challenges. People learn coping strategies from their parents, peers, and the circumstances life presents to them. People with a variety of life opportunities and supportive people in their lives have an advantage over those who lack them. Inadequate coping strategies can reflect a life in which a person has not had to respond to danger or lacks the necessary skills to do so. Exercise 20-2 helps you examine the many dimensions of coping strategies in your life.

Defensive coping strategies can present as avoidance, anger, or the use of ego defense mechanisms to reduce the anxiety associated with a difficult situation. Whether the situation exists in reality or is a perception of harm

Exercise 20-2 Coping

Purpose: To help students experience the wide range of adaptive and maladaptive coping strategies.

Procedure:

1. Identify all of the ways in which you handle stressful situations.
2. List three personal strategies that you have used successfully in coping with stress.
3. List one personal coping strategy that did not work, and identify your perceptions of the reasons it was inadequate or insufficient to reduce your stress level.
4. List on a chalkboard or flip chart the different coping strategies identified by students.

Discussion:

1. What common themes did you find in the ways people handle stress?
2. Were you surprised at the number and variety of ways in which people handle stress?
3. What new coping strategy might you use to reduce your stress level?
4. Are there any circumstances that increase or decrease your automatic reactions to stress?

when none is intended is immaterial. The impact of danger on the person is similar. **Ego defense mechanisms** (Table 20-1) are defined as protective coping strategies that work unconsciously to protect a person from intolerable anxiety by distorting a threat, substituting another reality, or completely blocking out the threat through denial. As a short-term strategy, they may prove beneficial. People need time to absorb the meaning of a serious stressor. As long-term coping strategies, ego defense mechanisms are ineffective when they serve as a smokescreen and deterrent to action. The nurse needs to respect a client's use of defensive coping strategies while at the same time moving the client toward more adaptive solutions. Providing new information or gently casting doubt can be helpful.

Case Example

Lynn was diagnosed as having a high cholesterol count and was advised to go on a low-fat diet. Her friends notice no change in her diet, and Lynn says she sees no reason to modify it. Lynn says she sees no purpose in going on a low-fat diet because "it's all in the genes." Both her parents had high cholesterol, and she claims there is nothing she can do about it, even though the physician has advised her differently.

Lynn's denial is a defense against feeling that she will die like her parents from heart disease. Her defensive coping strategy prevents her from taking action needed to reduce her risk for cardiovascular disease and can

Developing an Evidence-Based Practice

Drageset S, Lindstrom T, Christine MA: Coping with a possible breast cancer diagnosis: demographic factors and social support, *J Adv Nurs* 51(3):217-226, 2005.

The authors completed an exploratory study examining the relationships between demographic characteristics, social support, anxiety, coping, and defense among women with a possible breast cancer diagnosis. A survey design was used to elicit data from a nonprobabilistic convenience sample of 117 women who had recently undergone breast biopsy. Study instruments included the social provisions scale, state-trait anxiety scale, Utecht coping list, and defense mechanisms inventory. Demographic data were also collected. Data were analyzed using stepwise linear regression and statistical analysis methods.

Results: Study results indicated high internal reliability for the instruments used in the study. The social provisions scale was positively related to instrumental-oriented and emotion-focused coping and unrelated to cognitive defense and defensive hostility. Social support was most strongly correlated to coping style. There were positive correlations between education, attachment, and instrumental coping, with education emerging as the most important determinant. Family was also found to be an important source of social support. A defensive hostile style of relating was negatively related to social support.

Application to Your Clinical Practice: This study demonstrates the need to educate clients experiencing the stress of a new diagnosis about the benefits of social support. Defensive hostility is a behavior that often masks anxiety. How could you use this information to help clients experiencing the stress of a new diagnosis cope more effectively?

Table 20-1 Ego Defense Mechanisms

Ego Defense Mechanism	Clinical Example
Regression: returning to an earlier, more primitive form of behavior in the face of a threat to self-esteem	Julie was completely toilet trained by 2 years. When her younger brother was born, she began wetting her pants and wanting a pacifier at night.
Repression: unconscious forgetting of parts or all of an experience	Elizabeth has just lost her job. Her friends would not know from her behavior that she has any anxiety about it. She continues to spend money as if she were still getting a paycheck.
Denial: unconscious refusal to allow painful facts, feelings, or perceptions into awareness	Bill Marshall has had a massive heart attack. His physician advises him to exercise with caution. Bill continues to jog 6 miles a day.
Rationalization: offering a plausible explanation for unacceptable behavior	Annmarie tells her friends she is not an alcoholic even though she has blackouts, because she drinks only on weekends and when she is not working.
Projection: attributing unacceptable feelings, facts, behaviors, or attitudes to others; usually expressed as blame	Ruby just received a critical performance evaluation from her supervisor. She tells her friends that her supervisor does not like her and feels competitive with her.
Displacement: redirecting feelings onto an object or person considered less of a threat than the original object or person	Mrs. Jones took Mary to the doctor for bronchitis. She is not satisfied with the doctor's explanation and feels he was condescending, but says nothing. When she gets to the nurse's desk to make the appointment, she yells at her for not having the prescription ready and taking too much time to set the next appointment.
Intellectualization: unconscious focusing on only the intellectual and not the emotional aspects of a situation or circumstance	Johnnie has been badly hurt in a car accident. There is reason to believe he will not survive surgery. His father, waiting for his son to return to the intensive care unit, asks the nurse many questions about the equipment, and philosophizes about the meaning of life and death.
Reaction formation: unconscious assuming of traits opposite of undesirable behaviors	John has a strong family history of alcoholism on both sides. He abstains from liquor and is known in the community as an advocate of prohibition.
Sublimation: redirecting socially unacceptable unconscious thoughts and feelings into socially approved outlets	Bob has a lot of aggressive tendencies. He decided to become a butcher and thoroughly enjoys his work.
Undoing: verbal expression or actions representing one feeling, followed by expression of the direct opposite	Barbara criticizes her subordinate, Carol, before a large group of people. Later, she sees Carol on the street and tells her how important she is to the organization.

result in a heart attack or death. Here the nurse might provide the client with information about the link among diet, exercise, and heart disease and inquire about her parents' lifestyle.

APPLICATIONS

Sources of Stress in Health Care

Even under the best circumstances, the experience of hospitalization creates stress. Physical discomfort, strange noises and lights, unfamiliar people asking personal questions, and strange equipment heighten the stress most clients already feel coping with their health needs. Clients and their families often can experience extreme anxiety with transfer to the ICU, again when they are preparing to a step-down or regular unit, and again when they are transitioning to home (Chaboyer, James, & Kendall, 2005). Providing immediate practical and emotional support during each of these transitions can be extremely helpful in mitigating stress responses. Other stressors can include fear of death, uncertainty about outcome, changes in roles, disruption of family life, and financial concerns created by the hospitalization (Leske, 1998). These stressors affect not only the hospitalized client but

Box 20-3 Assessment/Intervention Tool

Assessment

A. Perception of stressors
 1. Major stress area or health concern
 2. Present circumstances related to usual pattern
 3. Experienced similar problem? How was it handled?
 4. Anticipation of future consequences
 5. Expectations of self
 6. Expectations of caregivers

B. Intrapersonal factors
 1. Physical (mobility, body function)
 2. Psychosociocultural (attitudes, values, coping patterns)
 3. Developmental (age, factors related to present situation)
 4. Spiritual belief system (hope and sustaining factors)

C. Interpersonal factors
 1. Resources and relationship of family or significant other(s) as they relate to or influence interpersonal factors

D. Environmental factors
 1. Resources and relationships of community as they relate to or influence interpersonal factors

Prevention as Intervention

A. Primary
 1. Classify stressor
 2. Provide information to maintain or strengthen strengths
 3. Support positive coping mechanisms
 4. Educate client and family

B. Secondary
 1. Mobilize resources
 2. Motivate, educate, involve client in health care goals
 3. Facilitate appropriate interventions; refer to external resources as needed
 4. Provide information on primary prevention or intervention as needed

C. Tertiary
 1. Attain/maintain wellness
 2. Educate or reeducate as needed
 3. Coordinate resources
 4. Provide information about primary and secondary interventions

Developed by J. Conrad, University of Maryland School of Nursing, 1993.

also the family. With experience, the nurse can anticipate stress reactions and help to minimize their impact through caring interventions, particularly the giving of relevant information.

Nurses also experience high levels of stress when working in critical care settings. Since they often serve as the link between other members of the multidisciplinary health team and the client, and the link between client and family, it is easy for conversations to be misinterpreted. Box 20-3 identifies strategies that can be used for conversations that take place when emotions run high and decisions are critical (Triola, 2006).

Special Issues for Children

Stress creates special problems for children because they lack the words and life experience to sort out the meaning of illness, either their own or that of a parent (Compas, Connor-Smith, Saltzman et al., 2001; Greene & Walker, 1997). Often the adults in their environment make the decision not to tell them much, assuming that they either won't understand or will be frightened by the explanation. Most children, however, know something is wrong even if they don't voice their concern. Stomachaches and headaches can alert the nurse to the discomfort of unvoiced stress.

Asking children what they know about their illness and how they think they are doing prompts them to voice significant fears and concerns. To obtain more detail, the nurse might ask the child how other people (e.g., parents, grandparents, or siblings) think they are doing. Small children can be encouraged to express their feelings through drawings and manipulating puppets. All children need to have their questions answered simply and honestly. When children are given false information or reassurance, they don't know what to believe because their intuition and/or body symptoms provide contradictory information.

Children who have a parent suffering from cancer or other serious illness face special challenges that may go unrecognized by their overstressed parents. Parents need help with communicating information about serious illness, with thinking through their children's reactions, and with advice on ways to break bad news to their children based on detailed knowledge of child development. Nurses with a strong understanding of child development can be particularly helpful to parents in interpreting information to small children who need an explanation about their own or a parent's illness. Hearing the information from someone they trust is very important in modifying the uncertainty of a serious illness.

Uncertainty is a difficult issue for both parents and children (Stewart & Mishel, 2000). Nurses are often placed in the difficult position of helping a child understand what is happening with a seriously ill parent while at the same time helping the parent cope with altered parenting skills (Lewandowski, 1996). In a study of stress and coping of parents of children in a pediatric intensive care unit, the most common stressors identified were loss of parenting role, uncertainty about outcome, and information need, all of which are amenable to stress reduction through empathetic, problem-focused nursing intervention (LaMontagne & Pawlak, 1990).

Special Issues for the Frail Elderly

In the frail elderly, stress occurs when meaning is lost. Life is experienced as a prolonged, meaningless existence in a body that no longer responds to their commands and with the loss of almost all that matters (e.g., family, home, and work). The frail elderly commonly mourn the social death they experience, and instead of fearing physical death, they long for it. Theirs is a chronic stress, often unrelieved by the presence of a social support system that their younger counterparts have at their disposal. The nurse is in a unique position to help frail elderly clients fill this gap, often with the simple strategy of asking questions about the client's life. Engaging in a life review reestablishes the sense of worth and contribution to society that each of us needs for fulfillment. (See Chapter 19 for other strategies.)

Hidden Stressors

Nurses who are reluctant to ask questions about the impact of an illness on personal relationships and family function do their clients a disservice. Clients need to talk about these sensitive areas, and the nurse can open the door to discussion. Sometimes the worry is about what will happen next, how to explain the illness, or what the client or family could have done differently to change the situation. Family members may wonder, "How will I manage?" "Was it my fault?" "Could I have done more?" The nurse who is astute enough to pick up on the client's or family's stress can prompt discussion of these hidden fears. For example, the nurse might say to the wife of a recent paraplegic, "Seeing your husband like this must be a terrible shock. I would think you might be wondering how you are going to live with John immobilized like this." This type of statement normalizes feelings and allows the client to describe an unexpressed, perhaps personally unacceptable, thought and to draw more reasonable conclusions.

It is difficult to answer client questions like "Have I got cancer?" "Will this surgery make me impotent?" or "Am I going to die?" Usually it is useful to ask the client what prompted the question and to have a good idea of the client's level of knowledge before answering. The answer can be tentative and should reflect the nurse's level of knowledge about the client as well as the condition. In framing a response, the nurse might reflect on the following:

- What type of information would be most helpful to this particular client at this particular time, given what the client has told me?
- How would I feel if I was in this person's position, and what would I want to know that might bring me comfort in this situation?

Using the Nursing Process in Stressful Situations

Assessment

Understanding stress from the client's perspective is essential in understanding a client's behavior in stressful situations (Hoff, 2001). If the nurse can assess the person's perception of a stressful situation accurately, then the nurse's response can mirror the client's experience. For example, stress perceived as a threat stimulates anxiety, but stress as a loss presents as depression and grief. The strategies the nurse would use to help clients reduce their stress would differ in each of these situations. In the first case, the nurse might suggest stress management techniques; in the second, the nurse would help the client acknowledge the loss and work through the grieving process.

It is helpful to put yourself in the client's or family's position and put into words how you might feel in a similar situation. It is also useful to caution clients not to pass negative judgment on themselves based on one incident. Statements such as, "Most people would feel anxious in this situation" or, "It would be hard for anyone to have all the answers in a situation like this" remind clients and families to accept the human limitations we all possess.

Data Analysis. The nurse needs to assess and analyze the factors that influence the impact of stress. These include suddenness of onset, the magnitude of change the stressor presents, the number and meaning of concurrent stressors in the family, and the biopsychosocial status of the individual and family before the onset of the current situation. In addition, the nurse needs to gather data about the impact of the stress on other family members and to identify likely sources of social support. Listening for relevant themes is important, but so are the communication patterns and what is not being said (see Box 20-3). The nurse might include the following observations as part of a database:

- Are family members and the client communicating with each other?
- What are the family's and client's expectations?
- What does the family or client need from you? From each other?
- Is there a family spokesperson?
- What are the client's cultural, religious, and family values concerning the meaning of the stressor?

The nurse also needs to know what coping strategies the client has used in the past and where the client perceives the greatest difficulty with coping. Assessment of past coping strategies may include questions such as the following:

- What kinds of things increase your stress?
- Are any of your activities limited by your stress level?
- What kinds of leisure activities do you engage in?
- What do you do to relieve your stress?
- What are your usual methods of coping when you do not feel stressed?

Nurses can ask these questions using an informal conversational format. The client's reactions will serve as a guide as to how much and how quickly the information can be gathered.

Diagnosis

Nursing diagnoses related to anxiety, grief, and ineffective coping strategies of individuals and families are familiar correlates of stress in health care settings. Lazarus and Folkman (1984) describe the following five coping tasks that clients in health care settings must address:

- Reducing toxic environmental conditions
- Tolerating and adjusting to new and negative realities
- Sustaining a positive self-image
- Maintaining emotional equilibrium
- Maintaining satisfying interpersonal relationships with significant others

Implementation

Nurses can use several simple measures to help their clients feel less stressed in health care situations, the first of which is to call the client by name and engage the client in a respectful manner (Arnold, Virvan, & Kizilay, 1998). This reinforces the client's identity and respects individuality. Orient the client and family to the unit, and provide enough information to familiarize but not overwhelm them as to what they might expect from health care. Take time to explain the following to the client:

- What will happen during tests or surgery
- Who is likely to interview the client
- How the client can best cooperate or assist in his or her treatment process

Family Involvement. Families suffer significant stress when a family member is critically ill or injured. Coping with the disruptions that such an event produces is difficult and stressful for even the most functional family (Leske, 1998). Families experiencing other stressors just prior to the injury or critical illness can become totally overwhelmed by it. Family involvement is critical to client stress reduction at all stages of the process for the following reasons: (a) the family is a constant presence in the client's life, whereas health care providers usually have more limited involvement; (b) family members know the client best and can provide valuable data that can affect the type and implementation of treatment; (c) the family will have to be intimately involved with the client's care at home; and (d) providing opportunities for family members to help will promote self-confidence and skill development (Whetsell & Larrabee, 1988).

Families feel helpless when all decisions are made by the health care team without consulting them. Holding regularly scheduled family conferences helps reduce family stress. Using a team approach when possible, the nurse, physician, social worker, and chaplain can meet with the family to discuss the client's care. These conferences offer the opportunity for two-way communication between the health care team and the client and family (Ceronsky, 1983). A family conference can be scheduled around any change in the client's condition or in the family's ability to cope. Family conferences help families feel they are partners in the care of their loved ones and provide a unique forum for giving information simultaneously to those most involved with the client's well-being.

Less-formal interventions act as a buffer to stress experienced by families. Provide information about visiting hours and the timing of tests and procedures; this allows family members and clients to plan and, in the process, to gain control over at least some aspects of the hospitalization. Some of the sources of stress for families include "fear of death, uncertain outcome, emotional turmoil, financial concerns, role changes, disruption of routines, and unfamiliar hospital environments" (Leske, 2002).

Encourage family and friends to visit, but monitor the client's response. If the client seems bothered or tired by the visit, the client will usually appreciate the nurse intervening. The nurse can act as a sounding board and reality tester related to the family's perception of the stressor and its personalized impact.

The nurse should prepare family members beforehand for their first visit with a client with a visible disfigurement, marked physical or psychological deterioration, or presence of technical apparatus, for example, "Your father will look as though he is sleeping, but he can still hear what you are saying." Another helpful intervention is to furnish the family with an initial verbal statement: "You might want to identify yourself and tell your father you are here with him." Offering such descriptions gives family members permission to ask questions and time to become more comfortable with undesired circumstances surrounding someone they care about deeply.

Offering self as support can be highly reassuring. The presence of the nurse during the initial encounter lessens the shock of a marked change in appearance or function. Sometimes the sight of a family member on a ventilator or with serious injuries overwhelms family members. Accompanying the client's family to the bedside for the first visit strengthens them during the initial shock of seeing their family member in such a condition. If the client is intubated, family members should be advised that he or she will not be able to speak.

The nurse may serve as a role model in initiating conversation with a seriously ill or comatose client (e.g., "Hello, Mr. James, I have brought your daughter in to see you."). By modeling a normal greeting, the nurse indirectly encourages the family to act in their usual manner with the client. Family members also appreciate a suggestion that if they feel uncomfortable, they should feel free to leave the bedside and return when they feel better.

Help family members conserve their strength. This will enable them to be more responsive to the client. Family members in critical care situations often feel that they need to be in constant attendance, and as a result become physically and emotionally exhausted (Leske, 2000). A useful strategy is to suggest that the family members take short breaks. Family members may need "permission" to go to a movie or eat in a restaurant outside the hospital. The family needs assurance that they will be called should there be any change in the client's condition.

Providing simple, practical suggestions helps the family feel more competent. Coaching can relieve stress by helping family members feel like they are "doing something" for the client. In the process, they develop a sense of competency and mastery over at least part of their environment. For example, providing guidelines for families to participate actively in caring for their loved one helps dispel feelings of helplessness. Families can provide simple loving actions, such as moistening the client's lips or stroking the client's hair or hand. The nurse may need to let the family know that these gestures are okay. Leske (2002) provides an evidence-based protocol for assisting families in the acute care environment (Table 20-2).

Stress Reduction Strategies

Taking Control

Taking control of one's life is perhaps the most important stress reduction strategy. In difficult situations, this coping strategy often becomes lost. Beckingham and Baumann (1990) suggest that it is not simply the identified problem but the accompanying feelings of helplessness and functional immobilization that create a stress state. People use a variety of coping mechanisms (e.g., negotiation, specific actions, seeking advice, and rearranging their priorities) to develop different perspectives and modify difficult stressful situations through direct action.

Clients should be encouraged to participate in all aspects of their care planning to whatever extent possible. This simple nursing action conveys the idea that the nurse considers the client a necessary partner in health care. Sample measures include the following:

- Developing a realistic plan to offset stress
- Dealing directly with obstacles as they emerge
- Evaluating action steps
- Making needed modifications in the plan and often lifestyle

Table 20-2 Suggested Nursing Protocol for Decreasing Family Anxiety

Recommendation	Rationale for Recommendation
Identify a family spokesperson and support persons.	Provides continuity of interventions.
Identify a primary nursing contact for the family.	Assists the family in understanding the client's condition.
Establish the mechanism for family access to the client. Open visitation Contract visitation Specific rules—are any adjustments needed? Unit telephone numbers	Assists in discharge planning. Fosters a trusting relationship.
Promote access to the patient and ensure staff consistency in adhering to unit policies.	
Establish a mechanism to contact the family. Telephone numbers Beeper system	Promotes family participation in client recovery.
Provide information based on family needs. Care conferences Video tapes Information booklets Attendance at bedside rounds Support groups Nurse advocacy—connects family with physicians and other members of the multidisciplinary team	Promotes family satisfaction and understanding of the situation.
Ensure support services are available.	Provides resources as needed.
Explain all procedures using understandable terms.	
Offer an ICU tour.	Reduces anxiety resulting from the environment.
Include family in providing direct care. Assist in performing activities of daily living. Provide a diversion with audiotapes, videotapes, music, pictures, reading stories. Assist with care activities as appropriate.	Allows family participation as indicated.
Include family in end-of-life planning and implementation.	Aligns family expectations.
Provide palliative care and support for terminally ill clients and families.	
Provide a comfortable environment for family. Volunteer support in waiting area Quiet room available Easy access to telephones and restrooms Resources to arrange accommodations for out-of-town family members	Promotes meeting the family's basic needs for rest, communication, and solitude.
Establish a system to update family on changes in client's condition.	Promotes family communication.
Refer to specialized supportive services as needed (chaplain, social worker, financial officer, clinical nurse specialist, support group).	Reduces family anxiety.

Modified from Leske J: Interventions to decrease family anxiety, *Crit Care Nurs* 22(6):62-63, 2002.

The nurse will need to reassure clients and their families that any change will probably provoke feelings of uncertainty, and that these feelings will pass as the person develops more familiarity with the changed expectations (Wurzbach, 1992).

Case Example

Sam Hamilton received a diagnosis of prostate cancer on a routine physical exam. His way of coping included obtaining as much information on the disease as possible. He researched the most up-to-date material on treatment options and sought advice from physician friends as to which surgeons had the most experience with this type of surgery. As he shared his diagnosis with friends and colleagues, he found several men who had successfully survived without a cancer recurrence. Sam used the time between diagnosis and surgery to finish projects and delegate work responsibilities. He attended a support group with his wife and was able to obtain valuable advice on handling his emotional responses to what would happen. When the time came for his surgery, Sam was still apprehensive, but he felt as though he had done everything humanly possible to prepare for it. The actions he took before surgery reduced his stress.

Venting Feelings

In stressful situations, black-and-white thinking can replace normal thought processes and leave little room for negotiation. Clients experiencing stress should be given the opportunity to express their feelings, thoughts, and worries. Crying, anger, and magical thinking are normal reactions to situations that one cannot control.

If there is no immediate jeopardy to treatment, it is best to support the client's right to process a stressful event in his or her own way. Helpful statements can include, "This must be very difficult for you to absorb. Can you tell me what you are experiencing right now as you think about…?" This response allows the client to put concerns into words and offers clues about the role of denial in the current situation. If the client tells the nurse, "I think I'm losing my mind," the nurse might respond, "Many people feel that way. You are not losing your mind. What really is happening is that you are feeling disoriented because of the sudden and unbelievable nature of what is happening here. Can you identify what worries you the most?" By acknowledging the legitimacy of the client's feelings and labeling the nature of it, the nurse reinforces the client's self-integrity and begins to help the client put boundaries on the anxiety by identifying important concerns.

In the process of helping clients express important feelings, the nurse can suggest actions clients can take to increase mastery. Allowing clients to control areas and issues that are not of critical importance to a protocol and helping clients discover the real causes of their frustration can reduce destructive behaviors. Encouraging clients to take one day at a time in their expectations and recovery activities and suggesting referral and concrete resources are helpful strategies the nurse can use to assist clients to take needed action.

Providing Anticipatory Guidance

Fear of the unknown intensifies the impact of a stressor. When people do not understand what is happening, they often try to fill in the gaps, usually with inaccuracies. **Anticipatory guidance** (i.e., helping the client foresee and predict potential difficulties) helps the client cope more effectively with the unknown. Exercise 20-3 provides role-playing practice in handling stressful situations.

Anticipatory guidance is particularly useful as a nursing strategy when something new is about to happen (e.g., a test, examination, or first visitation). Nurses can anticipate the need for information and proactively explain every procedure in detail, using terminology the client understands. For example, the nurse might go through the steps of a procedure, explaining sensations the client can expect to feel at each step. The nurse should take care to repeat important points at intervals. This is particularly important with elderly clients, who have the double stress of adjusting to a change in setting and the stress of an unfamiliar procedure.

Anticipatory guidance and reassurance can come from other clients as well as from the nurse. Arranging for a client to talk with someone who has survived a similar stressful experience is helpful. Talking with someone who has successfully adjusted and gone on with life can make all the difference for someone who feels life will never be normal again. A word of caution: always check with the other client first. Some people, even those with highly successful outcomes, are not ready to talk about their problems.

The nurse can frame the suggestion in the form of a question, leading the client to explore possible alter-

Exercise 20-3 Role-Play: Handling Stressful Situations

Purpose: To give students experience in responding to stressful situations.

Procedure:

Use the following case study as the basis for this exercise.

Dave is a 66-year-old man with colon cancer. In the past, he had a colostomy. Recently, he was readmitted to your unit and had an exploratory laparotomy for small bowel obstruction. Very little can be done for him because the cancer has spread. He is in pain, and he has to have a feeding tube. His family has many questions for the nurse: "Why is he vomiting?" "How come the pain medication isn't working?" "Why isn't he feeling any better than he did before the surgery?" You have just entered the client's room; his family is sitting near him, and they want answers now!

1. Have different members of your group role-play the client, the nurse, the son, the daughter-in-law, and the wife. One person should act as observer.
2. Identify the factors that will need to be clarified in this situation to help the nurse provide the most appropriate intervention.
3. Using the strategies suggested in this chapter, intervene to help the client and the family reduce their anxiety.
4. Role-play the situation for 10 to 15 minutes.

Discussion:

1. Have each player identify the interventions that were most helpful.
2. From the nurse's perspective, which parts of the client and family stress were hardest to handle?
3. How could you use what you learned from doing this exercise in your clinical practice?

natives and responding with simple counsel. A starting point is to ask the client what he or she anticipates will be the result of sharing difficult feelings—"What is the worst thing you can imagine happening if you tell your (mother, wife, child) about…?"—followed by another question about the best way to respond to this concern.

The nurse bears the responsibility to be knowledgeable as well as trustworthy in providing practical suggestions. Do not offer more than what the situation dictates. Encourage the client to expand on the suggestion rather than provide a full plan. The ability of the client to set priorities, to develop a meaningful plan to meet goals, and to establish milestones in the evaluation process stimulates self-confidence and decreases stress.

Repeating Information

In stressful situations, most people have difficulty concentrating. Information and directions given in the first 48 hours of an admission should be repeated, maybe more than once, because this is the time of highest stress. Providing written instructions that can be discussed and then left with the client or family enhances understanding. Allowing time to answer questions and providing the client's family with a person's name and telephone number to call if other issues arise is helpful.

Setting Priorities

When people feel stressed, normal problem-solving skills vanish into thin air. Clients need support and encouragement to rework old patterns that compromise the quality of their lives, and they do not always know where to start. The nurse needs to help the client identify the concrete tasks needed to achieve treatment goals, including the people involved, the necessary contacts, the amount of time each task will take, and specific hours or days for each task. Some tasks are more important than others in stressful situations. A helpful suggestion might be, "Let's see what you need to do right now and what can wait until tomorrow." Tasks that someone else can do and those that are not essential to the achievement of goals should be eliminated or ignored. The client should identify a time frame in which to accomplish each short-term goal.

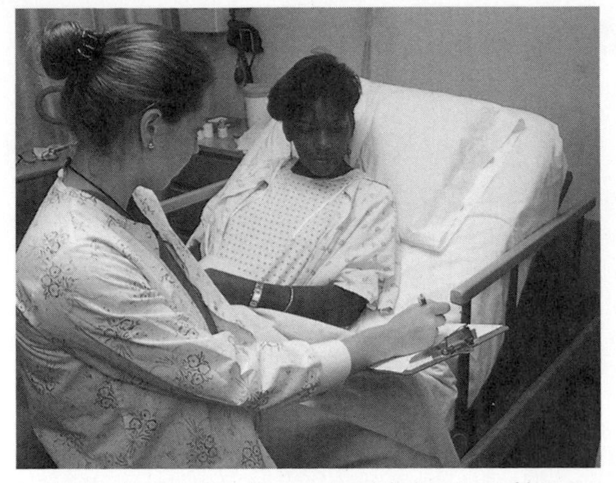

A calm approach and repetition of instructions can help clients in stressful situations relax enough to hear important instructions. (From Harkreader H: *Fundamentals of nursing: caring and clinical judgment*, Philadelphia, 2000, Saunders.)

Priority setting also helps reduce hesitation. Putting off tasks and decisions increases stress in health care as well as in personal situations. Most of the time, procrastination occurs when the client or family perceives a task or decision as potentially overwhelming. The nurse can help a client or family think through the elements of a situation and consider which elements are critical and which can be addressed later. Tasks that are appropriate but too overwhelming can be divided into manageable smaller segments. The most important tasks should be scheduled during times when the client or family has the most energy and freedom from interruption.

Sources of Strength and Hope

In times of stress, people reach out to others for solace and direction. Some people turn to their God, others to family and friends, and still others without these resources turn to community resources. Religion can take on new meaning in times of stress; some people use it to facilitate acceptance of a reality that cannot be changed, whereas others question its validity in the wake of unfavorable news. Some clients experience a spiritual void in times of stress. For many people, belief in a personal God provides an incomparable resource that helps them cope with shattered dreams and incomprehensible life crises. Additionally, religious end-of-life rituals may be extremely helpful in assisting families to experience healing. Carson (1998) notes that "spiritual services staff minister to the emotional, relational and spiritual needs of an individual, recognizing the importance of healing people, not diseases" (p. 1077).

Social support is an essential component of stress management (Lepore, Evans, & Schneider, 1991). Having contact with other human beings is a resource that most people depend on to help them reduce stress. Social support provides three distinct functions: validation, emotional support, and correction of distorted thinking. Validating the legitimacy of anger, frustration, and helplessness prevents the tunnel vision many clients experience under stress. Emotional support allows a person to feel loved and cared about. Informational support and feedback help a client correct distortions and maintain morale.

Community resources in the form of support groups, social services, and other public health agencies can help clients and families reduce stress. For example, a family caregiver of an Alzheimer's disease victim might find episodic respite care beneficial in reducing the ongoing stress of caring associated with this disorder. The nurse is in a unique position to help clients assess the type of aid they need and the most appropriate community resources (Logsdon & Davis, 1998). Sometimes it is difficult for clients to find community agencies and access their services. The more knowledgeable the nurse is about community resources, the better the client is served. Exercise 20-4 is designed to help you become better acquainted with resources in your community.

Mind/Body Therapies

Mind/body therapies are coping strategies designed to lessen the intensity of the stressor on a person once the stress response has occurred (Pearlin & Schooler, 1978). The purpose of mind/body therapies is twofold: to direct a person away from external stressors, and to refocus nonproductive physical and psychological energy in a positive, health-producing way. In the process of altering physiological reactions such as blood pressure, heart rate, muscle tension, and respiratory rate, most people experience greater calm and peace of mind (Luskin, Newell, Griffith et al., 1998). Regular practice of these techniques can improve physical and emotional well-being.

Meditation. Meditation is a stress-reduction strategy dating back to early Christian times. Early mystics and holy men used the practice to obtain an altered sense of consciousness that allowed them to experience the

Exercise 20-4 Community Resources for Stress Management

Purpose: To help students become aware of the community resources available in the community for stress management.

Procedure:

1. Contact a community agency, social services group, or support group in your community that you believe can help clients cope with a particularly stressful situation. Look in the newspaper for ideas.
2. Find out how a person might access the resource, what kinds of cases are treated, what types of treatment are offered, the costs involved, and what you as a nurse can do to help people take advantage of the resource.

Discussion:

1. How did you decide which community agency to choose?
2. How difficult or easy was it to access the information about the agency?
3. What information about the community resource did you find out that surprised or perplexed you?
4. In what ways could you use this exercise in planning care for your clients?

presence of God and to transcend the stresses of daily life. In modern times, meditation is used by many people to develop a sense of inner peace and tranquility. The practice of meditation requires four essential elements: a quiet place, a passive attitude, an object or word symbol to focus on, and a comfortable position (Benson, 1975). A guide to meditation is provided in Box 20-4.

Biofeedback. **Biofeedback** is a treatment modality in which people are trained to voluntarily take control over a variety of physiologic activities such as their brain activity, blood pressure, heart rate, pain, migraine or tension headaches, and other bodily functions as a means to improve their health. Biofeedback provides awareness of minute-by-minute changes in biologic activity. This feedback establishes a psychophysiological feedback loop.

Box 20-4 Meditation Techniques

1. Choose a quiet, calm environment with as few distractions as possible.
2. Get in a comfortable position, preferably a sitting position.
3. To shift the mind from logical, externally oriented thought, use a constant stimulus: a sound, word, phrase, or object. The eyes are closed if a repetitive sound or word is used.
4. Pay attention to the rhythm of your breathing.
5. When distracting thoughts occur, they are discarded and attention is redirected to the repetition of the word or gazing at the object. Distracting thoughts will occur and do not mean you are performing the techniques incorrectly. Do not worry about how you are doing. Redirect your focus to the constant stimulus and assume a passive attitude.

Adapted from Benson H: *The relaxation response,* New York, 1975, Morrow.

Equipment used with biofeedback includes the electroencephalogram; skin temperature devices; blood pressure measures; galvanic skin resistance measurements; and the electromyogram, which measures muscle tension. Each device monitors physical information from the client. The data are converted to visual or auditory signals that are reported back to the subject.

Biofeedback has an important role in management of clients with chronic stress responses affecting individual body systems (e.g., essential hypertension, migraine headaches, Raynaud's disease, and ulcerative colitis). The major disadvantages of biofeedback are the cost of the equipment, the availability of trained personnel, and the complexity of the stress response in most people.

Progressive Relaxation. Most people cannot relax on demand. Just wanting to relax and have relief from stress is not enough (Mast, Meyer, & Urbanski, 1987a, 1987b). Progressive relaxation is a technique that focuses the client's attention on conscious control of voluntary skeletal muscles. Originally developed by Jacobson (1938), a physiologist physician, the technique consists of alternately tensing and relaxing muscle groups. The client

Exercise 20-5 Progressive Relaxation

Purpose: To help students experience the beneficial effects of progressive relaxation in reducing tension.

Procedure:

This exercise consists of alternately tensing and relaxing skeletal muscles.

1. Sit in a comfortable chair with arm supports. Place the arms on the arm supports, and sit in a comfortable upright position with legs uncrossed and feet flat on the floor.
2. Close your eyes and take 10 deep breaths, concentrating on inhaling and exhaling.
3. Your instructor or a member of group should give the following instructions, and you should follow them exactly.

- I want you to focus on your feet and to tense the muscles in your feet. Feel the tension in your feet. Hold it, and now let go. Feel the tension leaving your feet.
- I would like you to tense the muscles in your calves. Feel the tension in your calves and hold it. Now let go and feel the tension leaving your calves. Experience how that feels.
- Tense the muscles in your thighs. Most people do this by pressing their thighs against the chair. Feel the tension in your muscles and experience how that feels. Now release the tension and experience how that feels.
- I would like you to feel the tension in your abdomen. Tense the muscles in your abdomen and hold it. Hold it for a few more seconds. Now release those muscles and experience how that feels.
- Tense the muscles in your chest. The only way you can really do this is to take a very deep breath and hold it. (The guide counts to 10.) Concentrate on feeling how that feels. Now let it go and experience how that feels.
- I would like you to tense your muscles in your hands. Clench your fist and hold it as hard as you can. Harder, harder. Now release it and concentrate on how that feels.
- Tense the muscles in your arms. You can do this by pressing down as hard as you can on the arm supports. Feel the tension in your arms and continue pressing. Now let go and experience how that feels.
- I would like to you to feel the tension in your shoulders. Tense your shoulders as hard as you can and hold it. Concentrate on how that feels. Now release your shoulder muscles and experience the feeling.
- Feel the tension in your jaw. Clench your jaw and teeth as hard as you can. Feel the tension in your jaw and hold it. Now let it go and feel the tension leave your jaw.
- Now that you are in this relaxed state, keep your eyes closed and think of a time when you were really happy. Let the images and sounds surround you. Imagine yourself back in that situation. What were you thinking? What are you feeling?
- Open your eyes. Students who feel comfortable may share the images that emerged in the relaxed state.

Discussion:

1. What are your impressions in doing this exercise?
2. Do you feel more relaxed after doing this exercise?
3. If applicable, after doing the exercise, in what ways do you feel differently?
4. Were you surprised at the images that emerged in your relaxed state?
5. In what ways do you think you could use this exercise in your nursing practice?

sits in a relaxed position in a chair with arm supports. Feet should be on the ground and legs placed side by side. To experience the progressive relaxation technique, see Exercise 20-5.

Guided Imagery. Guided imagery is a technique often used with other forms of interventions to help relieve the stress of pain (Papantonio, 1998). Imagery techniques use the client's imagination to stimulate mental pictures in ways that alter consciousness and promote distraction from painful effects or procedures. The guide may use the relaxation techniques described previously to prepare the client for imagery. Positive mental images are associated with improved functioning and reduced pain in clients suffering from intractable pain, cancer, depression, and hypertension.

Effects of Stress on the Nurse

Although the primary focus of this chapter is on interventions to reduce stress levels in clients, this portion of the chapter focuses on interventions for the professional nurses who regularly cope with the stress of caregiving. Caring for terminally ill, obnoxious, cognitively impaired, or out-of-control clients places a severe strain on the dedicated caregiver. Yet often nurses do not attend to their own level of stress or that of their co-workers (David, 1991). Nurses sometimes leave the profession because they view this as their only option in managing the unrelenting stress of caring for others. Alternatively, they may remain in nursing despite low energy and buried resentments; this results in a poorer quality of nursing care (Gray & Diers, 1992; Schaefer & Peterson, 1992).

Road to Burnout

Physical, emotional, and spiritual exhaustion among caregivers is sometimes called **burnout**. Nurses are at high risk for burnout because they care. The development of burnout often begins insidiously (Freudenberger, 1985). It occurs more often in people who have excessive expectations of themselves and who feel they need to do everything right, and nurses are especially prone to this determinant. So strong is the need to be the exemplary nurse and expert clinician that the compulsion to do the highest-quality job takes over at the expense of health and well-being.

The need to be perfect does not allow for error or reserve the right to correct for unexpected events (Porter-O'Grady, 1998). There is a story about Babe Ruth that applies also to how the professional nurse might approach tasks. Ruth was coaching a young, aspiring ball player, and he asked the boy how he was planning to pitch the ball. The boy answered, "I'm going to throw it with all my might and get it right where it needs to go. I'm going to give it 110 percent." Ruth, however, had different advice: "Throw the ball with 80 percent of your might. You will need the reserve to correct for any mistakes." Nurses need the same reserve to correct for the inevitable curve balls of life. Exercise 20-6 can help you assess your own burnout potential.

Symptoms of Burnout

Physiological, emotional, and spiritual symptoms of burnout are identified in Figure 20-3. Physical symptoms in the form of increased smoking, drinking, or eating; skipping meals; eating compulsively on the run; and sleep disturbances are all warning signals of stress. The potential burnout victim begins to feel emotionally drained, constantly tired, "like a robot," or in a constant state of hyperarousal, in which much of life seems irritating.

Conscientiousness becomes confused with the fear of losing control. It becomes increasingly difficult to delegate responsibility, because others might not do a task as well. Time begins to slip away, and the nurse finds little time for replenishing the self. Nor is there time for others (e.g., family or friends). Every demand on one's time seems like an intrusion. The person is always tired and preoccupied with work (Vernarec, 2001). Emotional pleasures become a thing of the past.

Personal needs are put on a back burner with rationalizations such as, "As soon as I get the unit staffed . . ."; "As soon as my child finishes college . . ."; or "As soon as I get my degree . . .". Despite working harder and enjoying it less, the nurse feels alone and isolated, misunderstood, and unappreciated. Repressed self-needs find maladaptive expression in overeating, overspending, snapping at family, or avoiding friends. Insomnia during the week, preoccupation with tasks, and utter exhaustion on the weekend or days off suggest a serious imbalance in lifestyle.

Burnout Prevention Strategies

Burnout is contagious and can spread quickly in health care settings. Taking the steps outlined in the following sections can help prevent burnout (Arnold, 1989).

Exercise 20-6 Burnout Assessment

Purpose: To help students understand the symptoms of burnout.

Procedure:

Consider your life over the past year. Complete the questionnaire by answering with a 5 if the situation is a constant occurrence, 4 if it occurs most of the time, 3 if it occurs occasionally, 2 if it has occurred once or twice during the last 6 months, and 1 if it is not a problem at all. Scores ranging from 60 to 75 indicate burnout. Scores ranging from 45 to 60 indicate you are stressed and in danger of developing burnout. Scores ranging from 20 to 44 indicate a normal stress level, and scores of less than 20 suggest you are not a candidate for burnout.

1. Do you find yourself taking on other people's problems and responsibilities?
2. Do you feel resentful about the amount of claims on your time?
3. Do you find you have less time for social activities?
4. Have you lost your sense of humor?
5. Are you having trouble sleeping?
6. Do you find you are more impatient and less tolerant of others?
7. Is it difficult for you to say no?
8. Are the things that used to be important to you slipping away from you?
9. Do you feel a sense of urgency and not enough time to complete tasks?
10. Are you forgetting appointments, friends' birthdays?
11. Do you feel overwhelmed and unable to pace yourself?
12. Have you lost interest in sex?
13. Are you overeating, or have you begun to skip meals?
14. Is it difficult to feel enthusiastic about your work?
15. Do you feel it is difficult to make real contact with others?

Tally up your scores and compare your scores with your classmates. Nursing school is a strong breeding ground for the development of burnout (demands exceed resources). To offset the possibility of developing burnout symptoms, do the following:

1. Think about the last time you took time for yourself. If you cannot think of a time, you really need to do this exercise.
2. Identify a leisure activity that you can do during the next week to break the cycle of burnout.
3. Describe the steps you will need to take to implement the activity.
4. Identify the time required for this activity and what other activities will need rearrangement to make it possible.
5. Describe any obstacles to implementing your activity and how you might resolve them.

Discussion:

1. Was it difficult for you to come up with an activity? If so, why?
2. Were you able to develop a logical way to implement your activity?
3. Were the activities chosen by others surprising or helpful to you in any way?
4. How might you be able to use this exercise in your future practice?

Awareness. The first step in burnout prevention is awareness. Deliberately reflecting on the stress in your life immediately puts boundaries on it. If you are in doubt, ask your colleagues to tell you how they experience you. Solutions become possible once the problem is defined appropriately. As you examine your stress behavior, note differences in the way you feel about important people in your life. To what extent have your

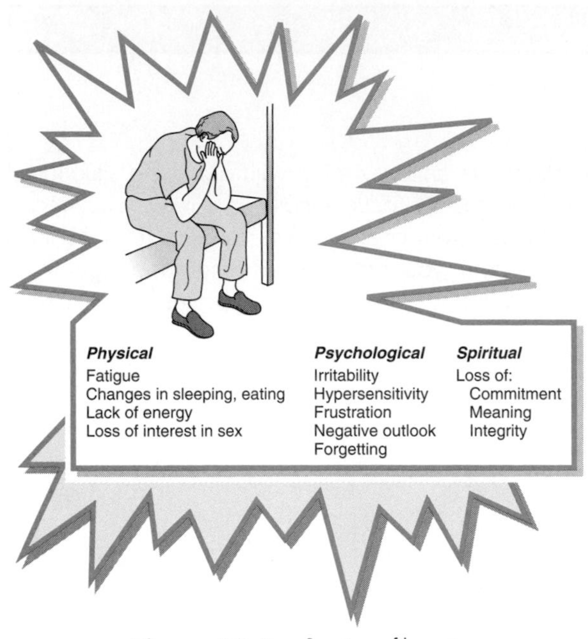

Figure 20-3 • Symptoms of burnout.

life, your attitudes, and your thinking become rigid or meaningless?

Emotional awareness requires that you look at the extent to which your ego is involved in the outcome and the extent to which ego involvement is useful. Who are you trying to please, and for what reasons? Most often our ego involvement gets in the way. Think about your feelings. Talk to someone who is able to offer you the support and sensitivity you need to become aware of what is going on in your life. Take into consideration what others are telling you about your behavior. A useful exercise is to imagine yourself a year from now and ask yourself how important the conflictive issue would be at that future date.

Balance. The second step, and perhaps the most important one, is restoring balance in your life. A healthy balance among work, family, leisure, and lifelong learning enhances personal judgments, satisfaction, and productivity. Actively scheduling time for each of these activities is the only way to achieve balance. Anything else falls short of the mark. Good intentions will never cure burnout; only deliberate actions will provide relief.

Choice. People experiencing the burnout syndrome usually do not think they have any choice other than to keep doing what they have been doing, but life is a series of choices and negotiations. All human beings have choices, and the choices we make create the fabric of our lives. Refusing to delegate work because someone else cannot do it as well, or not going out to dinner with friends because you have too much work to do are choices on your part. Making a different choice actually can enhance your productivity, even though this is difficult to appreciate in the throes of a burnout situation. Everyone needs emotional support to nourish the spirit.

Detachment. The fourth step, detachment, differs from disengagement. With disengagement, there is a withdrawal of excess emotional energy. Detachment allows full emotional involvement in a task or relationship, but not to the degree that it compromises the person's quality of life, values, or needs. It means focusing on a job or project to the best of one's ability and then, at the end of the day or time designated to the project, dropping it completely. Saying to oneself that something is "sufficient for the day" is a stress management strategy that puts boundaries on life tasks.

Emotional detachment means dropping ego involvement when it interferes with balance and integrity. Nothing is so important that friends, co-workers, family, and even oneself should be sacrificed on the altar of achievement. When someone asked Mother Teresa how she was able to remain so energetic and hopeful in the midst of the suffering she encountered in Calcutta, she replied that it was because she did the best she could, realizing that it was important to do her best and not at all important to worry about the outcome. She could not control the outcome, but she could regulate the quality of her work.

(Altruistic) Egoism. Potential burnout victims generally put everyone and everything ahead of themselves. Their own needs are ignored or taken for granted. Altruistic egoism simply means paying as much attention to your own personal needs as you do to the needs of others. Although this seems obvious, many nurses consider attention to their own needs as being selfish. Nothing is further from the truth. In the long run, a balance between self-needs and the needs of others enhances the quality of care one can give to others.

Focus. People who are focused achieve their goals. Those who are not may reach a goal, but usually it takes longer and it is not as certain. Focusing full energy on one thing at a time and finishing one project before starting another has several benefits. First, it is more likely that you will enjoy each activity more. Your full attention will make for a better product. A powerful contributor to the development of burnout is several unfinished projects, all demanding similar space in your mind.

Goals. This seventh step is closely aligned with focus as regards an emphasis on outcome. Identifying goals that are realistic, achievable, and in line with your personal values is an excellent burnout prevention strategy. If you want to go to New York, you do not buy a ticket to California. The same is true of life. Knowing where you want to go and what it takes to get there enhances your chances. It is important to know where you do want to go with your life and to have a realistic sense of what you will find when you get there. Too often people consider only the former and are disappointed when they find it is not where they really want to be!

Hope. People who feel burned out experience helplessness and hopelessness about ever changing their situation. The despair that accompanies emptiness and futility can be reversed by simply seeking out connections with empathetic others. Their advice and caring support, even in one encounter, can prove a powerful antidote to inner emptiness. It is important, however, to seek support from people who will work with you on developing solutions and not merely commiserate with how horrible the situation is. A solution-focused, rather than problem-oriented, approach is essential to the development of hope.

Integrity. The final step in reversing burnout is to restore your personal integrity. Burnout always leads to some loss of personal integrity in the sense that important values are ignored or devalued. When you begin to forget who you are and try to become what everyone else expects of you, you are in trouble. Reclaim yourself! Taking responsibility for yourself and doing what is important to you helps to reverse burnout. Take the risk to be all that you are as well as all that you can be! Nurses working in high-acuity settings and in chronic care facilities find professional support groups highly effective in providing needed time to reflect on their experience and in finding nurturance from others who understand (Parish, Bradley, & Franks, 1997).

Ethical Dilemma ■ *What Would You Do?*

The mother of a client with AIDS does not know her son's diagnosis because her son doesn't want to worry her and fears her disapproval if she knows he is gay. The mother asks the nurse if the family should have an oncology consult because she doesn't understand why, if her son has leukemia, an oncologist is not seeing him. What should the nurse do?

SUMMARY

This chapter presents a comprehensive overview of basic concepts related to stress, coping, and crisis. Stress is defined as a physiological and psychological response to the presence of a stressor. A stressor is defined as any demand, situation, internal stimulus, or circumstance threatening a person's personal security and balance. This sense of personal security and balance is referred to as homeostasis or dynamic equilibrium. Three theoretical models of stress are presented: stress as a stimulus, stress as a physiological response, and stress as a transaction. Factors influencing the development of a stress reaction include the nature of the stressor, the personal interpretation of its meaning, the number of previous and concurrent stressors, previous experiences with similar stressors, and the availability of support systems and personal coping abilities. Hidden stressors can be uncovered if a holistic approach to stress assessment is used.

Coping is defined as any response to external life strains that serves to prevent, avoid, or control emotional distress. People use three types of coping strategies to deal with stressful situations: change the stressful situation, change the meaning of the stressor, and relax enough to take the stress in stride. Accurate assessment allows the nurse flexibility in choosing the most appropriate intervention.

Burnout is a form of stress that commonly occurs in nurses. To reduce the possibilities of burnout, nurses must develop awareness and balance, make appropriate choices, maintain focus, and allow time for self.

REFERENCES

Antai-Otong D: Creative stress management for self-renewal, *Dermatol Nurs* 13(1):31–32, 35–39, 2001.

Arnold E: Burnout as a spiritual issue. In Carson V, editor, *Spiritual dimensions of nursing practice*, Philadelphia, 1989, Saunders.

Arnold E: The stress connection: women and coronary heart disease, *Crit Care Nurs Clin North Am* 9(4):565–575, 1997.

Arnold E, Virvan D, Kizilay P: Concepts of basic communication. In Leahy J, Kizilay P, editors, *Foundations of nursing practice: a nursing process approach*, Philadelphia, 1998, Saunders.

Beckingham A, Baumann A: The aging family in crisis: assessment and decision making models, *J Adv Nurs* 15:782–787, 1990.

Ben-Schlomo Y, Chaturvedi N: Stress and Graves' disease, *Lancet* 339:427, 1992.

Benson H: *The relaxation response*, New York, 1975, Morrow.

Bluhm J: Helping families in crisis hold on, *Nursing* 17(10):44–46, 1987.

Cannon WB: The emergency function of the adrenal medulla in pain and the major emotions, *Am J Physiol* 33:356–372, 1914.

Caplan G: Mastery of stress: psychosocial aspects, *Am J Psychiatry* 13(8):41, 1981.

Carson V: Spirituality. In Leahy J, Kizilay P, editors, *Foundations of nursing practice: a nursing process approach*, Philadelphia, 1998, Saunders.

Ceronsky C: Family/staff conferences open communication, resolve problems, *Hosp Prog* 64(8):58–59, 1983.

Chaboyer W, James H, Kendall M: Transitional care after the intensive care unit, *Crit Care Nurse* 25(3):16–27, 2005.

Compas B, Connor-Smith JK, Saltzman H et al.: Coping with stress during childhood and adolescence: problems, progress, and potential in theory and research, *Psychol Bull* 127(1):87–127, 2001.

Dantzer R: Stress and immunity: what have we learned from psychoimmunology? *Acta Physiol Scand Suppl* 640:43–46, 1997.

David J: How well do nurses care for their own? *J Adv Nurs* 16(8):887–888, 1991.

Dossey B: Awakening the inner healer, *Am J Nurs* 91(8):31–34, 1991.

Edens J, Larkin K, Abel J: The effect of social support and physical touch on cardiovascular reactions to mental stress, *J Psychosom Res* 36(4):371–381, 1992.

Freudenberger H: *Women's burnout*, New York, 1985, Doubleday.

Gadzella B, Ginther D, Tomcala M et al.: Differences between men and women on stress producers and coping strategies, *Psychol Rep* 69(2):561–562, 1991.

Gelent MD, Hochman JS: Acute myocardial infarction triggered by emotional stress, *Am J Cardiol* 69(17):1512–1513, 1992.

Gray S, Diers D: The effect of staff stress on patient behavior, *Arch Psychiatr Nurs* 6(1):26–34, 1992.

Greene J, Walker L: Psychosomatic problems and stress in adolescence, *Pediatr Clin North Am* 44(6):1557–1572, 1997.

Hoff LA: *People in crisis: clinical and public health perspectives*, ed 5, Menlo Park, CA, 2001, Addison-Wesley.

Holmes T, Rahe R: The social readjustment rating scale, *J Psychosom Res* 11:213–218, 1967.

Hull MM: Hospice nurses: caring support for caregiving families, *Cancer Nurs* 14(2):63–70, 1991.

Jacobson E: *Progressive relaxation*, Chicago, 1938, University of Chicago Press.

Johnson A: Death in the PICU: caring for the "other" families, *J Pediatr Nurs* 12(5):273–277, 1997.

LaMontagne L, Pawlak R: Stress and coping of parents of children in a pediatric intensive care unit, *Heart Lung* 19(4):416–421, 1990.

Lazarus RS: *Emotion and adaptation*, New York, 1991, Oxford University Press.

Lazarus R, Folkman S: *Stress, appraisal and coping*, New York, 1984, Springer.

Leininger M: *Culture theory: diversity and universality* (Pub. no. 152402), New York, 1991, National League for Nursing.

Lepore S, Evans G, Schneider M: Dynamic role of social support in the link between chronic stress and psychological distress, *J Pers Soc Psychol* 61(6):899–909, 1991.

Leske J: Treatment for family members in crisis after critical injury, *AACN Clin Issues* 9(1):129–139, 1998.

Leske J: Family stresses, strengths, and outcomes after critical injury, *Crit Care Nurs Clin North Am* 12(2):237–244, 2000.

Leske J: Interventions to decrease family anxiety, *Crit Care Nurs* 22(6):61–65, 2002.

Lewandowski L: A parent has cancer: needs and responses of children, *Pediatr Nurs* 22(6):518–521, 1996.

Logsdon M, Davis D: Guiding mothers of high risk infants in obtaining social support, *MCN Am J Matern Child Nurs* 23(4):195–199, 1998.

Luskin F, Newell K, Griffith M et al.: A review of mind-body therapies in the treatment of cardiovascular disease, *Altern Ther Health Med* 4(3):46–61, 1998.

Mast D, Meyer J, Urbanski A: Relaxation techniques: a self-learning module for nurses: unit I, *Cancer Nurs* 10:141–147, 1987a.

Mast D, Meyer J, Urbanski A: Relaxation techniques: a self-learning module for nurses: unit II, *Cancer Nurs* 10:217–225, 1987b.

Michalenko C: The odyssey of Marian the brave: a biopsychosocial fairy tale, *Clin Nurse Spec* 12(1):22–26, 1998.

Niaura R, Goldstein MG: Psychological factors affecting physical condition: cardiovascular disease literature review, *Psychosomatics* 33(2):146–155, 1992.

Papantonio C: Alternative medicine and wound healing, *Ostomy Wound Manage* 44(4):44–46, 48, 50, 1998.

Parish C, Bradley L, Franks V: Managing the stress of caring in ITU: a reflective practice group, *Br J Nurs* 6(20): 1192–1196, 1997.

Pearlin LI, Schooler C: The structure of coping, *J Health Soc Behav* 19:2–21, 1978.

Porter-O'Grady T: A glimpse over the horizon: choosing our future, *Orthop Nurse* 17(supp 2):53–60, 1998.

Rushton CH: Strategies for family centered care in the critical care setting, *Pediatr Nurs* 16(2):195–199, 1990.

Schaefer K, Peterson K: Effectiveness of coping strategies among critical care nurses, *Dimens Crit Care Nurs* 11(1): 28–34, 1992.

Schneiderman N, Antoni M, Saab P et al.: Health psychology: psychosocial and biobehavioral aspects of chronic disease management, *Annu Rev Psychol* 52:555–580, 2001.

Selye H: The general adaptation syndrome and the diseases of adaptation, *J Clin Endocrinol* 6(2):117–230, 1946.

Selye H: *The stress of life*, New York, 1956, McGraw-Hill.

Selye H: History and present status of the stress concept. In Goldberger L, Breznitz S, editors, *Handbook of stress: theoretical and clinical aspects*, New York, 1982, Free Press.

Steptoe A: Invited review: the links between stress and illness, *J Psychosom Res* 35(6):633–644, 1991.

Stewart JL, Mishel MH: Uncertainty in childhood illness: a synthesis of the parent and child literature, *Sch Inq Nurs Pract* 14(4):299–319, discussion 321–326, 2000.

Triola N: Dialogue and discourse: are we having the right conversations? *Crit Care Nurse* 26(1):60–66, 2006.

Vernarec E: How to cope with job stress, *RN* 64(3):44–46, 2001.

Whetsell M, Larrabee M: Using guilt constructively in the NICU to affirm parental coping, *Neonatal Netw* 6(4): 21–27, 1988.

Wurzbach ME: Assessment and intervention for certainty and uncertainty, *Nurs Forum* 27(2):29–35, 1992.

Chapter 21

Communicating with Clients in Crisis

Elizabeth Arnold

OUTLINE

OBJECTIVES

At the end of the chapter, the reader will be able to:

1. Define crisis and identify its characteristics in health care.
2. Identify theoretical frameworks for the study of crisis.
3. Identify two types of crises.
4. Define crisis intervention.
5. Apply the nursing process to the care of the client in crisis.
6. Identify issues and strategies for families in crisis.
7. Describe nursing care modifications with families in crisis.
8. Explain the nature of crisis intervention in disaster management.

Families come to us, the nurses, scared and seeking, at times not knowing themselves how to sort through what they fear or need most. This is often their first experience of this kind that involves a loved one.

(Kleeman, 1989)

Chapter 21 describes the nature of crisis and provides practical guidelines nurses can use with clients in crisis and in disaster management. Included in the chapter are theoretical frameworks to guide the process of crisis intervention and practical strategies nurses can use to work with clients and their families coping with an unexpected crisis event. Guidelines are provided for working with crisis mental health emergencies. Finally, as our world becomes more uncertain as a result of natural and human-made disasters, nurses will become increasingly involved in disaster management activities.

BASIC CONCEPTS

Crisis comes from the Greek word *krisis*, meaning turning point. The Chinese character word for crisis is composed of two character symbols, one meaning "danger," the other "opportunity." Flannery and Everly (2000) state that "a crisis occurs when a stressful life event overwhelms an individual's ability to cope effectively in the face of a perceived challenge or threat" (p. 119), which results in some level of functional impairment.

Roberts (2000) differentiates between two categories of crisis events. The first, a *private* crisis, affects individuals and families but not the community at large. Examples include suicide, a terminal diagnosis, a car crash, or the death of a family member. The second category is a *public* crisis event, more commonly referred to as a disaster. A disaster has an effect on the whole community and on large groups of people simultaneously.

Characteristics of the Crisis State

In a crisis situation, the client experiences the overwhelming emotional pain of an actual or perceived assault on self-concept, or the loss of something important, a loss that threatens to exceed the person's coping capacities. The *crisis state* represents an overwhelming internal reaction to stressors that conventional coping measures can no longer address. The resulting tension continues to increase, creating major personality disorganization and a crisis state.

A crisis state is a response, not an event (Everly, 2000). It is a *normal* human response to severely abnormal circumstances; it is *not* a mental illness. The client needs to be reassured that a crisis state is not in itself pathological. Because a crisis state is a personalized response to a crisis situation, two people experiencing the same crisis event can respond very differently to it. Thus, understanding the *person* who is experiencing the crisis rather than the objective crisis stressor is critical to successful intervention.

The behaviors seen in clients experiencing a crisis state appear significantly different from a person's regular pattern of coping and may appear to show evidence of scattered, erratic thinking processes. Such clients usually experience physical changes in eating habits, sleep disturbance, and feelings of "leaden paralysis." A person in crisis can experience a temporary disconnect from attachment to others, loss of meaning, and disruption of previous mastery skills (Flannery & Everly, 2000).

An individual's response to a crisis event can be either adaptive or maladaptive. An adaptive response results in fresh appraisals of life's priorities and offers a second chance to make significant life changes more aligned with personal goals. Working through the crisis strengthens people's coping responses, allowing them to cope with future stressful situations more effectively. Maladaptive responses can result in the development of acute stress disorder or posttraumatic stress disorder, both of which can require more extensive professional treatment. During the heightened state of vulnerability of a crisis state, individuals may be more open to making significant changes in their lives so health care providers have a unique opportunity to help clients shape their responses in a positive framework.

Theoretical Frameworks

Theoretical constructs about crisis intervention emerged from the pioneering work of Erich Lindemann and Gerald Caplan in the 1940s and 1950s. Lindemann and his associates developed their theory based on their observations of survivors following the Boston Coconut Grove fire, in which 493 people died. Their study of the grief process and what is needed to restore function following a significant loss was used as a prototype for helping clients complete grief work (see Chapter 8). Caplan extended Lindemann's work to include developmental crisis and personal crisis (Roberts, 2005).

Caplan's (1964) model of preventive psychiatry still forms the basis for much of our current thinking about crisis and crisis intervention. According to Caplan, a crisis will resolve itself in 4 to 6 weeks. The most current thinking is that 6-8 weeks is the time frame needed to initially recover from a crisis event, but full recovery can take a much longer period of time (Callahan, 1998), particularly from the emotional fallout of a disaster crisis (Salzer & Bickman, 1999). The outcome of crisis can be either a growth-enhancing or a limiting life experience, depending on the person's interpretation of the crisis within his or her life, the perception of coping ability, and the quality of human support the person receives to resolve the crisis. Caplan applied concepts of primary, secondary, and tertiary prevention to crisis intervention and viewed the nurse as a key figure in intervention.

Caplan (1964) describes four steps critical to the development of a crisis state: (a) rise in tension and use of problem-solving strategies; (b) coping strategies that are insufficient to resolve the problem, resulting in increased discomfort; (c) emergency coping strategies that are used whereby the problem is redefined and avoided or goals are relinquished; and (d) if emergency strategies do not work, tension increases and crisis results. Typically, people respond to a crisis state by moving through stages of shock, seen at the time of impact. When people are in shock, they display a wide range of behaviors, such as laughing, crying, anger, hysteria, withdrawal, or overcontrol (Slaikeu, 1990).

Then follows an extended period of adjustment, a period of recoil, which can last from 2 to 3 weeks and during which client behaviors can appear normal to outsiders. However, the crisis victim often describes nightmares, phobic reactions, and flashbacks of the crisis event. Over time, there is a period of *restoration* or reconstruction, which involves an adjustment to a new reality and return to normal functioning. With a positive adjustment, a person begins to take constructive action to rebuild a shattered dream and reestablish identity. Negative adjustments involve self-destructive coping strategies such as substance abuse, violence, or avoidance.

Aguilera (1997) and her colleagues developed a nursing crisis intervention model that is in common use today. These theorists believe that a crisis state occurs in response to a potentially life-changing event because of either a distorted perception of a situation or because the client lacks the resources to cope successfully with it. Balancing factors include a realistic perception of the event, the client's internal resources (beliefs or attitudes), and the client's external (environmental) supports. These factors can reduce the impact of the stressor, leading to the resolution of the crisis, and can help minimize overreactions. The absence of adequate situational support and coping skills or a distorted perception of the crisis event can result in a crisis state, leaving individuals and families feeling overwhelmed and unable to cope. The focus of intervention with this model is to increase the quality and quantity of balancing factors, which can help restore the client's equilibrium. Exercise 21-1 provides practice in using crisis intervention models.

Types of Crises

Developmental Crises

Developmental crises occur as an internal process that arises in connection with maturational changes.

Exercise 21-1 Understanding the Nature of Crisis

Purpose: To help students understand crisis in preparation for assessing and planning communication strategies in crisis situations.

Procedure:

1. Describe a crisis you experienced in your life. There are no right or wrong definitions of a crisis, and it does not matter whether the crisis would be considered a crisis in someone else's life.
2. Identify how the crisis changed your roles, routines, relationships, and assumptions about yourself.
3. Apply a crisis model to the situation you are describing.
4. Identify the strategies you used to cope with the crisis.
5. Describe the ways in which your personal crisis strengthened or weakened your self-concept and increased your options and your understanding of life.

Discussion:

What did you learn from doing this exercise that you can use in your clinical practice?

Erikson's (1982) theory of developmental psychosocial crises provides a basis for understanding the role of psychosocial crises at every life stage. A developmental view of crisis takes into consideration interpersonal challenges and stressors that occur at transitional crisis points in the life cycle. Examples of developmental crisis events include conflicts with teachers or parents, unwanted pregnancy, going away to college, marriage, a first job, and caring for aging parents (Slaikeu, 1990).

Situational Crises

A situational crisis represents an external event or environmental influence. It can be a random event, an unexpected illness or injury, a sudden change of role, or a move to a new area. In contrast to developmental crises, situational life crises can affect large numbers of people simultaneously, for example, acts of terror such as those that took place in New York and Washington, D.C. on September 11, 2001.

A situational crisis may be superimposed on a developmental crisis. For example, a woman losing a spouse at the same time she is going through menopause can feel the double impact of a situational crisis on a maturational crisis.

Crisis Intervention

Crisis intervention is defined as "the systematic application of problem-solving techniques, based on crisis theory, designed to help the client move through the crisis process as swiftly and as painlessly as possible and thereby achieve at least the same level of psychological comfort as he or she experienced before the crisis" (Kus, 1985). Although the literature contains a wealth of information on crisis intervention strategies, nursing actions must be adapted to fit each client's individual situation. People in crisis are very vulnerable. They need to feel that the nurse cares about them and wants to understand their situation.

The goals of crisis intervention are the following:

- Stabilize the client's physical condition and emotional state.
- Reduce symptoms of disorganization with a well-defined action plan.
- Help restore individuals to their pre-crisis state functional level.
- Facilitate access to continued care, if needed.

Crisis intervention is a *time-limited* intervention (usually 6 to 8 weeks). Treatment strategies are focused on immediate problem solving and strengthening the personal resources of clients and their families. In helping clients manage crisis situations, the nurse acts as advocate, resource, partner, and guide in the crisis intervention, with a strong focus on helping clients mobilize personal resources and use support resources effectively (Hoff, 1995).

Developing an Evidence-Based Practice

Dirkzwager A, Kerssens J, Yzermans C: Health problems in children and adolescents before and after a man-made disaster, *J Am Acad Child Adolesc Psychiatry* 45(1):94–103, 2006.

The authors completed an exploratory study designed to examine the health problems of children age 4–12 and adolescents age 13–18 before and after exposure to a man-made fireworks disaster, and to compare these with a control group of children and adolescents who had not experienced this disaster. Longitudinal data was collected from electronic medical records of family practitioners related to health problems from 1 year predisaster until 2 years postdisaster (N = 1628 for victims; N = 2856 for the control group). Prevalence rates of health problems were calculated for the two age groups related to psychological and social problems; medically unexplained physical symptoms; and gastrointestinal, musculoskeletal, respiratory, and skin problems.

Results: Study results indicated that postdisaster increases in health problems were significantly higher for the post-disaster group related to psychological and musculoskeletal problems and stress reactions. Children in the 4–12 age group experienced significantly higher rates of sleep problems than the control group, while adolescents 13–18 showed larger increases in anxiety problems than the controls. Significant predictors for postdisaster psychological problems included being relocated, low socioeconomic status, and having psychological problems predisaster.

Application to Your Clinical Practice: This study strongly suggests that young victims of disaster experience significant and long-lasting sequelae following a disaster. Particularly at risk are those who must be relocated. What implications do you see in your nursing practice for promoting the health and well-being of children and adolescents exposed to a disaster?

APPLICATIONS

Crisis Intervention Strategies

James and Gilliland (2004) identified a six-step model of crisis intervention, which can be used to guide the crisis intervention process in the nurse-client relationship, as described below.

1. Ensuring Client Safety

Safety is the first consideration in any crisis situation. Nursing interventions need to be clear and focused, with a balance between establishing a trusting relationship with the client and protecting the needs of others within the environment. Some clients need protection from their own impulses as well; they need to be in a safe holding environment that is free from extraneous stimulation, quiet, and well lighted. Your initial assessment should be to determine the severity of the crisis and the client's current danger potential—both to self and to others. Suicide and violence are psychiatric emergencies that present regularly in the emergency department. If the person in crisis is violent or physically injured, the crisis is treated as a medical emergency first, and then as a psychiatric emergency.

The nurse needs to evaluate the client's mental status before attempting crisis intervention. Clients who are psychotic, under the influence of drugs, organically impaired, or temporarily out of control require immediate triage to stabilize their physical condition. One-to-one observation is critical until the situation is brought under control. This type of observation has two advantages: it helps protect the client and others, and it provides the opportunity to maintain reduced stimulation in the environment. Table 21-1 provides guidelines for communicating with a client who is unable to cooperate because of an organically related health crisis. In the meantime, a family member or the person accompanying the client can provide assessment data related to the current crisis state (e.g., documenting changes in behavior, ingestion of drugs, or medical history).

2. Defining the Problem

In a crisis situation, time is of the essence, so what is needed is an accurate assessment of all the presenting issues as quickly as possible (Mitchell, 1999). Clients in crisis look to the professional to structure the interaction. It is important to model calmness and competence. The focus of assessment and intervention is on the present.

The following are guidelines for engaging the client and defining the problem:

- In the early stages of crisis, *people need to be listened to* rather than to be given much information (Artean & Williams, 1998). It is a period of enormous

Table 21-1 Guidelines for Choosing Intervention with Different Stages of Aggressive Behavior in the Emergency Department

Stage	Client Behavior	Nurse Actions
1. Environmental trigger	Stress response	Encourage venting: avoid challenge; speak calmly, clearly; offer alternative
2. Escalation period	Movement toward loss of control	Take control: maintain safe distance, acknowledge behavior, medicate if appropriate, remove to quiet area, "show force" if necessary
3. Crisis period	Emotional/physical discharge	Apply external control: implement emergency protocol, initiate confinement, give focused intensive care
4. Recovery	Cool down	Reassure: support; no retaliation; encourage to discuss behavior and alternative; release when in control; assess reaction to environment; conduct sessions for staff to process all areas of incident
5. Postcrisis and letdown	Reconciliatory	Demonstrate acceptance while continuing clarification of unit standards and expectations

From Steele RL: Staff attitudes toward seclusion and restraint: anything new? *Perspect Psychiatr Care* 29(3):28, 1993. Reprinted with permission of Nursecom, Inc.

emotional turmoil, and people can absorb very little compared with their usual capabilities. Let clients tell you what they are experiencing. Clients experiencing a crisis need to tell their story in their own words at their own pace. Listen for both facts and feelings.

- Ask directed questions when needed to keep the client focused on the crisis story by asking first for general data, followed by a request for more specific details (e.g., ask who was involved, what happened, and when it happened), and finally asking about feelings associated with the immediate crisis. Keep questions short and relevant to the crisis. Some cultures view the asking of questions as an invasion of privacy. A simple statement of the nurse's need to ask questions to be able to help the client more quickly orients the culturally diverse client to the purpose of the questioning and how the information will be used.
- Use a reflective listening response that matches the client's emotional response to the crisis (e.g., "It sounds as if you are feeling very sad [angry, lonely] right now.") to develop a complete picture of the crisis situation.
- Respond to clients in brief, concise sentences, and do not explain a lot initially.
- Follow clients' descriptions; do not let them get ahead of you. Ask for clarification to understand their perspective, but do not anticipate the story. Note changes in expression, body posture, and vocal inflections as clients tell their story.
- Identify central emotional themes in the client's story (e.g., powerlessness, shame, hopelessness) to provide a focus for intervention. A useful strategy is to help the client attach feelings to specific events by linking the precipitating event with the observed client response (e.g., "I wonder if because you think your son is using drugs [*precipitating event*], you feel helpless and confused [*client emotional response*], and it seems you don't know what to do next [*client behavioral reaction*]."). It is important to ask the client to validate the accuracy of the theme and/or modify it so it represents the client's truth.
- Prioritize the problems as concretely and succinctly as possible, in terms of both urgency and immediate small steps to encourage stabilization.
- Periodically summarize content so that both parties simultaneously arrive at the same place with a comprehensive definition of the problem.

3. Providing Support

Clients and families experiencing a crisis state amenable to nursing intervention require a compassionate, flexible, but clearly controlled and calm approach from the nurse. The following guidelines can help you best serve the client in crisis.

Minimize the Number of Providers. Ideally, having one nurse as the primary contact and information giver is important in crisis situations. Throughout your encounter with a client, keep your communication simple by doing the following:

- Explaining what is going to happen
- Keeping instructions as clear and simple as possible
- Having the client repeat any instructions back to you to ensure understanding of what you have said
- Providing *written* discharge or follow-up instructions, with phone numbers to call for added help

Normalize Feelings and Reactions. Often clients in crisis feel that their emotional reactions to a situation are abnormal because these reactions are strange and unwelcome. It is important to point out to the client that a wide array of feelings is quite normal in crisis situations, and to suggest common feelings that should be present when they are not. Should the client respond by saying, "I feel numb" or not express feeling, the nurse can assure the client that this "shutdown" of feelings is a common reaction in crisis situations. Even if the client does not respond immediately, linking the crisis event with the feelings about it helps the person in crisis recognize difficult feelings related to a stressful event. Although it may seem obvious to the nurse, the client may be unaware of the connection. Legitimizing feelings of rage and betrayal helps the victim make meaning of a devastating experience. Nurses can reassure clients that their feelings will gradually decrease in intensity.

Help the Client Clarify Distortions. Distinguishing realistic from unrealistic fears helps clients put a crisis situation in perspective and forces them to look at what can be changed in a situation versus what cannot. For example, the mother of a premature or deformed baby blamed herself for a number of reasons (e.g., she smoked, she did not really want this baby so God is punishing her, she should not have lifted anything when she was pregnant). The nurse can help provide a more objective perspective by gently challenging the validity

Exercise 21-2 Interacting in Crisis Situations

Purpose: To give students experience in using the three-stage model of crisis intervention.

Procedure:

1. Break up into groups of three. One student should take the role of the client and one the role of the nurse; the third functions as observer.
2. Using one of the following role-plays, or one from your current clinical setting, engage the client and use the crisis intervention strategies presented in this chapter to frame your interventions.
3. The observer should provide feedback.
   (This exercise can also be handled as discussion points rather than a role-play, with small-group or class feedback as to how students would have handled the situations.)

Role-Play:

Julie is a 23-year-old graduate student who has been dating Dan for the past 3 years. They plan to marry within the next 6 months. Last summer she had a brief affair with another graduate student while Dan was away, but never told him. She is seeing you in the clinic having just found out that she has herpes from that encounter.

Sally is a 59-year-old postmenopausal woman admitted for diagnostic testing and possible surgery. She has just found out that her tests reveal a malignancy in her colon with possible metastasis to her liver. You are the nurse responsible for caring for her.

Bill's mother was admitted last night to the ICU with sepsis. She is on life support and intravenous antibiotics. Bill had a close relationship with his mother earlier in his life, but he has not seen her in the past year. You are the nurse for the shift, but do not yet know her well.

Discussion:

1. What would you want to do differently as a result of this exercise when communicating with the client in crisis?
2. What was the effect of using the three-stage model of crisis intervention as a way of organizing your approach to the crisis situation?

of her assumptions and providing accurate information about the causes of fetal abnormalities.

Exercise 21-2 offers an opportunity to understand the versatility of reflection as a listening response in crisis situations.

Provide Truth in Information. Being truthful about the circumstances and letting clients know as much as possible about progress, treatment, and consequences of choosing different alternatives allows clients to make informed decisions and reduces the heightened anxiety associated with a crisis situation. Clients appreciate this and often give information they might otherwise not offer. Keep an updated resource file with contact numbers and services offered. Write them down for the client and explain their utility in providing support that the client may need at this time.

Recognize Personal Strengths. In a time of crisis, there is a tendency for both nurse and client to focus on what is wrong. By learning about the client's or family's personal and interpersonal strengths, capacities, competencies, and resources, the nurse can help the client incorporate the additional supports needed to resolve a crisis. For example, having a job, financial resources, knowledge, and experience with accessing health care services are all important assets in crisis situations that clients and families may not always recognize in the heat of the moment. Reinforce strengths as you observe them or as the client identifies them. Exercise 21-3 provides an opportunity to experience the power of getting in touch with personal strengths.

Use Simple Words and Repeat Them. The words the nurse uses are important, because clients are likely to

Exercise 21-3 Personal Support Systems

Purpose: To help students appreciate the breadth and importance of personal support systems in stressful situations.

Procedure:

All of us have support systems we can use in times of stress (e.g., church, friends, family, co-workers, clubs, recreational groups).

1. Identify a support person or system you could or do use in times of stress.
2. What does this personal support system or person do for you (e.g., listen without judgment; provide honest, objective feedback; challenge you to think; broaden your perspective; give unconditional support; share your perceptions)? List everything you can think of.
3. What factors go into choosing your personal support system (e.g., availability, expertise, perception of support)? Which is the most important factor?
4. How did you develop your personal support system?

Discussion:

1. What types of support systems were most commonly used by class or group members?
2. What were the most common reasons for selecting a support person or system?
3. After doing this exercise, what strategies would you advise for enlarging a personal support system?
4. What applications do you see in this exercise for your nursing practice?

misinterpret them in a crisis state. Sufficient time should be allowed for both processing and asking questions. Including significant others in discussion of the crisis helps by giving clients a resource that can confirm or correct what was heard. This inclusion needs the approval of the client. Remember that in a crisis situation, the client's anxiety prevents free comprehension of information. You may need to repeat information for full comprehension at different time intervals.

Link Crisis Content with Its Associated Emotional Response. People do not always link the event to specific feelings they are experiencing as emotional responses to a crisis. In the following clinical example, notice the difference when the nurse listens and responds to both the content (experience and thoughts) and the latent feelings in the message. The third response captures the full message content and intent.

Case Example

Client: It's my wife: she's dying. I'm afraid to go in there and see her. I can't act cheerful, and it won't do her any good to see me upset.

Nurse (responding to the content of the statement): You don't want your wife to see you're upset because she's dying?

Nurse (responding to the speaker's feelings): You're worried that you can't disguise your feelings of sadness?

Nurse (responding to the content and feelings expressed by the speaker): You're afraid of getting upset in front of your wife and unsettling her?

4. Developing Alternatives

Developing new options is key to the resolution of a crisis state (Perfetti, 1982; Roberts, 2005). Crisis intervention is action-oriented and goal-directed toward the urgent need to restore an individual to a precrisis functional state. Finding viable solutions helps bring closure to the crisis. Problems not related to the crisis need to be handled later. The nurse can use these guidelines to help the client identify a specific plan of action to cope with the crisis.

Give the Client as Much Control as Possible. Obviously, the nurse must take control when the client presents a danger to self or others, but when this is not the case, the locus of control should remain with the client to whatever extent possible. Usually clients in crisis feel powerless and need to feel as though they have more control of their lives. Allowing choices encourages clients to take charge of their actions and to take responsibility for the consequences of their choices.

Examine Potential Consequences. Helping a client examine the consequences of proposed solutions and breaking tasks down into small, achievable parts empowers clients. Proposed solutions should fit both the problem and the resources of the client. Part of the solution process includes discussing the consequences of one action versus another (e.g., "What would happen if you choose this course of action as compared to...?" or "What is the worst that could happen if you decided to...?"). Using common sense and knowledge of human behavior as a guide for developing solutions, the nurse may provide some alternative actions the client has not yet considered.

Enlarge Perspective. When the facts of a crisis event are overwhelming and cannot be changed, it still is possible to recast their meaning in supportive ways. For example, the loss of an infant at childbirth is undoubtedly one of life's greatest crises. The reality of the child's death cannot be reversed, but the nurse can help the parents integrate the tragic event into their lives in a meaningful way by dressing the child in an infant shirt and diaper, wrapping it in a blanket, and encouraging the family to see the child. Even if the infant is macerated or deformed, the external wrappings can emphasize the normal aspects of the infant, and the nurse, through his or her words, can emphasize the positive features. Arranging for baptism or religious support acknowledges the existence of the child and is a major source of comfort to many parents.

Strengthen the Client's Natural Social Support System. People in crisis have a tendency to withdraw from their natural support system. Social support for individuals in crisis represents a primary human coping resource for most individuals. This is particularly true for culturally diverse clients in crisis situations. A healthy, supportive family or a good friend is without peer in the resolution of almost any crisis. Social support can provide a sense of security, offer encouragement, and provide practical alternatives to the strong feelings of despair and confusion that most people experience in a crisis situation. Positive social supports and available community resources act as a buffer to the intensity of a crisis state. Friends and support groups provide practical advice and reaffirm a person's worth during the period of personal questioning that accompanies a crisis. The nurse needs to know what family and social support systems the client has available. Questions the nurse can ask about family and social supports are presented in Box 21-1.

Box 21-1 Questions About Family Support

- Does the client have close family ties?
- Does the client have close friends?
- Is the client a member in a social organization (e.g., church, social club)?
- Who currently is the most important person in the client's life?
- What is the impact of the crisis event on the client's social relationships (e.g., spouse, children, friends)?
- Who in the social network can be approached to help the client work through the crisis?
- Who in the client's network might hinder successful crisis resolution?

From Slaikeu K: *Crisis intervention: a handbook for practice and research,* Boston, 1984, Allyn & Bacon, pp. 130-132.

5. Making Plans

Helping a client assume responsibility for working on immediate goals related to resolving the crisis is essential to its resolution. Planning in crisis situations should be very concentrated, with a practical, here-and-now, therapeutic, short-term focus. Keep in mind the overarching goal of crisis intervention: to restore the functional capabilities of the individual to his or her precrisis state.

Begin with the Present. Help the client to think in terms of short time intervals (e.g. "What can you do with the rest of today just to get through it better, for example, getting more information, gathering data, taking a walk, calling a family member"). You can also ask, "What else do you feel you need to do right now? It can be as simple as giving yourself permission to do something for yourself or letting another help carry your burden." When people begin to take even the smallest step, it gives them a sense of control and stimulates hope for future mastery of the crisis situation.

Incorporate Previously Successful Coping Strategies. People who have demonstrated resiliency and creativity in other aspects of their lives are more likely to weather a crisis satisfactorily. Looking at past coping strategies implemented in other crises in clients' lives can reveal skills that can be used in a current crisis situation. Recalling past successes can offer hope to clients that the current crisis also is resolvable. On the other hand, drug use and major psychiatric illness make a person more vulnerable to the effects of a crisis situation. Factors in the environment (e.g., limited availability of resources, other life responsibilities, legal charges, marital problems, financial concerns) can intensify a crisis for individuals and their families.

The nurse should ask about tension-reducing strategies the client has used in the past (e.g., aerobics, Bible study, calling a friend). For example, you might ask, "What do you usually do when you have a problem?" or, "To whom do you turn when you are in trouble?" If the client seems immobilized and unable to give an answer about usual coping strategies, the nurse can offer prompts such as, "Some people talk to their friends, bang walls, pray, go to a bar…". Usually, with verbal encouragement, most people will identify characteristic coping mechanisms that they can use to cope with the current crisis.

Mutually Develop Small, Realistic Goals. Identifying specific, realistic goals is a critical component of crisis intervention. Here you would incorporate client strengths in planning actions that the client can achieve. Achievable goals give clients and families hope that they can get to a different place with their emotional and physical pain. Crisis offers clients an opportunity to discover and develop new skills. In helping clients develop goals, the client needs to have the full freedom to choose his or her own goals and action.

Select Achievable Tasks to Meet Small Goals. Achievable tasks can be as simple as getting more information or making time for self. You can suggest, "How about making a list of things that need to be done right now?" or, "Let's look at what you might be able to do quickly." These types of comments can help with the feelings of helplessness that so commonly accompany a crisis.

Mobilize Community Resources. Mobilizing resources in the community often is necessary in helping clients achieve mastery of the crisis. Neighborhood and agency resources can provide the client with needed secondary supports. An important piece of information is whether or not the client is willing to use outside resources, and if so, which ones. Some clients are reluctant to use social services, medications, or mental health services, even short-term, because of the stigma they feel about their use.

6. Getting Commitment

Plans without action are ineffective. When people experience a crisis, they often fear that they will never be able to resolve the level of emotional pain they are feeling in the height of their crisis state so that they will be able to fully function again. Nurses can help by letting clients validate their experience of loss while also giving them permission to move on and supporting their efforts to integrate the crisis as they begin a renewed life. Questions the nurse can ask include, "How do you see yourself right now?" or, "What have you been saying to yourself after you explain to someone what has happened to you?"

Setting time lines and monitoring task achievement is important. Nurses need to take an active role in supporting clients as they perform the tasks that will move them forward, providing necessary structure and helping them generate alternative options when the original one needs modifications. Slaikeu (1990) advises, "A comparison of crisis functioning in the behavioral and interpersonal modalities with pre-crisis functioning will serve as a guide in identifying the specific client activities necessary to negotiate this task" (p. 176).

Establish Follow-Up Mechanisms. Although the crisis state may have resolved, many clients will need follow-up for problems that cannot be resolved within the crisis intervention time frame of six to eight weeks. The nurse can facilitate the referral process by sharing information and giving the client enough information to follow through on getting the extra assistance. Exercise 21-4 provides an opportunity to practice crisis intervention skills.

Families in Crisis

A crisis can be a family event, experienced collectively as a direct hit when disaster strikes, or as a more individualized response to the illness or injury of a family member. Domestic abuse can create significant crisis for a family, affecting one or more family members for a lifetime if left untreated. Bluhm (1987) suggests an image of a family in crisis as "a group of people standing

Exercise 21-4 Using Reflective Responses in a Crisis Situation

Purpose: To provide students with a means of appreciating the multipurpose uses of reflection as a listening response in crisis situations.

Procedure:
Have one student role-play a client in an emergency room situation involving a common crisis situation (e.g., fire, heart attack, auto accident). After this person talks about the crisis situation for 3-4 minutes, have each student write down a reflective listening response that they would use with the client in crisis. Have each student read their reflective response to the class. (This can also be done in small groups of students if the class is large.)

Discussion:
1. Were you surprised at the variety of reflective themes found in the students' responses?
2. In what ways could differences in the wording or emphasis of a reflective response influence the flow of information?
3. In what ways do reflective responses validate the client's experience?
4. How could you use what you learned from doing this exercise in your clinical practice?

together, with arms interlocked. What happens if one family member becomes seriously ill and can no longer stand? The other family members will attempt to carry their loved one, each person shifting his weight to accommodate the additional burden" (p. 44).

A family's perception of a client's critical illness or injury is a subjective one, colored by the client's role in the family as well as by previous coping, past experience, current support systems, and family traditions (Reeder, 1991). Emotional symptoms of a family in crisis include anxiety, anger, shock, denial, guilt, grief, and hopelessness. These feelings are difficult for most people to put into words for fear of adding to the crisis. How do you tell your family you are afraid you will never walk again when your family does not want to hear such news?

The nurse needs to remember that even the most functional family system falters in the face of a critical illness or injury (Leske & Heidrich, 1996). Nurses can help clients voice their concerns within the safety of the nurse-client relationship and can assist family members to develop meaningful ways to communicate effectively with their loved one (Leske, 1998).

Various family members will experience the crisis in different ways, so different levels of information and support will be required. Diagrams, simulations, and pictures can sometimes help families understand what is happening better than words alone. If the client is capable of understanding, all explanations given to the family should also be given to the client. In a research study of family needs and coping strategies during illness crisis, family members identified the need to know the client's prognosis as being most important. Other needs were for information about the client, being able to stay with the client, close emotional support, and periodic assurance from the nurse (Twibell, 1998).

Observation of the family's physical state is important. Family members may need the nurse's encouragement to take time out and return before giving or receiving more information. Written information about unit rules may be read at home and used as an ongoing reference. The family should be given the telephone number of a primary caregiver, because a simple telephone call can relieve hours of potential worry.

Giving Information

Receiving bad news typically creates a crisis for the patient and the family and is usually accompanied by intense anxiety, uncertainty, confusion, helplessness, and fear of losing control (Baile & Beale, 2001). Identifying a primary health care contact is important because families often feel confused about what they hear, particularly if they receive incomplete or contradictory information. Similarly, the nurse can advise families to designate one contact person within the family to give information to outsiders and family friends. This intervention helps reinforce the family as the primary unit for

Box 21-2 Interventions for Initial Family Responses to Crises

Anxiety, Shock, Fear

- Give information that is brief, concise, explicit, and concrete.
- Repeat information and frequently reinforce; encourage families to record important facts in writing.
- Ascertain comprehension by asking family to repeat back to you what information they have been given.
- Provide for and encourage or allow expression of feelings, even if they are extreme.
- Maintain constant, nonanxious presence in the face of a highly anxious family.
- Inform family as to the potential range of behaviors and feelings that are within the "norm" for crisis.
- Maximize control within hospital environment, as possible.

Denial

- Identify what purpose denial is serving for family (e.g., is it buying them "psychological time" for future coping and mobilization of resources?).
- Evaluate appropriateness of use of denial in terms of time; denial becomes inappropriate when it inhibits the family from taking necessary actions or when it is impinging on the course of treatment.
- Do not actively support denial, but don't dash hopes for the future (e.g., "It must be very difficult for you to believe your son is nonresponsive and in a trauma unit.").
- If denial is prolonged and dysfunctional, more direct and specific factual representation may be essential.

Anger, Hostility, Distrust

- Allow for venting of angry feelings, clarifying what thoughts, fears, and beliefs are behind the anger; let the family know it is okay to be angry.
- Do not personalize family's expressions of these strong emotions.
- Institute family control within the hospital environment when possible (e.g., arrange for set times and set person to give them information in reference to the patient and answer their questions).
- Remain available to families during their venting of these emotions.
- Ask families how they can take the energy in their anger and put it to positive use for themselves, for the patient, and for the situation.

Remorse and Guilt

- Do not try to "rationalize away" guilt for families.
- Listen, support their expression of feeling and verbalizations (e.g., "I can understand how or why you might feel that way; however…").
- Follow the "howevers" with careful, reality-oriented statements or questions (e.g., "None of us can truly control another's behavior"; "Kids make their own choices despite what parents think and want"; "How successful were you when you tried to control ___________'s behavior with that before?"; "So many things have happened for which there are no absolute answers").

Grief and Depression

- Acknowledge family's grief and depression.
- Encourage them to be precise about what it is they are grieving and depressed about; give grief and depression a context.
- Allow the family appropriate time for grief.
- Recognize that this is an essential step for future adaptation; do not try to rush the grief process.
- Remain sensitive to your own unfinished business and, hence, comfort or discomfort with family's grieving and depression.

Hope

- Clarify with families their hopes, individually and with one another.
- Clarify with families their worst fears in reference to the situation; are the hopes/fears congruent? Realistic? Unrealistic?
- Support realistic hope.
- Offer gentle factual information to reframe unrealistic hope (e.g., "With the information you have or the observations you have made, do you think that is still possible?").
- Assist families in reframing unrealistic hope in some other fashion (e.g., "What do you think others will have learned from ____________ if he doesn't make it?" "How do you think ____________ would like for you to remember him/her?").

Adapted from Kleeman K: Families in crisis due to multiple trauma, *Crit Care Nurs Clin North Am* 1(1):25, 1989.

information and reduces the possibility of unnecessary or unauthorized calls to the unit. It also reduces the chance of misinterpretation; the more people involved in the information loop, the greater the possibility of misinformation in time of crisis.

Informing the family of a negative change in their loved one's condition—unless it is immediate and profound—should be introduced in incremental stages and in everyday language the client and family can understand. Sometimes it is helpful to mentally rehearse what you will say, particularly if you have not had much experience with delivering bad news (Vandekieft, 2001). Many decisions the family needs to make (e.g., related to surgery, placement of the family member in an alternative treatment center, use or discontinuance of extraordinary measures, and organ donation) have long-term emotional ramifications. It is important for the nurse to support the family's right to make the decision and to offer honest and compassionate information so that family members can make an informed decision. The client's physical and mental condition should be presented in a matter-of-fact, constructive manner with neither a pessimistic nor overly optimistic picture. Consequences of choosing one treatment alternative versus another can be helpful as the nurse gently leads involved family members in developing their own sense of the truth and the best way to proceed (Brant, 1998). Communication strategies the nurse can use to help families in crisis are presented in Box 21-2.

Emergency Mental Health

Callahan (1998) differentiates between crisis and emergency mental health situations. Emergency mental health situations are defined as "an unpredictable, acute situation, which requires an immediate response" (p. 167). Whereas crisis intervention represents a short-term response, a mental health emergency requires an *immediate* coordinated response designed to mitigate the symptoms as soon as possible. He identifies three types of mental health emergencies in health care: violence, suicide, and a psychotic break.

Violence

Violence is a special form of crisis in that it involves the use of physical force and demands an immediate response for the client's protection as well as that of others in the client's path (Cahill, Stuart, Laraia et al., 1991). It is a psychosocial emergency that can be just as critical as a life-threatening medical emergency. Violence is associated with anxiety and control; usually the perpetrator feels powerless or out of control, and the behavior is a maladaptive attempt to restore emotional balance.

When violence occurs in the emergency room or in a structured health care setting, more often than not the cause of violent behavior is organic, and the nurse should assume there is an organic component until otherwise indicated. Delirium, drugs, or alcohol most often are implicated. The violent client must be stabilized immediately for the protection of himself and others. Perry and Jagger (2003) advise that at least two health care providers be present at the bedside for all procedures if the client is suicidal or under the influence of drugs or alcohol.

The client's body language often offers the nurse clues to escalating anxiety, which can end in violent behavior if left unchecked. Table 21-2 presents characteristic indicators of increasing tension leading to violence. A recent history of violence, childhood abuse, a history of substance abuse, mental retardation, problems with impulse control, and psychosis, particularly when accompanied by command hallucinations, are common contributing factors.

Treatment of violent clients obviously consists of providing a safe, nonstimulating environment for the client. Sometimes the environment is overstimulating, and the client calms down if taken to an area that pro-

Table 21-2 Indicators of Potential Violence

Behavioral Categories	Suggested Indications
Mental status	Confused Paranoid ideation Evidence of drug involvement Organic impairment
Motor behavior	Agitated Pacing
Body language	Eyes darting Spitting Menacing posture
Speech patterns	Rapid Incoherent Menacing tones Verbal threats
Affect	Belligerent Labile

vides less sensory input. The client should be checked thoroughly for potential weapons and physically disarmed, if necessary. If there is any reason to suspect that a client has a weapon or is about to become violent, do not try to subdue him or remove the weapon by yourself. Instead, say you will be right back as calmly as possible, and get immediate help.

Prevention of escalating violent behavior is possible. The nurse can use simple strategies such as calling the client by name; using a low, calm tone of voice; or presenting a show of force if necessary to help the client defuse tension. Encouraging the client to physically walk and to vent emotions verbally can be helpful. Table 21-3 presents some useful guidelines for com-

Table 21-3 Don'ts and Dos in Dealing with an Impaired Violent Client

Don'ts	Dos
Don't overlook your feeling that your client is growing hostile and showing inappropriate anger.	Document your observations (even though your client has not behaved in an overtly dangerous way), and share your feelings and suspicions with the staff and the nursing administration. Request medication as needed (medication prescribed early enough and in adequate doses can help prevent violence). Review your client's history, searching purposefully for signs of alcoholism, drug addiction, reaction to a change of medication, or a metabolic or emotional disturbance.
Don't undervalue what others (family or staff) tell you about your client's behavior in the belief that the client will be different with you or that you can handle it.	Use what the family and other staff members already know about the client. This information is significant, especially information about previous violence, about what is apt to provoke the client, and how the client behaves when provoked.
Don't continue with a treatment or interview if a client is obviously growing more and more agitated. Don't touch or move toward the client. The client may misinterpret your gesture and react with physical aggression.	Ask the client why he or she is angry or agitated and what's making him or her act this way. Also ask the client how he or she handles such feelings ordinarily and what others can do to help. You want the client to know that his or her feelings and point of view are being respected so the client will feel less powerless and less victimized. Be sure the client understands that violence will not be tolerated.
Don't isolate yourself with a client who has a record of or potential for violence. Don't corner yourself in a setting without a clear exit. (Elevators may prove particularly troublesome because you have no instant exit.)	Put the client in a room near the nurses' station, not at the end of a long, relatively unprotected corridor. Keep the door open when working with the client and face the client (or align yourself literally and figuratively beside him or her) rather than turn your back.
Don't disturb the client (with treatments or taking vital signs) any more than is necessary. The client may need his or her own territory.	Arrange opportunities for physical activities if these seem to help the client siphon off excess energies. Arrange for time out of the room if this seems appropriate and the client agrees to it.
Don't assign a timid, inexperienced nurse to a potentially violent client.	Assign a mature, easy-going, experienced nurse to care for the client. (In this kind of powder keg situation, it is axiomatic that there should be only one anxious person in the room: the client.)
Don't overlook the significance of gender in the assignment of a nurse to this client.	Consider assigning a male staff nurse to the female client who is potentially violent, and a female nurse to the male client. Observers have learned that a woman client may be inclined to react negatively to another woman, but positively to a male staff member. This gender crossing also works for the male client, who might hesitate to strike or injure a female nurse.

Developed by J. Wallskog, PhD, RN, Marquette University, Milwaukee, WI, 1994.

municating with a potentially violent client. Organically impaired clients often perceive necessary medical procedures as being intrusive and threatening. Perry and Jagger (2003) advise that, before you start any procedure, you tell the client exactly what you are going to do and why the procedure is necessary, with a request to cooperate. If the client refuses, don't insist, but explain the reason for doing the procedure in a calm, quiet voice. They suggest that if you help your client regain a sense of control, he or she will be more likely to cooperate with you.

Working with violent clients and with those who experience violence takes a toll on the nurse. The emotionally laden trauma of the original violence cannot help but affect the nurse, arousing emotions and distress that may require consultation, supervision, or debriefing (Hartman, 1995).

Suicide

Suicide is the ultimate personal crisis because there can be no return to function. People turn to suicide as an option when they believe there are no other alternatives. It is a myth that people who talk about harming themselves are at less risk. Every suicidal statement, however indirect, should be taken seriously. Even in clients who have indicated that they are "just kidding," the fact that they have verbalized the threat places them at greater risk. Verbal indicators of potential suicide include statements such as "I don't think I can go on without . . ."; "I sometimes wish I wasn't here"; or "People would be better off without me." Less direct indicators include statements like "I don't see anything good in my life." Any of these statements requires further clarification (e.g., "You say you can't go on any longer. Can you tell me more about what you mean?"). Inquiring if the client has a plan is essential and, if a plan is present, constitutes an immediate suicidal threat.

Behavioral indicators of hopelessness include giving away possessions, apologizing for previous behavior, writing letters to significant people, more intense sharing of personal data, and frequent accidents. Irrational statements and command hallucinations, abuse of drugs or alcohol, previous suicide gestures, and verbal threats are always matters of concern, as is a sudden mood change from vegetative expressions of depression to significantly more energy. The client who verbalizes or behaviorally demonstrates "a weight being lifted off the shoulders" should be watched carefully.

Clients will usually admit to feelings of suicide if they are having them. Having a plan, especially one that could be implemented, no support system, and distorted feelings or thoughts about what the suicide attempt would accomplish increase the risk of suicide (Slaikeu, 1990). The nurse should ask the following questions:

- Are you thinking of hurting yourself?
- Do you have a plan? (If the client does have a plan, you should further explore seriousness of intent by examining the deadliness of the chosen method, availability of the method, and whether the plan seems detailed or vague.)
- What do you hope to accomplish with the suicide attempt?
- Have you thought about when you might do this?
- Who are you able to turn to when you are in trouble?

If the client has a concrete plan and an available method and expresses feelings of hopelessness, lacks an identifiable support system, and has a history of precious attempts, he or she may be at high risk for suicide. The client should be referred for psychiatric evaluation, and other precautions may be needed to ensure his or her safety. The client may need to be hospitalized, and should not be left alone if he or she meets the criteria for high risk.

Most clients are ambivalent about ending their life and experience relief that the decision has been taken out of their hands. The nurse should explain the reason for the referral with tact and an emphasis on the behaviors that led the nurse to make the referral: "I'm worried that you might harm yourself because of the way you say you are feeling. You have a plan in mind and you have several of the factors that place you at high risk for suicide. I would like you to see Dr. Jones for an evaluation." The nurse should try to address any of the client's reservations while simultaneously reinforcing the idea that the client has little to lose by having the evaluation. If the client declines treatment evaluation, this should be noted, with the time and date of refusal written on the chart.

When the nurse has reason to believe that the client is a danger to self or others, there is a legal and moral responsibility to disclose the information to appropriate parties. Confidentiality is secondary to the goal of saving human life. It is important, however, to inform the client about the disclosure of information and to whom the information will be given (e.g., "I may need to act on your behalf until your situation is stabilized, and that includes talking with your family and your doctor about what we have just discussed.").

The actively suicidal client should never be left alone, and all potential weapons (e.g., mirrors, belts, razors, and glass frames) should be confiscated. When taking these items, the nurse should explain in a calm, com-

Table 21-4 Sample of Level of Supervision Warranted by Suicidal Clients

Off checks	Verbalizes no suicidal ideation Congruence shown in verbal and behavioral information 100% compliance with treatment plan Has perception of support in community Verbalizes concerns on a feeling level to present nurse
Observations every 30 minutes	Verbalizes suicidal ideation Verbalizes no plan Verbalizes no intention Cooperative with treatment plan Withdrawn, low Multiple previous attempts Verbalizes superficially to present nurse
Observations every 15 minutes	Verbalizes suicidal ideation with plan and/or intent No perception of support Little compliance with treatment plan Subjective or objective frustration Anger Labile affect or mood Mute or decreased amount of verbalization Avoidance of staff and others Withdrawn, high Intoxicated Impaired reality testing Hyperactive Demonstrates limited problem-solving ability
Close observation every 5–10 minutes	Verbalizes suicidal ideation with plan and/or intent No perception of support Little compliance with treatment plan Subjective or objective frustration Anger Labile affect or mood Mute or decreased amount of verbalization Avoidance of staff and others Withdrawn, high Intoxicated Impaired reality testing Hyperactive Demonstrates limited problem-solving ability
1:1 restriction	Sudden change in activity level; not chronic anxiety Unable to agree not to (attempt) suicide Makes suicidal gesture currently
Restraint or seclusion	Attempt made to kill self in front of staff (i.e., even 1:1 cannot resist impulse to kill self)

From Bydlow-Brown B, Billman R: At risk for suicide. In Ismeurt R, Arnold E, Carson V, editors, *Readings in concepts fundamental to nursing*, Springhouse, PA, 1990, Springhouse Publishing. Reprinted with permission.

passionate manner the reason the items should not be in the client's possession and where they will be kept. The client should be assured that the items would be returned when the danger of self-harm resolves. Most people who attempt suicide feel ambivalence about their desire to end their lives. A major part of the intervention is directed toward helping suicidal clients better understand the reasons that led up to the suicide attempt and assisting them to develop alternative strategies. Acceptance of the client is a critical element of rapport. Helping people to reestablish a reason for living and getting others involved as a support system are critical interventions. Table 21-4 displays the level of supervision warranted by clients demonstrating suicidal behaviors.

If the circumstances are favorable and the client does not have a significant organic impairment, the nurse can establish a no-suicide contract with the client and can help the client develop a prevention plan for responding to difficult life issues. A no-suicide contract does not wipe out the need for other assessment and intervention strategies, but it provides another safeguard for the client because it forces him or her to consider the commitment to life. No-suicide contracts are contraindicated with clients demonstrating organic involvement (e.g., overtly psychotic or drug-abusing behaviors). If a client is actively suicidal, the nurse must stay within arm's length of the client at all times.

Crisis Management in Disaster and Mass Trauma Situations

Recent years have borne witness to more unprecedented natural disasters, terrorism, and barbaric war than the world has seen in recent times. Examples include the Indian Ocean tsunami, the September 11 attack on the World Trade Center, the wars in Iraq and Darfur, the attack on the *USS Cole*, the Oklahoma City bombing, Hurricane Katrina, the Tokyo subway sarin nerve gas attack, and violent earthquakes throughout the world. Myer and Moore (2006) argue that crisis theory must move beyond working only with the individual to include the social context of intervention. They advise that "crises do not happen in a vacuum, but are shaped by the cultural and social contexts in which they occur" (p. 139). The idea that both the individual and the social context in which a crisis occurs influence each other in explaining the impact of a crisis is consistent with Martha Roger's conceptualization of energy fields influencing one another in tandem. Webb (2004) identifies the components of mass trauma events in Table 21-5.

Table 21-5 Components of Mass Trauma Events

Variable	Example
Single versus recurring traumatic event	Type I (acute) trauma Type II (chronic or ongoing) trauma
Proximity to the traumatic event	On site On the periphery Through the media
Extent of exposure to violence/injury/pain	Witnessed and/or experienced
Nature of losses/death/destruction	Personal, community, and/or symbolic loss Danger, loss, and/or responsibility traumas Loved one "missing"/no physical evidence Death determined by retrieval of body or fragment Loss of status/employment/family income Loss of a predictable future
Attribution of causality	Random "Act of God" or deliberate Human-made

From Webb N: The impact of traumatic stress and loss on children and families. In Webb N, *Mass trauma and violence: helping families and children cope*, New York, 2004, The Guilford Press, p. 6. Reprinted with permission.

The level of direct involvement, degree of uncertainty about outcome, nature of the loss and relationship with the lost person or object, level of social support, and personal resiliency of the individual and family will affect the impact of the trauma or disaster event, both short- and long-term.

Fullerton, Ursan, Norwood et al. (2003) assert that the behavioral and psychological responses are not random, but occur in a sequential manner that can be described. During the initial *emergency* phase, defined as the immediate period after disaster strikes, the main emotion survivors experience is fear. Helping interventions should focus on providing a safe and secure place apart from the destruction in which survivors can begin to regain a sense of equilibrium. You should simultaneously ensure your own safety. Triaging high-risk individuals helps reduce their vulnerability. Padfield, Ursano, and Norwood (2003) state that "a sensible working principle in the immediate postincident phase is to expect normal recovery" (p. 104).

Critical Incident

With the September 11 terrorist attack on the United States and with Hurricane Katrina, which demolished a thriving city in a matter of days, came a fresh awareness of the need for community and national planned responses to critical incidents that can happen anywhere, and at any time, to innocent masses of people. Flannery and Everly (2000) use the term **critical incident** to describe a unique, overwhelming stressor event, capable of creating a crisis response in many individuals at the same time. They are random events producing permanent changes in people's lives and shaking their perception of being in charge of their lives. Examples of critical incidents include airplane crashes, acts of mass violence, civilian casualties in combat operations, earthquakes, plagues, or biological contamination confined to a particular area.

The effects of a critical incident can be devastating for both victims and health care providers. Because of their magnitude, critical incidents present a more complicated coping process for family survivors and the community at large (Flannery, 1999). Research also indicates that individuals, including health care providers who assist or witness critical incidents, are vulnerable to experiencing "secondary traumatization" similar to that experienced by direct victims of the incident.

Survivors of disaster experience personal response patterns similar to those described earlier in the chapter, and in addition they can experience what Lahad (2000) terms "breaks in continuity." Lahad suggests that victims, their families, and those secondarily exposed to a disaster are subject to a sudden, serious break in their belief in the continuity of their personal lives that is difficult to ease. He categorizes the immediate chaotic personal reactions to such breaks in continuity as the following (Lahad, 2000):

- I don't understand what is happening (*cognitive continuity*).
- I don't know myself (*historical continuity*).
- I don't know what to do, how to act here, what it is to be a bereaved person/an injured or wounded person (*role continuity*).
- Where is everyone? I am so alone. Where are my loved ones? (*social continuity*).

When considering the impact of the life-changing events inherent in a disaster, you should avoid assuming that the disaster involves the same type of intensity and experience for all survivors. Each survivor brings to the experience a unique personal history with its interpersonal strengths and deficits, and each interprets the meaning of the crisis differently. The availability of resources and individual, family, and community beliefs about its etiology and meaning also will influence each person's response to an overwhelming event.

Community Response Patterns

When disaster strikes, the existence and function of the community is significantly impaired and in danger of extinction. The community response to disaster characteristically consists of four phases (Call & Pfefferbaum, 1999; Jacobs & Kulkarni, 1999):

- Heroic phase
- Honeymoon phase
- Disillusionment phase
- Reconstruction phase

The *heroic phase* typically lasts through at least the first week postdisaster. The focus of intervention during this phase is to ensure the public health safety of the victims by establishing an infrastructure to support the immediate needs of the population. The most critical services to put in place include water, sanitation, food supplies, and insect and rodent control (Campos-Outcalt, 2006).

The shock of the disaster pulls people together, and emotions are strong. Large amounts of energy are expended in rescue efforts, providing shelter, and community emergency stabilization. Emergency medical teams, neighbors, and friends rally around the survivors, offering emotional support and tangible supplies needed for recovery. Bowenkamp (2000) notes that the *honeymoon phase* occurs when the "community pulls together and outside resources are brought in" after the initial search and recovery phase (p. 159). The honeymoon phase typically lasts up to 6 months postdisaster. Sharing the experience of the trauma with others and tangible evidence of continuing support are crucial.

The *disillusionment phase* usually appears as the initial emergency response starts to subside. People start to realize the extent of their losses. Survivors can experience anger, resentment, and bitterness at the loss of support, particularly if it is sudden and complete. Kaplan, Iancu, and Bodner (2000) suggest that opportunities for psychological debriefing sessions should continue for a period well beyond the initial disaster experience for victims of extreme stress.

The final *reconstruction phase* occurs when the survivors begin to take the primary responsibility for rebuilding their life. Ongoing support is required as survivors learn to cope with new roles and responsibilities and to develop new alternatives to living a full life posttrauma. Although the disaster experience recedes in memory, it is never lost, and the person never again fully trusts in the continuity of life.

Disaster management requires immediate emotional first aid and collection of data as the basis for informed decision making. In a disaster response situation, Noji (2000) identifies four goals to guide disaster management that the nurse can use:

- Assess the needs of disaster-affected populations.
- Match available resources to those needs.
- Prevent further adverse health effects; implement disease control strategies for well-defined problems.
- Evaluate the effectiveness of disaster relief programs and improve contingency plans for various types of future disasters.

Critical Incident Stress Debriefing

Critical incidents in health care affect the personnel who respond to them. If there is no opportunity to process the meaning of a critical situation, the nurse can become a psychological casualty. **Critical incident stress debriefing (CISD)** is a crisis intervention strategy designed to reduce the impact of a crisis event on professional staff and others involved in the crisis situation by processing it as soon as possible after it occurs. This is a group intervention for individuals following exposure to trauma or disaster in their work situation, designed to reduce the initial distress of the situation and avert subsequent pathology. A CISD offers people an opportunity to externalize a traumatic experience through being able to vent feelings, discuss their role in the situation, develop a realistic sense of the big picture, and receive peer support in putting a crisis event in perspective (Curtis, 1995).

Critical incident debriefing also is useful with families witnessing a tragedy involving one of their family members (Ragaisis, 1994). The leader uses a group discussion format to provide a safe place in which nurses and those intimately involved with a critical incident can talk about what happened. A specially trained professional generally leads the debriefing. Only those actively involved in the critical incident can attend the debriefing session.

The leader introduces the purpose of the group and assures the participants that everything said in the session will be kept confidential. People are asked to identify who they are and what happened from their perspective, including the role they played in the incident. After these preliminary data emerge, the leader might ask the participants to recall the first thing they remember thinking or feeling about the incident. Participants are asked to discuss any stress symptoms they may have related to the incident. This part of the session is followed by psychoeducational strategies to reduce stress. Any lingering questions are answered, and the leader summarizes the high points of the critical incident debriefing for the group (Rubin, 1990).

SUMMARY

Crisis is defined as an unexpected, sudden turn of events or set of circumstances that requires an immediate human response. A crisis is an event that can occur with anyone; it does not respect age, socioeconomic, or cultural differences. People experience a crisis as overwhelming, traumatic, and personally intrusive. It is an unexpected life event challenging a person's sense of self and his or her place in the world. Common crisis situations in

Ethical Dilemma ■ *What Would You Do?*

Sara Murdano was only 20 when she came to the mobile intensive care unit (MICU), but this is not her first hospital admission. She has been treated for depression previously. She states she is determined to kill herself because she has nothing to live for, and that is her right to do so because she is no longer a minor. As she describes her life to date, you can't help but think that she really doesn't have a lot to live for. How would you respond to this client from an ethical perspective?

health care settings include violence against others or against the self, rape, life-threatening illness, and severe injury.

The outcome of a crisis state can be either positive or negative, with long-range effects on a person's mental health and consequent behaviors.

Two types of crises are identified: developmental crises, which parallel psychosocial stages of ego development; and situational crises, which occur as unanticipated episodic events unrelated to human development. Crisis must be considered within the social context in which it occurs. Crisis intervention is a time-limited treatment that focuses only on the immediate problem and its resolution. Roberts's six-step model of intervention provides useful guidelines that include ensuring safety, defining the problem, exploring alternatives, planning, taking action, and follow-up monitoring.

Family members often experience a crisis state when someone close to them is dying or is critically ill, and nurses can be helpful in helping them interpret and respond effectively in crisis situations. Guidelines for communication with clients experiencing mental health emergencies (e.g., violence and suicide) focus on safety and rapid stabilization of the client's behavior. As the world becomes more dynamically unstable, nurses will need to understand the dimensions of disaster management and develop the skills to respond effectively in disaster situations. Critical incident debriefing is a crisis intervention strategy designed to help nurses process critical incidents in health care, thereby reducing the possibility of symptoms occurring.

REFERENCES

Aguilera D: *Crisis intervention: theory and methodology*, ed 7, St Louis, 1997, Mosby.

Artean C, Williams L: What we learned from the Oklahoma City bombing, *Nursing* 28(3):52–55, 1998.

Baile W, Beale E: Giving bad news to cancer patients: matching process and content, *J Clin Oncol* 19(9):2575–2577, 2001.

Bluhm J: Helping families in crisis hold on, *Nursing* 17(10):44–46, 1987.

Bowenkamp C: Coordination of mental health and community agencies in disaster response, *Int J Emerg Ment Health* 2(3):159–165, 2000.

Brant JM: The art of palliative care: living with hope, dying with dignity, *Oncol Nurs Forum* 25(2):137–143, 1998.

Cahill C, Stuart G, Laraia M et al.: Inpatient management of violent behavior: nursing prevention and intervention, *Issues Ment Health Nurs* 12:239–252, 1991.

Call JA, Pfefferbaum B: Lessons from the first two years of Project Heartland: Oklahoma's mental health response to the 1995 bombing, *Psychiatr Serv* 50(7):953–955, 1999.

Callahan I: Crisis theory and crisis intervention in emergencies. In Kleespies PM, editor, *Emergencies in mental health: evaluation and management*, New York, 1998, Guilford Press.

Campos-Outcalt D: Disaster medical response: maximizing your effectiveness, *Fam Pract* 55(2):113–115, 2006.

Caplan G: *Principles of preventive psychiatry*, New York, 1964, Basic Books.

Curtis J: Elements of critical incident debriefing, *Psychol Rep* 77(1):91–96, 1995.

Dirkzwager A, Kerssens J, Yzermans C: Health problems in children and adolescents before and after a man-made disaster, *J Am Acad Child Adolesc Psychiatry* 45(1):94–103, 2006.

Erikson E: *The life cycle completed*, New York, 1982, Norton.

Everly G: Principles of crisis intervention: reducing the risk of premature crisis intervention, *Int J Emerg Ment Health* 2(1):1–4, 2000.

Flannery R: Treating family survivors of mass casualties: a CISM family crisis intervention approach, *Int J Emerg Ment Health* 1(4):243–250, 1999.

Flannery RB Jr, Everly GS Jr: Crisis intervention: a review, *Int J Emerg Ment Health* 2(2):119–125, 2000.

Fullerton C, Ursano R, Norwood A, Holloway HC. In Ursano RJ, Fullerton C, Norwood A (editors): *Terror and disaster: Individual and community mental health interventions*, Cambridge, MA, 2003, Cambridge University Press.

Hartman CR: The nurse-patient relationship and victims of violence, *Sch Inq Nurs Pract* 9:175–192, 1995.

Hoff L: *People in crisis: understanding and helping*, ed 4, Menlo Park, CA, 1995, Jossey-Bass.

Jacobs GA, Kulkarni N: Mental health responses to terrorism, *Psychiatr Ann* 29(6):376–380, 1999.

James R, Gilliland B: *Crisis intervention strategies*, ed 5, Belmont, CA, 2004, Thomson Brooks/Cole.

Kaplan Z, Iancu I, Bodner E: A review of psychological debriefing after extreme stress, *Psychiatr Serv* 52(6): 824–827, 2000.

Kleeman K: Families in crisis due to multiple trauma, *Crit Care Nurs Clin North Am* 1(1):25, 1989.

Kus R: Crisis intervention. In Bulechek G, McCloskey J, editors, *Nursing interventions: treatments for nursing diagnoses*, Philadelphia, 1985, WB Saunders.

Lahad M: Darkness over the abyss: supervising crisis intervention teams following disaster [online article], *Traumatology* 6(4), 2000; available online: http://www.fsu.edu/~trauma/v6i4/v6i4a4.html.

Leske J: Treatment for family members in crisis after critical injury, *AACN Clin Issues* 9(1):129–139, 1998.

Leske J, Heidrich S: Interventions for aged families, *Crit Care Nurs Clin North Am* 8(1):91–102, 1996.

Mitchell J: *The dynamics of crisis intervention: loss as the common denominator*, Springfield, IL, 1999, Charles C Thomas.

Myer R, Moore H: Crisis in context theory: an ecological model, *J Counsel Dev* 84:139–148, 2006.

Noji EK: The public health consequences of disasters, *Prehospital Disaster Med* 15(4):21–31, 2000.

Padfield P, Norwood A, Ursano R: *Trauma and disaster: Responses and management*, Arlington, VA, 2003, American Psychiatric Publishing.

Perfetti T: *Training manual for crisis counselors*, Bethesda, MD, 1982, Montgomery County Crisis Center.

Perry J, Jagger J: Reducing risks from combative patients, *Nursing* 33(10):28, 2003.

Ragaisis K: Critical incident stress debriefing: a family nursing intervention, *Arch Psychiatr Nurs* 8(1):38–43, 1994.

Reeder J: Family perception: a key to intervention, *AACN Clin Issues Crit Care Nurs* 2(2):188–194, 1991.

Roberts A: *Crisis intervention handbook: assessment, treatment and research*, New York, 2005, Oxford University Press.

Rubin J: Critical incident stress debriefing: helping the helpers, *J Emerg Nurs* 16(4):255–258, 1990.

Salzer M, Bickman L: The short and long term psychological impact of disaster: Implications for mental health intervention. In Gist R, Lubin B, editors, *Response to disaster: psychological, community and ecological approaches*, Philadelphia, 1999, Brunner/Mazel.

Slaikeu K: *Crisis intervention: a handbook for practice and research*, ed 2, Boston, 1990, Allyn & Bacon.

Twibell R: Family coping during critical illness, *Dimens Crit Care Nurs* 17(2):100–112, 1998.

Vandekieft G: Breaking bad news, *Am Fam Physician* 64(12):1975–1980, 2001.

Webb, NB (editor): *Mass trauma and violence: Helping families and children cope*, New York, 2004, Guilford Press.

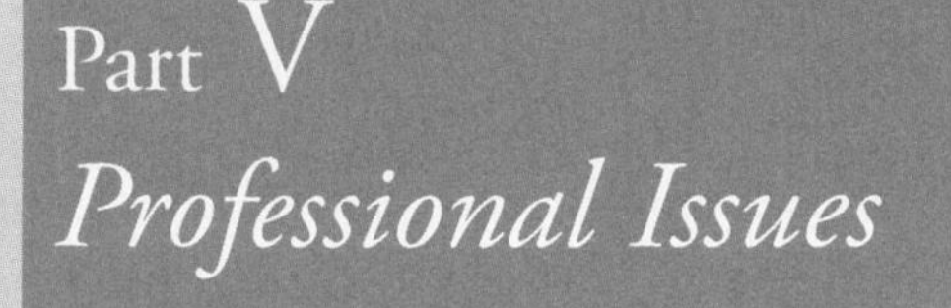

Chapter 22

Communicating with Other Health Professionals

Kathleen Underman Boggs

OUTLINE

OBJECTIVES

At the end of the chapter, the reader will be able to:

1. Identify concepts in professional relationships.
2. Describe methods to handle conflict through interpersonal negotiation when it occurs.
3. Discuss methods for communicating effectively in organizational settings.
4. Apply group communication principles to work groups.
5. Discuss application of one research study to clinical practice.

While the context and scope of nursing practice is changing significantly, the role of the beginning professional nurse continues to encompass: provider of care to individuals, families, groups, communities and populations . . . To implement this fully the nurse must (. . . among other things) communicate, collaborate, and negotiate; serve as a member and leader within interdisciplinary health teams; form partnerships with patient and with other health care professionals . . .

American Association of Colleges of Nursing, 1998

Chapter 22 focuses on the development of collegial relationships with other health team members using principles of communication. Specific bridges to communication with other health professionals are described, along with strategies to remove communication barriers.

To be effective as a nursing professional, it is not enough to be deeply committed to the client. Ultimately, the workplace's corporate climate will have an effect on the relationship that takes place between you and your client. Failures in communication among health care providers are among the most common factors contributing to adverse client outcomes and nurse dissatisfaction (Coeling & Cukr, 2000; Rosenstein & O'Daniel, 2005; Tschannen, 2004). Commitment to collaboration in working relationships with other professionals helps sustain a high quality of client care.

BASIC CONCEPTS

Delegation

Delegation is defined as the transfer of responsibility for the performance of an activity from one individual to another while retaining accountability for the outcome. Whether delegating to a peer or unlicensed assistive personnel (UAP), the nurse is only transferring the responsibility for the performance of the activity, not the professional accountability for the overall care (American Nurses Association, 1994). In earlier times, delegating and trusting went hand in hand, because the nurse was transferring responsibility to a peer and had some assurance of the skills and knowledge of that peer. The present health care environment poses a much different reality because the nurse is no longer sure of the skills and knowledge of the person to whom he or she is delegating. Some UAPs possess minimal experience, skills, or knowledge.

Supervision of UAPs is a newly emerging and important aspect of the professional nurse's role and responsibilities. The challenges of maintaining professional integrity and concurrently surviving in today's health care arena are felt by nurses in all settings. Effective and appropriate use of delegation can facilitate the nurse's ability to meet these challenges.

More often than not, novice nurses are inadequately prepared for the demands of delegating much of their nursing tasks to UAPs while retaining responsibility for interpreting patient outcomes. However, the novice nurse is not alone in feeling inadequate; experienced nurses are facing the same dilemmas. Findings from a 1997 study revealed that registered nurses were dissatisfied with UAPs' ability to perform delegated nursing tasks, communicate pertinent information, and provide more time for professional nursing activities (Barter, McLaughlin, & Thomas, 1997).

Inherent in effective delegation is an adequate understanding of the skills and knowledge of UAPs as well as of the Nurse Practice Act of the state in which the nurse is practicing (Johnson, 1996). Within each state's Nurse Practice Act are specific guidelines describing what nursing actions can and cannot be delegated and what type of personnel these actions can be delegated to. In addition to knowing nurse practice guidelines and the skills and knowledge level of UAPs, the nurse must educate and reinforce the UAPs' knowledge base, assess the UAPs' readiness for delegation, delegate appropriately, oversee the task, and evaluate and record the outcomes (Adams, 1995; Boucher, 1998). The appropriate implementation of these principles (e.g., educating, assessing, overseeing, and evaluating) is a costly process both in time and energy. Practice Exercise 22-1 to facilitate your understanding of the principles. The following case example highlights one particular principle.

Case Example

After receiving the report on her client assignments, Monica Lewis, RN, assigns a newly hired UAP to provide routine care (e.g., morning care, assistance with meals, vital signs, finger sticks for glucose, and reporting of any changes) to Mrs. Jones, who was recently admitted for exacerbation of her type 2 diabetes. While on routine rounds, during lunch, Monica finds Mrs. Jones unresponsive, with cold, clammy skin, a heart rate of 110, and a finger stick reading of 60 mg/dL, which the UAP had obtained. Thinking Mrs. Jones was experiencing hypoglycemia, Monica requested the UAP to obtain another blood glucose. While administering high-glucose intravenous solutions to raise Mrs. Jones' blood sugar, Monica observed the UAP violate a number of basic principles in obtaining an accurate blood glucose. Upon further questioning, the UAP admitted never having been taught the proper procedure and thought reading the directions was sufficient. Monica had wrongly assumed all UAPs underwent training on the principles of obtaining blood glucose finger sticks.

Exercise 22-1 **Applying Principles of Delegation**

Purpose: To help students differentiate between delegating nursing tasks and evaluating client outcomes.

Procedure:

Divide the class into two groups: A and B. The following case study is a typical day for a charge nurse in an extended-care facility. After reading the case study, Group A is to describe the nursing tasks they would delegate and instructions they would give the nursing assistants and certified medicine aides (CMAs). Group B is to describe the professional nursing responsibilities related to the delegated tasks. The two groups then share their reports.

Situation:

Anne Marie Roache is the day shift charge nurse on one of the units at Shadyside Nursing and Rehabilitation Facility. On this particular day, her census is 24, and her staff includes four nursing assistants and two CMAs who are allowed to administer all oral and topical medications. Her nursing assistants are qualified to perform morning care: assist with feedings; obtain and record vital signs, fluid intake and output, and blood glucose finger sticks; turn and position residents; assist with ambulation; and perform decubitus dressing changes. Of the residents, 12 are bedridden, requiring complete bed baths and some degree of assistance with feeding. The remaining 12 require varying degrees of assistance with their morning baths and assistance to the dining rooms for their meals. Nine of the residents are diabetics requiring pre-meal blood glucose finger sticks; seven are recovering from cerebrovascular accidents and display varying degrees of right- or left-sided weakness; three require care of their sacral decubiti; and all of the residents are at risk for falling because of varying degrees of confusion, disorientation, or general weakness. The night shift reported that all the residents' conditions were stable and they had slept well. Ms. Roache is ready to assign her staff.

Discussion:

Entire class can identify client goals.

APPLICATIONS

Conflict Resolution

Conflicts will inevitably arise in the work setting. Refer to Box 22-1. Aside from the nurse-client conflicts described in Chapter 14, most workplace conflicts occur between the nurse and authority figures. In a study published in *Nursing Times*, 30% of nurses surveyed reported being harassed or bullied on the job, but only 6% made a formal complaint (Shah, 2001). Another form of conflict may arise from agency employee policies. Internal employee-management disputes detract from the agency's health care mission and from its financial bottom line (Miller & Wax, 1999).

Many of the same strategies for conflict resolution discussed in Chapter 14 for conflict between client and nurse can be applied to conflicts between the nurse and other health care workers. Review the principles of conflict management in Figure 14-1. You need to think through the possible causes of the conflict, as well as your own feelings about it, and respond appropriately, even if the response is a deliberate choice not to respond verbally. Interpersonal conflicts that are not dealt with leave residual feelings that reappear unexpectedly and affect your ability to respond realistically and responsibly in future interactions.

As mentioned, conflict is not necessarily detrimental to productivity and job satisfaction. Successful resolution often has a positive effect on both outcomes. Thus, the primary goal in dealing with workplace conflict is to find a high-quality, mutually acceptable solution: a win-win strategy. In many instances, a different type of relationship can be developed through the use of conflict management communication techniques (Bacal, n.d.; Cascardo, 2001). Reframe a clinical situation as a cooperative process in which the health goals and not the status relations of the health care providers become the focal object by following these steps:

Developing an Evidence-Based Practice

Olade RA: Evidence-based practice and research utilization activities among rural nurses, *J Nurs Scholarsh* 36(3):220-225, 2004.

The author designed a descriptive research study to determine the extent to which rural nurses utilize evidence-based guidelines from research in their practice. An additional purpose was to identify the barriers these nurses encountered in evidence-based practice. The sample was 106 rural nurses who answered open-ended questionnaires.

Results: Findings indicated that only 20.8% of these nurses were currently involved in research utilization. The two areas of greatest evidence-based practice were management of pain and management of pressure ulcers. Identified barriers included isolation and lack of access to nursing research consultants.

Application to Your Clinical Practice: Nursing administrators could model the value of evidence-based practice by budgeting for brief consultant visits. Each agency's Quality Assurance/Improvement committee could collect data about the extent to which nursing practice in their agency is evidence-based. First, though, each nurse needs to value scientific research-based practice. How would you convince a fellow staff nurse that he or she would get better outcomes for the client if evidence-based practice guidelines were followed?

Box 22-1 Interpersonal Sources of Conflict in the Critical Area

- Being asked to do something you know would be irresponsible or unsafe
- Having your feelings or opinions ridiculed or discounted
- Being asked to do something to a client that is in conflict with your personal or professional moral values
- Getting pressure to give more time or attention than you are able to give
- Being asked to give more information than you feel comfortable sharing
- Maintaining a sense of self in the face of hostility or sexual harassment

- *Identify your goal.* A clear idea of the outcome you wish to achieve is a necessary first step in the process. Remember the issue is the conflict, not your co-worker.
- *Obtain factual data.* It is important to do your homework by obtaining all relevant information about the specific issues involved—and about the client's behavioral responses to a health care issue—before engaging in negotiation.
- *Consider the other's viewpoint.* Having some idea of what issues might be relevant from the other person's perspective provides important information about the best interpersonal approach to use.
- *Intervene early.* The best time to resolve problems is before they escalate to a conflict. Create a forum for two-way communication, preferably meeting periodically.

Avoiding Barriers to Resolution

Refer to Box 22-2 for tips on how to turn conflict into collaboration. Much of the individual behavior was discussed in Chapter 14, such as avoiding the use of negative or inflammatory, anger-provoking words. Also avoiding phrases that imply coercion or than are patronizing. Examples include "We must insist that..." or "You claim that...". Most individuals react to anger directed at them with a fight-or-flight response. Other barriers to successful negotiation include the following:

- Becoming emotional, rather than focusing on the issue
- Blaming others
- Viewing negotiation as confrontational
- Not trying to understand the perspective of others

Conflict situations among colleagues or among departments become negative when not dealt with. When effectively addressed, there is a tendency for the team to become stronger and to function more effectively.

Box 22-2 How to Turn Conflict into Collaboration

- Take the initiative to discuss problems.
- Use active listening skills (refrain from simultaneous activities that interrupt communication).
- Present documented data relevant to the issue.
- Propose resolutions.
- Create a climate in which participants view negotiation as a collaborative effort.
- Use a brief summary to provide feedback.
- Record all decisions in writing.

Physician-Nurse Conflict Resolution

Nurses influence physician-client communication. The Williams and Gossett (2001) study showed that nurses assess what physicians tell clients, encourage clients to seek clarification, encourage second opinions, and spend time defending the physician's competence. Smooth collaboration between nurses and physicians improves the quality of client care (Coeling & Cukr, 2000). Yet there will be occasions when you have collaboration difficulties. Articles addressing the nursing shortage focus on factors that lead to job dissatisfaction. One major factor related to job satisfaction and job retention currently being openly discussed in the literature is "disruptive" communication between other professionals, especially physician-nurse interactions. Case law defines disruptive physician behavior as conduct that "disrupts the operation of the hospital, affects the ability of others to get their jobs done, creates a hostile work environment" (Harmon & Pomm, 2004). Perhaps interactional dysfunction occurs because the professional health care alliance has changed from a traditional notion of the nurse as "handmaiden to the physician" to a concept of the nurse as an autonomous professional who collaborates with the physician to maximize client health goals. According to Rosenstein and O'Daniel (2005), studies demonstrate that disruptive behavior has a negative impact on client health outcomes.

The relationship between the doctor and the nurse remains an evolving process. Consultants note that changes in the physician-nurse communication process are occurring as nurses become more empowered, in contrast to a historical oppression of both women and nurses. The majority of nurses occasionally encounter problems in the physician-nurse relationship. The differences in power, perspective, education, pay, status, class, and sometimes gender are cited as contributing factors (Salvage & Smith, 2000). Contemporary society is redefining traditional gender role behavior, negating some of the traditional "nurse as subservient female" stereotypical behaviors. Reflect on content presented on gender differences in communication to determine whether your current situation might be related to gender differences in communication styles rather than a more serious problem. Some doctors are reluctant to be challenged; some nurses are quick to feel slighted. Some physician-nurse relationships are marked with conflict, mistrust, and disrespect. Although these feelings are changing, it is slow, and some physicians still regard themselves as the only legitimate authority in health care, seeing the professional nurse as an accessory. An attitude that excludes the nurse as a professional partner in health care promotion benefits no one and is increasingly challenged as being costly to professionals and clients alike. Changes in physician-nurse relationships are driven not only by more assertive, better-educated nurses but also by broader changes in society and in the health care system. Tips for clear communication are listed in Box 22-3.

Box 22-3 Tips to Clarify Requests to Physicians

1. Identify all names.
   - State the physician's name.
   - State your name and position.
   - Identify client and client's diagnosis or other people involved in the problem by name.
2. Summarize the problem.
   - Be brief and list factual data about the current problem.
3. State your goal.
4. Suggest a solution.
   - List interventions already attempted.
   - Cite any relevant clinical practice guideline solutions.
5. Write a conclusion.
   - Clarify who will be responsible for the implementation.
   - Summarize the new order, especially if this is a phone conversation.
   - Specify the time frame.

The most common factor in adversarial relations is communication failure. You can use skills taught in this book to improve both the clarity of message content and the emotional tone of interactions. You can apply the same principles of conflict resolution discussed in Chapter 14 when dealing with a physician-nurse conflict. Make a commitment to open dialogue. Listening should constitute at least half of a communication interaction. Foster a feeling of collegiality. Use strategies from that chapter to defuse anger. During your negotiation, discussion should begin with a statement of either the commonalities of purpose or the points of agreement about the issue (e.g., "I thoroughly agree Mr. Smith will do much better at home. However, we need to contact social services and make a home care referral before we actually discharge him; otherwise, he will be right back in the hospital again."). Points of disagreement should always follow rather than precede points of agreement.

Empathy and a genuine desire to understand the issues from the other's perspective enhance communication and the likelihood of a successful resolution.

It is important to remain flexible yet not to yield on important, essential dimensions of the issue. Sometimes it is difficult to listen carefully to the other person's position without automatically formulating your next point or response, but it is important to keep an open mind and to examine the issue from a number of perspectives before selecting alternative options. The communication process should not be prematurely concluded.

The authors feel that nurses have a responsibility to foster good physician-client communication. This is especially true when it becomes obvious to you from content, tone, or body language that antagonism is developing. Do you think it is ever appropriate for a nurse to criticize a physician's actions to a client? A common underlying factor in at least 25% of all malpractice suits is an inadvertent or deliberate critical comment by another health care professional concerning a colleague's actions. So think before you speak!

Solutions that take into consideration the needs and human dignity of all parties are more likely to be considered as viable alternatives. Backing another health professional into a psychological corner by using intimidation, coercion, or blaming is simply counterproductive. More often than not, solutions developed through such tactics never get implemented. Usually there are a number of reasons for this phenomenon, but the basic issues have to do with how the problem was originally defined and the control issues that were never actually dealt with in the problem-solving discussion. The final solution derived through fair negotiation is often better than the one arrived at alone by the nurse, the physician, the client, or another health care provider.

Outcomes for clients can be moderately improved when physician and nurse develop collaborative relationships. One study of hospital admissions found that using daily team rounds with joint decision making resulted in a shortened average length of hospital stay and lower hospital charges (Zwarenstein & Bryant, 2000).

Nurse-to-Nurse Conflict Resolution

The nurse-physician relationship is not the only source of workplace conflict. While it is inevitable that you will encounter some communication problems with nurse colleagues, remember that, if managed appropriately, these conflicts can lead to innovative solutions and improved relationships (Smith-Trudeau, 2002).

Negotiating with Nursing Authority Figures. Negotiating can be even more threatening with a nursing supervisor or an instructor who has direct authority, because these people have some control over your future as a staff nurse or student. Supervision implies a shared responsibility in the overall professional goal of providing high-quality nursing care to clients. The wise supervisor is able to promote a nonthreatening environment in which all of the aspects of professionalism are allowed to emerge and prosper. In a supervisor-nurse relationship, conflict may arise when expectations for performance are unclear or when the nurse is unable to perform at the desired level. Communication of expectations often occurs after the fact, within the context of an employee performance evaluation. To effectively manage requires that performance expectations are known from the beginning. The supervisor needs to advise you about the need for improvement as part of an ongoing, constructive, interpersonal relationship. When the supervisor must give constructive criticism, it should be given in a nonthreatening and genuinely caring manner.

Managing Nursing Staff Problems. Improving how nurses deal with conflict is an investment in co-workers, our organization, and ultimately in improved client outcomes. Nonaction has been identified as the most common repressive management strategy (Bacal, 2005a). Nurse managers have learned that ignoring conflict among staff does not solve problems. Avoidance perpetuates the status quo or leads to an escalation (Ohio Nurses Foundation, 2003). When managed appropriately, you reduce time wasted by staff in griping, defending, and so on, as illustrated in the following case, adapted from "Workplace Issues" in *Nursing News* (New Hampshire Nurses Association, 2002) and Ohio Nurses Foundation (2003). Use the steps in Box 22-4 to analyze this case.

Case Example

Two nursing teams work the day shift on a busy medical unit. As nurse manager, Ms. Libby notices that both teams are arguing over use of the computer, have become unwilling to help cover the other team's client, are taking longer to complete assigned work, and so on. To achieve a more harmonious work environment, she arranges a staff meeting to get the teams communica-

Box 22-4 Steps to Promote Conflict Resolution Among Groups of Health Care Workers

- Set the stage for collaborative communication (privacy, etc.).
- Meet, bringing together all involved groups.
- Solicit the perspectives of each.
- Define the problem issue clearly:
  - Identify the key points.
- Have an objective or a goal clearly in mind.
- Maintain respect:
  - Respect the values and dignity of all parties.
  - Group members can be assertive but not manipulative.
  - Remember to criticize ideas, not people.
- Discuss solutions:
  - Identify the merits/drawbacks of each solution.
  - Be open to alternative solutions in which all parties can meet essential needs.
  - Depersonalize conflict situations.
  - Avoid emotion.
- Decide to implement the best solution:
  - Specify persons responsible for implementation.
  - Establish time line.
  - Decide on the evaluation method.

ting. Rather than just issues about sharing the computer, several problem issues arise suggesting inadequate time management and overload. Ms. Libby listens actively, responds with empathy, and provides positive regard and feedback for solutions proposed by the group. She asks the group to decide on two prioritized solutions. Recognizing that her staff feel unappreciated and knowing that compromise is a strategy that produces behavior change, she resolves to offer more frequent performance feedback. She herself assumes responsibility for requesting an immediate second computer purchase under her unit budget's emergency funding allocation. A team member who is on the employee relations committee assumes responsibility for requesting that the Human Services Department schedule an inservice training on time management and stress reduction within the next month. The group agrees to meet in six weeks to evaluate.

Giving constructive criticism and receiving criticism is difficult for most people (Box 22-5). When a supervisor gives constructive criticism, some type of response from the person receiving it is indicated.

Box 22-5 Steps in Giving Constructive Criticism

1. Express sympathy.
   Sample statement: "I understand that things are difficult at home."
2. Describe the behavior.
   Sample statement: "But I see that you have been late coming to work three times during this pay period."
3. State expectations.
   Sample statement: "It is necessary for you to be here on time from now on."
4. List consequences.
   Sample statement: "If you get here on time, we'll all start off the shift better. If you are late again, I will have to report you to the personnel department."

Initially, it is crucial that the conflict problem be clearly defined and acknowledged. To help handle constructive criticism, nurses can do the following:

- Schedule a time when you are calm.
- Request that supervisory meetings be in a place that allows privacy.
- Defuse personal anxiety.
- Listen carefully to the criticism and then paraphrase it.
- Acknowledge that you take suggestions for improvement seriously.
- Discuss the facts of the situation but avoid becoming defensive.
- Develop a plan for dealing with similar situations; become proactive rather than reactive.

In studying approaches to authority figures, you are encouraged to analyze your overall personal responses to authority, as in Exercise 22-2.

Collaborating with Peers. The nurse-client relationship occurs within the larger context of the professional relationship with other health disciplines. How the nurse relates to other members of the health team will affect the level and nature of the interactions that transpire between nurse and client. Interpersonal conflict between health team members periodically is concealed from awareness and projected onto client behaviors.

Case Example

On a psychiatric nursing unit, the nursing staff found Mr. Tomkins's behavior highly disruptive. At an inter-

Exercise 22-2 Feelings About Authority

Purpose: To have students recognize their feelings about authority.

Procedure:

1. Lean back in your chair, close your eyes, and think of the word "authority."
2. Who is the first person that comes to mind when thinking of that word?
3. Describe how this person signifies authority to you. Next, think of an incident in which this person exerted authority and how you reacted to it.
4. After you have visualized the memory, answer the following questions:
   a. What were your feelings about the incident after it was over?
   b. What changes of feelings occurred from the start of the incident until it was over?
   c. Was there anything about the authority figure that reminded you of yourself?
   d. Was there anything about the authority figure that reminded you of someone else with whom you once had a strong relationship (if the memory viewed is not mother or father)?
   e. How could you have handled the incident more assertively?
   f. Can you see any patterns in yourself that might help you handle interactions with authority figures?
   g. What about those patterns that are not assertive?
   h. How could those patterns be improved to be more assertive?

Adapted from Levy R: *Self-revelation through relationships*, Englewood Cliffs, NJ, 1972, Prentice Hall.

disciplinary conference attended by representatives from all shifts, there was general agreement that Mr. Tomkins would spend 1 hour in the seclusion room each time his agitated behavior occurred. The order was written into his care plan. The plan was implemented for a week with a noticeable reduction in client symptoms. During the second week, however, Mr. Tomkins would be placed in the seclusion room for the reasons just mentioned, but the evening staff would release him after 5 or 10 minutes if he was quiet and well-behaved.

The client's agitated behavior began to escalate again, and another interdisciplinary conference was called. Although the stated focus of the dialogue was on constructive ways to help Mr. Tomkins cope with disruptive anxiety, the underlying issues related to the strong feelings of the day nursing staff that their interventions were being undermined. Equally strong was the conviction of the evening staff that they were acting in the client's best interest by letting him out of the seclusion room as soon as his behavior normalized. Until the underlying behaviors could be resolved satisfactorily at the staff level, the client continued to act out the staff's anxiety as well as his own.

Similar types of issues arise now and again when there is no input from different work shifts in developing a comprehensive nursing care plan. The shift staff may not agree with specific interventions, but instead of talking the discrepancy through in regularly scheduled staff conferences, they may act it out, unconsciously undoing the work of the other shifts.

Occasionally you may have to work with a peer with whom you develop a "personality conflict." Stop and consider what led up to the current situation. Generally it is due to an accumulation of small annoyances that occurred over time. The best method to avoid such situations is to verbalize occurrences rather than ignoring them until they become a major problem. Avoid the "blame game" and discuss in a private, calm moment what you *both* can do to make things better.

Case Example

"Jane, we seem to disagree about the best way to teach Mr. Santos about his.... He seems to be getting confused about our two different approaches. Let's talk about how we might be able to work more effectively together. What is the most important point you want to teach him?" ***(Use active listening skills to really pay attention to what Jane says. Do a self-inventory to eli-***

minate any nonverbal behavior that is triggering Jane's reaction and eliminate it. Ask yourself, "Do I want to win, or do I want to fix this problem?" Then state your expectations in a calm tone.)

Whenever there is covert conflict among nursing staff or between members of different health disciplines, it is the client who ultimately suffers the repercussions. The level of trust the client may have established in the professional relationship is compromised until the staff conflict can be resolved.

Delegation or Supervision of Unlicensed Personnel. As mentioned earlier in the concepts section of this chapter, nursing organizations have identified trends toward increased use of unlicensed workers in agencies wishing to reduce costs. Such organizations speak out about the burden this places on registered nurses. Becoming active in your state nurses association or professional specialty organization allows you to add your voice to this debate. Obtain a copy of your state's Nurse Practice Act. Usually these can be downloaded from your state Board of Nursing's website. This document will spell out what you, as a registered nurse, can delegate and to whom.

Even as a beginning staff nurse you will be expected to delegate some client care duties to others. You are responsible for the completeness, quality, and accuracy of this care. To do so, you need to be clear about the rules and regulations of your state and agency. What may this person legally do? For example, while most states allow a physician to delegate any care activity he or she chooses, some states forbid unlicensed persons receiving verbal orders from a physician. Most states explicitly forbid unlicensed persons from administering medications. To avoid conflicts in delegating client care, clearly state your expectations. It is your responsibility to ensure that care was given correctly.

Removing Barriers to Communication with Other Professionals

Responding to Putdowns

At some time in your professional career, you will run into unwarranted putdowns and destructive criticisms. Generally, they have but one intent: to decrease your status and enhance the status of the person delivering the putdown. The putdown or criticism may be handed out because the speaker is feeling inadequate or threatened. Often it has little to do with the actual behavior of the nurse to whom it is delivered. Other times the criticism may be valid, but the time and place of delivery are grossly inappropriate (e.g., in the middle of the nurses' station or in the client's presence). In either case, the automatic response of many nurses is to become defensive and embarrassed and in some way actually begin to feel inadequate, thus allowing the speaker to project unwarranted feelings onto the nurse.

Recognizing a putdown or unwarranted criticism is the first step toward dealing effectively with it. If a comment from a co-worker or authority figure generates defensiveness, embarrassment, and doubt about one's professional ability to perform the nursing role, it is likely that the comment represents more than just factual information about performance. If the comment made by the speaker contains legitimate information to help improve one's skill and is delivered in a private and constructive manner, it represents a learning response and cannot be considered a putdown. Learning to differentiate between the two types of communication helps the nurse to "separate the wheat from the chaff."

Case Example

You examine a crying child's inner ears and note that the tympanic membranes (eardrums) are red. You report to your supervisor that the child may have an ear infection.

A. *Response:* When a child is crying, the drums often swell and redden. How about checking again when the child is calm? (*Learning response*)

Or

B. *Response:* Of course they are red when the child is crying. Didn't you learn that in nursing school? I haven't got time to answer such basic questions! (*Putdown response*)

Which response would you prefer to receive? Why?

Whereas the first response allows the nurse to learn useful information to incorporate into practice, the second response serves to antagonize, and it is doubtful much learning takes place. What will happen is that the nurse will be more hesitant about approaching the supervisor again for clinical information. Again, it is the client who ultimately suffers.

Once a putdown is recognized as such, the nurse needs to respond verbally in an assertive manner as soon as possible after the incident has taken place. Waiting an appreciable length of time is likely to cause resentment in the nurse toward the other person, leaving the staff nurse with feelings of lost self-respect. Furthermore, it may be more difficult later for the other person to remember the details of the incident. At the same time, if the nurse's own anger, not the problem behavior, is likely to dominate the response, it is better to wait for the anger to cool a little and then to present the message in a more dignified and reasoned manner.

The Process for Responding to Putdowns. In responding to putdowns, the nature of the relationship should be considered. Attitudes are important. Respect for the value of each individual as a person should be evidenced throughout the interaction. Try to determine how to respond to this person in a productive way so that you are on speaking terms but still get your point across. Even if you do not fully succeed in your initial tries, you probably will have learned something valuable in the process.

Address the objectionable or disrespectful behaviors first. Briefly state the behavior and its impact on you. It is important to deliver a succinct verbal message without getting lost in detail and without sounding apologetic or defensive. Do not try to give a prolonged explanation of your behavior at this point in the interaction, and do not suggest possible motivations.

Emphasize the specifics of the putdown behavior. Once the putdown has been dealt with, you can discuss any criticism of your behavior on its own merits. Refer only to the behaviors identified, and do not encourage the other person to amplify the putdown.

Prepare a few standard responses. Because putdowns often catch one by surprise, it is useful to have a standard set of opening replies ready. Examples of openers might include the following:

- "I think it was out of line for you to criticize me in front of the client."
- "I found your comments very disturbing and insulting."
- "I experienced what you said as an attack that wasn't called for by my actions."
- "I thought that was an intolerable remark."

A reply that is specific to the putdown delivered is essential. The tone of voice needs to be even and firm. In the clinical example given previously, the nurse might have said to the head nurse: "My school is not an issue, and your criticism is unnecessary" or, "It seems to me that the assessment of the child's ears, not my school, is the issue, and your superior tone is uncalled for."

An important aspect of putdowns is that they get in the way of the nurse's professional goal of providing high-quality nursing care to clients. The effect of the head nurse's second response is for both nurses to assume the reddened eardrums are from crying and not to reevaluate the child's eardrums. Feeling resentful and less sure of his or her clinical skills, the staff nurse is less likely to risk stirring up such feelings again. If fewer questions are asked, important information goes unshared. In the clinical example just cited, a possible ear infection might not be detected.

Peer Negotiation

As students, you will encounter situations in which the behavior of a colleague causes a variety of unexpressed differences or disagreement because the colleague's interpretation of a situation or meaning of behavior is so different from yours. The conflict behaviors can occur as a result of differences in values, philosophical approaches to life, ways of handling problems, lifestyles, definitions of a problem, goals, or strategies to resolve a problem. Nevertheless, these differences cause friction and turn relationships from collaborative to competitive.

Recognizing the existence of a conflict is the first step toward peer negotiation. Generally, conflict increases anxiety. When interaction with a certain peer or peer group stimulates anxious or angry feelings, the presence of conflict should be considered. Once it is determined that conflict is present, look for the basis of the conflict and label it as personal or professional. If it is personal in nature, it may not be appropriate to seek peer negotiation. It might be better to go back through the self-awareness exercises presented in previous chapters and locate the nature of the conflict through self-examination.

Sharing feelings about a conflict with others helps to reduce its intensity. It is confusing, for example, when nursing students first enter a nursing program or clinical rotation, but this confusion does not get discussed, and students commonly believe they should not feel confused or uncertain. As a nursing student, you face complex interpersonal situations. These situations may

Exercise 22-3 Applying Principles of Confrontation

Purpose: To help students understand the importance of using specific principles of confrontation to resolve a conflict.

Procedure:

1. Divide the class into two groups: Group A is the day shift (7 AM–7 PM), and Group B is the night shift (7 PM–7 AM).
2. The following case study is an example of some problems between the night and day shifts resulting in mistrust and general tension between the two groups. After reading the case study, each group is to use three principles as identified in the text (i.e., identify concerns; clarify assumptions; and identify real issue). The two groups then share their concerns, assumptions, and what they believe to be the real issue. Finally, both groups are to apply the fourth principle, collaboratively identifying a solution or solutions that satisfy both groups.

Situation:

The night shift's (Group B) responsibilities include completing as many bed baths as possible and the taping report as close to the shift change (7 AM) as possible. The day shift (Group A) finds that very few, if any, of the bed baths are completed and that the taped report is usually done at about 5 AM, reflecting very few of the client changes that occurred between 5 AM and 7 AM. The day shift is angry with the night shift, feeling they are not assuming their fair share of the workload. The night shift feels the day shift does not understand their responsibilities; they believe they are contributing more than their fair share of work.

Discussion:

Instructor might role-play the part of the nurse manager who acts to facilitate resolution of this conflict.

lead you to experience loneliness or self-doubt about your nursing skills compared with those of your peers. These feelings are universal in humans at the beginning of any new experience. By sharing them with one or two peers, one usually finds that others have had parallel experiences. In reviewing Exercise 22-3, think of a conflict or problem that has implications for your practice of nursing, one you would be willing to share with your peers.

Self-awareness is beneficial in assessing the meaning of a professional conflict. For instance, if the nurse's major response to the conflict is emotional, one can be reasonably certain the conflict raises personal feelings from a previous experience. This assumption does not negate the legitimacy of the conflict issue, but it suggests that the personal material needs to be recognized, worked through, and removed from the peer negotiation process. Concrete, observable facts related to the issue should be the focus of discussion; conflicted personal feelings should be discussed elsewhere, except as they directly affect the current situation. Now that you have had an opportunity to study different types of conflict, work on Exercise 22-4.

Developing a Support System

Collegial relationships are an important determinant of success as professional men and women entering nursing practice. Although there is no substitute for outcomes that demonstrate professional competence, interpersonal strategies can facilitate the process. Integrity, respect for others, dependability, a good sense of humor, and an openness to sharing with others are communication qualities people look for in developing a support system.

Forming a reliable support system at work to share information, ideas, and strategies with colleagues adds a collective strength to personal efforts and minimizes the possibility of misunderstanding. With problem or conflict situations, getting ideas from trusted colleagues beforehand enhances the probability of accomplishing outcomes more effectively. An Australian study of 157 registered nurses working in a private hospital found that support lowered job-related stress and increased job satisfaction. Support was given to nurses by supervisors and other nurses (Bartram, Joiner, & Stanton, 2004).

Exercise 22-4 Barriers to Interprofessional Communication

Purpose: To help students understand the basic concepts of client advocacy, communication barriers, and peer negotiation in simulated nursing situations.

Procedure:

1. Following are two examples of situations in which interprofessional communication barriers exist. Refamiliarize yourself with the concepts of professionalism, client advocacy, communication barriers, and peer negotiation.
2. Formulate a response to each example.
3. Compare your responses with those of your classmates, and discuss the implications of common and disparate answers. Sometimes dissimilar answers provide another important dimension of a problem situation.

Case A

Dr. Tanlow interrupts Ms. Serf as she is preparing pain medication for 68-year-old Mrs. Gould. It is already 15 minutes late. Dr. Tanlow says he needs Ms. Serf immediately in Room 20C to assist with a drainage and dressing change. Knowing that Mrs. Gould, a diabetic, will respond to prolonged pain with vomiting, Ms. Serf replies that she will be available to help Dr. Tanlow in 10 minutes (during which time she will have administered Mrs. Gould's pain medication). Dr. Tanlow, already on his way to Room 20C, whirls around, stating loudly, "When I say I need assistance, I mean now. I am a busy man, in case you hadn't noticed."

If you were Ms. Serf, what would be an appropriate response?

Case B

A newly hired nurse is helping a resident draw femoral blood. The nurse states that although she has never assisted with this procedure, she is thoroughly familiar with the procedure through the hospital manual. The nurse requests that, if the resident requires anything different from the manual, he should tell her so. The resident responds, "You should have practiced this with someone else. I shouldn't be stuck with a neophyte. Ha ha! Get it? Neophyte, instead of needle."

How should the nurse respond?

Discussion:

These cases could be discussed in class, assigned as a term paper, or used as an essay exam.

Professional Support Groups. One of the meanings of the word *comfort* is "to strengthen." Nurses need to take time to strengthen personal resources, and one way to do this is to seek comfort and understanding in a professional support group. A professional support group composed of individuals with similar work experience is designed to provide emotional and cognitive support, enabling nurses to work more effectively in high-risk nursing situations. Often, family and friends have a limited understanding of the emotional impact of such experiences or the heart-rending toll it takes over time on the individual nurse. Talking things through with other nurses is comforting.

Professional organizations don't usually have the primary purpose of providing emotional support; however, small subgroups within professional organizations may be used for personal support. Another support source may be a nursing chat group on the Internet. Often membership in these is based on clinical specialty interests.

Guidelines for Communication

Guidelines for managing communication problems with colleagues are the same as those used when you have a communication problem with a client. Strategies described in Chapter 14 can be readily applied to communication problems with colleagues. Often a person is not directly aware of personal communication blocks in professional relationships. Asking for feedback and engaging in self-reflection give the nurse an honest appraisal of personal communication strategies in professional situations.

When communicating with other members of the health care organization, it is advisable to consider the ego of the other person. Negative comments can affect the self-esteem of the receiver. Even when the critical statements are valid (e.g., "You do..." or "You make me feel..."), they should be replaced with "I" statements that define the sender's position. Otherwise, the meaning of the communication will be lost as the individual strives to defend against a personally felt attack. Statements discounting the value of the person can prevent you from achieving professional objectives. For example, verbal expressions using dogmatic language or derogatory adjectives, violating confidences, interrupting a conversation, and asking loaded or offensive questions usually diminish the other person's feelings of personal power and self-esteem. Nonverbal behaviors (e.g., lateness or withdrawal) serve to disconfirm the importance of the other person. Any behavior that makes an individual feel small or less significant is counterproductive. These stimulate needless hostility and, in the end, sabotage the legitimate goals of the communication.

Strategies

Understand the Organizational System. Whenever you work in an organization, either as student or professional, you automatically become a part of an organizational system with established political norms of acceptable behavior. Each organizational system defines its own chain of command and rules about social processes in professional communication. Even though your idea may be excellent, failure to understand the chain of command or an unwillingness to form the positive alliances needed to accomplish your objective dilutes the impact. For example, if your instructor has been defined as your first line of contact, then it is not in your best interest to seek out staff personnel or other students without also checking with the instructor.

Although sidestepping the identified chain of command and going to a higher or more tangential resource in the hierarchy may appear less threatening initially, the benefits of such action may not resolve the difficulty. Furthermore, the trust needed for serious discussion becomes limited. Some of the reasons for avoiding positive interactions stem from an internal circular process

Table 22-1 Examples of Unclear Communication Processes That Block the Development of Cooperative and Receptive Influencing Skills

Situation	Communication Process
Low self-disclosure	No one knows my real thoughts, feelings, and needs. *Consequently:* I think no one cares about me or recognizes my needs.
	Others see me as self-sufficient and are unaware that I have a problem. *Consequently:* Others are unable to respond to my needs.
Reluctance to delegate tasks	Other people think I don't believe that they can do the job as well as I can. *Consequently:* The others work at a minimum level.
	I don't expect or ask others to be involved. *Consequently:* Other people don't volunteer to help me. *Consequently:* I feel resentful, and others feel undervalued and dispensable.
Making unnecessary demands	I expect more from others than they think is reasonable. *Consequently:* I feel the others are lazy and uncommitted, and I must push harder.
	Others see me as manipulative and dehumanizing. *Consequently:* Others assume a low profile and don't contribute their ideas. *Consequently:* Work production is mediocre. Morale is low. Everyone, including me, feels disempowered.

of faulty thinking. Because communication is viewed as part of a process, the sender and receiver act on the information received, which may or may not represent the reality of the situation. Examples of the circular processes that block the development of cooperative and receptive influencing skills in organizational settings are presented in Table 22-1.

Use Interprofessional Collaboration. A recent study in a Norwegian hospital explored cooperation among health professionals (Skjorshammer, 2001). As described in Chapter 14, these new findings show that nurses continue to use avoidance as their major method of conflict management. As discussed in the section on conflict with clients, the more effective strategy would be negotiation.

Identify the Most Appropriate Communication Style. In addition to the tips provided in Chapter 14, there are some strategies that apply to communication within large organizations. It is useful to use the most appropriate method. Some people prefer written communication over verbal discussion; others respond better with more informal interaction. In an organization, written communication may be the best method of successful professional communication.

Use a Focused Opening Statement. A focused opening statement gives the receiver of the message an overview of the issue to be discussed. This is made in general terms, without initially getting into detailed specifics or tangential issues. Such an overview can be accomplished by using an initial focus statement capturing the essence of the communicated message. For example, a nursing student might approach an instructor to discuss problems with the development of a care plan with the focus statement, "I'd like to discuss my care plan with you, and more specifically, how to individualize my behavioral objectives before I start my next care plan." This type of statement is preferable to an interpersonal approach that shows little forethought (e.g., "I'm not sure what you want from me on this care plan.").

Keep Your Options Open. Avoid getting locked into an either/or type of discussion. Having more than one option usually gives both the sender and the receiver a greater feeling of flexibility and personal control in responding. It allows the person to respond rather than to react. The best way to keep your options open is to consider the issue from a variety of perspectives and to listen. Talking situations through with an impartial, trusted colleague or mentor beforehand decreases anxiety and allows the person initiating the dialogue an opportunity to look at the issues from more than one perspective.

Approaching the dialogue with an open mind about which path to take increases the probability of developing a more satisfactory solution. Approaching a person as a mystery waiting to unfold is useful in that the final answers may be quite different from what either of you might have projected as possibilities.

Professional Work Groups

Throughout a professional nursing career, nurses are involved in peer work-related groups of many kinds. Multiple group membership is a fact of life in most organizations. Groups found in organizational settings (e.g., standing committees, ad hoc task forces, and quality circles) accomplish a wide range of tasks related to the goals of the organization. Nurses traditionally use task and support groups for goal accomplishment in health care settings.

Every organization develops permanent and temporary task groups to do the work necessary for the agency to accomplish its mission. In work groups, just as in therapy groups, there are two main elements: content and process. In contrast with therapy groups, task group content is predetermined by an assignment or charge given to the group. Work groups center their attention on a task to be accomplished or the resolution of difficult interpersonal issues specifically related to the professional work setting.

Emotional issues, except as they relate to the accomplishment of group goals, are not addressed. Successful groups make this distinction because a work group is not designed to be a personal growth or therapy group. The goal is to complete the assigned task. Personal growth may be an important by-product of task accomplishment, but it cannot become the primary concern of the group. Failure to understand the differences between the purposes of a work group and a therapeutic group can be a disruptive sidetrack for the group and a personally devastating experience for individual group members.

Leadership Style

Flexibility of leadership style is an essential characteristic of successful work groups. Effective leadership develops from leader characteristics, situational features, and member needs in combination with each other. Successful leadership in one group situation does not guarantee similar success in other group situations (Sullivan & Decker, 1997). Different groups require different leadership behaviors. Leadership is contingent on a proper match between a group situation and the leadership style.

The three basic types of leadership styles found in groups are authoritarian, democratic, and laissez-faire. Of the three leadership styles, the authoritarian style is the most structured.

Leaders demonstrating an **authoritarian leadership** style take full responsibility for group direction and control group interaction. Dissenting opinions are squelched. The leader makes little attempt to encourage team effort, and decision making is accomplished through authority rule. Authoritarian leadership styles work best when the group needs structure and there is limited time to reach a decision. Most mature groups resist an authoritarian leadership style.

Democratic leadership involves members in active discussion and decision making. The leader encourages open expression of feelings and ideas while providing support and encouragement. Democratic leaders are goal-directed but allow flexibility in how group objectives and goals are met. In general, a democratic leadership style offers the group structure while preserving individual member autonomy. Member satisfaction is highest in groups with a democratic leadership. A variation of a democratic leadership style is a **participatory leadership** style. Here the group leader maintains final control but actively solicits and uses group member input.

The third leadership style studied is referred to as **laissez-faire**. Leaders with a laissez-faire style, although physically present, provide little or no structure and essentially abdicate their leadership responsibilities. Group members are free to decide the direction of the group interaction without leader input or structure. Groups with a laissez-faire leader are likely to be less productive and less satisfying to group members. The committee members may get mired in discussions that prevent them from completing their assigned task.

Leadership Responsibilities

The activities of a responsible, successful work group leader include the following:

- Form the committee structure.
- Establish the agenda.
- Clarify the work group's tasks and goals (providing background data and material if needed).
- Notify each member of meeting dates, times, place, and other parameters. It is best to do this in written format (e.g., by memo or via e-mail).
- Keep the group members focused on their tasks.
- Adhere to time limits.
- Conclude each meeting by summarizing progress and allocating assignments to be completed for the next meeting.

Member Responsibilities

Sensitivity to group process and acceptance of personal responsibility as a group member make a person a more effective group participant. Teamwork enhances the probability of goal achievement, as well as personal satisfaction with group outcomes and one's own participation (Sheafor, 1991). In a professional work-related group, each group member assumes individual responsibility for the overall functioning of the group and the achievement of group task goals. Effective professional groups need the cooperation of all members. The functional goals in a professional group cannot be dictated by others; they need to emerge from the member roles and responsibilities created in group interaction.

The primary purpose of using a group format is to benefit problem resolution by generating new ideas. A second purpose is to involve key individuals directly in clarifying work-related or difficult interpersonal problems and in seeking workable answers to concrete problems. Personal ownership of problem definition and change are essential to successful implementation. Each member is equally responsible for the success or failure of the achievement of the group purposes. As you begin membership in a professional group, understanding the nature of the group task enables you to take personal responsibility for your own actions and learning in a group situation. Responsibilities of a work group member include the following:

- Coming prepared to all meetings
- Demonstrating respect for other group members' ideas
- Examining problems objectively and impersonally
- Analyzing the problem
- Developing several options for solutions and comparing alternatives

- Taking an active participatory role to facilitate decision making and choose the best solution
- Implementing and then evaluating outcome

Task Identification in Different Group Phases

Pregroup Tasks. Before the group starts, participants should have a clear idea of what the group task commitment will entail in terms of time, effort, and knowledge. Group members should have enough in common to engage in meaningful communication, a willingness to make a contribution to the group solution, and the ability to complete the task. A strong commitment to the group goal is not always a prerequisite, because this may develop as part of the group process, but a commitment to engage constructively in the development of a viable solution is essential. Including participants with complementary views on task group issues, rather than the same views, ensures a more lively discussion and a potentially stronger outcome.

Forming. Clear goal identification is important because the objectives and specific nature of the group problem will determine the number of members required to accomplish the task. The leader responsible for convening the group explains the group's purpose and structural components (e.g., time, place, and commitment) in detail. Group members take personal responsibility for clarifying and modifying group goals. A task group with vague or poorly understood goals can breed boredom or frustration and lead to power struggles and inadequate task resolution. Members must hold the belief that they will, as a group, reach a mutually acceptable solution.

Norming. Member responsibilities are outlined clearly and understood by all members. To be successful, a work group must foster free exchange of ideas. Each member must feel that his or her idea is as valuable as another's. In general, all data developed within the group context should be kept confidential until officially ready for publication. Otherwise, the "grapevine" is likely to distort information and sabotage the efforts of the group.

Members need to be held accountable for regular attendance. If administrative staff is part of the group membership, it is essential that they attend every meeting. Few circumstances are more threatening to a work-related group than having a supervisor enter and exit the task group at will.

Performing. Once norms are in place, attention turns directly to the designated work of the group. Leader interventions should be consistent and well defined. By fulfilling the responsibilities of leader and member already described, the group works to develop an understanding of the problem and achieve resolution.

After identification of basic data relevant to the work of the group, the group members begin to analyze possible solutions. Brainstorming is a strategy used to generate ideas quickly. In addition to creating innovative ideas, brainstorming usually is a stimulating and pleasant experience for group members. The following are some guidelines for brainstorming:

- All ideas are entertained without censure.
- The more promising ideas are tested for legitimacy.
- For each idea chosen, possible consequences are explored.
- Personnel and resources are identified (need for and availability).
- A final group solution is developed.

Group members are partners in the brainstorming process. The process of pulling diverse ideas together in a group means that each member has a clear understanding of the problem and personal satisfaction of contributing to the group goals. Exercise 22-5 provides practice in the use of brainstorming.

Group formats are particularly useful for facilitating changes in organizational life. Sufficient time and administrative support for proposals are essential components of successful group work. Most of the failed efforts to implement change occur because of a lack of understanding of the processes needed to effect change, insufficient administrative support, unclear expectations, and poor communication with those who are affected by the change. See Box 22-6 for suggestions on how to overcome these obstacles. Although it is beyond the scope of this text to describe all dimensions of the organizational change process, Box 22-7 summarizes guidelines that nurses can use in groups responsible for developing changes in organizational settings.

Termination Phase. Termination in professional groups can be either an experience that all members share when the group task is accomplished and there is no further need for the group, or it can take place for one individual leaving the group. For the single individual leaving an intact group, it is important for that person to

Exercise 22-5 **Brainstorming: A Family Dilemma**

Purpose: To increase self-awareness and provide practical experience with the use of brainstorming as a group activity.

Procedure:

1. Using the format on brainstorming identified in this chapter, consider the following clinical problem:
   Mrs. Joan Smith is an 80-year-old woman living in Florida. Her husband recently suffered a stroke, which has affected his speech. All he is able to say to his wife is that he loves her, although he seems to understand her words to him. He is paralyzed on one side. When he tried to get out of bed, he fell and broke his hip, so he is confined to a wheelchair. No longer able to care for him, Mrs. Smith moved to Virginia to be close to her daughter, and Mr. Smith is being cared for in a nearby nursing home. Mrs. Smith is living temporarily in her daughter's home, sleeping on the couch because her daughter has a 15-year-old boy and a 3-year-old girl occupying the bedrooms.
   Mrs. Smith visits her husband every day and entertains the idea that he will get well enough that they will be able to return to Florida. She tries to be there at mealtime because she thinks no one will feed him if she doesn't, and he can't eat by himself. Now that the evenings are getting darker, her daughter fears her driving after dark. She hesitates to bring up the idea of selling the house in Florida for fear it will distress her mother. Mrs. Smith is not sleeping at night and seems driven to be with her husband. Her daughter worries that her mother will collapse if she keeps up her current pace. Meanwhile, the house in Florida remains empty, her mother has taken no steps to secure legal advice, and the current living situation is becoming more permanent by default.
2. Divide the class into groups of three to six students, depending on class size.
3. Each group should identify a spokesperson to the larger group. Use a flip chart or board to record ideas.
4. Brainstorm to generate ideas for a practical solution to the Smith family's problem. Allow 15 minutes for the first part of the exercise and 20 minutes for the brainstorming section.
5. Describe your group's solution and give the rationale for your selection.

Discussion:

In the larger group, each spokesperson presents the smaller group's solution to the Smith family's problem.

1. How did your group's answers compare with those of other groups?
2. What did you learn about the brainstorming process as a problem-solving format?
3. What was the most difficult part of the process for your group?
4. As you listen to how other groups implemented the process, what ideas came to mind?
5. How might you use this format in your nursing practice?

know that he or she was valued as a group member. The remaining group members need an opportunity to express their feelings of loss to and about the departing member. If the termination is unplanned and affects the work of the group, the group may need to discuss the matter further after the loss of the member.

Usually it is better to overestimate rather than underestimate the extent of relationship in groups. Although most people will not deny that an important work-related group is ending, they often ignore or minimize their feelings about it. It seems harder to acknowledge that important interactions with our peers are ending than it is to admit this with our clients. As a result, it is not unusual for group members to allow one of their peers to leave without saying a genuine good-bye.

Box 22-6 Effective Staff-Level Interventions

Strategies to help staff include the following:

- Arranging a group meeting of caregivers
- Using a consultant
- Venting feelings, with a focus on their own reactions and feelings, not on complaints about the client's behavior
- Elevating awareness of their own feelings of anger and other emotions, showing that these are common reactions exhibited by several nurses in the group
- Developing increased awareness among staff of the cause of the client's unacceptable behavior
- Developing a plan for handling the client's unacceptable behavior, perhaps behavior modification strategies
- Obtaining consensus (for all shifts to use)
- Committing the plan to writing

Ethical Dilemma ■ *What Would You Do?*

You are working a 12-hour shift on a labor and delivery unit. Today Mrs. Kalim is one of your assigned clients. She is fully dilated and effaced, but contractions are still 2 minutes apart after 10 hours of labor. Mrs. Kalim, her obstetrician Dr. Mary, and you have agreed on her plan to have a fully natural delivery without medication. However, her obstetrician's partner is handling day shift today and Dr. Mary goes home. This new obstetrician orders you to administer several medications to Mrs. Kalim to strengthen contractions and speed up delivery, because he has another patient across town to deliver. Your unit adheres to an empowering model of practice that believes in client advocacy. How will you handle this potential physician conflict? Is this a true moral dilemma?

For a similar case example, refer to Sleutel MR: Intrapartum nursing care, *Birth* 27(1):38–45, 2000.

Box 22-7 Guidelines for Groups Planning Organizational Changes

1. Clarify plans.
   - Make one person responsible for implementation plans.
   - Formulate clear, simple, time-bound goals.
   - Make specific plans with milestones and outcomes.
   - Make plans public.
   - Give and solicit frequent face-to-face feedback.
2. Integrate new practices.
   - Limit the amount of change introduced at any one time.
   - Slow the change process.
   - Introduce the change to receptive users first.
   - Ensure that the rationale and procedure for change are well known.
3. Provide education.
   - Involve the end users and incorporate their experience.
   - Provide "hands-on" training whenever possible.
   - Design training from the end-user's perspective.
   - Train motivated or key end-users first.
   - Evaluate the effects of training or work practices and end-users' attitudes.
4. Foster ownership.
   - Ensure that the change improves end-users' ability to accomplish work.
   - Provide incentives for end-users applying the change.
   - Specify milestones for obtaining end-user feedback.
   - Incorporate end-user suggestions in the implementation plans.
   - Publicize end-user suggestions.
5. Give feedback.
   - Document and communicate the expected outcomes of the change.
   - Ensure frequent face-to-face feedback.
   - Identify clear milestones.
   - Make sure feedback includes the large organization.
   - Acknowledge key successes.

From Schoonover S, Dalziel M: Developing leadership for change. In Cathcart R, Samovar L, editors, *Small group communication: a reader*, ed 5, Dubuque, IA, 1988, WC Brown.

SUMMARY

In this chapter, the same principles of communication used in the nurse-client relationship are broadened to examine the nature of communication among health professionals. Most nurses will experience conflicts with co-workers at some time during their careers. The same elements of thoughtful purpose, authenticity, empathy, active listening, and respect for the dignity of others that underscore successful nurse-client relationships are needed in relations with other health professionals. Building bridges to professional communication with colleagues involves concepts of collaboration, coordination, and networking. Modification of barriers to professional communication includes negotiation and conflict resolution. Learning is a lifelong process, not only for nursing care skills but also for communication skills. These will develop as you continue to gain experience working as part of an interdisciplinary group.

Work groups are an important part of organizational life. Although the focus is different from client-centered groups, work groups follow a similar pattern of growth and development. Content from this chapter can be reviewed and used throughout your nursing career.

REFERENCES

Adams D: Teaching the process of delegation, *Semin Nurse Manag* 3(4):171–174, 1995.

American Association of Colleges of Nursing: *The essentials of baccalaureate nursing education*, Washington, DC, 1998, Author.

American Nurses Association: *Registered professional nurses and unlicensed assistive personnel*, Washington, DC, 1994, Author.

Bacal R: Dealing with angry employees [online article], n.d.; available online: http://work911.com/articles/angrye.htm.

Bacal R: Organizational conflict: the good, the bad & the ugly [online article], n.d.; available online: http://work911.com/articles/orgconflict.htm.

Barter M, McLaughlin FE, Thomas SA: Registered nurse role changes and satisfaction with unlicensed assistive personnel, *J Nurs Adm* 27(1):29–38, 1997.

Bartram T, Joiner TA, Stanton P: Factors affecting the job stress and job satisfaction of Australian nurses: implications for recruitment and retention, *Contemp Nurse* 17(3): 293–304, 2004.

Boucher MA: Delegation alert! *Am J Nurs* 98(2):26–33, 1998.

Cascardo DC: Resolve billing problems before they start, *Medscape Money & Medicine* 2(1), 2001; available online: http://www.medscape.com/viewarticle/408348_1.

Coeling HV, Cukr PL: Communication styles that promote perceptions of collaboration, quality, and nurse satisfaction, *J Nurs Care Qual* 14(2):63–74, 2000.

Harmon L, Pomm RM: Evaluation, treatment, and monitoring of disruptive physician behavior, *Psychiatr Ann* 34(10):770–774, 2004.

Johnson SH: Teaching nursing delegation, *J Contin Educ Nurs* 27(2):52–58, 1996.

Miller M, Wax D: Instilling a mediation-based conflict resolution culture, *Physician Exec* 25(4):45–51, 1999.

New Hampshire Nurses Association: Workplace issues, *Nurs News* 26(3), 2002.

Ohio Nurses Foundation: ONF: turning conflict into cooperation, *ISNA Bulletin* 29 (2):1–7, February 1, 2003; retrieved 12/19/04 from http://web36.epnet.com

Olade RA: Evidence-based practice and research utilization activities among rural nurses, *J Nurs Scholarsh* 36(3):220–225, 2004.

Rosenstein AH, O'Daniel M: Disruptive behavior and clinical outcomes: perceptions of nurses and physicians, *Am J Nurs* 105(1):54–64, 2005.

Salvage J, Smith R: Doctors and nurses: doing it differently, *BMJ* 320(7241):1019–1020, 2000.

Shah B: One in six nurses "bullied at work," *Nurs Times,* May 30, 2001.

Sheafor M: Productive work groups in complex hospital units: proposed contributions of the nurse executive, *J Nurs Adm* 21(5):25–30, 1991.

Skjorshammer M: Co-operation and conflict in a hospital, *J Interprof Care* 15(1):7–18, 2001.

Smith-Trudeau P: Diversity consciousness: from conflict to collaboration, *Vermont Nurse Connection* 5(1):3–5, 2002.

Sullivan E, Decker P: *Effective management in nursing*, ed 4, Redwood City, CA, 1997, Addison-Wesley.

Tschannen D: The effect of individual characteristics on perceptions of collaboration in the work environment, *Medsurg Nursing* 13(5):312–319, 2004.

Williams CA, Gossett MT: Nursing communication: advocacy for the patient or physician? *Clin Nurs Res* 10(3):332–335, 2001.

Workplace issues, *Nurs News* 26: 3, 2002.

Zwarenstein M, Bryant W: Interventions to promote collaboration between nurses and doctors, *Cochrane Database Syst Rev* 2:1–15, 2000.

Chapter 23

Documentation in the Age of the Electronic Health Record

Kathleen Underman Boggs

OUTLINE

OBJECTIVES

At the end of the chapter, the reader will be able to:

1. Identify five purposes for documentation.
2. Define electronic health records (EHRs) as part of computer information systems.
3. Describe advantages and disadvantages of electronic health records.
4. Discuss the advantages and disadvantages of various charting formats.
5. Identify legal aspects of charting.
6. Discuss application of basic rules for writing professional forms of documentation.
7. Discuss how evidence-based clinical practice may change the way nursing is practiced and documented.

Documentation is the key element of communication between the provider of services and the third party payer.

(Baeten, 1997)

When standardized language is used to document practice, we can compare and evaluate effectiveness of [our] care.

(Dochterman & Bulechek, 2004)

The process of obtaining, organizing, and conveying client health information to others in print or electronic format is referred to as **documentation**. As illustrated in Figure 23-1, documentation serves the following five purposes:

1. Provides a record of care received
2. Shows pertinent information about the client's condition and response to treatment interventions
3. Substantiates the quality of care by showing adherence to care standards
4. Provides evidence for reimbursement
5. Serves as a means of aggregating client care information to research and establish interventions to establish "best practice" for effective care

This chapter focuses on electronic health records (EHRs) and documenting client care. Regulatory and ethical implications of documentation are also discussed. The newest technology devices for medical communication will be discussed in Chapter 24.

Box 23-1 Reasons Nurses Document

- To communicate to others what you know about a client in order to facilitate care planning and delivery
- To record individual patterns or norms so that deviation from these is noted as soon as possible
- To communicate to other caregivers what is done or still needs to be done
- To document evidence as to how you individualized your client's care
- To record client's health outcomes after care
- To contribute information to a database so aggregated total data can be analyzed to identify best interventions
- To protect yourself and your employer from threats of malpractice
- To provide a record on which to base the billed cost to the client
- To provide evidence of acuity to make decisions about staffing
- To provide evidence of adherence to established standards of care (of JCAHO and other regulatory bodies)

Modified from Iowa Intervention Project: Proposal to bring nursing into the information age, *Image* 29(3):275, 1997.

BASIC CONCEPTS

Documenting Client Information

Documentation of client care must be complete and accurate. Standards of documentation must meet the specifications of government, health care agency and professional standards of practice, accreditation standards, third-party payers, and the courts. Box 23-1 outlines the reasons that nurses document care. Every health care agency has its own version of forms and procedures guiding clinical documentation. In most organizations this clinical documentation, whether in written or electronic format, includes a client history (a database that often includes a summary list of health problems and needs), a client-centered nursing care plan (NCP), daily records of client progress, and evaluation of outcomes. These daily records often run many pages and may include flow sheets, nursing notes, intake and output forms, and medication records. Computerization of this client care information makes information more accessible and allows graphing of ongoing outcome measures, such as vital signs and diagnostic test results.

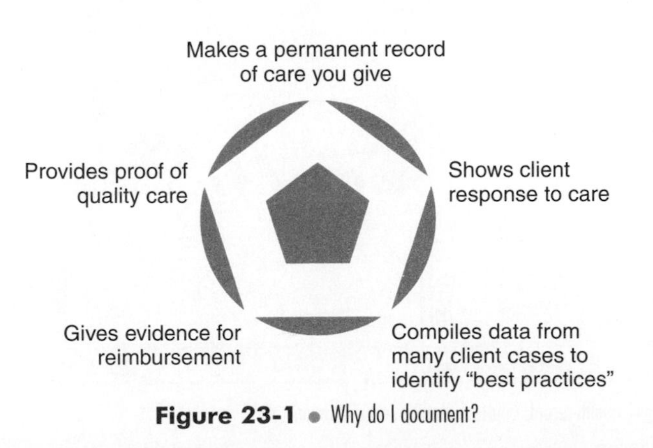

Figure 23-1 • Why do I document?

The Computerized Patient Electronic Health Record

There is a major communication revolution occurring right now in health care, made possible by the increased use of computers. In their 1995 position statement, the American Nurses Association (ANA) said that computerization offers opportunities to improve the quality of health care and to reduce its cost (ANA, 1995). Also in 1995, the Institute of Medicine (IOM) wrote that the use of EHRs is "essential." In the evolving new health care system, this means a fundamental change in information gathering, use of, and access to client records (ANA, 1995). This involves creating a whole new system, not just putting the 100-year-old existing paper charting system on a computer. Chapters 23 and 24 describe some aspects of the new system, with a focus on the role of the nurse.

While the computerized patient **electronic health record (EHR)** is rapidly becoming the accepted process for documenting, some agencies still use paper records. Transition is expensive and will take a while. Implementation is best done in stages, according to a carefully planned timeline. For example, most agencies have already put their billing process online. As new departments are computerized, it is vital that computer programs are compatible within the entire agency. Eventually, use of compatible software, a "common platform," will also permit interfacing across different agencies. EHRs are also referred to as electronic clinical records, electronic patient records, person-centered health records, or electronic medical records (Figure 23-2).

Advantages of Computerized Patient Electronic Health Records. The full potential of electronic health records is just beginning to be realized. The EHR is not just a version of the paper record available on the computer (Hebda, Czar, & Mascara, 2001); it is part of an entire information technology computerized system designed to support the multiple information needs required by today's complex client care. A client's EHR may be stored so that it is assessable to all of a client's care providers. Electronic records support telehealth, for example, in the case of a fully computerized medical record that includes graphic files (e.g., sonograms, x-rays, and other diagnostic imaging) that can be sent and analyzed by specialists hundreds of miles away. Information is instantly available to a variety of users. Results of your client's laboratory tests, posted in the lab, can be

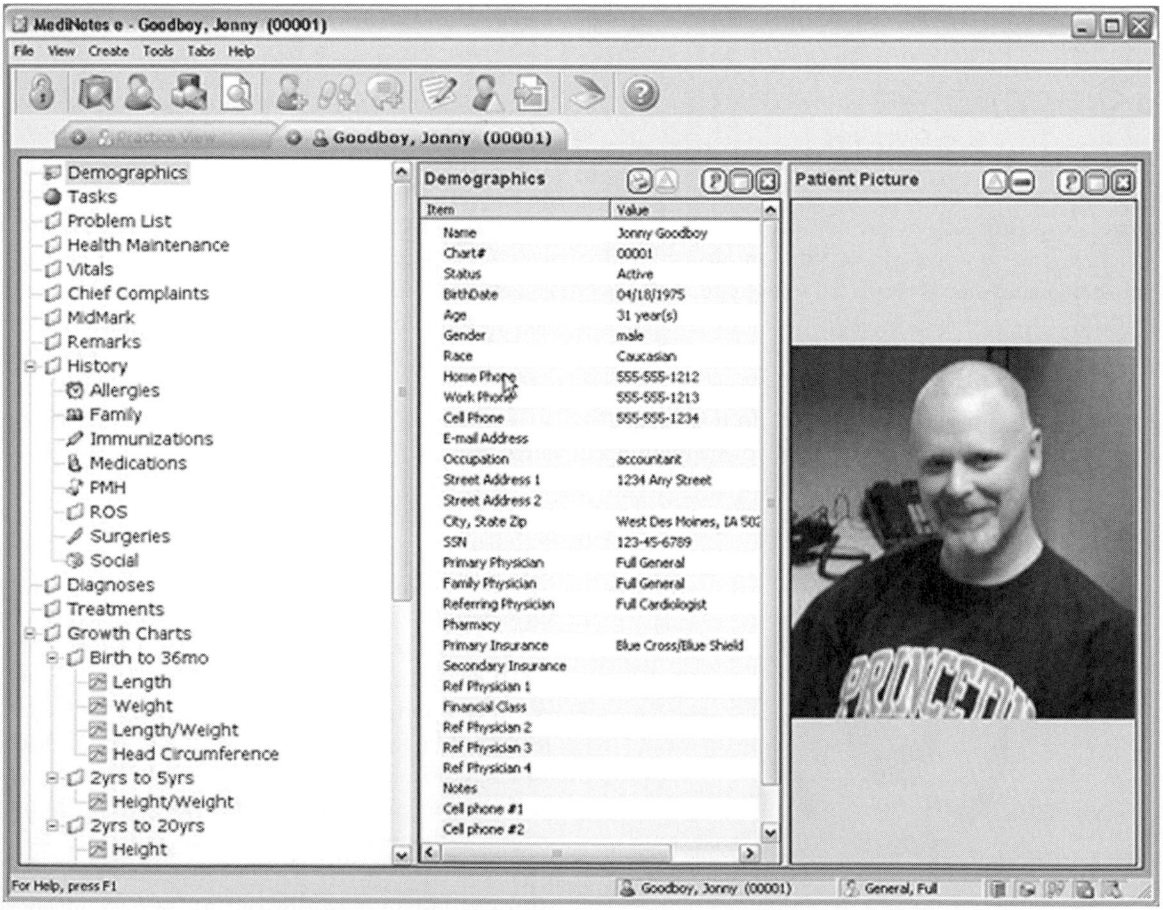

Figure 23-2 • Example of an electronic health record. Courtesy MediNotes Corporation.

accessed by you from the client's inpatient unit, by the community health nurse, and by the primary physician's office as soon as the lab tech enters them into the hospital computer system.

Electronic records are more durable than paper charting and easily transferable. For example, during Hurricane Katrina in 2005, the New Orleans Veterans Administration was able to send their 50,000 client health records to a secure site, while untold thousands of paper records at other hospitals were destroyed by flood waters.

Efficiency and Ease of Use. Computer-assisted charting facilitates the recording of nursing notes. It also has the potential to eliminate duplication in charting. In a study by Moody, Slocumb, Berg, and colleagues (2004), 75% of nurses reported that the EHR had improved the quality of charting. Your terminal may be located at the nurse's station, in your client's room, or it may be portable where ever you go, including to a client's home or a community clinic. When charting, you type in your password/identification number, scan your identity card, or scan your fingerprint. Then you enter data into the client's computer file. Most systems use a mouse or light pen to select from a menu of standard groupings or categories in documenting client care information.

Enhanced Quality of Care. The adoption of a comprehensive computer information system changes the way information flows through the health care delivery system. Communication is more rapid. For example, after the client's admission to an acute care hospital, a physician's orders entered into the computer are transmitted simultaneously to the pharmacy, the laboratory, and the nursing unit.

EHR systems "prompt" you to do complete care and then to chart comprehensively. This prompt enhances the quality of care by reminding you about the specific standards of care that may apply to the client you are currently charting about. Most electronic client monitors, such as those recording blood pressure, pulse, oxygenation, record this information directly into the client's electronic health record. This saves charting time, eliminates transcription errors, and allows the computer to provide "alerts" notifying you about possible abnormalities.

Safety. One of the most important reasons for computerizing is to reduce errors. Computers force standardization of nursing terminology, eliminating use of inappropriate abbreviations. In this way they improve accurate communication. Cornell (2001) notes that this technology not only can save time, but can reduce errors due to illegible handwriting. The Institute of Medicine's report (Kohn, Corrigan, & Donaldson, 2000) on deaths from medication errors has accelerated the movement toward creating safer care and preventing mistakes. This has further encouraged agencies to computerize. Will this significantly prevent errors? Is it worth the cost? More outcome data are needed.

Beyond eliminating errors due to sloppy handwriting, computers also prevent errors by assisting with drug calculations, performing checks in real time (of drug incompatibility, allergies, etc.), assisting with decision support, and providing feedback (Bates & Gawande, 2003). A study by Marshall and Chin (1998) showed that health care workers perceived that use of such a computerized system led to improved client care, improved interactions, faster access to laboratory test results, more timely referrals, and reduced medication errors.

Cost Reduction. Administrators estimate that the cost of using paper records in an agency is 25% of total health care costs. In addition to the actual paper and printing costs, there are costs involved in record filing, storage, and retrieval of information. Improved access time occurs with computerized information. Using paper files, Quality Assurance (QA) auditing done by the agency, as well as written record audits by insurance companies, researchers, and others, involved laborious hand searches through stacks of paper. Cost decreases occur over the long term when computerized records permit easy data entry, analysis, and retrieval.

Ability to Aggregate Data. Computerized client information offers ease of access in order to aggregate (combine together) information from many clients for reports and other purposes. Keepnews, Capitman, and Rosati (2004) demonstrated that one computer charting system, OASIS, can be used to obtain reports about predictors of client outcomes in home health care. For example, you can easily get information identifying the most effective specific nursing interventions to establish best practice and identify other interventions that need to be changed. (OASIS is discussed later in this chapter.)

Data from many clients are combined to produce external reports. For example, public health agencies analyze information about illness to generate epidemiological information such as the spread of influenza across the country and across the world.

Disadvantages of Computerized Patient Electronic Health Records. There are barriers to adoption of the EHR, not the least of which are the high start-up costs. Future changes in technologies associated with your client care will necessitate that the EHR software format be periodically revised. There will be significant costs associated with these upgrades. Other barriers include the following.

User Resistance. Staff face a learning curve challenge, particularly those who work in multiple agencies having different computer systems, such as physicians who admit to three different hospitals or temporary agency nurses who float to several hospitals. Any new addition or upgrade to a system requires an adjustment period as staff learn. Also, all computers require "downtime" for storing records on backup software or while technicians service system hardware. Any time the computer is unavailable for entering your documentation, you need alternative documentation forms.

Lack of Legal Guidelines. Few nations have adequate laws governing information misuse of EHRs. In the United States, government HIPAA regulations provide some privacy guidelines for your client's records, limiting who you can share this information with. When computers are located at the bedside, the screen displays EHR information to anyone who stops by the bedside. You need to be alert to this potential violation of your client's privacy.

Lack of Uniform Standards and Universal Client Identifier Numbers. While many countries have solved the problem of all agencies using the same universal number to identify the client, in the United States, clients often have multiple identity numbers across agencies. Proposals for using one's social security number have received criticism, with some favoring a separate national identification number. During the transitional phase-in stage, some information is still in paper charts while other data are in a computer.

Problems with System Function. When there is a dysfunction or glitch and your computer crashes, you get frustrated. Imagine what would happen if an entire hospital computer system malfunctioned! Of course your files are routinely backed up at least once a day. For electronic records to be used to their potential, there must be compatible software. Then the EHR must be integrated in multiple departments such as pharmacy, radiology, physical therapy, and nursing. Problem statements, interventions, and outcomes must be recorded using a uniform and standard language. Lee (2005) has raised concerns about the need for staff training to maintain work efficiency.

Confidentiality Issues. Confidentiality and legal issues are by far the biggest areas of concern. Whenever there are multiple users, there are risks that others not involved in a client's care may access confidential information. This is particularly true for computerized data, but is also a concern with any data transmitted electronically (e.g., information sent by fax or through telehealth networks). Ensuring privacy and developing security safeguards have become a requirement for electronic records. Procedures requiring passwords, preset log-on time limitations, and internal computer system safeguards to prevent tampering with or unauthorized access to client data are now routine expectations of nursing documentation. Confidentiality and privacy issues are discussed later.

Transition Considerations. Some governments, such as the provincial government in Alberta, Canada, have already made the transition to EHRs. In the United States, the federal government's goal is to move to a paperless system by 2015, while some state groups set earlier goals. Transition problems are being encountered. Cost is a significant drawback of these information systems. Changing systems within an agency also requires significant investment of time and money to reeducate the staff and implement the new system. Incompatibility of software within a health care facility would make it difficult to follow care from acute treatment to rehabilitation to home care. The lack of standardized data terminology and classification has also been a key barrier to electronic health record information sharing. As with the medical profession, the nursing profession has been intensely engaged in developing standardized languages for their practice.

Classification of Care

To input information into a computer, alphanumerical letters and numbers are used to classify health information. Beyond supplying information to those caring for a specific client, this allows us to generate a variety of administrative or external reports.

Goal for the Classification of Nursing Care

Like other professionals in health care, nurses must be able to communicate and demonstrate the value and effectiveness of care. In the past, nursing has been unable to describe the units of care and establish a cost for its contributions to client care. Nowhere on a client's hospital bill does the cost of our nursing care appear. It traditionally has been part of the "room charge." The goal of developing standardized terminology and classification codes is to make nursing practice visible within (computerized) health information systems.

The nursing profession has been very active in developing **coding systems** for the classification of nursing care. If nursing cannot categorically classify the care provided and the outcomes of that care, there is little hope that the profession will be able to effectively communicate or get reimbursed for its essential role in the health care of the individual, family, and community.

Developing Classifications for Coding

As client documentation becomes computerized, the numerous nursing interventions need to be standardized so that they can be assigned code numbers, allowing them to be entered into the computer.

Use of a standardized nursing language can save time by clearly describing clients' needs, interventions used, and the outcomes of care; by improving communication among staff members and in writing nursing care plans and nursing notes; and in conferring with health team members across the continuum of primary care, acute care, and home care practices. It can also be instrumental in describing nursing practice. The time spent teaching, providing support, and assisting in grieving are the types of nursing activities that nurses spend considerable time doing, yet they rarely show up in the medical record. In a study of documented care in home health, Lee and Mills (2000) found that nurses most often identified nursing problems or diagnoses related to the medical diagnosis, but spent most of their care in client teaching.

Standardized Language Terminology in Nursing

The challenge for nursing is to move toward a common language—an accepted standardized language or classification system that can be used to describe nursing practices and their outcomes. This terminology would be used in communication and comparisons across health care settings and providers. So far the international nursing community has not agreed on one common terminology. The International Council of Nurses (ICN) has developed one of these taxonomies. Currently the American Nurses Association recognizes seven different taxonomies for describing nursing care. The ANA has specific criteria, important to the process of refining and developing the language of nursing, that taxonomies must meet to be initially approved or to continue to be approved. Box 23-2 outlines the major approval criteria standardized nursing languages must meet. Four of the most commonly used nursing taxonomies are briefly discussed below.

Box 23-2 Criteria for ANA Approval of Standardized Nursing Language

- Validated as clinically useful in practice
- Terms precisely defined
- Tested for reliability
- Documentation of systematic methodology for further development
- Process of periodic review and provisions for revision
- Taxonomic structure is conceptually coherent
- Terms are associated with unique identifiers or codes
- Coded so it is computer compatible
- Specifies defining characteristics

Modified from Young K: *Informatics for healthcare professionals*, Philadelphia, 2000, FA Davis.

North American Nursing Diagnosis Association. **NANDA** was one of the earliest to develop standardized nursing languages. The domains are based on Gordon's Functional Health Patterns (NANDA, 2001). As the taxonomy has evolved, slight changes have occurred. The domains are health promotion, nutrition, elimination, rest/activity, perception/cognition, self-perception, role relationships, sexuality, coping-stress tolerance, life principles, safety/protection, comfort, and growth and development. NANDA has approved for clinical testing and refinement more than 150 standardized terms to describe nursing diagnoses. Initially designed to classify the problems of hospitalized ill clients, nursing diagnoses have been expanded to include community nursing, especially in areas used by home health nurse (see Online Resources).

A nursing diagnosis is not another name for a medical diagnosis; rather, it delineates areas of independent nursing functions. When a physician orders a primary intervention, the nursing actions are collaborative, secondary interventions that include monitoring and managing physician-prescribed interventions. A sample of the syntax for describing a NANDA diagnosis

Box 23-3 Sample Nursing Diagnoses

Nursing Diagnosis Problem Statement Relevant to Interpersonal Relationships

Directions: When writing a diagnostic statement for an actual nursing diagnosis (which describes a human response the nurse can treat), the nurse should use the PES formula, stating the *P*roblem, the *E*tiology, and the *S*ymptoms or signs of risk factors that validate the diagnosis. Take any of the case studies in this book and practice writing a diagnosis.

Example: Impaired verbal communication related to inability to speak English as evidenced by inability to follow instructions in English and verbalizing requests in Spanish

Sample Diagnosis

1. Re: role (interpersonal) relationships
   Impaired parenting (associated with . . .)
   Sexual dysfunction
   Social isolation (related to . . .)
   Interrupted family processes (related to . . .)
   Ineffective role performance (related to . . .)
   Parental role conflict (associated with . . .)
2. Re: perceiving
   Disturbed sensory perception: visual (associated with . . .)
   Disturbed thought processes (associated with . . .)

is provided in Box 23-3 with the intent of generating enough material for application in the accompanying learning exercises. The reader should refer to books on nursing diagnoses for complete information on the use of nursing diagnoses. Writing nursing diagnoses takes practice.

The Omaha System. In the 1970s, Omaha System research was initiated to address the needs of community health nurses, managers, and administrators. Recently revised, **the Omaha System** is a comprehensive practice, documentation, and information management tool used by nurses and other health providers (Martin, 2005). Studies show it can also be used in acute care situations. Categories cover common transitional care problems as clients move from hospitalized care to long-term or home care. Transitional care problems include categories such as nutrition, communication, pain, physical activity, and medication administration. Bowles (2000) reviewed the medical records of 30 clients hospitalized from home care using the Omaha System and found that it coded 97% of the problems, was easy to use, and was highly reliable. Expansion of the Omaha System into acute care could standardize and improve communication between home care and the hospital.

The Omaha System includes an assessment, or Problem Classification Scheme. This consists of four levels: (a) the major domains (environmental, psychosocial, physiological, and health-related behaviors); (b) specific problems; (c) modifiers; and (d) signs and symptoms. The Intervention Scheme is similarly organized into categories: (a) teaching guidance and counseling; (b) treatments and procedures; (c) case management; and (d) surveillance. Each domain has targets of the intervention. Lastly it has an outcome component, the Problem Rating Scale for Outcomes. This consists of a five-point ordinal scale assessing the client's knowledge, behavior, and condition (the status or symptoms of the identified problem). The outcomes rating scale can be applied as a baseline and then reevaluated after the intervention to measure change in knowledge, related behaviors, and symptoms of the originally identified problem (Martin, 2005). Figure 23-3 illustrates a case example using the Omaha System.

Nursing Interventions Classification. **Nursing Interventions Classification (NIC)** was developed as a standardized language describing direct and indirect care that nurses perform in settings relevant to illness prevention, illness treatment, and health promotion. The fourth edition of the NIC text (Dochterman & Bulechek, 2004) identifies 514 nursing interventions that are classified in seven domains. The domains are physiologic basic, physiologic complex, behavioral, safety, family, health systems, and community. Under each domain are classes, and under the classes are the specific interventions. For example, in the domain of physiologic basic there is a class called "immobility management." Specific intervention activities include bedrest care, cast care maintenance, physical restraint, positioning, splinting, traction, and transport. You can use or modify these interventions to meet your client's need. Each nursing intervention has a unique code number and thus can be computerized and potentially used to reimburse the nurse. The following case example demonstrates how NIC is used.

Case Example

Barbara, 64 yrs, 1 day post-operation for heart valve replacement

Sadiya M: Woman With Active Tuberculosis

By Luanne S. Crinion, RN, MS; and Beth B. Patterson, RN, MN; as published in Martin, KS (2005).

Sadiya M. was a 55-year-old woman who emigrated from Somalia 1 year ago with her daughter and other relatives. She was recently diagnosed with active pulmonary tuberculosis; she had a history of hypertension and congestive heart failure. The referral indicated that she was not taking her cardiac medications as prescribed.

The public health nurse wore a protective particulate air respirator to give Sadiya her first dose of oral medications as part of directly observed therapy (DOT). DOT is recommended as the standard protocol for active tuberculosis, and includes administration of isoniazid (INH), rifampin, pyrazinamide, and ethambutol. For at least the first 8 weeks, public health nurses visit clients 5 days a week and set up their 4 medications in a reminder box for the weekends.

Sadiya did not speak or understand English. In order for Sadiya and the nurse to converse, an interpreter joined the conversation by telephone. Sadiya had a productive cough during the visit; the nurse complimented her for appropriate tissue disposal and washing her hands. The nurse took Sadiya's vital signs and blood pressure, and listened to her lung sounds and recorded that they were within normal limits. They reviewed infection precaution guidelines, the risk to her family and close contacts, and why the nurse wore a respirator. The nurse described the sputum specimen that would be part of the next visit. Previously, Sadiya had received translated written information; she and the nurse reviewed this with the interpreter's assistance. The information described the disease, transmission, DOT treatment, potential toxic effects of the medications, medical care, and when to contact providers. The nurse also described the need to avoid alcohol and restrict social activity temporarily. Based on Sadiya's comments, the nurse questioned if she understood tuberculosis and the health care system in this country.

Sadiya showed the public health nurse the three medications prescribed for her congestive heart failure and hypertension. She shrugged her shoulders when asked about the pill schedule but agreed to take them as prescribed. She said she did not want to return to the primary care clinic but did not say why not. When the visit began, Sadiya had given the nurse a note from her daughter, indicating that the nurse could call her at work. The nurse called the daughter; they decided to meet during the next DOT appointment to review Sadiya's treatment plan. The nurse also wanted to determine if Sadiya took her cardiac medications as prescribed and if she could read.

Application of the Omaha System

Using her laptop the nurse charts several problems, including the following:

DOMAIN: PSYCHOSOCIAL [02]

Problem: Communication with community resources [06] (high priority)

Problem Classification Scheme

Modifiers: Individual and Actual

SIGNS/SYMPTOMS OF ACTUAL

- Difficulty understanding roles/regulation of service providers [02]
- Language barrier [05]
- Cultural barrier [08]

Intervention Scheme

Category: Case Management

TARGETS AND CLIENT-SPECIFIC INFORMATION

- Communication (scheduled appointment with daughter to check on Sadiya's coping with treatment regimen, and ability to read/understand materials)
- Interpreter/translator services (scheduled/used interpreter by telephone)

Category: Surveillance

TARGETS AND CLIENT-SPECIFIC INFORMATION

- Continuity of care (facilitate communication between Sadiya, family, interpreter, providers)

Problem Rating Scale for Outcomes

Knowledge: 3-basic knowledge (may not understand/be overwhelmed by health care system)

Behavior: 3-inconsistently appropriate behavior (needed nurse to arrange interpreter; does not want to return to primary care clinic)

Status: 3-moderate signs/symptoms (barriers for communication and obtaining services)

Additional problems identified in this case study are Communicable/Infectious condition and Medication regimen (high priority).

For complete discussion refer to Martin, KS (2005). The Omaha System: A Key to Practice, Documentation, and Information Management. St. Louis: Elsevier, p395-396. Used with permission.

Figure 23-3 • Case example of Sadiya M., a woman with active tuberculosis. Case example by Luanne S. Crinion, RN, MS, and Beth B. Patterson, RN, MN. As published in Martin KS: *The Omaha System: a key to practice, documentation, and information management*, St Louis, 2005, Mosby, pp. 395-396. Used with permission.

Domain: Physiological
Class: 1 (Respiratory management: ventilation adequate to maintain arterial blood gases within normal limits)
Intervention:
Label: Airway management [#3140]
Definition: Facilitation of patency
Activities: Monitor rate, rhythm, depth and effort of respirations q4h; instruct how to cough effectively and assess ability; note changes in SaO_2 and arterial blood Gases.
(Dochterman & Bulechek, 2004; Henry, Holzemer, Randell et al., 1997)

McCloskey, Bulechek, and Donahue (1998) conducted a survey and identified 34 core interventions. A partial list of these core interventions is presented in Box 23-4. Identification of core interventions provides nurse educators and clinicians with a focus for developing entry-level competencies for nursing practice. Findings from a study by Henry and associates (1997) suggest that NIC is superior to Current Procedural Terminology (CPT) for categorizing nursing activities because it describes nursing activities more fully.

Nursing Outcomes Classification. **Nursing outcomes classification (NOC)** was developed in an effort to identify and classify client outcomes due to health care. NOC complements NANDA and NIC and provides a language and coding numbers for evaluating the nursing process. The third edition of the NOC text (Moorhead, Johnson, & Maas, 2004) identifies 330 nursing-sensitive outcomes. An outcome assesses the client's actual status on specific behaviors (indicators) using a five-point scale, ranging from #1 = severely compromised function, to #5 = not compromised (see Online Resources).

Box 23-4 Sample Core NIC Interventions

For Medical-Surgical Nursing
- Documentation
- Electrolyte Management
- Emotional Support
- Medication Administration (*with specified route*)
- Pain Management
- Teaching: Individual

For Psychiatric Nursing
- Active Listening
- Anger Control Assistance
- Anxiety Reduction
- Coping Enhancement
- Crisis Intervention

For a complete listing of interventions for each of 43 nursing specialty areas of practice, see Dochterman JM, Bulechek GM: *Nursing interventions classification (NIC)*, St Louis, 2004, Mosby.

Case Example

Mr. Lee, 46 years old, is admitted with right-sided paralysis. The nursing diagnosis is impaired verbal communication related to a left hemisphere bleed as evidenced by expressive aphasia. Using NOC we get a code number (0903), Communication: Expressive Ability, and rate him as #1 = severely compromised on seven indicators listed. A student is assigned to his care. Her interventions to increase his expressive communication ability as listed in NOC include naming things aloud as she gives care, encouraging speech, encouraging nonverbal gestures, introducing a board displaying the pictures and words for several common needs for him to point at. After 2 days of care, Mr. Lee is assessed on the seven indicators. His use of spoken language is still rated as #1 = severely compromised.

Changing this case to add additional information, suppose a nurse assesses two of the other listed indicators (his use of nonverbal language and ability to point to the picture board to communicate) as having progressed to #4, mildly compromised. This shows a specific change in Mr. Lee's status after specific nursing interventions. It is numerical and thus can be coded.

(Adapted from Moorhead and colleagues, 2004, p. 812; case written by nursing student Krista Lukes.)

Advantages of Nursing Classification Systems

Nursing classification systems provide a standard and common language for nursing care so that nursing contributions to client care become visible and define professional practice. The ANA has issued a position statement stating that standards for terminology are an essential requirement for a computer-based patient record (see Online Resources). A standardized language of nursing can help develop realistic standards of care. Groups of client records can be analyzed to describe the client population (e.g., to discover the most common inter-

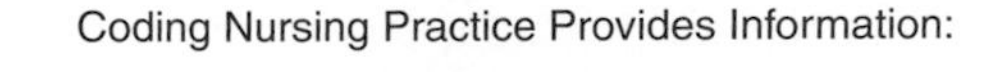

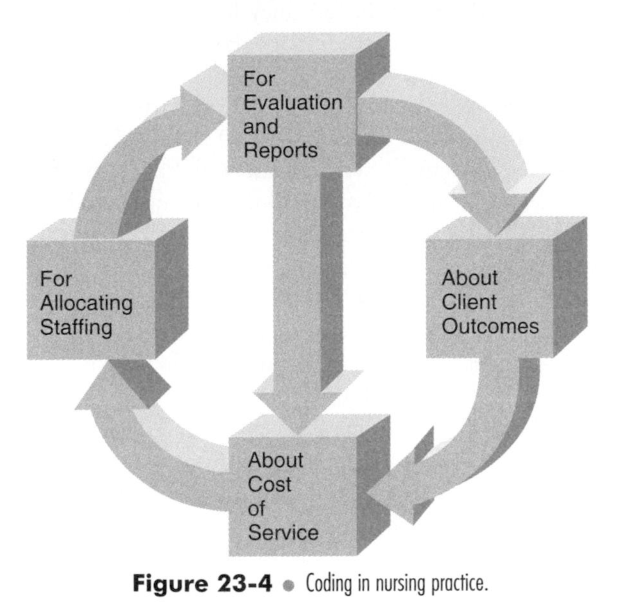

Figure 23-4 ● Coding in nursing practice.

ventions used for a specific nursing diagnosis). Analyzing client records in this way can lead to developing benchmarks that set the desired outcomes for a condition or diagnosis and then measure the client's actual level of achievement. Agencies could use a nursing classification system to bill for specific nursing care and build further accountability into the care and its documentation. Figure 23-4 shows how coding allows a client's data to be easily aggregated with other cases to produce a larger picture describing health care delivered by the agency (Cimino, 1996).

Work has begun on linking NANDA, NIC, and NOC (NNN) to create relationships between nursing diagnoses, interventions, and specific outcome evaluation criteria (Johnson, Bulechek, Dochterman et al., 2001). The formal linking of these independently developed systems creates a systematic schema for implementing the nursing process. Table 23-1 presents an example of the linkages for the nursing diagnosis of chronic pain. Linking nursing diagnosis, intervention, and outcome aids in developing computerized records so that for each diagnosis there are specific interventions and outcomes that can be selected and saved into a client database.

Table 23-1 Linkages of NANDA, NIC, and NOC with Selected Characteristics

Nursing Diagnosis	Nursing Outcome	Nursing Intervention
Chronic Pain *Defining Characteristics*	*Pain Control* *Indicators:* • Recognizes pain onset • Uses analgesics appropriately • Reports symptoms to provider • Reports pain controlled *Pain: Disruptive Effects* *Indicators:* • Impaired role performance • Compromised work • Disrupted sleep • Lack of appetite *Pain Level* *Indicators:* • Frequency of pain • Duration of pain episode • Oral expressions of pain • Facial expressions of pain • Protective body positioning	*Pain Management* *Nursing Activities:* • Determine impact of pain on quality of life. • Evaluate effectiveness of past pain control measures. • Select and implement pharmacology and nonpharmacology measures. • Teach client nonpharmacologic techniques of pain control. • Use pain control measures before pain increases. • Promote adequate rest. • Teach client to monitor own pain.

Modified from Johnson M, Bulechek G, Dochterman JM et al: *Nursing diagnosis, outcomes, and interventions: NANDA, NOC, and NIC linkages*, St Louis, 2001, Mosby.

Disadvantages of Nursing Classification Systems

Standardized nursing languages need to convince the business and medical interests managing health care agencies of the need to incorporate nursing classification codes as part of their information technology systems. The greatest problem has been that nursing classifications have not yet been thoroughly incorporated into many agency clinical records. Other difficulties include awkward syntax, lack of completeness, and problems with portability to other cultures.

Implementation can be expensive, and training nursing staff is time-consuming. Some research has shown that implementing a nursing information system does not immediately increase the accuracy of charting. In a study by Larrabee, Boldrighini, Elder-Sorrells, and associates (2001), documentation of nursing assessment, interventions, and blood pressure measurements did not improve six months after implementation of a new computerized documentation system. However, with continued training, there was a significant improvement in documentation by 18 months. As is true of medical classification systems, nursing classification systems continue to evolve and develop as they are used in practice.

Other Coding Systems in Health Care

The National Library of Medicine maintains a metathesaurus for a unified medical language. But because of the complexity of health care and the variety of providers involved, multiple medical classification systems have emerged. Often providers use several in combination. A major drawback for nursing is that use of computerized documentation systems based on medical code numbers often forces nurses to use classification systems designed to describe medical practice instead of describing nursing assessment and care of clients. In doing so, the richness of the nursing care provided often goes undocumented. Four common medical classification and coding systems are described here.

ICD-9-CM, ICD-10-CM, and ICD-10-PCS Codes. One of the most common medical coding systems is the ICD codes. The World Health Organization (WHO) publishes this International Statistical Classification of Disease and Related Health Problems for coding mortality and morbidity diagnoses. It has become the international standard for diagnostic classification (see online resources). Generally, diseases are classified according to body system. For example, in ICD-9, circulatory diseases all have numbers ranging from 390 to 459. An additional fourth and fifth digit may be added to describe the diagnosis more specifically. For example, hypertensive heart disease is coded 402, but by adding a fourth digit to make the code 402.1, we further define it as benign; by adding a fifth digit, 402.11, we know it is benign hypertensive heart disease with congestive failure. Many insurance corporations will not reimburse unless the information is coded to its highest level of specificity.

WHO published a revised 10th edition of these codes in 1994. While the United States continues to use ICD-9 codes, more than 100 other developed countries upgraded to using ICD-10 codes (WHO, NHSIA, CDC NCHS, 2005; see Online Resources). ICD-10 codes are better suited for use in EHRs than prior codes, providing better data to support quality care, improve bioterrorism monitoring, and provide more accuracy for reimbursement (American Health Information Management Association [AHIMA]; see Online Resources). ICD-10 can be expanded with new codes as needed. The U.S. National Center for Health Statistics does use ICD-10 codes to report causes of death.

ICD-10 uses a four-digit alphanumeric code that begins with a letter to record diagnosis and care interventions and has 3,000 more categories than ICD-9, which used a four-digit numeric code. For example, respiratory diseases are all classified beginning with the letter *J* (AHRQ). Pneumonia is listed in this grouping. Death from pneumonia and influenza is classified under ICD-9 as 480, but under ICD-10 code it is J10.

Current Procedural Terminology Codes. The American Medical Society developed CPT codes to provide coding for diagnostic procedures. The client's record must provide sufficient information about a diagnosis so that the insurance company computer accepts the diagnostic test as relevant and necessary for reaching a correct diagnosis. For example, the ordering of a digoxin level by a provider would be appropriate related to a diagnosis with a code for hypertension with congestive failure, but would not be appropriate or reimbursable for a diagnosis code for epilepsy.

Diagnosis Related Groups. These were originally developed for use in prospective payment for the Medicare program. DRG coding provided a small number of codes for classifying client hospitalizations based on diagnosis and severity of illness.

DSM-IV-TR. The *Diagnostic and Statistical Manual of Mental Disorders, fourth edition, text revision* (*DSM-IV-TR*) is the standardized diagnostic classification for mental illness. The *DSM-IV-TR* is organized using five axes describing psychiatric diagnosis and functional status. It provides a comprehensive assessment and labeling of psychiatric and mental health–related conditions. The five axes are clinical disorders, personality disorders, general medical conditions, psychosocial and environmental problems, and global assessment of functioning (American Psychiatric Association, 2000).

JCAHO Computerized Documentation Guidelines. Electronic Clinical Information Systems (CISs) promote entry, storage, and linkage of *all* information about a client's health care. Ideally, any CIS allows ease of access to one client's information as inputted by any of the client's health care providers, including the hospital and community. The Joint Commission on Accreditation of Healthcare Organizations, which accredits health care organizations, has developed standards for uniform data for agencies it accredits. In the past, JCAHO required that nurses repeat information recorded by the physician. Now, documentation may consist merely of completing and updating an intake history form supplied by the agency.

The OASIS System. In 1998 and 1999, home care agencies phased in a new requirement to complete a functional health assessment on all Medicare clients before they begin care. The results of the assessment feed into a standardized database. The Health Care Financing Administration (HCFA) developed the OASIS assessment for the purpose of describing home care clients, developing outcome benchmarks, and providing feedback regarding quality of care to home health agencies. OASIS stands for *O*utcome and *AS*sessment *I*nformation *S*et.

The OASIS assessment is required for home health agencies to receive reimbursement for the care provided to Medicare recipients. Home health care agencies are sent reports comparing their client populations and functions to benchmarks established through analysis of multiple home health agency clients. OASIS can be used to establish standards of quality. The report can also be used by individual home health agencies to monitor and improve outcomes of care. The components of OASIS are essential items for documenting a comprehensive assessment of functional health status of adult home care clients. The assessment documentation is used by HCFA to analyze the health status and needs of Medicare recipients.

OASIS data items include the sociodemographic, environmental, support system, health status, and functional status attributes of nonmaternity adult clients, as well as the attributes of health service utilization. OASIS was not developed as a comprehensive health assessment tool, and home care agencies need to supplement the assessment items. The items of OASIS have evolved over a 10-year period and are the result of a national research program funded by HCFA and cofunded by the Robert Wood Johnson Foundation.

Home health agencies are required to submit OASIS data to a designated state site. The state agency then has the responsibility of collecting OASIS data that can be retrieved from a central repository. These data provide a national picture of health status, outcome, and cost of Medicare enrollees who require home health care. To learn more, visit HCFA's Medicare website (see Online Resources).

Charting Formats for Documenting Nursing Care

Problem-Oriented Record

In the **problem-oriented record (POR)**, the focus is on the client's identified list of health problems. A problem list typically consists of medical diagnoses. In POR, nurses refer to the problem list and chart their observations by referring to the listed problem by number or by name or both. Information about the client's progress in each problem area is supposed to be documented only when some measurable change occurs.

Using the SOAP Format. A specific format (called **SOAP**) is used to record data relevant to each problem. The first part of the suggested four-step method of documentation lists client's subjective comments (*S*) relevant to the identified problem. The second section lists all the current objective information (*O*) noted by the nurse. Under the next part (*A*) is listed the medical and nursing diagnoses, the nurse's analysis of the problem, or the client's current progress. Finally, there is a list of plans or intended future interventions (*P*).

Case Example

Problem 4: Impaired skin integrity: decubitus related to immobility as evidenced by excoriation and drainage

S: "My leg looks better today; it doesn't hurt."

O: 4 cm excoriation on outer aspect of left thigh. Minimal serous drainage. Sensitive to touch. Unable to note skin color due to purple staining from gentian violet treatments. Peripheral area red and puffy.

A: Decreased drainage; less peripheral inflammation; healing decubitus.

P: Continue applications of 1:1 H_2O_2/NS every 4 hr. Apply gentian violet every 8 hr; cover with DSD, monitor for signs of infection. 1400: K. DiPalo, SN

Advantages. SOAP notes focus on the status of the client's progress in terms of identified problems.

Disadvantages. There is a tendency to focus on medical diagnoses only.

Using the PIE Format. **PIE** started as an expanded variation of the SOAP format (known as SOAPIE), with additional information about implementation interventions and evaluation of outcome. More recently, use of PIE in the inpatient setting usually combines use of a daily client assessment flow sheet with notations containing the following: (*P*), problems identified (label each problem number); (*I*), interventions documented; and (*E*), evaluation of outcome.

Case Example

3/12/07 1300 (P): sudden onset of generalized itching and rash, RR 28, wheezing, B/P 140/80, HR 112. (problem #1)

1305 #1: (I) infusion of erythromycin stopped, Dr. Smith notified. Benedryl 50 mg given po.

1430 #1: (E) RR 18, no wheezing, lung sounds clear, no rash, HR 78. M. Puritis, RN

Focus Charting

Focus charting is similar to POR except that the "focus" may be positive instead of a problem. It is a quick description of the client's current status, a brief statement about what is happening to the client. The SOAP is replaced by DAR, which stands for *D*ata, *A*ction, and *R*esponse.

Data lists subjective and objective assessment information, client behaviors, client status, and nursing observations to substantiate the problem or strength (the focus). *Action* is the nursing plan and interventions and the nursing orders for the identified focus. *Response* includes evaluation of client's response. This method is supplemented by a client database, flow sheets, graphs for vital signs, and checklists, because only relevant data are selected for documentation. The focused charting method streamlines documentation in some cases and has the advantage of capturing the critical-thinking and decision-making processes of the professional nurse.

Case Example

6/15/07 Pain

D: RR 32, c/o leg pain 9 on scale 0-10.

A: Demerol 75 mg, IV

R: Immediately stated relief of pain. M. Traywick, RN

Advantages. The use of focus charting has been shown to take less time than the methods previously discussed.

Disadvantages. This technique is not used by medical staff. There are legal questions regarding its lack of comprehensiveness.

Charting by Exception

The **charting by exception** method is based on a system of predetermined standards of care protocols. It requires a clear understanding of standards of care. This method is well suited to use with clinical pathways. Charting by exception uses **flow sheets** with predefined client progress parameters based on written standards with preprinted categories of information. They contain daily assessments of normal findings. For example, in assessing lung sounds, the nurse needs to merely check or circle "clear" if that information is normal. Deviations from norm must be charted either in narrative notes or in some space on the form designated for this format. By marking a flow sheet, you are saying all care was performed according to existing agency protocols. The best example of this format is known as critical pathways or clinical pathways.

Clinical pathways are a comprehensive documentation system that is based on standardized plans of care

Patient Name ____________________ Date ____________

DRG# ____________________ Expected LOS <23 hours

	Preprocedure	Preoperative	Intraoperative	Postoperative Phase I PACU	Postoperative PHASE II PACU	Discharge	Postoperative PHASE II PACU
Medication	Review medical history	Start IV	Administer meperidine	Administer naloxone, flumazenil pm	Pain med prn	Start on Rx omeprazole	Continue medications
Diagnostic tests	H & P chest x-ray, ECG, blood work	Review tests	Endoscopy procedure	None, unless complications	None	None	None
Diet	Regular	NPO	NPO	NPO	Clear liquids & progress	Regular	Regular
Activity	Not restricted	Ambulate	None	Turn, cough, and deep breathe	Increase activity to ambulation	Normal ambulation	Not restricted
Nursing action	Assessment	Vital signs	Vital signs, O_2 saturation	Vital signs, level of consciousness, O_2 saturation	Monitor as before	Prepare for discharge	Follow-up evaluation via phone
Teaching/ discharge planning	Phone call	Patient education about procedure	Transport to PACU	Discharge when Aldrete criteria I met	Discharge when Aldrete criteria II met	Instructions reviewed	Phone call for follow-up

Figure 23-5 • Clinical pathway for endoscopy. *DRG*, Diagnosis-related group; *LOS*, length of stay; *PACU*, postanesthesia care unit; *IV*, intravenous; *prn*, as needed; *H&P*, history and physical; *ECG*, electrocardiogram; *NPO*, nothing by mouth; O_2, oxygen. (From Monahan FD, Neighbors M: *Medical-surgical nursing: foundations of clinical practice*, ed 2, Philadelphia, 1998, Saunders.)

resulting from aggregating computerized assessment and outcome data from client records. A "pathway" is created, with benchmark milestones clients are expected to achieve within an identified time frame. Each specific disease or procedure has a standard path developed by an interdisciplinary team. The path describes expected care for each day and also permits the nurse to record care given.

The trend toward more streamlined yet comprehensive and meaningful charting is exemplified in clinical pathways. The goals are to provide a structured tool for planning the highest quality of care; encourage interdisciplinary communication; decrease the time spent charting, because you are charting by exception; focus care on expected client outcomes; and facilitate quality assurance evaluations. Most agencies give the client a copy of the pathway at the time of admission, so that he or she understands what is expected each day (Figure 23-5). Thus, the pathway becomes a teaching tool for client education and a tool to measure quality.

Unlike the POR, the clinical pathway is truly an *interdisciplinary tool.* It allows the entire health team to monitor the client's progress compared with a standard time frame for progress. A variance or exception occurs when a client does not progress as anticipated or an expected outcome does not occur. A variance is a red flag, alerting staff of a need for further action to assist the client.

Advantages. Charting by exception can be efficient and time-saving. Use of clinical pathways provides a concise method for documenting routine care. Nurses direct attention to abnormal or significant findings, rather than spending time detailing normal findings. This documentation method may cut charting time in half. Short (1997) found that charting by exception integrated with clinical pathways took an average 0.82 hours per shift in charting time, as compared with other forms, which required up to 2.5 hours. Other studies show use of pathways can reduce hospital stays.

Disadvantages. Charting by exception does not allow for qualitative information. If you fail to perform even one step of the protocol, you are guilty of falsifying the client's record. Legal decisions in the early 1990s found that certain nurses charting by exception were negligent by virtue of items not charted. Clinical pathways are labor-intensive to develop, and they require "buy-in" by physicians and nursing staff, because in the current malpractice climate nurses tend to repeat flow sheet information in the "Nursing Notes" section.

Documenting Nursing at the Point of Care

The technology supporting electronic documentation and access to client health records is revolutionizing nursing documentation. Wireless Internet access and use of laptop computers or handheld devices has made documentation at the point of care, such as the client's home, possible.

Ethical, Regulatory, and Professional Standards

The use of electronic medical records and storage of personal health information in computer databases has refocused attention on ethical and security issues of privacy and confidentiality. For example, a nurse in one unit of a hospital who accesses the electronic medical record of a client who is in another unit and for whom the nurse has no responsibilities for care is violating confidentiality. Ethical professional practice requires that you do not allow others to use your access log-on.

Confidentiality and Privacy

The Institute of Medicine defines **confidentiality** as the act of limiting disclosure of private matters appropriately; maintaining the trust that an individual has placed in an agent entrusted with private matters. In the United States, most states have laws that grant the client ownership rights to the information contained in the client's health record. Electronic storage and transmission of medical records have sparked intense scrutiny over privacy protection. Violations of confidentiality due to unauthorized access or distribution of sensitive health information can have severe consequences for clients. It may lead to discrimination at the workplace, loss of job opportunities, or disqualification for health insurance. Issues of privacy will dominate how nurses and other health care providers address clinical documentation in the years ahead. Currently a personal medical identification number is used on client records. To prevent unauthorized access, hardware safeguards such as workstation security, keyed lock hard drives, and automatic log-offs are used in addition to user identification and passwords.

Box 23-5 Overview of Federal HIPAA Guidelines Protecting Client Confidentiality

- All medical records and other individually identifiable health information used or disclosed in any form, whether electronically, on paper, or orally, are covered by the final rule.
- Providers and health plans will be required to give clients a clear written explanation of how their health information may be used and disclosed. (Under current law, agencies are not required to get written permission from clients to use this information.)
- Clients are able to see and get copies of their records and request amendments. In addition, a history of nonroutine disclosures must be made accessible to clients.
- Health care providers will be required to obtain client consent before sharing their information for treatment, payment, and health care operations. In addition, separate client authorization must be obtained for nonroutine disclosures and most non–health care purposes. Clients will have the right to request restrictions on the uses and disclosures of their information.
- People will have the right to file a formal complaint with a covered provider or health plan, or with the U.S. Department of Health and Human Services (HHS), about violations of the provisions of this rule or the policies and procedures of the covered entity.
- Health information covered by the rule generally may not be used for purposes not related to health care (e.g., disclosures to employers to make personnel decisions or to financial institutions) without explicit authorization from the individual.
- In general, disclosure of information is limited to the minimum necessary for the purpose of the disclosure. However, this provision does not apply to the disclosure of medical records for treatment purposes, payment, or limited operations such as Quality Assessment reviews, credentialing, or "national priority" activities.
- Written privacy procedures must be in place to cover anyone who has access to protected information, how the information will be used within the organization, and when the information may be disclosed. Covered organizations need to take steps to ensure that their business associates protect the privacy of health information.
- Covered organizations need to train their employees in their privacy procedures and must designate an individual to be responsible for ensuring the procedures are followed.
- Health plans, providers, and clearinghouses that violate these standards will be subject to civil liability. Civil monetary penalties are $100 per violation, up to $25,000 per person, per year, for each requirement or prohibition violated. Congress also established criminal penalties for knowingly violating client privacy. Criminal penalties are up to $50,000 and 1 year in prison for obtaining or disclosing protected health information; up to $100,000 and up to 5 years in prison for obtaining protected health information under "false pretenses"; and up to $250,000 and up to 10 years in prison for obtaining or disclosing protected health information with the intent to sell, transfer, or use it for commercial advantage, personal gain, or malicious harm.

From HIPAA Guidelines: www.hhs.gov/ocr/hipaa.

HIPAA: Federal Medical Record Privacy Regulations. In the United States, the first federal legislation dealing with privacy of medical records was part of P.L. 104-191, the **Health Insurance Portability and Accountability Act** of 1996 (HIPAA; see Online Resources). The rules and regulations in this legislation protect the client's medical record confidentiality. Improper disclosure of medical information is punishable by fines or imprisonment. The regulations were developed by the U.S. Department of Health and Human Services and are enforced by the Office of Civil Rights. The legislation requires that health care providers get authorization from clients before disclosing or sharing any personal medical information. The major elements of the HIPAA privacy regulations are presented in Box 23-5.

Client authorization is not required in situations concerning the public's health (e.g., when clients with tuberculosis are reported to local public health authorities), criminal and legal matters, quality assurance, and record reviews for accreditation. Agencies face severe penalties for violations of a client's private health information. Most nurses are required to complete annual training in confidentiality procedures and sign documents promising compliance to agency policies. Study your agency's policies to determine to whom and under what conditions personal health information can be released. More information can be obtained through the website of the Office of Civil Rights.

Other ethical issues are on the horizon as computer systems begin automating care plans based on the assessment and outcome data that nurses collect and enter. Who is responsible for the computer-generated care decisions?

Other Legal Aspects of Charting

Management literature emphasizes the need for less repetitive, less time-consuming methods of documentation that still reflect the nursing process. At the same time, documentation must be legally sound. The legal assumption is that the care was not given unless it is documented in the client's record. Malpractice settlements have approached the multimillion-dollar mark for individuals whose charts failed to document safe, effective care. Aside from issues of legal liability, third-party reimbursement depends on accurate recording of care given. Major insurance companies audit charts and contest any charges that are not documented in the written record.

If It Was Not Charted, It Was Not Done. This statement stems from a legal case (Kolesar v. Jeffries) heard before Canada's Supreme Court, in which a nurse failed to document the care of a client on a Stryker frame before he died. Because the purpose of the medical record is to list care given and client outcomes, any information that is clinically significant must be included. Legally all care must be documented. Cone, Anderson, and Johnson (1996) state, "Since documenting is fundamental to continuity and quality of care, care delivered but not documented is, from a legal perspective, care not done." Murray (2005) says that conscious practice and documentation is not enough and that since society is so litigious, every nurse should anticipate having their clients' records subpoenaed at some time during their nursing career.

Any method of charting that provides comprehensive, factual information is legally acceptable. This includes graphs, checklists, and all of the types of charting discussed earlier in this chapter. Long narrative paragraphs should rarely be a part of charting; however, by initialing a protocol, the nurse is documenting that every step was carried out. If a protocol exists in a health care agency, you are legally responsible for carrying it out.

Correcting errors to the medical record should be done in such a way that the incorrect information is still legible and never obliterated. In the preferred method of correction, the nurse draws a line through the incorrect entry and adds his or her initials and the date. Additions to existing charting, even if added shortly afterward, are not a problem in the courtroom. Additions that occur after the defendant has been notified that the client is contemplating legal action are difficult to defend in court.

Box 23-6 lists recommended rules for charting to keep you legally safe, as well as common charting mistakes to avoid. Contact the American Nurses Association's marketing division for a copy of *Liability Prevention and You: What Nurses and Employers Need to Know*.

Box 23-6 Charting Rules

Content

- Chart promptly, but never ahead of time. Do not wait until end of shift.
- Document complete care reflecting the nursing process.
- Document all noncooperative or bizarre behavior.
- Document all refusals of ordered treatments.
- Document teaching (information you gave the client and/or family).
- When care or medicine is omitted, document action and rationale (who was notified and what was said).
- Document all significant changes in the client's condition and who was notified, as well as your nursing interventions.

Mistakes to Avoid

- Failing to record complete, pertinent health information
- Making subjective conclusions rather than recording objective data (Do not describe the client in derogatory terms. A client has a legal right to read health records if a lawyer obtains them, and angry clients are more likely to sue.)
- Not charting in a legible manner, or erasing or using correction fluid to obliterate comments
- Using incorrect or obscure abbreviations
- Making "untimely" entries (e.g., charting after the fact, later than past the end of your day)
- Failing to record drug administration, route, outcome
- Not recording all nursing actions
- Recording on the wrong chart
- Failing to document a discontinued medication
- Failing to record outcome of an intervention such as a medicine
- Writing about incident reports in the client record (do not attach a copy to the chart)

Communicating Medical Orders

Written Orders. Nurses are required to question orders that they do not understand or those that seem to them to be unsafe. Failure to do so puts the nurse at *legal risk*. "Just following orders" is not an acceptable excuse. On the other hand, nurses can be held liable if they arbitrarily decide not to follow a legitimate order, such as choosing to withhold ordered pain medication (Shapiro, 2003). Reasons for such a decision would have to be explicitly documented. With computerization, it is possible to have standing orders, such as for administering vaccines (Dexter, Perkins, & Maharry, 2004). The computer is programmed to recognize the absence of a vaccination and then to automatically write an order for a nurse to administer. What might the legal implications be?

Persons licensed or certified by appropriate government agencies to conduct medical treatment acts include physicians, advance practice nurses, and physician assistants. These providers have their own prescribing number and must abide by government rules and restrictions. Nurse practitioners in most areas cannot prescribe controlled substances unless they obtain a Drug Enforcement Agency number. Consult your agency policy regarding who is allowed to write client orders for the nurse to carry out.

Faxed Orders. The physician or nurse practitioner may choose to send a faxed order. Because this is a form of written order, it has been shown to decrease the number of errors that occur when translating verbal or telephone orders. However, there is the risk of violating client confidentiality when faxing health-related information. See the American Health Information Management Association's general guidelines for faxing medical orders (Hughes, 2001).

Verbal Orders. Often, a change in client condition requires the nurse to telephone the primary physician or hospital staff resident to obtain new orders. The nurse transcribes these verbal orders onto the order sheet, adding a notation that these are verbal orders (v.o.). Legal requirements specify a time frame by which the physician, nurse practitioner, or physician assistant must personally sign these. Most primary providers work in group practices, so it is necessary to determine who is "on call" or who is covering your client when the primary provider is unavailable. It may be necessary to call for new orders if there is a significant change in the client's physical or mental condition as noted by vital signs, lab value reports, treatment or medication reactions, or response failure. Before calling for verbal orders, obtain the chart and familiarize yourself with current vital signs, medications, infusions, and other relevant data.

With the growth of unlicensed personnel, there is greater likelihood that a verbal order will be relayed through someone with this status. The legality is vague, but basically, if harm comes to the client through miscommunication of a verbal order, the licensed nurse will be held accountable.

Case Example

Tracy, the secretary on your unit, answers the telephone. Dr. Uganda gives her an order for a medication for a client. Tracy asks him to repeat the order as soon as she gets a registered nurse to take the call. If you cannot answer the telephone immediately, have her tell him you will call back in 5 minutes to verify the order.

Charting for Others. It is not a wise practice to chart for others, although sometimes you may be required to cosign an entry.

Case Example

Juanita Diaz worked day shift. At 6 PM she calls you and says she forgot to chart Mr. Reft's preoperative enema. She asks you to chart the procedure and his response to it. Can you just add it to your notes? In

Developing an Evidence-Based Practice

Makoul G, Curry R: The use of electronic medical records: communication patterns in outpatient encounters, *J Am Inform Assoc* 8(6):610-615, 2001.

The authors conducted an observational analysis of 204 videotaped physician-client encounters comparing communication by three physicians using computer charting with three physicians using traditional paper charting.

Results: Using electronic charting averaged a 38% longer time for initial visits; physicians were more active in clarifying information, obtaining complete information, and encouraging questions. Those using traditional charting gave more attention to exploring the client's agenda, the client's emotional issues, and finding out how illness affected the client's life.

Application to Your Clinical Practice: Spend time discussing how computer charting might affect your practice. What would using a computer add to your care? What might it sacrifice? Could you imagine a similar study examining nurse-client interactions?

court this would be portrayed as an inaccuracy. The correct solution is to chart "1800: Nurse Diaz called and reported . . ."

APPLICATIONS

Computer Literacy

To practice nursing in coming years, it is clear that all of us will need to be computer-literate. You will need skills such as data entry, data transmission, word processing, Internet accessing, spreadsheet entry, and use of standard language and codes describing practice. Voice recognition software may eventually revolutionize clinical documentation, making documentation easier for us.

Documenting on a Client's Health Record

Use Exercise 23-1 to stimulate discussion of appropriate documentation.

Confidentiality

Ethical and legal dilemmas inherent in use of computerized systems will require continued debate in the coming decades, especially regarding the concern of protecting client privacy. As cases come to court, a body of case law will provide some guidance. HIPAA regulations mandating clients' right to privacy are the current guidelines. You need to become aware of threats to privacy and your obligation to protect your clients' privacy where possible. Discuss the ethical dilemma provided at the end of this chapter.

Use of Universal Nursing Languages and Codes

The need for a uniform language about nursing practice seems self-evident. The need to identify and analyze outcomes of nursing practice requires computer-compatible frameworks. Adoption of one standard nursing intervention classification scheme would allow us to gather and analyze large amounts of information about which nursing interventions produce positive client outcomes. One universal coding scheme would provide a common language across health settings. Think about

Exercise 23-1 Charting Nursing Diagnoses

Purpose: To clarify diagnoses.

Procedure:

Discuss in small groups which of the following examples help provide a direction for independent nursing interventions.

Example 1

Incorrect: Inability to communicate related to deafness

Suggested: Impaired social interaction (00052) related to anatomical (auditory), as evidenced by refusal to interact with others

Discussion:

What additional information is provided in the correct diagnosis? Why would the first statement be incorrect? Are all people who are deaf unable to communicate?

Example 2

Incorrect: Acute lymphocytic leukemia

Suggested: Acute pain (00132) during ambulation related to leukemia disease process, as evidenced by limping, grimacing, and increased pulse

Discussion:

Could a nurse make any independent intervention based on the information provided by the diagnosis "acute lymphocytic leukemia"?

Exercise 23-2 **Application of NIC Finding**

Purpose: To make use of NIC meaningful.

Procedure:

Consider the following finding from Dochterman's study, then answer the questions.

On Day 3 of hospitalization, nurses averaged four intravenous therapy interventions for clients with a diagnosis of hip fracture but averaged only two interventions for (oral) fluid management.

1. How could you use this information to justify the need for skilled nursing care?
2. Suppose data showed that by Day 6, skilled care activities had been cut in half. How might the nurse manager readjust the client assignment for her nurse aides?

On Day 3, clients with hip fractures received three times as many nursing interventions encouraging proper coughing as were made for clients with congestive heart failure.

1. Speculate about why there was this difference.
2. Suppose hospital units with more nursing interventions to encourage coughing were shown to have greatly decreased rates of clients with pneumonia complications. Could this information be used to justify a better nurse-to-client ratio?

From Dochterman J, Titler M, Wang J et al. Describing use of nursing interventions for three groups of patients, *J Nurs Scholarsh* 37(1):57-66, 2005.

this "bigger picture" as you learn use of nursing terminology in your clinical practice.

Dochterman, Titler, Wang, and colleagues (2005) were among the first to demonstrate that NIC-coded patterns of nursing interventions can be analyzed. They examined three types of interventions for older adults in 13,758 acute care hospitalizations. Data were obtained for interventions for clients with diagnoses of heart failure and hip fracture, and for fall prevention interventions. Results demonstrated that interventions occurred throughout the hospitalization period, were individualized, and could be classified into daily patterns (and potentially could produce better health outcomes). Information describing the type and amount of nursing care delivered could also potentially help staff managers plan for amount and type of staff needed on a unit.

Standardization work is ongoing internationally, as evidenced by groups such as the Association for Common European Nursing Diagnoses, Interventions, and Outcomes. Try Exercise 23-2 to explore how you might apply information.

SUMMARY

This chapter focuses on the use of written communication in the nurse-client relationship. Documentation refers to the process of obtaining, organizing, and conveying information to others in a written format. Emphasis is placed on computerized documentation systems that reduce redundancy, increase time efficiency, reduce cost, decrease data errors, and force compliance with standards and policies. An electronic health record system is more than just a computerized version of written documentation of care. Chapter 24 will discuss technology that can facilitate communication among health care workers, increase client education, send reminders of appointments, assist the providers of health care with

Ethical Dilemma ■ *What Would You Do?*

You work in an organization with a computerized clinical documentation system. A co-worker mentions that Alice Jarvis, RN, has been admitted to the medical floor for some strange symptoms and that her lab results have just been posted, showing she is positive for hepatitis C, among other things.

1. Identify at least two alternative ways to deal with this ethical dilemma. (What response would you make to your co-worker who retrieved information from the computerized system? What else might you do?)
2. What ethical principle can you cite to support each answer?

From Sonya R. Hardin, RN, PhD, CCRN, University North Carolina, Charlotte.

decision-making prompts, monitor medications, and use Internet access to obtain information resources.

REFERENCES

American Nurses Association: *On access to patient data*, ANA Position Statement No. 12.22, 1995a; available online: http://nursingworld.org/readroom/position/joint/jtdata.htm.

American Nurses Association: *Position paper on computer-based patient record standards*, ANA Position Statement No. 12.20, 1995b; available online: http://nursingworld.org/readroom/position/joint/jtcpri1.htm.

American Psychiatric Association: *Diagnostic and statistical manual of mental disorders*, ed 4, text rev, Washington, DC, 2000, Author.

Baeten AM: Documentation: the reviewer perspective, *Top Geriatr Rehabil* 13(1):14–22, 1997.

Bates DW, Gawande AA: Improving safety with information technology, *N Engl J Med* 348:2526–2534, 2003.

Bowles KH: Application of the Omaha System in acute care, *Res Nurs Health* 23:93–105, 2000.

Cimino JJ: Review paper: coding systems in health care, *Methods Inf Med* 35:273–284, 1996.

Cone KJ, Anderson MA, Johnson J: Documentation of assessment in the emergency department, *Chart* 93(1):9, 1996.

Cornell S: Electronic prescribing, *Adv Nurse Pract* 9(6): 107–108, 2001.

Dexter PR, Perkins SM, Maharry KS: Inpatient computer-based standing orders vs. physician reminders to increase influenza and pneumococcal vaccination rates, *JAMA* 292(19):2366–2371, 2004.

Dochterman JM, Bulechek GM, editors: *Nursing interventions classification (NIC)*, ed 4, St Louis, 2004, Mosby.

Dochterman J, Titler M, Wang J et al.: Describing use of nursing interventions for three groups of patients, *J Nurs Scholarsh* 37(1):57–66, 2005.

Hebda T, Czar P, Mascara C: *Handbook of informatics for nurses and health care professionals*, ed 2, Upper Saddle River, NJ, 2001, Prentice Hall.

Henry SB, Holzemer WL, Randell CR et al.: Comparison of nursing interventions classification and current procedural terminology codes for categorizing nursing activities, *Image* 29(2):133–138, 1997.

Hughes G: *Practice brief: facsimile transmission of health information (updated)*, AHIMA Practice Brief, *J AHIMA* 72(6): 64E–64F, 2001; available online: http://library.ahima.org/xpedio/groups/public/documents/ahima/bok2_000116.hcsp?dDocName=bok2_000116

Iowa Intervention Project: Proposal to bring nursing into the information age, *Image* 29(3):275, 1997.

Johnson M, Bulechek G, Dochterman JM et al.: *Nursing diagnosis, outcomes, and interventions: NANDA, NOC, and NIC linkages*, St Louis, 2001, Mosby.

Keepnews D, Capitman JA, Rosati RJ: Measuring patient-level clinical outcomes of home health care, *J Nurs Scholarsh* 35(1):79–85, 2004.

Kohn LT, Corrigan JM, Donaldson MS: *To err is human: building a safer health system*, Washington, DC, 2000, National Academies Press.

Larrabee JH, Boldrighini S, Elder-Sorrells K et al.: Evaluation of documentation before and after implementation of a nursing information system in an acute care hospital, *Comput Nurs* 19:56–65, 2001.

Lee T: Nurses' concerns about using information systems: analysis of comments on a computerized nursing care plan system in Taiwan, *J Clin Nurs* 14(3):344–353, 2005.

Lee T, Mills ME: The relationship among medical diagnosis, nursing diagnosis, and nursing interventions and the implications for home health care, *J Prof Nurs* 21(2):84–91, 2000.

Makoul G, Curry RH, Tang PC: The use of Electronic Medical Records: communication patterns in outpatient encounters, *J Am Med Inform Assoc* 8(6):610–615, 2001.

Marshall PD, Chin HL: The effects of an Electronic Medical Record on patient care: clinician attitudes at a large HMO, *Proc AMIA Symp* 150–154, 1998.

Martin KS: *The Omaha System: a key to practice, documentation and information management*, ed 2, St Louis, 2005, Elsevier [Saunders].

McCloskey JC, Bulechek GM, Donahue W: Nursing interventions core to specialty practice, *Nurs Outlook* 46:67–76, 1998.

Moody LE, Slocumb E, Berg B et al.: Electronic health records documentation in nursing: nurses' perceptions, attitudes and preferences, *Comput Inform Nurs* 22(6): 337–344, 2004.

Moorhead S, Johnson M, Maas M: *Nursing outcomes classification (NOC)*, ed 3, St Louis, 2004, Mosby.

Murray RB: The subpoena and day in court: guidelines for nurses, *J Psychosoc Nurs Ment Health Serv* 43(3):38–44, 2005.

North American Nursing Diagnosis Association: *Nursing diagnoses: definitions and classifications 2001–2002*, Philadelphia, 2001, Author.

Shapiro RS: Health care providers' liability exposure for inappropriate pain management, *J Law Med Ethics* 24(4):360–364, 2003.

Short MS: Charting by exception on a clinical pathway, *Nurs Manage* 28(8):45–46, 1997.

Young K: *Informatics for healthcare professionals*, Philadelphia, 2000, FA Davis.

Chapter 24

Communicating in the Age of e-Health Technology

Kathleen Underman Boggs

OUTLINE

Basic Concepts
- Wireless Technology in Health Care: Access to Information at the Point of Care
  - *Personal Digital Assistant (PDA)*
  - *Mobile/Cellular Telephones and Pagers*
  - *Laptop Computers*
- Computers Providing Automated Decision Support
  - *Telemedicine/Telehealth*
  - *Electronic-Mail Communication (E-Mail)*
  - *Interactive Computer Programs for Health Education, Support, and Assessment*
  - *Websites*
  - *Client Health Monitor Data Transmission*

Applications
- *Example: Developing an Evidence-Based Practice*
- Education via Computer
- Cautions or Barriers to Application of New Technologics
- Wireless Handheld Computer Use
- Use of Wireless/Cellular Telephones and Advanced Capability "Smart Phones"
- Bar Coding for Client Safety: Technology Application
- Skill Mastery: Documenting Student-Client Interactions Using Interpersonal Process Records
  - *Written Interpersonal Process Record (IPR)*
  - *Using Electronic Recordings of Student-Client Interactions for Analysis*

Summary

OBJECTIVES

At the end of the chapter, the reader will be able to:

1. Identify types of wireless technologies of use in decentralized health care.
2. Discuss the advantages and disadvantages of various assistive technologies for continual communication.
3. Describe barriers to use of continual communication technologies in health care.
4. Discuss application of technology in professional documentation at the point of care.
5. Demonstrate mastery of all communication skills by describing and analyzing interactions between nurse and client in written process recordings or analysis of videotaped interactions.

The U.S. government has articulated the necessity of implementing the use of handheld computers [at] the point of care.

(Thompson, 2005)

The sustained growth of evidence-based practice and ongoing assessment of the efficacy of our communication approaches will serve as important underpinnings to successfully blending new modalities, such as information technology, with our more traditional communication patterns.

(Miller, 2004)

This chapter focuses on using new technology to enhance communication between nurse and client, nurse and other professional health care providers, and nurse and reference information. Decentralized access to documentation is transforming health care. Emerging wireless electronic technologies are discussed as they relate to communication and nursing care. Also in this chapter, information is provided about the use of interpersonal process records as a way for students to develop and demonstrate mastery of communication skills discussed in this book.

BASIC CONCEPTS

Three major transformations are occurring due to technology use in nursing care (Figure 24-1). In addition to the electronic health record discussed in Chapter 23, new devices allow nurses decentralized access to client records. Nursing practice now incorporates continual use of updated client information and reference material at any client location (the point-of-care information) via the Internet. This is called "real-time bedside nurse charting" (Nelson, Evans, Samore et al., 2005).

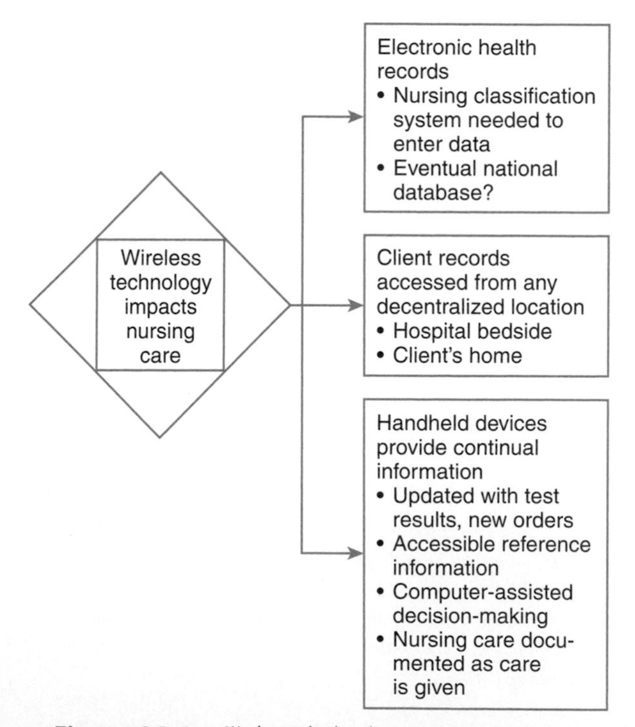

Figure 24-1 • Wireless technology has an impact on nursing care.

Development of technology is advancing hundreds of times faster than at any previous time in history. This chapter describes a few of the current choices. Governmental agencies in many countries have been funding use of electronic technology and giving incentives to providers of high-quality care (Institute of Medicine, 2001). According to Roland (2004), the use of clinical information technology computing systems will result in improved health outcomes.

Many medical errors result from inadequate access to clinical data (Bates & Gawande, 2003), but more are medication errors. According to the landmark Institute of Medicine study (Kohn, Corrigan, & Donaldson, 2000) of hospitalized client deaths, up to 98,000 clients in the United States die each year from preventable causes. In this retrospective study, more than 11% died due to wrong drug name, 11.1% from wrong dosage due to errors in calculation, and 10.8% due to unclear dosage directions. From computers come printed orders, verification of client identity via bar code checks, and automatic dosage checks (sort of like spell check!). Computers also provide reminders about standard protocols for care, integrated into the agency's e-health technology.

Unlike the banking industry, health care was slow to adopt new e-technology (Thompson, 2005). But now that wireless handheld devices with Internet access are commonly used, the transition to e-health is making rapid progress.

Consumers also are willing to access to the Internet to meet their health care needs. Resources are available for health education. The Pew Internet and American Life Project (2005) found that about 80% of Internet users search for health information, especially on specific medical problems, wellness information, or treatment procedures, on the Internet. Clients with electronic health records may have the ability to view parts of their records such as test results, make appointments, and receive follow-up care directions.

Box 24-1 presents a summary of advantages and disadvantages of the use of wireless technology by nurses. As a new generation of wireless technology comes into common use, communication is improving. Not only will it reduce the cost of health care and improve quality, but also continual wireless access to client records will become a crucial factor in reducing errors. As Thompson (2005) says, it has the power to transform nursing care.

Box 24-1 Use of Wireless Handheld Computers

Advantages

- Easily portable; can be used at the point of care (client's bedside, in the home, etc.)
- Quick charting when nurse enters information by tapping menu selections
- Can contain reference resources about treatment, for medication dosage, etc., if uploaded
- May provide dictionary, reminders about standards of care
- When accompanied by Internet access, provides quick communication (e.g., nurse is signaled by beep regarding receipt of new orders)
- Provides quick access to client records

Disadvantages

- Possible threats to client's legal privacy rights
- Long learning curve; may take awhile to become familiar with how to use
- Nurse does not have a printed copy of information (until downloaded to agency printer)
- Small screen does not allow you to view entire page of information
- Technical problem may result in dysfunction/downtime

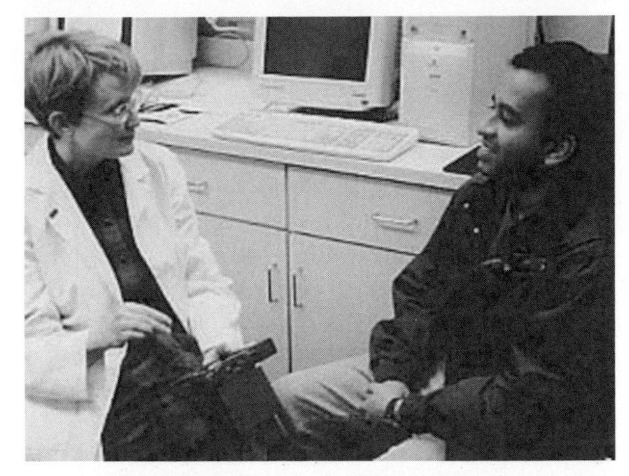

Personal digital assistants (PDAs) are handheld electronic devices that may contain multiple databases, possibly including a language translator for use when interviewing a patient from another culture. With these devices, data can be entered at the point of care, whether it is in a clinic or a patient's home, then transmitted wirelessly to a central agency computer or printer. (Photo courtesy of Adam Boggs.)

Wireless Technology in Health Care: Access to Information at the Point of Care

Personal Digital Assistant (PDA)

PDA is a generic term for any of several brands of small, handheld computerized electronic devices that fit in the palm of the nurse's hand. First introduced in the mid-1990s as the U.S. Robotics Pilot (Palm Pilot), PDAs reduce paperwork and help the nurse save time tracking down client information, leaving more time to focus on client care (George & Davidson, 2005). PDA applications can check for drug interactions, calculate dosages, analyze lab results, schedule procedures, and order prescriptions, among other functions. It is easy to periodically upload reference sources, such as the latest medication information or disease treatment protocols, making them akin to a portable medical and nursing library. PDAs can be taken to where the client is, allowing data access and documentation at that "point of care" so often referred to in the literature.

All PDA operating systems incorporate various types of handwriting recognition, allowing the user to tap, draw, or write on the screen using a stylus. The great advantage of PDAs over laptop computers is they are small, lightweight, and easy to carry. Because they are wireless, they can be used in the client's hospital room, in an outpatient clinic, or in the community, including in the client's home. Most PDAs can send stored information to another PDA, to the agency computer, or directly to a printer.

PDAs are used to record client data. You can enter your client's history, make a problem list, update assessment data, and write nursing notes. Your wireless handheld device can also be used to track information such as client's medications and dosages or lab test results in a flow sheet format. In addition, handhelds can serve as a dictionary or a calculator.

By 2002, more than 25% of residency training programs required physicians to have PDAs. Nursing programs are slower to do so, although many nurse practitioner students find PDAs a very useful tool (Craig, 2002). Emergency department nurses in Australia also report finding PDAs useful in their practice (Gururajan, 2004). In the community, PDAs with Internet capability can be used to access client records. For example, a nurse practitioner using a PDA can call up a client's previous prescriptions, renew them at a touch, record this new information in the agency mainframe computer, correctly calculate the dosage of a new medication, write the order, and send this prescription to the client's pharmacy instantly—all without writing anything on paper (Cornell, 2001).

There are a number of brands of hardware available to run operating systems like Palm OS or Windows CE Pocket PC. Downloadable software is available (e.g., free drug information programs like ePocrates), as are programs that support the computerized documentation of client care data. Limited battery life and incompatibility of software uploadable programs are limitations that need to be considered prior to adoption.

Devices similar to "smart phones" can provide nurses with improved wireless access via the Internet to client information, new lab results, and physician orders. They may even provide computer-assisted decision support as described above.

Mobile/Cellular Telephones and Pagers

Mobile/cellular telephones can be used for improved wireless access to physicians and health team members. Some hospitals are issuing cell phones for staff nurses to use at work to directly contact physicians or other hospital departments from the client's bedside, to give condition updates, or to obtain verbal orders. Taylor, Coakley, Reardon, and colleagues (2004) say this use of cell phones has improved nurse communications. Nurses working in the community are likely to benefit from use of mobile phones to contact clients on the way to give home care. Mobile telephones provide easy access from the field back to the agency, to the client's primary physician, and to other resources. Some community nurses prefer pagers, which notify them of telephone messages so they can return calls.

Cellular phones equipped with cameras and picture transmission capability have potential for long distance diagnosis, a "snapshot" version of telemedicine/telehealth interactive video and vocal transmissions. Home health nurses may someday use these to obtain expert consulting for their client while the client remains at home, just as physicians successfully do to obtain expert consultations (Tsai, Pong, Liang et al., 2004). Phones may also increase direct access to health care for the client. One company, TelaDoc, provides a physician's advice or treatment by telephone to its members for a nominal fee ("These docs...", 2005).

Laptop Computers

Laptop computers are more powerful than PDAs yet are still small and portable enough to be taken into the client's home. They are used to chart the client's care and send information over a phone line or via wireless networks directly to an agency, physician, pharmacist, and so on via a local server. One example is the Nightingale Tracker. If a laptop with a networking card is near a wireless Internet transmitter, information can be sent in a wireless fashion. Many urban areas such as Philadelphia have or plan to have these transmitters in place atop lampposts. Otherwise, you can use a telephone to transmit your nursing documentation.

Computers Providing Automated Decision Support

With the advent of computerized client information technology systems, another potential asset is the development of computerized "cues" or prompts to assist in clinical decision making. One example is the computer program for medication dispensing used by pharmacists. All the medications prescribed for a specific client are stored in the database. When a new drug is entered, the program not only alerts the provider about whether the prescribed dose exceeds maximum standard safety margins, but the program also compares the new medicine with those the client is already taking to cross-check for potential drug interactions.

Im and Chee (2003) describe a computer software program designed to assist nurses in making decisions about treating cancer pain. Wireless technology extends decision support into the client's home. For example, nurses working with pediatric clients have long used calculators to determine correct fractional dosage based on the child's weight. Now an automated support system could be employed that automatically predetermines the correct doses.

Telemedicine/Telehealth

Telemedicine/telehealth is defined as the use of telecommunication technology to facilitate health care. Specifically it provides live transmissions from one doctor to another or to a client located in a remote site. It allows for the transmission of digitized audio, video, and still images. This technology was hailed as a boon to rural practitioners, facilitating long-distance consultations by expert specialists. Potentially it could deliver these services into the client's home. It requires expensive hardware equipment at both ends of the transmission, as well as the infrastructure to support its use.

Electronic-Mail Communication (E-Mail)

According to the American Medical Association (AMA, 2004), e-mail can be a convenient, inexpensive method of communicating follow-up instructions, test results, and educational information to the client in his or her home. Almost all clients express a desire to communicate with their health care providers via e-mail, but only a small percentage of physicians actually use e-mail for scheduling appointments, providing prescription refills, and other routine tasks (Gerstle & AAP Task Force on Medical Informatics, 2004). Physicians express concern about lack of income generation, confidentiality, malpractice, and the belief that it would be too time-consuming (Bauchner, Adams, & Burstin, 2002; Gerstle & AAP Task Force on Medical Informatics, 2004; Kleiner, Akers, Burke et al., 2002). However, in a study by Goldman (2005), physicians were in favor of using e-mail to obtain feedback from emergency departments as a follow-up to treatment the department provided to their patients. Nurses could use e-mail as a way to communicate with clients, for example, in tracking the response of clients who are on new medication, instead of waiting until their next office appointment (Abrahamsen, 2003).

AMA guidelines (2004) suggest that electronic or paper copies be made of e-mail messages sent to patients; the use of auto-reply messages; and parameters for messages from clients such as turnaround time, need for brevity, and so on.

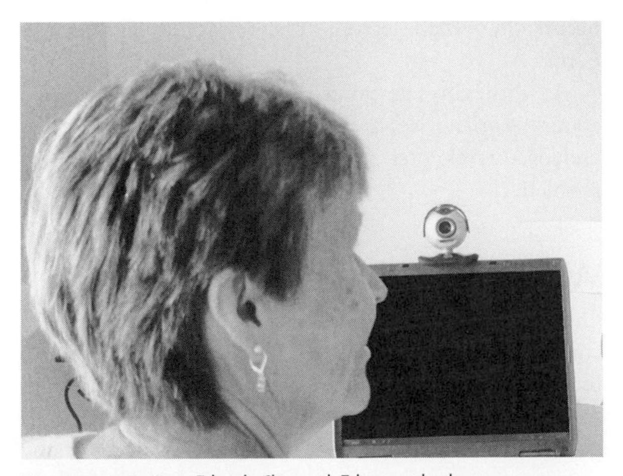

Figure 24-2 • Teleweb: Client with Telecam at her home computer conversing with nurse at the hospital. Note the "eyeball"-size camera mounted above the computer.

Interactive Computer Programs for Health Education, Support, and Assessment

Clients have a hunger to learn more about their illness (Malpani, 2001). The literature suggests there is strong potential for improved health learning associated with interactive computer teaching programs. Using webcam technology real-time (synchronous) communication between health teacher and client can deliver health maintenance information and provide answers to illness-related questions (Figure 24-2).

The Internet has also been used to organize client or family support groups. A study by Baum (2004) found that this activity not only provided needed social support but also improved parent relationships with their special needs children.

Websites

A personalized website can be used by an agency for far broader functions than providing business hours or travel directions. In an American Hospital Association study report, O'Dell (2005) says that nearly all health care organizations now have their own websites. Such sites can include health assessment tools and allow clients to schedule appointments. Another primary function is to provide health information. Websites can have hyperlinks embedded that the client can use to access general information about his or her condition, medications, or treatment. They can also contain an e-mail link so that clients can directly contact the nurse responsible for patient education.

Client Health Monitor for Data Transmission

A variety of monitors worn by clients can periodically transmit data directly to a primary provider or nurse in a health agency via ground telephone lines or even using wireless technology (Yao, Schmitz, & Warren, 2005). Such devices include 24-hour heart monitors, pacemakers, uterine contraction monitors, and respiratory function peak-flow readings, among others. Nurses are assuming increased responsibilities for interpretation of these data and for instituting interventions.

APPLICATIONS

In 2004, the National Coordinator for Health Information Technology set several goals, including the need to use new technology to improve health by facilitating quality of care monitoring and quickly disseminating

Developing an Evidence-Based Practice

Nelson NC, Evans RS, Samore MH et al.: Detection and prevention of medication errors using real-time bedside nurse charting, *J Am Med Inform Assoc* 12(4):390-397, 2005.

This quasiexperimental pre and post study was conducted to measure nurses' use of real-time computerized charting on two 40-bed surgical units. The researchers hypothesized that an educational intervention emphasizing that real-time charting reduces errors would increase use of this type of charting.

Results: After 12 weeks of intervention education, the experimental group increased their use of real-time charting by 14%.

Application to Your Clinical Practice: Discuss your feelings about carrying a handheld wireless device versus using a laptop bedside computer terminal each time you chart in a client's hospital room. How likely are you to do real-time charting at the bedside on a computer with decision support features if you know this program will help you avoid errors?

research findings into practice (Thompson, 2005). Wireless entry of data at the point of care may improve the way we compile information for analysis.

There are few sound studies supporting better client outcomes from the use of wireless technology. In a qualitative study of physicians using handheld computers, users perceived that they increased productivity and improved care (McAlearney, Schweikhart, & Medow, 2004). Certainly, more data are needed to support all the assertions in the literature that e-health technology will decrease costs while improving care.

Education via Computer

Education programs using the Internet have been popular. Entire master's and doctoral programs are now offered online. Initially designed as distance education programs, courses at local nursing programs now use computer-based or computer-enhanced courses in response to student demand. Students say they prefer asynchronous (not in real time) courses that they can access at their convenience. After graduation, would you prefer this method to earn continuing education credits as required for your relicensure or recertification? Gross and Gross (2005) also suggest using the asynchronous format for meetings, especially when content is controversial or has emotional aspects; this format increases participation.

Teaching clients about preventive health promotion or about their disease conditions might also be done effectively using the Internet. Commercial companies produce many software packages that nurses could use to supplement their own teaching. Client learning would need to be evaluated. Outcome studies show some clients learn more from computer-based programs than from traditional teaching. One example is the HIV/AIDS program described by Marsch and Bickel (2004). Refer to Chapter 16 for in-depth discussion of health education.

Cautions or Barriers to Application of New Technologies

Outcomes need to be carefully evaluated to determine the effectiveness of use of these new communication technologies. Their expense will only be justified if outcome measures show significant positive improvement in client/consumer health status. *Illiteracy* could be a barrier to use. More than 40 million Americans have significant literacy deficits, and more than 20% of Americans read at or below 5th grade level. (National Institute for Literacy, 2000).

Use of the Internet presents many questions about how to maximize its communication potential with an increasingly diverse population (Miller, 2004). *Liability* and regulatory issues are outmoded, relevant to the century gone by. For example, if transmission (and treatment) crosses state lines, in which region does the provider need to be licensed? If malpractice occurs, in which region or state would legal action occur?

As with any computer use, we are also concerned about *security*. See the Ethical Dilemma box at the end of this chapter for an exercise that explores this problem.

Wireless Handheld Computer Use

Guidelines are available for physician use of e-mail to communicate with clients (AMA, 2004); these guidelines are also appropriate for nurses. While some colleges are now requiring all students to have laptop-type computers with Internet access, no one knows how many nurses are accustomed to using wireless technology devices in their care of clients. Guidelines for their use in giving client care need to be developed.

Use of Wireless/Cellular Telephones and Advanced Capability "Smart Phones"

While just about every nursing student has seen or used a wireless or cellular telephone, not everyone has used them as an aid to giving client care. Nursing is just beginning to deal with guidelines for use of wireless telephones in these situations.

Bar Coding for Client Safety: Technology Application

The increased attention on client safety has increased the application of established bar coding technology to health care. Bar codes on name bands allow for verification of client identity via checking by a bar code reader prior to administering a medication. Laboratory specimens labeled with the computer-generated bar codes prevent mix-ups. The Veterans Administration Hospital System instituted a national bar code system in 1999. When a new medication is ordered by a physician, it is transmitted to the pharmacy, where it is labeled with the same bar code as is on the client's name band. The nurse administering that medication must first verify both codes by scanning with the battery-operated bar code reader, just as a grocery store employee scans merchandise. According to Wright and Katz (2005), this resulted in a 24% decrease in medication administration errors. Radiofrequency identification (RFID) is an emerging technology allowing you to locate a certain nurse, identify a patient, or even locate an individual medication. According to Thompson (2005), RFID may be able to be incorporated into the nurse's handheld computer.

Skill Mastery: Documenting Student-Client Interactions Using Interpersonal Process Records

Often in a relationship, interactions occur that either help or hinder the progression of the relationship. Many times, however, we remain unaware of exactly what helped move us along or what disrupted communication. The skills described in this book can be self-assessed. Two methods are described here.

Written Interpersonal Process Record (IPR)

This is a tool to help analyze interpersonal communication. There are three essential parts to the process record. First, a written anecdotal record is made of both the client's words and the nurse's words, along with notes about their nonverbal behaviors. Second, a written analysis of the interaction process is done, identifying specific communication skills and interventions used. This analysis is an evaluation of the effectiveness of the nurse's communication skills in fostering the goals of the interaction. The goal of analyzing a process record is to promote use of more effective nursing interventions, so the third component of the process is to add written suggestions for making more effective comments. The writer either suggests alternative communication responses that might enhance the therapeutic interaction or identifies why a strategy did not work.

Use of the written process record is a time-consuming but effective process. To obtain maximum benefit from this learning tool, you need to record a series of nurse-client interactions, conduct a self-analysis, and obtain feedback for each interaction from a reader. Confidentiality must be maintained at all times to protect the client and the therapeutic nature of the nurse-client relationship. Anonymity can be ensured on the process record by using only client initials, rather than full names, and by omitting identifying demographic information.

Instructions for Using Process Records for Learning. To be able to review an interaction objectively, it is necessary first to record the content of the conversation. The written process record is designed for use after you finish interacting with a client. Taking notes during the interaction may be disruptive to the conversation.

Find a quiet, private spot as soon after the interaction as possible and write down the content of the interaction. An example of this content is provided in Columns 1 and 2 of Figure 24-3. Because this form is a tool for learning, space is provided for self-analysis of the therapeutic components of the interaction. Any interaction between a nurse and a client can be recorded and analyzed to learn better communication skills. Travelbee (1971) notes that no nurse is without some degree of skill in being able to purposefully use the communication process; neither is any nurse a communication expert in the sense that he or she cannot develop further skill.

Date: 1/18/07–9:23 a.m. Intake interview in clinic, private exam room. Mrs. Sams's second visit for weight reduction.

Client	*Nurse*	*Analysis*
Hello, Ms. Foy.	Hello, Mrs. Sams. I brought you those booklets on dieting I promised you.	
Thank you.	I'd like to spend time today talking about them with you.	Establishing trust
I've been on every diet published in every magazine. I gain on them all.	You have tried dieting several times before?	Tried to clarify
Yes, I've had a weight problem for five years. Diets don't help. *(loud voice, sad face)* I get disgusted with them after two or three weeks.	You've had trouble actually losing weight on these diets?	Paraphrased to verify
Yes, I'd like to be slimmer. For years I pictured myself as a lump in a bathing suit but every time I resolve to diet, I end up stuffing myself. I always reward myself with a treat when I've had a hard day at work like I'm a big nothing…just a weak-willed slob. *(started crying)*	You find dieting discouraging. *(attentive posture)*	Reflection
	(I began to feel uncomfortable when she got off into these negatives.)	Silence
	Well, I see it upsets you. Let's review these booklets now. I have a lot to cover today.	Acknowledgement of nonbehavioral feelings but changed subject; my own anxiety led me to focus on my own needs
(No comments; avoided eye contact, slumped in chair)	Mrs. Sams, you look like this conversation is getting you down. Maybe we should talk about how you're feeling and discuss the exchanges later. You've mentioned that being overweight makes you feel bad about yourself. What is it about the weight that bothers you most?	Attempt to salvage discussion by refocusing on client's problem Open-ended question to facilitate communication
I find it most depressing to fail on a diet because of the way it makes me feel, but I also can't accept not fitting into a size less than 16.	Okay, Mrs. Sams, I think I have a better idea of how you feel. You feel equally bad being overweight and failing to successfully lose weight on a diet. To help me better understand your usual eating patterns, I'd like you to fill out this daily record of food intake. With each meal entry, also list a rating of 1 to 10, bad to good, of how you feel. Next week when you come for your appointment, we'll go over this notebook together and look for clues to help you succeed in losing weight.	Summarization
Thanks, I'll be glad to try something constructive. Good-bye.	*(I felt great!)*	Summary: Figured I'd really turned around a bad situation. Her mood change let me know I might be on the right track. (1) She needs to develop insight into her eating patterns. (2) Participating in the process of selecting her diet may be a more effective plan than teaching exchange groups.

Figure 24-3 ● A sample process recording. This example illustrates beginning-level student analysis appropriate for a communications course. A more in-depth analysis would be expected of an advanced student practicing in a psychiatric clinical setting.

A form similar to that shown in Figure 24-3 can be used to list interpersonal interactions. The process record should list information about any preceding event, such as medication for pain with a strong narcotic, that might have affected the client response.

A complete listing should be made of all comments. Notes about tone of voice may also be made. This record should be as accurate as possible. You should resist the natural inclination to edit or "improve" the comments made to the client. The list should record the conversation in the order in which it occurred. Because it is often difficult to recall extensive information, limit the actual interaction to be described on the process recording to 10 to 15 minutes.

Because nonverbal behaviors can significantly affect the nature of a communication, all relevant nonverbal behaviors exhibited by either of you are also listed along with verbal responses. Of particular interest are comments about your thoughts and feelings listed in parentheses (see Column 2 of Figure 24-3).

The last column in Figure 24-3 is for analysis of the meaning of the interaction. Write your interpretation of events. Specific communication skills should be identified, along with the rationale for using them and a critique of their effectiveness. Commentary about transitions in the conversation, such as the rationale for changing the subject, should be entered. A brief analysis of identified emotions should be recorded in the third column, as well as the effects of personal values.

Exercise 24-1 A Process Record

Purpose: To provide students with practice in writing process records.

Procedure:

1. Conduct a 10-minute interaction with a client.
2. Write down the actual interaction as soon as possible after your contact with the client (see the example interaction in Figure 24-3). Fill in any needed data about the client, time, or place of the interaction. Identify your goal for the interaction (i.e., what you intended to accomplish). Then fill out only the first two columns, listing raw data (e.g., all the comments made by both the client [Column 1] and the nurse [Column 2] in the order in which they occurred). Some inaccuracies will naturally occur, but try to write as faithful a record as you can recollect. In parentheses, note nonverbal behaviors observed in the client or any feeling you recall that accompanied your conversation with the client.
3. After recording all the raw data, begin your analysis (Column 3). Read through each exchange between you and the client (usually, an initial exchange comprises only one or two sentences from each of you). The analysis should be guided by the purpose for doing the process recording. Essential components usually are development of communication skills and identification of client problems requiring nursing assessment and intervention.
   a. Identify each communication skill used.
   b. Describe your rationale for using each skill in your responses. Suggest alternative skills for areas in which the listed skill did not achieve the desired results.
   c. Describe relevant feelings not previously identified in Column 2, particularly if they are related to your choice of the next intervention.
   d. Make comments about what you think went on in the process of the conversation. List any opinions, tentative interpretations, or hypotheses you can make about the recorded behavior. In particular, highlight your interpretation of the client's behavior. Apply principles from communication theory to help identify the underlying process that occurred during the interaction.
   e. Conclude with a statement summarizing those aspects in the process that seem relevant for your future interactions with the client (e.g., certain inferences made from this record may need to be checked or validated with the client in your next interaction).

Exercise 24-2 The Interpersonal Process: Related Concepts

Purpose: To help students analyze interpersonal responses in process records. Process recording is an effective tool for developing increased awareness of process problems and use of communications skills. Alternatively, audio or video recordings may accomplish the same purpose. The following exercise may be used to supplement process records or may be used alternately with process records.

Procedure:
Answer the following questions after completing a nurse-client interaction.

1. Were your goals or objectives for the interaction achieved?
2. To what extent were they not achieved?
3. Cite evidence to document that your objective was achieved. (This is usually in the form of a behavioral change noted in the client.)
4. Identify why some goals were not achieved.
   a. Were your goals realistic?
   b. Were they mutual goals or just your goals as a nurse?
5. Were any client goals achieved or client needs fulfilled?
6. What were your preconceptions or feelings before this interaction? To what extent did they affect the outcome of the interaction?
7. What did you learn about the client that you were not aware of before?
8. What particular communication skills were you uncomfortable using? Which were ineffective?
9. What new nursing diagnoses or client problems did you identify after this interaction?

You should then make an overall critical analysis summary evaluating the effectiveness of your interventions and listing possible alternatives. Some of the most effective learning may occur as a result of analysis of less-than-perfect responses. Column 2 of Figure 24-3 clearly reveals errors made by the nurse during the course of the interaction. Many individuals have commented that some of their best learning has occurred when they "bomb." It can be threatening to write comments that may reveal us in an unfavorable light. This is particularly true for students when an instructor reads the process record and makes comments on it or grades it.

Exercise 24-1 is provided to give practice in writing process records and to help you further your understanding of process records.

Using Electronic Recordings of Student-Client Interactions for Analysis

New technology can be used to record an interaction between student and client, after obtaining required permission. Examples include digital video cameras, digital cameras with brief video capabilities, and wireless phones with similar video capabilities. These replace older, larger videotaping equipment. Recordings of an interaction, either a real-life situation or a case simulation, can be analyzed as described above. Try suggestions in Exercise 24-2 to write your self-analysis of a conversation with a client.

SUMMARY

This chapter focuses on the use of technology for communication in the nurse-client relationship. Written tools used in developing communication skills, transcribed documentation of the nursing process, and the reporting of client information in professional records. Learning to write process records and to provide clear written communication to other health professionals is an essential component of successful nurse-client relationships.

Ethical Dilemma ■ *What Would You Do?*

One of the largest health insurance companies/medical service providers routinely fills many of its 8.5 million clients' prescriptions over the Internet, so the system contains their identification numbers, their names, addresses, diagnoses, and so on. The agency's system also allows members to schedule appointments and seek health advice. After rebooting their system following a temporary shutdown to upgrade, a technician began replying to accumulated e-mails. Unfortunately these e-mails were sent to the wrong recipients. When he noticed this, the technician stopped sending e-mails but did not report the problem to agency administrators. Subscribers began to complain that they had been promised confidentiality of medical records as long as they did not give out their password, yet they were receiving e-mails containing other members' medical information.

In another case, a pharmacy chain replaced their computers. They then sold the older computers but neglected to wipe out customer medical information from the hard drives. Buyers were able access information, as in the above case, including information such as which customers had AIDS.

1. What safeguards could have prevented these violations of confidentiality?
2. If you were the nurse sending the "e-mails gone astray," what would you do? Are you responsible? Or is only the agency responsible?

Adapted from Anderson JG, Goodman KW: *Ethics and information technology: a case-based approach to a health care system in transition*, New York, 2002, Springer.

REFERENCES

Abrahamsen C: Patient safety: take the informatics challenge, *Nurs Manage* 34(4):48–51, 2003.

American Medical Association: Guidelines for physician-patient electronic communications [online article], 2004; available online: http://www.ama-assn.org/ama/pub/category/2386.html.

Anderson JG, Goodman KW: *Ethics and information technology: a case-based approach to a health care system in transition*, New York, 2002, Springer.

Bates DW, Gawande AA: Improving safety with information technology, *N Engl J Med* 348(25):2526–2534, 2003.

Bauchner H, Adams W, Burstin H: "You've got mail": issues in communicating with patients and their families by e-mail, *Pediatrics* 109(5):954–956, 2002.

Baum LS: Internet parent support groups for primary caregivers of a child with special health care needs, *Pediatr Nurs* 30(5):381–388, 2004.

Cornell S: Electronic prescribing, *Adv Nurse Pract* 9(6): 107–108, 2001.

Craig A: Personal digital assistant use: practical advice for the advanced practice nurse, *Topics in Advanced Practice Nursing eJournal* 2(4), 2002; available online: www.medscape.com/viewarticle/442736.

George L, Davidson L: PDA use in nursing education: prepared for today, poised for tomorrow, *Online Journal of Nursing Informatics* 9(2); available online: http://eaa-knowledge.com/ojni/ni/9_2/george.htm.

Gerstle RS, AAP Task Force on Medical Informatics: E-mail communication between pediatricians and their patients, *Pediatrics* 114(1):317–321, 2004.

Goldman RD: Community physicians' attitudes toward electronic follow-up after an emergency department visit, *Clin Pediatr (Phila)* 44(4):305–309, 2005.

Grebus C: (2002, 2005) *It's all in the palm of your hand: handheld computing in clinical settings*, presentation at National Nurse Practitioner Conference, Boston.

Gross D, Gross C: Impact of an electronic meeting system on the group decision-making process, *Comput Inform Nurs* 23(1):46–51, 2005.

Gururajan R: A study of the use of hand-held devices in an emergency department, *J Telemed Telecare* 10 Supplement 1: 33–35, 2004.

Im EO, Chee W: Decision support computer program for cancer pain management, *Comput Inform Nurs* 21(1): 12–21, 2003.

Institute of Medicine: *Crossing the quality chasm: a new health system for the 21st century*, Washington, DC, 2001, National Academy Press.

Kleiner KD, Akers R, Burke BL et al.: Parent and physician attitudes regarding electronic communication in pediatric practices, *Pediatrics* 109(5):740–744, 2002.

Kohn LT, Corrigan JM, Donaldson MS: *To err is human: building a safer health system*, Washington, DC, 2000, National Academies Press.

Malpani A: Doctor.com: why should a doctor have his own website? *J Postgrad Med* 47(1):40–41, 2001.

Marsch LA, Bickel WK: Efficacy of computer-based HIV/AIDS education for injection drug users, *Am J Health Behav* 28(4):316–327, 2004.

McAlearney AS, Schweikhart SB, Medow MA: Doctors' experience with handheld computers in clinical practice: a qualitative study, *Br Med J* 328(7449):1565, 2004.

Miller E: Making connections in a high-tech world, *Rehabil Nurs* 29(5):142, 153, 2004.

National Institute for Literacy: *Fact sheet: adult and family literacy*; April, 2000; available online: http://www.nifl.gov/nifl/policy/famlitfactsheet.doc.

Nelson NC, Evans RS, Samore MH et al.: Detection and prevention of medication errors using real-time bedside nurse charting, *J Am Med Inform Assoc* 12(4):390–397, 2005; available online: http://www.jamia.org/cgi/content/full/12/4/390.

O'Dell GJ: American Hospital Association environmental assessment, *Hosp Health Netw* 79(10):69–71, 2005.

Pew Internet and American Life Project Report: Doctor, doctor give me the Web, *Smart Computing in Plain English* 16(8):6, 2005.

Roland M: Linking physician's pay to the quality of care, *N Engl J Med* 351(14):1448–1454, 2004; available online: http://content.nejm.org/cgi/content/full/351/14/1448.

Taylor DP, Coakley A, Reardon G et al.: An analysis of inpatient nursing communication needs, *Medinfo* 2004:1393–1397, 2004.

These docs are literally on call: TelaDoc offers medical care that's a phone call away—but that's all, *USA Today* May 25, 2005, p. 3B.

Thompson BW: The transforming effect of handheld computers on nursing practice, *Nurs Adm Q* 29(4):308–314, 2005.

Travelbee J: *Interpersonal aspects of nursing*, Philadelphia, 1971, Davis.

Tsai HH, Pong YP, Liang CC et al.: Teleconsultation by using the mobile camera phone for remote management of the extremity wound: a pilot study, *Ann Plast Surg* 53(6):584–587, 2004.

Wright AA, Katz IT: Bar coding and patient safety, *N Engl J Med* 353(4):329–331, 2005.

Yao J, Schmitz R, Warren S: A wearable point-of-care system for home use that incorporates plug-and-play and wireless standards, *IEEE Trans Inf Technol Biomed* 9(3):363–371, 2005.

Glossary

Accommodation: A desire to smooth over a conflict through cooperative but nonassertive responses. **(ch. 14)**

Acculturation: A learning process by which members of one culture learn and accept the common attitudes, habits, language patterns and values of a new culture. **(ch. 11)**

Active listening: A dynamic interpersonal process whereby a person hears a message, decodes its meaning, and conveys an understanding about the meaning to the sender. **(ch. 10)**

Advance directive: Written legal statement executed by a competent adult that allows a client to express preferences regarding treatment options in the event that the client is unable to make valid decisions in the future. **(chs. 2, 8)**

Advanced practice nurse: Registered nurse with a baccalaureate degree in nursing and a Master's degree in a selected clinical specialty with relevant clinical experience. Certification and state licensing requirements vary according to the state for practice in advanced practice roles. **(ch. 7)**

Advocacy: Interceding or acting on behalf of the client to provide the highest quality of care obtainable. **(chs. 7, 19)**

Affective learning: Emotional learning; changes in attitude that inform and direct behaviors. **(ch. 16)**

Aggressive behavior: A response in which the individual acts to defend the self and to deflect the emotional impact of the perceived threat to the self through personal attack, blaming, or an extreme reaction to a tangential issue. **(ch. 14)**

Andragogy: The art and science of helping adults to learn. **(ch. 15)**

Anticipatory grief: An emotional response that occurs before the actual loss, for example, a terminal illness in a family member, an eviction, or projected job loss. **(ch. 8)**

Anticipatory guidance: Helping the client foresee and predict potential difficulties. **(chs. 10, 20)**

Anxiety: A vague, persistent sense of impending doom. **(chs. 6, 20)**

Aphasia: A neurological linguistic deficit that is most commonly associated with neurological trauma to the brain. **(ch. 17)**

Apraxia: The loss of ability or the inability to take purposeful action even when the muscles, senses, and vocabulary seem intact. **(ch. 19)**

Assertive behavior: Setting goals, acting on these goals in a clear and consistent manner, and taking responsibility for the consequences of one's actions. **(ch. 14)**

Assimilation: A person's adoption of common behaviors, customs, values, and language of the dominant or mainstream culture, such that the political or ethnic identification with the original culture virtually disappears. **(ch. 11)**

Authenticity: The capacity to be true to one's personality, spirit, and character in interacting with clients and others in the nurse-client relationships. **(ch. 5)**

Authoritarian leadership: A leadership style in which the leader takes full responsibility for group direction and controls group interaction. **(ch. 22)**

Autonomy: Ethical principle dealing with the client's right to decision-making power in his health care; the nurse supports autonomy by leaving decision making to the client whenever possible and by supporting the client's decisions unless there is a chance of harm to the client or others. **(chs. 3, 19)**

Avoidance: A withdrawal from conflict. **(ch. 14)**

Beneficence: Ethical principle guiding decisions, based on the concept of doing the greatest good and avoiding malfeasance; producing the least harm to the client. **(ch. 3)**

Biofeedback: Immediate and continuous information about a person's physiological responses; auditory and visual signals that increase one's response to external events. **(ch. 20)**

Body image: The physical dimension of self-concept; thoughts and feelings about one's physical appearance, body parts, movements, and body functions. **(chs. 3, 10)**

Body language: A system of communication that includes facial expressions, eye movements, body movements, posture, gestures, and proxemics. **(chs. 9, 10)**

Boundaries: Invisible limits within a relationship that help determine what is acceptable behavior. In a professional relationship, boundaries are dictated by legal, moral, and professional standards of nursing that respect nurse and client rights. **(chs. 2, 5, 7, 12, 13)**

Burnout: A state in which a person's physical, psychosocial, and spiritual resources are exhausted. **(ch. 20)**

Caring: An intentional human action characterized by commitment and a sufficient level of knowledge and skill that allows the nurse to support the basic integrity of the person being cared for. **(chs. 1, 6)**

Catastrophic reactions: Outbursts of a dementia victim that represent an angry, disorganized set of responses in reaction to real or perceived frustration. Warning signs may be restlessness, refusals, or general uncooperativeness. **(ch. 19)**

Charting by exception: A type of charting in which normal data are charted using check marks on flow sheets, with only abnormal/significant findings, called exceptions, being charted in a long-hand descriptive format. **(ch. 23)**

Circular questions: Questions that focus on the impact of a health situation on family relationships rather than the cause-effect sequence of linear questions. **(ch. 10)**

Clarification: A therapeutic active listening strategy designed to aid in understanding the message of the client by asking for more information or for elaboration on a point. **(ch. 10)**

Clinical pathway (*also* critical pathway)**:** A comprehensive documentation tool based on standardized plans of care resulting from aggregating computerized assessment and outcome data from client records. **(chs. 2, 23)**

Closed groups: Groups that have a defined membership with an expectation of regular attendance and time commitment, usually at least 12 sessions. **(ch. 12)**

Closed-ended question: A question that can be answered with *yes, no,* or another one-word answer. **(ch. 10)**

Coding systems: Numerical systems (e.g., ICD-9, CPT) for recording client diagnosis or treatment. **(ch. 23)**

Cognitive dissonance: The holding of two or more conflicting values at the same time. **(ch. 3)**

Cognitive distortions: Automatic thoughts related to a stressful situation that cause a person to interpret a neutral situation in an exaggerated, personalized, or negative way. **(ch. 1)**

Cognitive learning: Knowledge obtained from information a person did not have before. **(ch. 16)**

Cohesiveness: The degree of positive attachment and investment that members have for the group. **(ch. 12)**

Collaboration: Two or more people working together to solve a common problem and sharing responsibility for the process and outcome. **(chs. 7, 14)**

Communication: An interpersonal activity involving the transmission of messages by a source to a receiver for the purpose of influencing the receiver's behavior; a complex composite of verbal and nonverbal behaviors integrated for the purpose of sharing information. **(chs. 1, 9, 10)**

Competition: A response style characterized by domination; a contradictory style in which one party exercises power to achieve personal goals regardless of the needs of others. **(ch. 14)**

Complementary role relationships: Relationships that involve unequal distribution of power. **(ch. 1)**

Complicated grieving: An incapacitating form of grief (also called *morbid grief*) that is unusually long in duration and involves disorganized, depressed behaviors. **(ch. 8)**

Concrete operations period: Piaget's developmental stage in which a child can play cooperatively and employ complex rules. **(ch. 18)**

Confidentiality: The respect for another's privacy that involves holding and not divulging information given in confidence except in cases of suspected abuse, commission of a crime, or threat of harm to self or others. **(chs. 2, 6, 23)**

Confirming responses: The validation of the client as a person and of the client's thoughts and feelings in the context of the situation. **(ch. 10)**

Conflict: A mental struggle resulting from incompatible or opposing needs, drives, wishes, or internal demands; a hostile encounter. It may be *overt* (observable) or *covert* (hidden or buried). **(ch. 14)**

Connotation: The personalized meaning of a word or phrase. **(ch. 9)**

Coordination: Two or more people providing services to a client or program separately and keeping one another informed of all pertinent activities. **(ch. 7)**

Coping: Any response to external life strains that serves to prevent, avoid, or control emotional distress. **(ch. 20)**

Countertransference: The personal feelings or attitudes the helping person may feel toward a client that emerge as a reaction to the client's behavior or from the nurse's past life experiences. **(ch. 1)**

Crisis: A sudden, unanticipated, or unplanned event that necessitates immediate action to resolve the problem. A crisis may be *situational* (e.g., an external event or environmental influence) or *developmental* (e.g., an internal process that arises in connection with maturational changes). **(ch. 21)**

Crisis intervention: The systematic application of problem-solving techniques, based on crisis theory, designed to help the client move through the crisis process as swiftly and painlessly as possible and thereby achieve at least the same level of psychological comfort the client experienced before the crisis. **(ch. 21)**

Critical incident: A unique, overwhelming, random stressor event, capable of creating a crisis response in many individuals at the same time. **(ch. 21)**

Critical incident stress debriefing (CISD): A crisis intervention strategy designed to reduce the impact of a crisis event on professional staff and others involved in the crisis situation by processing it as soon as possible after it occurs. **(ch. 21)**

Critical thinking: A framework for problem solving by which a person can identify and analyze the assumptions underlying the actions, decisions, values, and judgments of the self and others. **(ch. 3)**

Cultural competence: A set of cultural behaviors and attitudes integrated into the practice methods of a system, agency, or its professionals that enables them to work effectively in cross-cultural situations. **(ch. 11)**

Cultural diversity: The differences among cultural groups. **(ch. 11)**

Cultural relativism: The belief that cultures are neither inferior nor superior to one another and that there is no single scale for measuring the value of a culture. **(ch. 11)**

Culture: The collective beliefs, values, and shared understandings and patterns of behavior of a designated group of people. **(ch. 11)**

Delegation: The transfer of responsibility for the performance of an activity from one individual to another while retaining accountability for the outcome. **(ch. 22)**

Democratic leadership: The leadership style in which the leader involves members in active discussion and decision making, encouraging open expression of feelings and ideas. **(ch. 22)**

Denial: An unconscious refusal to allow painful facts, feelings, and perceptions into conscious awareness. **(ch. 8)**

Denotation: The generalized meaning assigned to a word. **(ch. 9)**

Deontological (duty-based) model: A framework for making ethical decisions based on basic duties and moral worth. **(ch. 3)**

Dependent nursing interventions: Nursing actions that require an oral or written order from a physician. **(ch. 2)**

Discrimination: Situations and actions in which a person is denied legitimate opportunity offered to others because of bias or prejudice. **(ch. 6)**

Distress: A stress response capable of creating permanent pathological changes and even death. **(ch. 20)**

Documentation: The process of obtaining, organizing, and conveying information to others in a written or computerized format. **(ch. 23)**

Dysfunctional conflict: Conflict in which information is withheld, feelings are expressed too strongly, the problem is obscured by a double message, or feelings are denied or projected onto others. **(ch. 14)**

Ecomap: A diagram of a family member's relationship with people, agencies, and institutions outside the family. **(ch. 13)**

Ego defense mechanisms: The conscious and unconscious coping methods used by people to change the meaning of a situation in their minds. **(chs. 1, 20)**

Electronic health record (EHR): Various types of computerized client health records. **(ch. 23)**

Empathy: The capacity to understand another's world and to communicate that understanding; the ability of one person to perceive and understand another person's emotions accurately and to communicate the meaning of feelings to the other through verbal and nonverbal behaviors. **(chs. 5, 6)**

Empowerment: Helping a person become a self-advocate; an interpersonal process of providing the appropriate tools, resources, and environment to build, develop, and increase the ability of others to set and reach goals. **(chs. 5, 6, 7)**

End-of-life decision making: The process that healthcare providers, patients, and patients' families go through when considering what treatments will or will not be used to treat a life-threatening illness. **(ch. 8)**

Environment: All the cultural, developmental, physical, and psychosocial conditions external to an individual that influence a person's perception and involvement. **(ch. 1)**

Ethical dilemma (*also* moral dilemma)**:** The conflict of two or more moral issues; a situation in which there are two or more conflicting ways of looking at a situation. **(ch. 3)**

Ethnicity: A chosen awareness that reflects a person's commitment to a cultural identity; a personal awareness of certain symbolic elements that bind people together in a social context. **(ch. 11)**

Ethnic group: A social grouping of people who share a common racial, geographical, religious, or historical culture. **(ch. 11)**

Ethnocentrism: The belief that one's own culture is superior to others. **(ch. 11)**

Eustress: A moderate level of stress that acts as a positive stress response with protective and adaptive functions. **(ch. 20)**

Evidence-based practice: The conscientious explicit and judicious use of current best evidence in making decisions about the care of individual clients; utilization of research findings to create "best nursing practice." **(ch. 1)**

Exploitation phase: A component of the working phase of a therapeutic relationship in which the nurse helps the client use his or her personal strengths in conjunction with health and community resources to resolve health care issues. **(ch. 1)**

Facial expression: Facial configurations that convey feelings without words. **(ch. 9, 10)**

Family: A self-identified group of two or more individuals whose association is characterized by special terms, who may or may not be related by bloodlines or law, but who function in such a way that they consider themselves to be a family. **(ch. 13)**

Feedback: The response given by the receiver to the sender about the message. **(chs. 1, 10)**

Flow sheets: Charting by exception uses flow sheets with predefined client progress parameters based on written standards with preprinted categories of information. The best example of this format is known as critical or clinical pathways. **(ch. 23)**

Focus charting: A charting format using a focus (e.g., a sign or symptom, a nursing diagnosis, a behavior, a condition, a significant event, or an acute change in condition) and three steps: data, action, and response (DAR). **(ch. 23)**

Formal operations period: Piaget's developmental stage in which abstract reality and logical thought processes emerge and independent decisions can be made. **(ch. 18)**

Functional similarity: Group members have enough common intellectual, emotional, and experiential characteristics to interact with each other and to carry out the group objectives. **(ch. 12)**

Gender roles: A set of beliefs about or expectations of male and female behavior and experiences. **(ch. 13)**

General adaptation syndrome (GAS): A series of changes caused by the body's response to and compensation for stress, including: (1) *alarm phase,* the immediate biological response that includes increased breathing, muscle tension, and accelerated heart rate; (2) *resistance phase,* in which the body produces endorphins and the brain attempts to restore homeostasis; and (3) *exhaustion phase*, the result of unremitting stress, the stage during which serious physical symptoms, dangerous mental disorganization, physical collapse, and even death may occur. **(ch. 20)**

Genogram: A family diagram that records information about family members and their relationships for at least three generations. **(ch. 13)**

Grief: Mourning, bereavement, and the journey toward healing and recovering from the pain of a significant loss. **(ch. 8)**

Group: A gathering of two or more individuals who share a common purpose and meet over time in face-to-face interaction to achieve an identifiable goal. **(ch. 12)**

Group dynamics: All of the communication processes and behaviors that take place within a group. **(ch. 12)**

Group norms: Behavioral standards expected of group members. *Universal norms:* Behavioral standards held by most groups to be essential to the success of group life (e.g., confidentiality, regular attendance). *Group-specific norms:* Standards of behavior that represent the combined expectations, values, and needs of group members. **(ch. 12)**

Group process: The identifiable structural development of the group that is needed for a group to mature. **(ch. 12)**

Group think: A fear of expressing conflicting ideas and opinions because loyalty to the group and approval by other group members has become so important. **(ch. 12)**

Healing touch: An energy-based skilled listening response used to connect with a client when words would break a mood or verbalization would fail to convey the empathy or depth of feeling. **(ch. 10)**

Health: A broad concept that is used to describe an individual's state of well-being and level of functioning. **(ch. 1)**

Health care outcome: Change in an individual's health status between a baseline time point and a final time point. **(ch. 2)**

Health Insurance Portability and Accountability Act (HIPAA): Federal privacy standards enacted in 2003, designed to protect client records and other health information provided to health plans and other health care providers. These standards provide clients with access to their medical records and offer more control for clients over how their personal health information is used and disclosed. **(chs. 2, 23)**

Health literacy: The degree to which people have the capacity to obtain, process, and understand basic health information and services needed to make appropriate health decisions. **(ch. 15)**

Health promotion: In clinical practice, organized actions or efforts that enhance, support, or promote the well-being or health of individuals, families, groups, communities, or societies. **(ch. 15)**

Health teaching: A flexible, person-oriented process in which the helping person provides information and support to clients with a variety of health-related learning needs. **(ch. 16)**

Homeostasis (*also* dynamic equilibrium)**:** A person's sense of personal security and balance. **(ch. 20)**

Homogeneous group: A group in which the membership has a common denominator pertaining to all members of the group such as a diagnosis (e.g., breast cancer support group) or a personal characteristic such as age range or gender. **(ch. 12)**

Human rights–based model: A framework for making ethical decisions based on the belief that each client has basic rights. **(ch. 3)**

I-thou relationship: A relationship in which each individual responds to the other from his or her own uniqueness and is valued for that uniqueness in a direct, mutually respected, reciprocal alliance. **(ch. 1)**

Independent nursing interventions: Interventions that nurses can provide without a physician's order or direction from another health professional. **(ch. 2)**

Inference: An educated guess by the nurse about the meaning of a client behavior or statement. **(ch. 2)**

Informed consent: Assurance that the client fully understands what is happening or is about to happen in his or her health care and knowingly consents to care. **(chs. 2, 16)**

Intercultural communication: Communication in which the sender of a message is a member of one culture and the receiver is from a different culture. **(ch. 11)**

Interpersonal competence: The ability to interpret the content of a message from the point of view of each of the participants and the ability to use language and nonverbal behaviors strategically to achieve the goals of the interaction. **(ch. 9)**

Interpersonal process record: A three-part record of the nurse-client interaction, including: (1) a written anecdotal record of the client's and the nurse's words as well as their nonverbal behaviors; (2) a written analysis of the interaction, identifying communication skills and interventions; and (3) written suggestions for making more effective comments. **(ch. 24)**

Justice: Ethical principle guiding decision making. Justice is actually a legal term; however, in ethics it refers to being fair or impartial. **(ch. 3)**

Laissez faire: A hands-off approach. **(ch. 22)**

Leadership: Interpersonal influence that is exercised in situations and directed through the communication process toward attainment of a specified goal or goals. **(ch. 12)**

Loss: A generic term that signifies absence of an object, person, position, ability, or attribute of value to the client. **(ch. 8)**

Magnet status: ANA national program that recognizes quality patient care and nursing excellence in health care institutions and agencies and identifies them as work environments that act as a "magnet" for professional nurses desiring to work there because of their excellence. **(ch. 7)**

Maintenance functions: Group role functions that foster the emotional life of the group. **(ch. 12)**

Mentoring: A special type of professional relationship in which an experienced nurse or clinician (mentor) assumes a role responsibility for guiding the professional growth and advancement of a less experienced person (protégé). **(ch. 7)**

Message: A verbal or nonverbal expression of thoughts or feelings intended to convey information to the receiver and requiring interpretation by that person. **(ch. 1)**

Message competency: The ability to use language and nonverbal behaviors strategically to achieve the goals of interaction. **(ch. 9)**

Metacommunication: All verbal and nonverbal factors that influence how a message is received and interpreted. **(chs. 1, 9, 10)**

Minimal cues: The simple encouraging phrases, body actions, or words that communicate interest and encourage clients to continue with their story. **(ch. 10)**

Modeling: The transmission of values by presenting oneself in an attractive manner and living by a certain set of values, hoping that others will follow one's lead; teaching by performing a behavior that another observes. **(ch. 16)**

Moral distress: A feeling that occurs when one knows what is "right" but feels bound to do otherwise because of legal or institutional constraints. **(ch. 3)**

Moral uncertainty: A difficulty in deciding which moral rules (e.g., values or beliefs) apply to a given situation. **(ch. 3)**

Motivation: The forces that activate behavior and direct it toward one goal instead of another. **(ch. 15)**

Multiculturalism: A term to describe a heterogeneous society in which diverse cultural world views can coexist with some general characteristics shared by all cultural groups and some perspectives that are unique to each group. **(ch. 11)**

Mutuality: An agreement on problems and the means for resolving them; a commitment by both parties to enhance well-being. **(ch. 6)**

Networking: A form of peer collaboration whereby individuals take advantage of making and using contacts. **(ch. 7)**

Nonverbal gesture: A body movement that conveys a message without words. **(ch. 9)**

North American Nursing Diagnosis Association International (NANDA-I): A professional organization of registered nurses that promotes accepted nursing diagnoses. **(ch. 23)**

NNN: Abbreviation designating the combination of NANDA, NIC, and NOC. **(chs. 2, 23)**

Nurse Practice Acts: Legal documents developed at the state level that define professional nursing's scope of practice and outline the nurse's rights, responsibilities, and licensing requirements in providing care to individuals, families, and communities. **(ch. 2)**

Nursing: An involved interaction with persons in a caring mode. **(ch. 1)**

Nursing Interventions Classification (NIC): A standardized language describing direct and indirect care that nurses perform. NIC and Nursing Outcomes Classification (NOC) attempt to quantify nursing care so that it becomes visible and defines professional practice. **(chs. 2, 23)**

Nursing Outcomes Classification (NOC): The measure of how nursing care affects client outcomes. NOC and Nursing Interventions Classification (NIC) attempt to quantify nursing care so that it becomes visible and defines professional practice. **(chs. 2, 23)**

Objective data: Data that are directly observable or verifiable through physical examination or tests. **(ch. 2)**

The Omaha System: A comprehensive computerized information management system for documentation at the point of care (i.e., the client's location). **(ch. 23)**

Open groups: Groups that do not have a defined membership other than that imposed by the purpose and goals of the group. **(ch. 12)**

Open-ended question: A question that is open to interpretation and that cannot be answered by *yes, no,* or another one-word response. **(ch. 10)**

Optacon: A reading device that converts printed letters into a vibration that can be felt by the deaf-blind person. **(ch. 17)**

Orientation phase: The period in the nurse-client relationship when the nurse and client first meet and set the tone for the rest of their relationship, assessing the client's situation and setting goals. **(chs. 1, 5)**

Palliative care: A compassionate, clinical approach designed to improve the quality of life for clients and families coping with a life-threatening illness, beginning with a terminal illness diagnosis. **(ch. 8)**

Paradigm: A world view reflecting the knowledge developed about a phenomenon of interest within a scientific discipline. **(ch. 1)**

Paralanguage: The oral delivery of a verbal message expressed through tone of voice and inflection, sighing, or crying. **(ch. 9)**

Paraphrasing: Transforming the client's words into the nurse's words, keeping the meaning intact. **(ch. 10)**

Participatory leadership: A leadership style in which the leader maintains final control but actively solicits and uses the input of group members. **(ch. 22)**

Patterns of knowing: A unified form of knowledge embedded in nursing practice and grounded in empirical principles, intuitive personal responses, creative aesthetics used to connect with a client, and ethics, which the nurse uses to address the individualized needs of clients in health care situations. **(ch. 1)**

Perception: A personal identity construct by which a person transforms external sensory data into personalized images of reality. **(ch. 4)**

Person: A unitary concept that includes physiological, psychological, spiritual, and social elements. **(ch. 1)**

Personal digital assistant (PDA): A wireless electronic device containing databases that may also have the potential for electronic message transfer. **(ch. 24)**

Personal space: The invisible and changing boundary around an individual that provides a sense of comfort and protection to a person and that is defined by past experiences and culture. **(ch. 6)**

Personal value system: A set of values developed over a lifetime that has been extensively shaped by family, religious beliefs, and life experiences. **(ch. 3)**

PIE: A method for documentation that started as an expanded variation of the SOAP format with additional information about implementation interventions and evaluation of outcome, known as *SOAPIE.* Notations include the following: *(P)*, problems identified; *(I)*, document interventions; and *(E)*, evaluation of outcome. **(ch. 23)**

Point of care information: Client information and reference material that is updated via wireless Internet devices at any client location. **(ch. 24)**

Prejudices: Stereotypes based on strong emotions. **(ch. 6)**

Premack principle: An operant condition term, meaning that a desired activity can act as a reinforcer or reward for another behavior. Reinforcers that have meaning and value to the client offer the most effective reinforcement. Nurses need to choose activities and rewards that the client values (e.g., child must clean his room before he can watch television). **(ch. 16)**

Preoperational period: Piaget's developmental stage in which learning by the toddler is developed through concrete experiences and devices and the child is markedly egocentric. **(ch. 18)**

Prevention: A way of thinking and being that actively promotes responsible behavior and the adoption of lifestyles that are maximally conducive to good health. **(ch. 15)**

Primary group: A spontaneous group formation characterized by an informal structure and social process; it can be automatic, like a family, or based on a common interest; it has no defined time limit. **(ch. 12)**

Primary prevention: Actions taken to preclude illness or to prevent the natural course of illness from occurring; focus is on teaching people how to establish and maintain lifestyles conducive to optimal health. **(ch. 15)**

Problem-oriented record (POR): A chart containing four basic sections: (1) a database, (2) a list of the client's identified problems, (3) a treatment plan, and (4) progress notes. **(ch. 23)**

Profession: A calling requiring specialized knowledge and often long and intensive academic preparation. **(ch. 7)**

Professional boundaries: The invisible structures imposed by legal, moral, or professional standards of nursing that respect nurse and patient rights. **(ch. 5)**

Professional value system: A set of values that has been shaped by a person's education. **(ch. 3)**

Proxemics: The study of an individual's use of space. **(chs. 6, 9)**

Psychomotor learning: The process of learning a skill through "hands on" practice. **(ch. 16)**

Receiver: The recipient of a message, the person who decodes or translates the message into word symbols that make sense to the receiver. **(ch. 1)**

Reflection: A communication strategy linking the client's apparent emotion with the content of the client's message; it is used to clarify what the client is feeling and to affirm that the client's feelings are acceptable. **(ch. 10)**

Reframing: A strategy in which the nurse helps the client look at a situation in a new way. **(ch. 10)**

Reinforcement (*also* conditioning)**:** The consequences of performing identified behaviors; positive reinforcement increases the probability of a response, and negative reinforcement decreases the probability of a response. **(ch. 16)**

Restatement: An active listening strategy used by the nurse to broaden a client's perspective by repeating all or part of the client's statement. **(ch. 10)**

Role: A set of expected standards of behavior established by the society or community group to which a person belongs; role represents the social aspects of self-concept. **(ch. 7)**

Role ambiguity: A situation in which roles are not clearly defined. **(ch. 7)**

Role conflict: An incompatibility between one or more role expectations. **(ch. 7)**

Role performance: A person's capacity to function as expected in social roles, in sexual relations with a partner, in family, and in a job. **(ch. 7)**

Role pressures: The external or internal circumstances, capable of change, that interfere with role performance. **(ch. 7)**

Role stress: A subjective experience of mental, physical, and social fatigue often accompanied by a loss of meaning in what was previously important and exciting. **(ch. 7)**

Scope of practice: The legal boundaries of practice for professional nurses established by each state and defined in written state statutes. **(ch. 2)**

Secondary groups: Groups that are formally established to achieve certain agreed-on goals; they have a prescribed structure and a designated leader, and they last for a specified length of time. **(ch. 12)**

Secondary prevention: Interventions designed to promote early diagnosis of symptoms or timely treatment after the onset of the disease. **(ch. 15)**

Self-actualization: A level of development in which a person balances interdependence with individual self-awareness. **(ch. 1)**

Self-awareness: The means by which a person gains knowledge and understanding of all aspects of self-concept. **(chs. 4, 5, 7)**

Self-concept (*also* self, self-system)**:** An abstract structural construct that is used to describe the different images that make up the self in each person's mind; all of the psychological beliefs and attitudes people have about themselves: (e.g., perceptual, cognitive, emotional, and spiritual). **(ch. 4)**

Self-differentiation: The capacity to stay involved in one's family or group without losing one's identity. **(ch. 13)**

Self-esteem: The value and significance people place on their self-concepts; an emotional process of self-judgment; an orientation to the self, ranging on a continuum from feelings of self-efficacy and respect to feeling that one is fatally flawed as a person. **(ch. 4)**

Self-talk: A cognitive process that produces a thought or thoughts, which then lead to a feeling about a situation. **(ch. 4)**

Sender: The source or initiator of a message. **(ch. 1)**

Sensorimotor period: Piaget's developmental stage in which the infant explores its own body as a source of information about the world. **(ch. 18)**

Shaping: The process of changing a person's behavior through using simple behavioral steps to achieve a desired behavior. **(ch. 16)**

SOAP: A four-step method of documentation that lists all of the client's subjective *(S)* comments; all of the current objective *(O)* information noted by the nurse; the nurse's analysis or assessment *(A);* and future interventions or plans *(P)* for care. **(ch. 23)**

Social cognitive competency: The ability to interpret message content within interactions from the point of view of each participant. **(ch. 9)**

Social support: All of the social and environmental factors that contribute to a person's sense of well-being. **(ch. 20)**

Stereotyping (*also* bias)**:** Attributing characteristics or behaviors, generalized opinions, attitudes, and beliefs to a group of people as if all persons in the group possessed them. **(chs. 6, 11)**

Stress: The physiological and psychological response to the presence of a stressor. **(ch. 20)**

Stressor: Any demand, situation, internal stimulus, or circumstance that threatens a person's personal security and balance. **(ch. 20)**

Subculture: An ethnic, regional, or economic group of people who are joined together by distinguishing characteristics that differentiate the group from the predominant culture or society. **(ch. 11)**

Subjective data: A client's perception of the data and what the client says about the data. **(ch. 2)**

Subsystems: Member unit relationships within the family such as spousal, sibling, and child-parent subsystems. **(ch. 13)**

Summarization: The reworking of a lengthy interaction or discussion into a few succinct sentences. **(ch. 10)**

Symmetrical role relationships: Relationships in which each person has equal power and the exchanges mirror each other. **(ch. 1)**

Task functions: The group role functions that facilitate goal achievement. **(ch. 12)**

Telehealth: The use of telecommunications and information technology to provide access to health assessment, diagnosis, intervention, consultation, supervision, education, and information across distance. **(ch. 1)**

Tellatouch: A portable machine into which an individual can type a message that is then converted to Braille. **(ch. 17)**

Termination phase (*also* resolution)**:** A period in the nurse-client relationship when the nurse and client examine and evaluate their relationship and its goals and results; the time when they deal with the emotional content (if any) involved in saying good-bye. **(chs. 1, 5)**

Tertiary prevention: Rehabilitation strategies designed to minimize the handicapping effects of a disease. **(ch. 15)**

Theme: The underlying feeling associated with concrete facts a client presents (e.g., feelings of powerlessness, fear, abandonment, and helplessness). **(ch. 10)**

Theory: An organized, conceptual representation or explanation of a phenomenon. **(ch. 1)**

Therapeutic communication: The goal-directed, focused dialogue between nurse and client that is fitted to the needs of the client. **(chs. 1, 10)**

Therapeutic touch: The harnessing of energy fields to promote healing. **(chs. 9, 10)**

Transference: Behaviors in which the client projects irrational attitudes and feelings from the past onto people in the present. **(ch. 1)**

Triangle: A three-person emotional system in which there is tension between two members and a third person steps in to stabilize the relationship. **(ch. 13)**

Touch: Providing comfort and communication through purposeful contact. **(ch. 9)**

Trust: A reliance on the consistency, sameness, and continuity of experiences that are provided by an organized combination of familiar and predictable things and people. **(ch. 6)**

Utilitarian (goal-based) model: A framework for making ethical decisions in which the rights of the client and the duties of the nurse are determined by what will achieve maximum welfare. **(ch. 3)**

Validation: A form of feedback involving verbal and nonverbal confirmation that both participants have the same basic understanding of the message. **(chs. 1, 10)**

Values: A set of personal beliefs and attitudes about truth, beauty, and the worth of any thought, object, or behavior. Attitudes, beliefs, feelings, worries, or convictions that have not been clearly established are called *value indicators.* **(ch. 3)**

Values acquisitions: The conscious assumption of a new value. **(ch. 3)**

Values clarification: A process that encourages one to clarify one's own values by sorting them through, analyzing them, and setting priorities. **(ch. 3)**

Violence: Physical force used by one person against another. **(ch. 21)**

Well-being: A subjective experience associated with personal satisfaction in six personal dimensions: (1), intellectual, (2) physical, (3) emotional, (4) social, (5) occupational, and (6) spiritual. **(ch. 15)**

Working phase: The period in the nurse-client relationship when the focus is on communication strategies, interventions for problem resolution, and enhancement of self-concept. **(chs. 1, 5)**

Index

Page reference followed by b indicates box, e indicates exercise, f indicates figure or illustration, and t indicates table.

B

C

D

E

H

I

N

O

R

S

U

V

W

ONLINE RESOURCES

Chapter 1

American Association of Colleges of Nursing (AACN): www.aacn.org/
American Nurses Association (ANA): www.nursingworld.org
American Telemedicine Association: www.atmeda.org/
Florence Nightingale and other Nursing Leaders: www.NIGHcommunities.org
Nursing Theory: www.sandiego.edu/academics/nursing/theory/
Nursing Theory Link Page: www.healthsci.clayton.edu/eichelberger/nursing.htm
Sigma Theta Tau International Honor Society of Nursing: www.nursingsociety.org
Text from Nightingale's Notes on Nursing: http://digital.library.upenn.edu/women/nightingale/nursing/nursing.html
The Cochrane Collaboration: www.cochrane.org/
United States Department of Health & Human Services, Agency for Healthcare Research and Quality (AHRQ): www.ahrq.gov

Chapter 2

United States Department of Health & Human Services, HIPAA: www.hhs.gov/ocr/hipaa/
United States Department of Health & Human Services, Medical Privacy-National Standards: www.hhs.gov/ocr/hipaa/privacy.html
American Nurses Association Code of Ethics for Nurses: www.ana.org/ethics/chcode.htm
The Canadian Code of Ethics for Registered Nurses: www.cna-nurses.ca/CNA/practice/ethics/code/default_e.aspx
Joint Commission on Accreditation of Healthcare Organizations: www.jointcommission.org/
National Council for State Boards of Nursing: www.ncsbn.org
The Sara Cole Hirsh Institute for Best Nursing Practice Based on Evidence: http://fpb.cwru.edu/HirshInstitute
Academic Center for Evidence-Based Practice (ACE), University of Texas Health Science Center at San Antonio: www.acestar.uthscsa.edu
Evidence-Based Practice, University of Washington: http://healthlinks.washington.edu/ebp
Nursing Documentation, American Nurses Association Committee for the Nursing Practice Information Infrastructure: www.nursingworld.org/npii

Chapter 3

American Nurses Association Center for Ethics and Human Rights: www.nursingworld.org/ethics/
American Nurses Association Position Statements: Nursing and the Patient Self-Determination Acts: www.nursingworld.org/readroom/position/ethics/etsdet.htm
American Nurses Association Position Statements: Nursing Care and Do-Not-Resuscitate Decisions: www.nursingworld.org/readroom/position/ethics/etdnr.htm
American Society for Bioethics and Humanities: www.asbh.org
American Society of Law, Medicine & Ethics: www.aslme.org
American College of Physicians' Ethics Manual: www.acponline.org/ethics/ethics_man.hym?hp
American College of Surgeons' Statement on Principles: www.facs.org/fellows_info/statements/stonprin.html
American Medical Association's Code of Medical Ethics: www.ama-assn.org/ama/pub/category/2498.html
Markkula Center for Applied Ethics, Santa Clara University: www.scu.edu/ethics/practicing/focusareas/medical/

Chapter 5

American Psychiatric Nurses Association: www.apna.org
International Society for Interpersonal Psychotherapy: www.interpersonalpsychotherapy.org/index.html

Chapter 6

Communication Institute for Online Scholarship: www.cios.org
American Nurses Association: www.nursingworld.org

Chapter 7

Magnet Recognition Program, American Nurses Credentialing Center: www.nursingworld.org/ancc/magnet/index.html

Chapter 8

National Hospice and Palliative Care Organization: www.nho.org
Coalition on Donation: www.shareyourlife.org/

Chapter 9

Gender Differences in Communication: www.towson.edu/~vanfoss/wmcomm.htm
Nonviolent Communication: www.nonviolentcommunication.com

Chapter 10

American Academy on Communication in Healthcare: www.physicianpatient.org
Institute for Health Care Communication: www.bayerinstitute.org
Center for the Advancement of Health: www.cfah.org
Medical Outcomes Trust: www.outcomes-trust.org
Partnership for Clear Health Communication: www.askme3.org

Chapter 11

Association of Asian Pacific Community Health Organizations: www.aapcho.org
United States Department of Health & Human Services: Improving Health Care for Ethnic and Racial Minority Populations: www.ahrq.gov/research/minorhlth.htm
National Alliance for Hispanic Health: www.hispanichealth.org/
United States Department of Health & Human Services, Office of Minority Health: www.omhrc.gov/
Transcultural Nursing: www.culturediversity.org